Personalized Medicine in the Field of Inflammatory Skin Disorders

Personalized Medicine in the Field of Inflammatory Skin Disorders

Editors

Mircea Tampa
Monica Neagu
Constantin Caruntu
Simona Roxana Georgescu

MDPI • Basel • Beijing • Wuhan • Barcelona • Belgrade • Manchester • Tokyo • Cluj • Tianjin

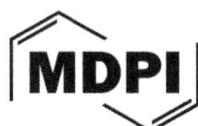

Editors

Mircea Tampa
Dermatology Department
"Carol Davila" University of Medicine and Pharmacy
Bucharest
Romania

Monica Neagu
Immunobiology Department
"Victor Babes" National Institute of Pathology
Bucharest
Romania

Constantin Caruntu
Department of Physiology
"Carol Davila" University of Medicine and Pharmacy
Bucharest
Romania

Simona Roxana Georgescu
Dermatology
"Carol Davila" University of Medicine and Pharmacy
Bucharest
Romania

Editorial Office
MDPI
St. Alban-Anlage 66
4052 Basel, Switzerland

This is a reprint of articles from the Special Issue published online in the open access journal *Journal of Personalized Medicine* (ISSN 2075-4426) (available at: www.mdpi.com/journal/jpm/special_issues/Inflammatory_Skin).

For citation purposes, cite each article independently as indicated on the article page online and as indicated below:

LastName, A.A.; LastName, B.B.; LastName, C.C. Article Title. *Journal Name* **Year**, *Volume Number*, Page Range.

ISBN 978-3-0365-3574-6 (Hbk)
ISBN 978-3-0365-3573-9 (PDF)

© 2022 by the authors. Articles in this book are Open Access and distributed under the Creative Commons Attribution (CC BY) license, which allows users to download, copy and build upon published articles, as long as the author and publisher are properly credited, which ensures maximum dissemination and a wider impact of our publications.

The book as a whole is distributed by MDPI under the terms and conditions of the Creative Commons license CC BY-NC-ND.

Contents

Preface to "Personalized Medicine in the Field of Inflammatory Skin Disorders" vii

Mircea Tampa, Monica Neagu, Constantin Caruntu and Simona Roxana Georgescu
Personalized Medicine in the Field of Inflammatory Skin Disorders
Reprinted from: *J. Pers. Med.* 2022, *12*, 426, doi:10.3390/jpm12030426 1

Hou-Ren Tsai, Jing-Wun Lu, Li-Yu Chen and Tai-Li Chen
Application of Janus Kinase Inhibitors in Atopic Dermatitis: An Updated Systematic Review and Meta-Analysis of Clinical Trials
Reprinted from: *J. Pers. Med.* 2021, *11*, 279, doi:10.3390/jpm11040279 5

Vladimir Sobolev, Anna Soboleva, Elena Denisova, Malika Denieva, Eugenia Dvoryankova and Elkhan Suleymanov et al.
Differential Expression of Estrogen-Responsive Genes in Women with Psoriasis
Reprinted from: *J. Pers. Med.* 2021, *11*, 925, doi:10.3390/jpm11090925 25

Paul Balanescu, Eugenia Balanescu, Cristian Baicus and Anca Balanescu
S100A6, Calumenin and Cytohesin 2 as Biomarkers for Cutaneous Involvement in Systemic Sclerosis Patients: A Case Control Study
Reprinted from: *J. Pers. Med.* 2021, *11*, 368, doi:10.3390/jpm11050368 45

Simona Roxana Georgescu, Andreea Amuzescu, Cristina Iulia Mitran, Madalina Irina Mitran, Clara Matei and Carolina Constantin et al.
Effectiveness of Platelet-Rich Plasma Therapy in Androgenic Alopeciamdash;A Meta-Analysis
Reprinted from: *J. Pers. Med.* 2022, *12*, 342, doi:10.3390/jpm12030342 55

Elena-Georgiana Dobre, Carolina Constantin, Marieta Costache and Monica Neagu
Interrogating Epigenome toward Personalized Approach in Cutaneous Melanoma
Reprinted from: *J. Pers. Med.* 2021, *11*, 901, doi:10.3390/jpm11090901 69

Marcella Ricardis May, Albert Rübben, Andrea Lennertz, Luk Vanstreels and Marike Leijs
Dealing with Corticosteroid and High-Dose Cyclosporine Therapy in a Pyoderma Gangrenosum Patient Contracting a COVID-19 Infection
Reprinted from: *J. Pers. Med.* 2022, *12*, 173, doi:10.3390/jpm12020173 109

Roxana Nedelcu, Alexandra Dobre, Alice Brinzea, Ionela Hulea, Razvan Andrei and Sabina Zurac et al.
Current Challenges in Deciphering Sutton Nevi—Literature Review and Personal Experience
Reprinted from: *J. Pers. Med.* 2021, *11*, 904, doi:10.3390/jpm11090904 119

Andreea Barbu, Bogdan Neamtu, Marius Zăhan, Gabriela Mariana Iancu, Ciprian Bacila and Vioara Mireșan
Current Trends in Advanced Alginate-Based Wound Dressings for Chronic Wounds
Reprinted from: *J. Pers. Med.* 2021, *11*, 890, doi:10.3390/jpm11090890 131

Mihaela Surcel, Adriana Munteanu, Gheorghita Isvoranu, Alef Ibram, Constantin Caruntu and Carolina Constantin et al.
Unconventional Therapy with IgY in a Psoriatic Mouse Model Targeting Gut Microbiome
Reprinted from: *J. Pers. Med.* 2021, *11*, 841, doi:10.3390/jpm11090841 151

Corina Daniela Ene, Simona Roxana Georgescu, Mircea Tampa, Clara Matei, Cristina Iulia Mitran and Madalina Irina Mitran et al.
Cellular Response against Oxidative Stress, a Novel Insight into Lupus Nephritis Pathogenesis
Reprinted from: *J. Pers. Med.* **2021**, *11*, 693, doi:10.3390/jpm11080693 . . . . **173**

Alin Codruț Nicolescu, Ștefana Bucur, Călin Giurcăneanu, Laura Gheucă-Solovăstru, Traian Constantin and Florentina Furtunescu et al.
Prevalence and Characteristics of Psoriasis in Romania—First Study in Overall Population
Reprinted from: *J. Pers. Med.* **2021**, *11*, 523, doi:10.3390/jpm11060523 . . . . **191**

Maria Dudau, Alexandra Catalina Vilceanu, Elena Codrici, Simona Mihai, Ionela Daniela Popescu and Lucian Albulescu et al.
Sea-Buckthorn Seed Oil Induces Proliferation of both Normal and Dysplastic Keratinocytes in Basal Conditions and under UVA Irradiation
Reprinted from: *J. Pers. Med.* **2021**, *11*, 278, doi:10.3390/jpm11040278 . . . . **203**

Mircea Tampa, Ilinca Nicolae, Cristina Iulia Mitran, Madalina Irina Mitran, Cosmin Ene and Clara Matei et al.
Serum Sialylation Changes in Actinic Keratosis and Cutaneous Squamous Cell Carcinoma Patients
Reprinted from: *J. Pers. Med.* **2021**, *11*, 1027, doi:10.3390/jpm11101027 . . . . **213**

Cristian Scheau, Constantin Caruntu, Ioana Anca Badarau, Andreea-Elena Scheau, Anca Oana Docea and Daniela Calina et al.
Cannabinoids and Inflammations of the Gut-Lung-Skin Barrier
Reprinted from: *J. Pers. Med.* **2021**, *11*, 494, doi:10.3390/jpm11060494 . . . . **227**

Preface to "Personalized Medicine in the Field of Inflammatory Skin Disorders"

Skin inflammation is associated with a wide range of conditions which represent major health issues worldwide. Skin and mucosal surfaces represent the primary interface between the human body and the environment, susceptible to numerous factors whose action results in diseases produced by chemical substances, mechanical trauma, microbial agents, radiation, etc. Inflammation, a complex network of interactions between soluble molecules and cells, represents the main modality of the skin's response to injuries. Numerous studies have revealed close links between chronic inflammation, oxidative stress, and carcinogenesis. Chronic inflammation induces the activation of various cell types and an increase in the production of reactive oxygen species, promoting the initiation of a malignant process. Identifying specific biomarkers is essential for understanding molecular mechanisms and developing therapies appropriate to the patient's characteristics.

Personalized medicine is an emerging field of medicine that has the potential to predict which therapy will be safe and efficacious for specific patients using an individual's genetic profile to guide decisions regarding the diagnosis, treatment, as well as prevention of disease. Personalized medicine stratifies patients based on molecular markers and enables the identification of the best possible solution for the patient. In this respect, inflammatory skin disorders are complex afflictions with a variable course, treatment response, and unpredictable outcome, and represent important candidates for personalized approaches.

This book gathers articles that present recent advancements in research involving the mechanisms that underlie the development of inflammatory skin disorders, skin and mucosal inflammation in general, as well as potential biomarkers for personalized treatment and prevention.

Mircea Tampa, Monica Neagu, Constantin Caruntu, and Simona Roxana Georgescu
Editors

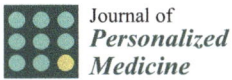

Editorial

Personalized Medicine in the Field of Inflammatory Skin Disorders

Mircea Tampa [1,2,*], Monica Neagu [3,4,*], Constantin Caruntu [5,*] and Simona Roxana Georgescu [1,2]

1. Department of Dermatology, "Carol Davila" University of Medicine and Pharmacy, 020021 Bucharest, Romania; srg.dermatology@gmail.com
2. Dermatology Department, "Victor Babes" Hospital of Infectious Diseases, 030303 Bucharest, Romania
3. "Victor Babes" National Institute of Pathology, 050096 Bucharest, Romania
4. Colentina University Hospital, 020125 Bucharest, Romania
5. Department of Physiology, "Carol Davila" University of Medicine and Pharmacy, 050474 Bucharest, Romania
* Correspondence: dermatology.mt@gmail.com (M.T.); neagu.monica@gmail.com (M.N.); costin.caruntu@gmail.com (C.C.)

Citation: Tampa, M.; Neagu, M.; Caruntu, C.; Georgescu, S.R. Personalized Medicine in the Field of Inflammatory Skin Disorders. *J. Pers. Med.* 2022, 12, 426. https://doi.org/10.3390/jpm12030426

Received: 7 March 2022
Accepted: 8 March 2022
Published: 9 March 2022

Publisher's Note: MDPI stays neutral with regard to jurisdictional claims in published maps and institutional affiliations.

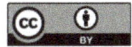

Copyright: © 2022 by the authors. Licensee MDPI, Basel, Switzerland. This article is an open access article distributed under the terms and conditions of the Creative Commons Attribution (CC BY) license (https://creativecommons.org/licenses/by/4.0/).

Inflammatory skin diseases occur after the onset of abnormal immune cell responses and the activation of various immune signaling pathways in the skin [1]. Inflammation may become a chronic process when the cause is not removed or the control mechanisms responsible for preventing the progress of the inflammatory process fail. A chronic inflammatory response can lead to cell mutation and proliferation, creating a microenvironment suitable for carcinogenesis [2]. Chronic inflammatory skin diseases are incurable but treatable. Targeted therapies need to be tailored according to the patient's characteristics. Personalized medicine requires the detection of reliable biomarkers of the pathways that are involved in disease pathogenesis [3]. Recent advances in the field of chronic inflammatory skin diseases have been achieved and are aimed to improve the management of these disorders. A broad range of studies that approach inflammation from several perspectives are available.

Psoriasis is probably the most representative chronic inflammatory skin disease. Psoriasis is a multifaceted and challenging immune disorder with a complex pathogenesis that mainly involves the alteration of the immune system [4]. Nicolescu et al. developed a questionnaire to estimate the national prevalence and risk factors associated with psoriasis. They obtained a 99.13% concordance between the diagnosis based on the questionnaire and the final diagnosis of psoriasis. This is the first study to attempt to identify the prevalence and characteristics of patients with psoriasis in Romania; therefore, these results may represent the starting point for the implementation of new programs including personalized recommendations based on population characteristics [5]. Sobolev et al. found a differential expression of six estrogen-controlled genes (HMOX1, KRT19, LDHA, HSPD1, MAPK1, and CA2) in the skin of female patients with psoriasis compared to male patients with psoriasis and concluded that these proteins may be involved in the defense of skin cells against inflammation damage. Considering that estrogens exert anti-inflammatory effects, low estrogen levels can influence the course of the disease in women with psoriasis [6]. Using a mouse model of induced psoriatic dermatitis, Surcel et al. obtained promising results after the administration of IgY, which led to the improvement in skin lesions and the normalization of immune parameters. IgY is involved in antibacterial and antiviral defense; therefore, these results are important since the skin microbiome participates in the pathogenesis of psoriasis [7].

In the treatment of atopic dermatitis, important advances are being made, and Janus kinase inhibitors (JAK) represent new treatment options. Tsai et al. conducted a systematic review and meta-analysis of the efficacy and safety of JAK inhibitors in atopic dermatitis. The analyzed data showed that JAK inhibitors are an effective therapy, and that side effects are tolerable [8]. This article provides a comprehensive review of the studies available until the time of publication and is welcome given that a few months later, in September 2021, the first topical JAK-1/JAK-2 inhibitor, ruxolitinib, was approved by the FDA, and in early 2022, in January, two oral JAK-1 inhibitors, upadacitinib and abrocitinib, were approved for patients with moderate to severe atopic dermatitis [9].

The identification of novel biomarkers in connective tissue diseases is currently ongoing and may provide new insights into the molecular mechanisms involved in these disorders [10]. Balanescu et al. showed that serum calumenin, S100A6, and cytohesin 2 could be used as biomarkers in systemic sclerosis. Regarding the characteristics of the patients, the most notable association was obtained between the serum levels of these biomarkers and severe skin involvement. Calumenin exhibited the best predictive capacity for cutaneous diffuse manifestation, and S100A6 was correlated with the presence of digital ulcers [11]. Ene et al. emphasized the role of the equilibrium between oxidants and antioxidants in the pathogenesis of lupus nephritis by evaluating markers of oxidative stress according to the four oxidative stress targets—lipids, proteins, nucleic acids, and carbohydrates—and antioxidant capacity. The authors concluded that the oxidant–antioxidant balance is altered in these patients. The most important changes included the impairment of the DNA repair mechanism via 8-oxoguanine DNA glycosylase (OGG1), low serum levels of soluble receptor for advanced glycation end products (sRAGE), which acts as a protective factor against the deleterious effects of inflammation and oxidative stress, the alteration in thiol–disulfide homeostasis, and high nitrotyrosination [12].

The close link between inflammation and skin tumors is well documented [13]. Mediators of inflammation exert pleiotropic effects on the onset and progression of a malignant tumor. Tampa et al. investigated patients with cutaneous squamous cell carcinoma (cSCC) and actinic keratosis and a control group and reported interesting results regarding aberrant sialylation in cSCC, which was associated with tumor aggressiveness. They identified elevated serum levels of total sialic acid (TSA), lipid-bound sialic acid (LSA), ST6GalI, and NEU3 in the cSCC group compared to the control group. Regarding actinic keratoses, only the serum TSA levels were significantly higher. They suggest that the serum ST6GalI/NEU3 level may be useful in differentiating patients with cSCC from noncancer patients [14]. Dudau et al. showed that sea buckthorn seed oil, a compound rich in long-chain fatty acids known to have beneficial effects on the skin, may promote the proliferation of normal and dysplastic keratinocytes under basal conditions and when they are exposed to UVA irradiation. Therefore, this study opens new perspectives on the involvement of lipids in health and disease [15]. Nedelcu et al. focused on recent knowledge regarding the etiology and pathogenesis of halo nevi. Their paper describes clinical aspects, dermoscopic features, immunohistochemical characteristics, and immunological mechanisms involved in the occurrence of halo nevi, which can be viewed as models for better understanding the antitumor human body response [16]. Dobre et al. conducted an extensive review of epigenetic modifications that are involved in the pathogenesis of cutaneous melanoma. In this review, the authors also discuss epigenetic modifications as a source of new therapies for cutaneous melanoma, including cases resistant to conventional therapies, and these data may be used to develop new therapeutic algorithms [17].

The recent literature presents data with clinical significance that can be used to improve the management of various inflammatory skin diseases. There is an increasing body of evidence on the role of cannabinoids in several pathologies [18]. The review by Scheau et al. comprehensively appraises the effects of natural and synthetic cannabinoids on the inflammation of the epithelia of the gut–lung–skin barrier and shows that, although human studies present conflicting data, some results are encouraging and additional studies are required to elucidate the role of cannabinoids in inflammation [19]. Barbu et al. performed an overview of the current status of advanced alginate-based wound dressings for chronic wounds. They present the properties and roles of alginates that make them one of the favorite therapies for chronic wounds. They focused mainly on hydrogels, nanofiber networks, 3D scaffolds and sponges able to capture different cells such as fibroblasts or keratinocytes, or drugs to be released on the wound surface [20]. Georgescu et al. conducted a meta-analysis that investigated the effectiveness of platelet-rich plasma therapy in androgenic alopecia. This is the first meta-analysis that identifies a significant positive correlation between the number of PRP treatments per month and the percentage change in hair density [21]. May et al. reported a challenging case of COVID-19 infection in a patient with pyoderma gangrenosum treated with corticosteroids and high-dose cyclosporine therapy [22].

Our Special Issue underlines personalized medicine as an emerging field of medicine that has the potential to predict which therapy will be safe and efficacious for individual patients using an individual's genetic profile to guide decisions regarding the diagnosis, treatment, and prevention of disease. Personalized medicine stratifies patients based on molecular markers and allows the identification of the best possible solution for the patient. In this respect, inflammatory skin disorders are complex afflictions with a variable course, treatment response, and unpredictable outcome and represent important candidates for a personalized approach.

Funding: This manuscript received no external funding.

Conflicts of Interest: The authors declare no conflict of interest.

References

1. Milando, R.; Friedman, A. Cannabinoids: Potential Role in Inflammatory and Neoplastic Skin Diseases. *Am. J. Clin. Dermatol.* **2019**, *20*, 167–180. [CrossRef] [PubMed]
2. Singh, N.; Baby, D.; Rajguru, J.P.; Patil, P.B.; Thakkannavar, S.S.; Pujari, V.B. Inflammation and Cancer. *Ann. Afr. Med.* **2019**, *18*, 121. [CrossRef] [PubMed]
3. Litman, T. Personalized Medicine—Concepts, Technologies, and Applications in Inflammatory Skin Diseases. *Apmis* **2019**, *127*, 386–424. [PubMed]
4. Casciaro, M.; Di Salvo, E.; Gangemi, S. HMGB-1 in Psoriasis. *Biomolecules* **2022**, *12*, 60. [CrossRef]
5. Nicolescu, A.C.; Bucur, Ș.; Giurcăneanu, C.; Gheucă-Solovăstru, L.; Constantin, T.; Furtunescu, F.; Ancuța, I.; Constantin, M.M. Prevalence and Characteristics of Psoriasis in Romania—First Study in Overall Population. *J. Pers. Med.* **2021**, *11*, 523. [CrossRef]
6. Sobolev, V.; Soboleva, A.; Denisova, E.; Denieva, M.; Dvoryankova, E.; Suleymanov, E.; Zhukova, O.V.; Potekaev, N.; Korsunskaya, I.; Mezentsev, A. Differential Expression of Estrogen-Responsive Genes in Women with Psoriasis. *J. Pers. Med.* **2021**, *11*, 925. [CrossRef]
7. Surcel, M.; Munteanu, A.; Isvoranu, G.; Ibram, A.; Caruntu, C.; Constantin, C.; Neagu, M. Unconventional Therapy with IgY in a Psoriatic Mouse Model Targeting Gut Microbiome. *J. Pers. Med.* **2021**, *11*, 841. [CrossRef]
8. Tsai, H.-R.; Lu, J.-W.; Chen, L.-Y.; Chen, T.-L. Application of Janus Kinase Inhibitors in Atopic Dermatitis: An Updated Systematic Review and Meta-Analysis of Clinical Trials. *J. Pers. Med.* **2021**, *11*, 279. [CrossRef]
9. Drug Approvals and Databases. Available online: https://www.fda.gov/drugs/development-approval-process-drugs/drug-approvals-and-databases (accessed on 2 March 2022).
10. Jog, N.R.; James, J.A. Biomarkers in Connective Tissue Diseases. *J. Allergy Clin. Immunol.* **2017**, *140*, 1473–1483. [CrossRef]
11. Balanescu, P.; Balanescu, E.; Baicus, C.; Balanescu, A. S100A6, Calumenin and Cytohesin 2 as Biomarkers for Cutaneous Involvement in Systemic Sclerosis Patients: A Case Control Study. *J. Pers. Med.* **2021**, *11*, 368. [CrossRef]
12. Ene, C.D.; Georgescu, S.R.; Tampa, M.; Matei, C.; Mitran, C.I.; Mitran, M.I.; Penescu, M.N.; Nicolae, I. Cellular Response against Oxidative Stress, a Novel Insight into Lupus Nephritis Pathogenesis. *J. Pers. Med.* **2021**, *11*, 693. [CrossRef] [PubMed]
13. Ciążyńska, M.; Olejniczak-Staruch, I.; Sobolewska-Sztychny, D.; Narbutt, J.; Skibińska, M.; Lesiak, A. Ultraviolet Radiation and Chronic Inflammation-Molecules and Mechanisms Involved in Skin Carcinogenesis: A Narrative Review. *Life* **2021**, *11*, 326. [CrossRef]
14. Tampa, M.; Nicolae, I.; Mitran, C.I.; Mitran, M.I.; Ene, C.; Matei, C.; Georgescu, S.R.; Ene, C.D. Serum Sialylation Changes in Actinic Keratosis and Cutaneous Squamous Cell Carcinoma Patients. *J. Pers. Med.* **2021**, *11*, 1027. [CrossRef] [PubMed]
15. Dudau, M.; Vilceanu, A.C.; Codrici, E.; Mihai, S.; Popescu, I.D.; Albulescu, L.; Tarcomnicu, I.; Moise, G.; Ceafalan, L.C.; Hinescu, M.E. Sea-Buckthorn Seed Oil Induces Proliferation of Both Normal and Dysplastic Keratinocytes in Basal Conditions and under UVA Irradiation. *J. Pers. Med.* **2021**, *11*, 278. [CrossRef] [PubMed]
16. Nedelcu, R.; Dobre, A.; Brinzea, A.; Hulea, I.; Andrei, R.; Zurac, S.; Balaban, M.; Antohe, M.; Manea, L.; Calinescu, A. Current Challenges in Deciphering Sutton Nevi—Literature Review and Personal Experience. *J. Pers. Med.* **2021**, *11*, 904. [CrossRef] [PubMed]
17. Dobre, E.-G.; Constantin, C.; Costache, M.; Neagu, M. Interrogating Epigenome toward Personalized Approach in Cutaneous Melanoma. *J. Pers. Med.* **2021**, *11*, 901. [CrossRef]
18. Fraguas-Sánchez, A.I.; Torres-Suárez, A.I. Medical Use of Cannabinoids. *Drugs* **2018**, *78*, 1665–1703. [CrossRef]
19. Scheau, C.; Caruntu, C.; Badarau, I.A.; Scheau, A.-E.; Docea, A.O.; Calina, D.; Caruntu, A. Cannabinoids and Inflammations of the Gut-Lung-Skin Barrier. *J. Pers. Med.* **2021**, *11*, 494. [CrossRef]

20. Barbu, A.; Neamtu, B.; Zăhan, M.; Iancu, G.M.; Bacila, C.; Mireșan, V. Current Trends in Advanced Alginate-Based Wound Dressings for Chronic Wounds. *J. Pers. Med.* **2021**, *11*, 890. [CrossRef]
21. Georgescu, S.R.; Amuzescu, A.; Mitran, C.I.; Mitran, M.I.; Matei, C.; Constantin, C.; Tampa, M.; Neagu, M. Effectiveness of Platelet-Rich Plasma Therapy in Androgenic Alopecia—A Meta-Analysis. *J. Pers. Med.* **2022**, *12*, 342. [CrossRef]
22. May, M.R.; Rübben, A.; Lennertz, A.; Vanstreels, L.; Leijs, M. Dealing with Corticosteroid and High-Dose Cyclosporine Therapy in a Pyoderma Gangrenosum Patient Contracting a COVID-19 Infection. *J. Pers. Med.* **2022**, *12*, 173. [CrossRef] [PubMed]

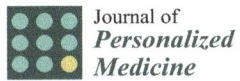

Review

Application of Janus Kinase Inhibitors in Atopic Dermatitis: An Updated Systematic Review and Meta-Analysis of Clinical Trials

Hou-Ren Tsai [1], Jing-Wun Lu [2], Li-Yu Chen [3] and Tai-Li Chen [1,4,*]

1. Department of Medical Education, Medical Administration Office, Hualien Tzu Chi Hospital, Buddhist Tzu Chi Medical Foundation, Hualien 970, Taiwan; melotsai0830@gmail.com
2. Department of Physical Medicine and Rehabilitation, Hualien Tzu Chi Hospital, Buddhist Tzu Chi Medical Foundation, Hualien 970, Taiwan; jingwunlu@gmail.com
3. Library of Hualien Tzu Chi Hospital, Buddhist Tzu Chi Medical Foundation, Hualien 970, Taiwan; rani37jason@gmail.com
4. School of Medicine, Tzu Chi University, Hualien 970, Taiwan
* Correspondence: terrychen.a@gmail.com; Tel.: +886-983-249-828

Abstract: Janus kinase (JAK) inhibitors are promising treatments for atopic dermatitis (AD). The aim of this study was to assess the efficacy and safety of JAK inhibitors for AD treatment via the "Grading of Recommendations Assessment, Development, and Evaluation" approach. We identified 15 randomized controlled trials comparing oral or topical JAK inhibitors against placebo to treat AD. A random-effects meta-analysis was performed, and the numbers-needed-to-treat (NNTs)/numbers-needed-to-harm (NNHs) were calculated. Patients treated with JAK inhibitors were associated with higher rates of achieving eczema area and severity index-75 (rate ratio (RR): 2.84; 95% confidence interval (CI): 2.20–3.67; I^2: 38.9%; NNT = 3.97), Investigator's Global Assessment response (RR: 2.99; 95% CI: 2.26–3.95; I^2: 0%; NNT = 5.72), and pruritus numerical rating scale response (RR: 2.52; 95% CI: 1.90–3.35; I^2: 39.4%; NNT = 4.91) than those treated with placebo. Moreover, patients treated with JAK inhibitors had a higher risk of treatment-emergent adverse events (RR: 1.14; 95% CI: 1.02–1.28; I^2: 52%; NNH = 14.80) but not adverse events leading to drug discontinuation. According to the evidence-based results, JAK inhibitors are potentially effective strategies (certainty of evidence: "moderate") for treating AD with tolerable side effects (certainty of evidence: "low"). Nevertheless, long-term follow-up is required.

Keywords: atopic dermatitis; eczema; JAK inhibitors; systematic review; meta-analysis; evidence-based medicine; immune-mediated skin diseases; target therapy; skin conditions and systemic inflammatory diseases

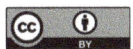

1. Introduction

Atopic dermatitis (AD) is the most common inflammatory skin disease affecting approximately 20% of children and 10% of adults worldwide [1,2]. This chronic condition is characterized by intense pruritus and recurrent eczematous lesions and has a considerable negative impact on patients' quality of life [3]. Moreover, AD patients may display different clinical patterns depending on their age, ethnicity, and underlying mechanisms [4]. There are three main types of AD patterns: the persistent form where AD appears in childhood and then persists into adulthood; the relapsing form, in which AD occurs in childhood and recurs in adulthood with a symptom-free interval; and the adult-onset AD, the most difficult type to detect, where the disease is firstly observed in adulthood [5]. Due to its various presentations, the diagnosis and treatment of AD remained a challenge for clinicians [6].

While topical interventions are the mainstay treatment of AD, systemic therapy is recommended for patients with inadequate treatment response [7–9]. Advances have been made in systemic AD therapy owing to an improved understanding of the molecular mechanism of AD [10]. Innovative treatment options are available, such as dupilumab (obstructing alpha subunit of the IL-4 receptors), crisaborole (blocking phosphodiesterase 4), and lebrikizumab (preventing IL-13Rα1/IL-4Rα heterodimerization) [11]. Of note, the upregulation of key cytokines (interleukin (IL)-4, IL-5, and IL-13) and subsequent activation of the Janus kinase/signal transducer and transcription (JAK/STAT) pathways play important roles in the complex mechanism of AD [12,13]. In a growing number of preclinical studies, the inhibition of intracellular JAK/STAT signal transmission has demonstrated therapeutic potential [14,15].

Since their first approval, JAK inhibitors have become a promising AD treatment option [16]. In randomized controlled trials (RCTs), several JAK inhibitors (oral/topical) have significantly improved the clinical outcomes of patients with inadequate responses to other therapies [17,18]. An integrated safety analysis indicated similar incidences of adverse events (AEs) between JAK inhibitor application and placebo [19]. An earlier meta-analysis showed that JAK inhibitors lowered the eczema area and severity index (EASI) and pruritus scores [20]. Nevertheless, the sample sizes of the enrolled studies were small, and no phase III RCTs were included [20]. Considering the rapid developments in this field of study, an updated literature review with a meta-analysis is warranted to improve statistical power and provide supporting evidence for current guidelines.

In the present study, we performed a systematic review and meta-analysis of RCTs to compile evidence on the application of JAK inhibitors in the management of AD. We also graded certainty of evidence (CoE) based on the "Grading of Recommendations Assessment, Development, and Evaluation" (GRADE) approach and calculated the numbers-needed-to-treat (NNTs) and numbers-needed-to-harm (NNHs) to facilitate decision-making in clinical practice.

2. Materials and Methods

This study was conducted in accordance with the recommendations of the Cochrane Handbook for Systematic Reviews of Interventions (v. 6.2) [21] and reported based on the Preferred Reporting Items for Systematic Reviews and Meta-Analyses (PRISMA) statement [22]. The methodology was prespecified and registered on the PROSPERO website (Registration No. CRD42020173098). Two reviewers (H.R. Tsai and J.W. Lu) independently searched for suitable records, extracted the data, and evaluated the quality of the included studies. In the event of any discrepancy, a third reviewer (T.L. Chen) provided consensus or contributed to the discussions.

2.1. Data Sources and Literature Search

Relevant publications indexed in electronic databases (MEDLINE, Embase, Cochrane Central Register of Controlled Trials, and Web of Science) between database inception and 1 February 2021 were searched. The keywords "atopic dermatitis" and "Janus kinase inhibitor" and their synonyms and derivatives were used for the search. Details of the search strategies are described in Table S1 in the Supplementary Materials. No language restriction was applied. To identify unpublished or ongoing trials, the trial registries of the US National Institutes of Health (https://clinicaltrials.gov/ accessed on 2 February 2021), International Clinical Trials Registry Platform (https://www.who.int/ictrp/en/ accessed on 2 February 2021), and European Union Drug Regulating Authorities Clinical Trials Database (https://eudract.ema.europa.eu/ accessed on 3 February 2021) were searched. The bibliographies of available review articles and meta-analyses were also examined to find additional candidate studies. The literature search was performed with the assistance of a librarian (L.Y. Chen) at Hualien Tzu Chi Hospital.

2.2. Study Selection and Eligibility

Only RCTs were enrolled to avoid potential selection and confounding bias [21,23]. Studies comparing oral/topical JAK inhibitors against placebo were included with no defined limitations on age, sex, ethnicity, AD severity, or treatment duration of participants. Case reports, letters, editorials, review articles, conference abstracts, and in vivo studies involving animals were excluded.

2.3. Data Extraction and Efficacy and Safety Outcomes

The extracted data comprised study information (first author, publication year, clinical trial identifier, study design, and study period), patient characteristics (sample size, age, definition criteria, and AD severity), details of the various JAK inhibitors and placebos used (administration route, dosage, frequency, mode of action, and endpoint), and outcomes (efficacy and safety). Potential conflicts of interest were also listed.

The efficacy outcomes included (1) a $\geq 75\%$ decrease in EASI from baseline (EASI-75 response), (2) an Investigator's Global Assessment (IGA) score of 0 (clear) or 1 (almost clear) with a $\geq$ 2-point reduction from baseline (IGA response), and (3) a $\geq$ 4-point decrease from baseline in pruritus numerical rating scale response (pruritus-NRS response). The safety outcomes included the development of treatment-emergent AEs (TEAEs) and AEs that lead to drug discontinuation.

2.4. Risk of Bias Assessment

The methodological quality of the RCTs was appraised using the Cochrane Risk of Bias Tool (RoB v. 2.0, The Cochrane Collaboration) [24].

2.5. Data Synthesis and Statistical Analyses

Pooled estimates and their confidence intervals (CIs) were obtained with a random-effects meta-analysis model (DerSimonian–Laird estimator) [21] based on the assumption of substantial clinical heterogeneity. Rate ratios or relative risks (RRs) and 95% CIs were used to evaluate the efficacy and safety outcomes. If the desired effect estimates were inadequate for data synthesis, the corresponding authors were contacted to obtain relevant information. Statistical significance was indicated by $p < 0.05$ and a CI not containing 1. All statistical analyses were conducted using Stata v.16 (StataCorp, College Station, TX, USA).

A pairwise meta-analysis comparing the effect of JAK inhibitors against placebos was conducted. However, when a multiple-arm RCT was enrolled, a unit-of-analysis error may arise if the same group of participants is included twice in the same meta-analysis (for example, if "dose 1 vs. placebo" and "dose 2 vs. placebo" are both included in the same analysis, with the same placebo patients in both comparisons) [25]. Therefore, when an enrolled RCT included more than two arms, the reported results were combined to create a single pairwise comparison against placebos [21]. This method had been utilized in previous studies [26,27].

Between-study heterogeneity was quantified using Cochran's Q and I^2 statistics [28]. $p < 0.01$ and $I^2 \geq 50\%$ indicated substantial heterogeneity. To identify the potential sources of heterogeneity, several subgroup analyses were conducted according to the administration route, AD severity, participant age, mode of action, and different JAK inhibitors at different time points. Meta-regression analyses were also performed to explore potential effect modifiers, which refer to the explanatory variables of the overall effect estimates that may contribute to the heterogeneity [21]. Visual inspection of the funnel plot and Egger's regression test were used to assess publication bias [21].

Concerning the possibility of producing false-positive results when using the DerSimonian–Laird method, we applied the Hartung–Knapp–Sidik–Jonkman (HKSJ) method for sensitivity analyses [29]. This method widens the CIs to reflect uncertainty in estimating between-study heterogeneity, especially when the study number is less than 20 [21,30]. The HKSJ method had been widely used in previous meta-analyses [31–33].

The GRADE approach was adopted to summarize the CoE at the outcome level [34] and judged by all authors. In the event of disagreement, discussions were undertaken to arrive at a consensus for each outcome. CoE, classified as high, moderate, low, or very low, refers to the confidence that the true effect lies in a particular range [34]. The CoE was downgraded by one level if a serious flaw was present in the domains of risk of bias, inconsistency, indirectness, imprecision, and publication bias [34]. The NNT and NNH were calculated to evaluate the evidence-based efficacy and safety of JAK inhibitors in the management of AD [34].

3. Results

3.1. Search Results

A PRISMA flowchart of the process of study selection is shown in Figure S1. Initially, a total of 1237 records were retrieved. After screening the titles, abstracts, and full texts, 14 original articles involving 15 RCTs were eligible for a quantitative meta-analysis. These comprised seven phase III trials [19,35–39], seven phase II trials [40–46], and one phase I trial [47].

3.2. Characteristics of Eligible Studies

The demographic data and relevant outcomes are summarized in Table 1. We included 4367 patients with AD in this meta-analysis and assessed seven different JAK inhibitors. Four of them (abrocitinib, baricitinib, gusacitinib, and upadacitinib) were orally administered, while the remaining three (delgocitinib, ruxolitinib, and tofacitinib) were topically administered. All eligible studies had participants with a documented history of inadequate treatment response to topical corticosteroids/calcineurin inhibitors. Guttman-Yassky et al. also recruited participants with a documented history of inadequate treatment response to systemic corticosteroids or immunosuppressants [42]. Most eligible studies did not report participants with failure of systemic treatment but a washout period for systemic steroid, immunosuppressive, and biologic treatments.

Most of the enrolled trials involved adult patients with moderate to severe AD. Three studies involved children or adolescents, while another three included patients with mild to moderate AD. All enrolled studies had declared their conflict of interest with an institution or a company.

3.3. Risk of Bias Assessment

We used the Risk-of-Bias VISualization tool to create "traffic light" plots of domain-level judgments [48]. Most of the enrolled RCTs were judged to have a "low" risk of bias (Figure S2).

3.4. Efficacy Outcomes

3.4.1. EASI-75 Response

Twelve studies (involving 3498 patients) reported EASI-75 response as the indicator of efficacy outcome. A random-effects meta-analysis showed that patients treated with JAK inhibitors (both oral and topical) were associated with higher rates of achieving EASI-75 response (RR = 2.84; 95% CI = 2.20–3.67) than those treated with placebo (Figure 1); no significant heterogeneity was observed (I^2 = 38.9%; P = 0.08).

Table 1. Characteristics of studies included in the meta-analysis.

Source	Clinical Trial Identifier	Study Design	Study Period	No. of Participants (Age)	Definition of AD	Severity of AD	Interventions	Mechanism of Inhibition	Endpoint	Efficacy Outcomes	Safety Outcomes	COI
Bissonnette 2016	NCT02201181	Phase II RCT	December 2013–September 2014	69 (18–60 y)	Hanifin and Rajka criteria	Mild to moderate	Treatment: topical tofacitinib, 2% twice daily Placebo: topical control vehicle twice daily	JAK1 and JAK3	Week 4	IGA, EASI, and BSA	TEAEs and SAEs	Yes
Bissonnette 2019	NCT03139981	Phase I RCT	April 2017–November 2017	36 (18–75 y)	AAD guideline	Moderate to severe	Treatment: oral gusacitinib, 20 mg, 40 mg, 80 mg once daily Placebo: oral vehicle once daily	JAK1, JAK2, JAK3, TYK2, and SYK	Week 4	IGA, EASI, pruritus NRS, and BSA	TEAEs, SAEs, and AEDC	Yes
Gooderham 2019	NCT02780167	Phase II RCT	April 2016–April 2017	267 (18–75 y)	AAD guideline	Moderate to severe	Treatment: oral abrocitinib, 10 mg, 30 mg, 100 mg, 200 mg once daily Placebo: oral control vehicle once daily	JAK1	Week 12	IGA, EASI, pruritus NRS, BSA, SCORAD, DLQI, HADS, and POEM	TEAEs and SAEs	Yes
Guttman-Yassky 2018	NCT02576938	Phase II RCT	February 2016–March 2017	124 (≥18 y)	Hanifin and Rajka criteria	Moderate to severe	Treatment: oral baricitinib, 2 mg and 4 mg once daily plus TCSPlacebo: oral control vehicle once daily	JAK1 and JAK2	Week 16	IGA, EASI, pruritus NRS, SCORAD, DLQI, and POEM	TEAEs, SAEs, and AEDC	Yes
Guttman-Yassky 2019	NCT02925117	Phase II RCT	November 2016–April 2017	167 (18–75 y)	Hanifin and Rajka criteria	Moderate to severe	Treatment: oral upadacitinib, 7.5 mg, 15 mg, 30 mg once daily Placebo: oral control vehicle once daily	JAK1	Week 16	IGA, EASI, pruritus NRS, BSA, SCORAD, and POEM	TEAEs, SAEs, and AEDC	Yes
Kim 2020	NCT03011892	Phase II RCT	January 2017–November 2017	307 (18–70 y)	NA	Mild to moderate	Treatment: topical ruxolitinib, 0.15%, 0.5%, 1.5% once daily, and 1.5% twice daily; Placebo: topical control vehicle twice daily	JAK1 and JAK2	Week 8	pruritus NRS, and Skindex-16	TEAEs, SAEs, and AEDC	Yes

Table 1. Cont.

Source	Clinical Trial Identifier	Study Design	Study Period	No. of Participants (Age)	Definition of AD	Severity of AD	Interventions	Mechanism of Inhibition	Endpoint	Efficacy Outcomes	Safety Outcomes	COI
Nakagawa 2017	JapicCTI-152887	Phase II RCT	April 2015–May 2016	327 (16–65 y)	JDA guideline	Moderate to severe	Treatment: topical delgocitinib, 0.25%, 0.5%, 1%, 3% twice daily Placebo: topical control vehicle twice daily	JAK1, JAK2, JAK3, and TYK2	Week 4	IGA, mEASI, pruritus NRS, and BSA	SAEs and AEDC	Yes
Nakagawa 2019	JapicCTI-173553	Phase II RCT	March 2017–February 2018	103 (2–15 y)	JDA guideline	Mild to moderate	Treatment: topical delgocitinib, 0.25%, 0.5% twice daily Placebo: topical control vehicle twice daily	JAK1, JAK2, JAK3, and TYK2	Week 4	IGA, mEASI, pruritus NRS, and BSA	SAEs and AEDC	Yes
Nakagawa 2020	JapicCTI-173554	Phase III RCT	March 2017–September 2018	158 (≥16 y)	JDA guideline	Moderate to severe	Treatment: topical delgocitinib, 0.5% twice daily Placebo: topical control vehicle twice daily	JAK1, JAK2, JAK3, and TYK2	Week 4	IGA, mEASI, pruritus NRS, BSA, and Skindex-16	TEAEs, SAEs, and AEDC	Yes
Reich 2020	NCT03733301 (BREEZE-AD7)	Phase III RCT	November 2018–August 2019	329 (≥18 y)	AAD guideline	Moderate to severe	Treatment: oral baricitinib, 2 mg, 4 mg once daily plus TCS Placebo: oral control vehicle once daily	JAK1 and JAK2	Week 16	IGA, EASI-50, EASI-75, EASI-90, pruritus NRS, pain NRS, SCORAD, ADSS, POEM, HADS, DLQI, and WPAI	TEAEs, SAEs, and AEDC	Yes
Silverberg 2020	NCT03575871 (JADE MONO-2)	Phase III RCT	June 2018–August 2019	391 (≥12 y)	Hanifin and Rajka criteria	Moderate to severe	Treatment: oral abrocitinib, 100 mg and 200 mg once daily Placebo: oral control vehicle once daily	JAK1	Week 12	IGA, EASI, pruritus NRS, PSAAD, DLQI, CDLQI, POEM, and HADS	SAEs and AEDC	Yes

Table 1. Cont.

Source	Clinical Trial Identifier	Study Design	Study Period	No. of Participants (Age)	Definition of AD	Severity of AD	Interventions	Mechanism of Inhibition	Endpoint	Efficacy Outcomes	Safety Outcomes	COI
Simpson 2020a	NCT03334396 (BREEZE-AD1)	Phase III RCT	November 2017–January 2019	624 (≥18 y)	AAD guideline	Moderate to severe	Treatment: oral baricitinib, 1 mg, 2 mg, 4 mg once daily Placebo: oral control vehicle once daily	JAK1 and JAK2	Week 16	IGA, EASI, pruritus NRS, pain NRS, SCORAD, and ADSS	TEAEs, SAEs, and AEDC	Yes
Simpson 2020b	NCT03334422 (BREEZE-AD2)	Phase III RCT	November 2017–December 2018	615 (≥18 y)	AAD guideline	Moderate to severe	Treatment: oral baricitinib, 1 mg, 2 mg, 4 mg once daily Placebo: oral control vehicle once daily	JAK1 and JAK2	Week 16	IGA, EASI, pruritus NRS, pain NRS, SCORAD, and ADSS	TEAEs, SAEs, and AEDC	Yes
Simpson 2020c	NCT03349060 (JADE MONO-1)	Phase III RCT	December 2017–March 2019	387 (≥12 y)	Hanifin and Rajka criteria	Moderate to severe	Treatment: oral abrocitinib, 100 mg and 200 mg once daily Placebo: oral control vehicle once daily	JAK1	Week 12	IGA, EASI, pruritus NRS, PSAAD, DLQI, CDLQI, and POEM	TEAEs, SAEs, and AEDC	Yes
BREEZE-AD4 2020 *	NCT03428100 (BREEZE-AD4)	Phase III RCT	May 2018	463 (≥18 y)	AAD guideline	Moderate to severe	Treatment: oral baricitinib, 1 mg, 2 mg, 4 mg once daily Placebo: oral control vehicle once daily	JAK1 and JAK2	Week 16	NA	TEAEs, SAEs, and AEDC	Yes

AAD, American Academy of Dermatology; AD, atopic dermatitis; ADSS, atopic dermatitis sleep scale; AE, adverse event; AEDC, adverse events leading to drug discontinuation; BSA, body surface area; CDLQI, children's dermatology life quality index; COI, conflict of interest; DLQI, dermatology life quality index; EASI, eczema area and severity index; HADS, hospital anxiety and depression scale; IGA, investigator global assessment; JAK, Janus kinase; JDA, Japanese Dermatological Association; mEASI, modified eczema area and severity index; NA, not applicable; NRS, numerical rating scale; POEM, patient-oriented eczema measure; PSAAD, pruritus and symptoms assessment for atopic dermatitis; RCT, randomized controlled trial; SAE, serious adverse event; SCORAD, scoring atopic dermatitis; SYK, spleen tyrosine kinase; TEAE, treatment-emergent adverse event; TYK: tyrosine kinase; WPAI, work productivity and activity impairment questionnaire * BREEZE-AD4 is an ongoing RCT. Its safety outcomes were presented in Bieber et al. (2020).

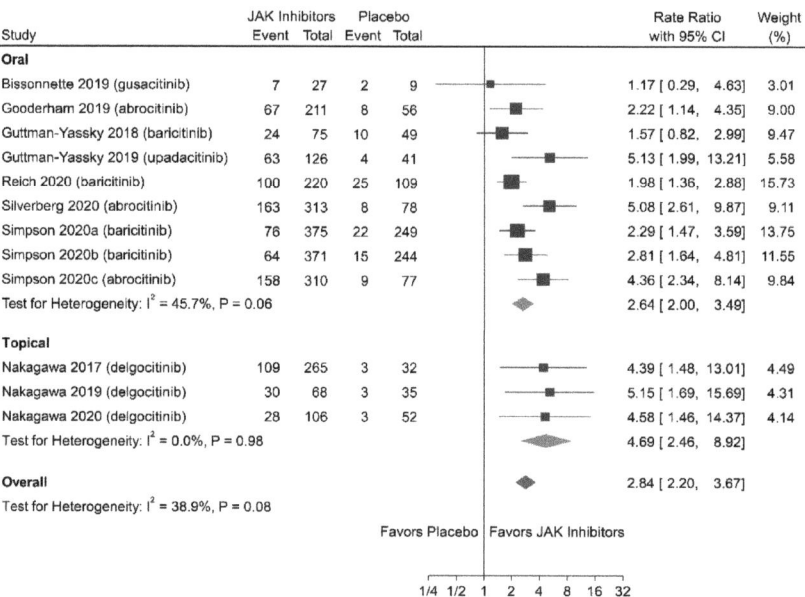

Figure 1. Association of Janus kinase (JAK) inhibitors versus placebo achieving at least a 75% improvement in Eczema Area and Severity Index (EASI) score from the baseline (EASI-75 response). CI, confidence interval.

3.4.2. IGA Response

Eleven studies (involving 2417 patients) reported IGA responses. Figure 2 shows that patients treated with JAK inhibitors (both oral and topical) were associated with higher rates of achieving IGA responses (RR = 2.99; 95% CI = 2.26–3.95) than those treated with placebo; no significant heterogeneity was observed ($I^2 = 0\%$; $P = 0.60$).

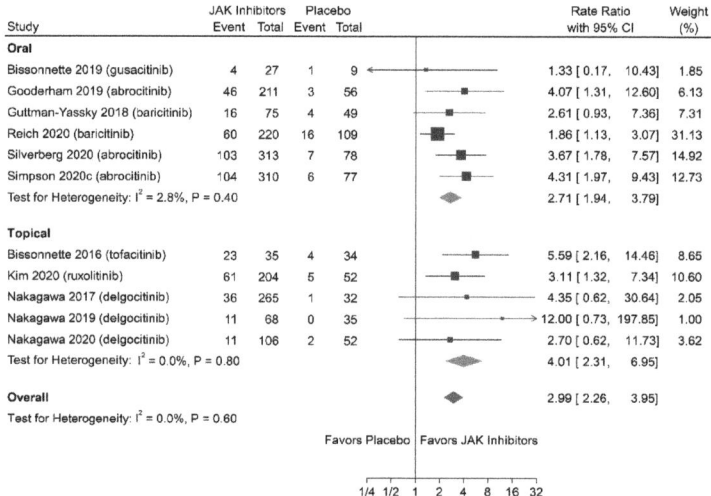

Figure 2. Association of Janus kinase (JAK) inhibitors versus placebo achieving of an Investigator Global Assessment (IGA) of 0 (clear) or 1 (almost clear) with at least a two-point reduction from the baseline (IGA response). CI, confidence interval.

3.4.3. Pruritus-NRS Response

Eight studies (involving 3036 patients) reported pruritus-NRS responses. The meta-analysis revealed that patients treated with JAK inhibitors were associated with higher rates of achieving pruritus-NRS responses (RR = 2.52; 95% CI = 1.90–3.35) compared with those treated with placebo (Figure 3). No significant heterogeneity was observed ($I^2 = 39.4\%$; $P = 0.12$).

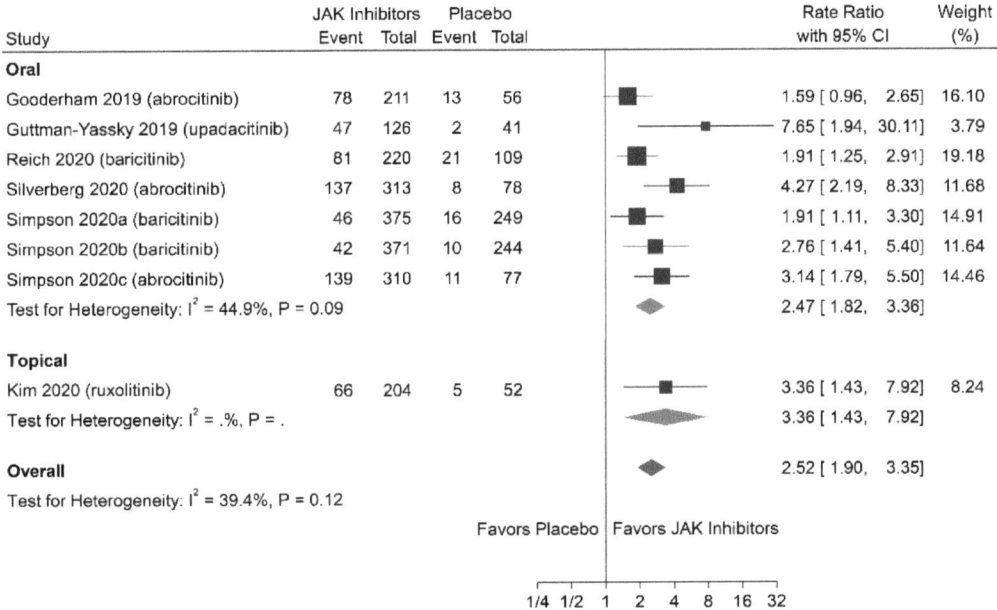

Figure 3. Association of Janus kinase (JAK) inhibitors versus placebo achieving at least a four-point improvement in pruritus Numerical Rating Scale (NRS) score from the baseline (pruritus-NRS response). CI, confidence interval.

3.4.4. Subgroup Analyses and Meta-Regression of Efficacy Outcomes

The subgroup analyses indicated that JAK inhibitors improved AD. From the meta-regression analyses, we identified age as a potential effect modifier of EASI-75 responses. Studies involving children and adolescents showed a higher RR of achieving an EASI-75 response than those exclusively involving adults (Table S2). According to the subgroup analyses of different JAK inhibitors at different time points, gusacitinib was unlikely to achieve EASI-75 and IGA responses (Table S3).

3.5. Safety Outcomes

3.5.1. TEAEs

Twelve studies (involving 3402 patients) were included in the analysis of TEAEs. AD patients treated with JAK inhibitors had relatively higher risks of developing TEAEs (RR = 1.14; 95% CI = 1.02–1.28) than those treated with placebo (Table 2). Most TEAEs were tolerable; nasopharyngitis was the most reported event (Table 3), followed by upper respiratory tract infection, headache, nausea, diarrhea, elevated blood creatine phosphokinase levels, and acne. Herpesvirus infection was reported in patients treated with abrocitinib or baricitinib. However, substantial heterogeneity was observed among studies ($I^2 = 52\%$; $P = 0.023$). Table 2 shows several potential effect modifiers accounting for the considerable heterogeneity among the TEAEs, including administration route, AD severity, and treatment duration. Patients who were administered oral JAK inhibitors experienced moderate to severe AD at baseline. Those treated with JAK inhibitors for >12 weeks were more likely to develop TEAEs.

3.5.2. AEs Leading to Drug Discontinuation

Fourteen studies (involving 3926 patients) were included in the analysis of AEs that led to drug discontinuation. Table 2 shows that patients who were administered with JAK inhibitors were unlikely to have higher risks of developing AEs (RR = 0.89; 95% CI = 0.57–1.38) than those treated with placebo. No significant heterogeneity was detected ($I^2 = 0\%$; $P = 0.62$).

3.5.3. Sensitivity Analyses

As shown in Table S4, a sensitivity analysis of the overall effects on each outcome before and after the application of modified HKSJ adjustment yielded similar results, demonstrating the robustness of the findings.

3.6. Publication Bias

No publication bias was detected after the visual inspection of the funnel plot or Egger's regression test except for the pruritus-NRS response outcome (Figure S3).

3.7. GRADE Approach for CoE

We presented the CoE using a modified GRADE evidence profile (Table 4) on the GRADEpro website (https://gdt.gradepro.org/ accessed on 23 February 2021). The GRADE guidelines [49] indicated that publication bias levels were downgraded for studies that identified conflicts of interest. The overall CoE of the efficacy outcomes was deemed "moderate." Owing to the "high" bias risk of BREEZE-AD4 2020, the overall CoE of the safety outcomes was considered "low." The NNTs for patients achieving IGA, EASI-75, and pruritus-NRS response were 3.97, 5.72, and 4.91, respectively. The NNH for patients experiencing TEAEs was 14.80.

Table 2. Safety outcomes of Janus kinase inhibitors.

Subgroups	Treatment-Emergent Adverse Events				Meta-Regression		Adverse Events Leading to Drug Discontinuation				Meta-Regression	
	No. of Studies	Pooled RR (95% CI)	p-Value	I^2 (%)	τ^2	p-Value	No. of Studies	Pooled RR (95% CI)	p-Value	I^2 (%)	τ^2	p-Value
Overall	12	1.14 (1.02 to 1.28) *	0.023	52.0			14	0.89 (0.57 to 1.38)	0.621	0.0		
Route of administration					0.013	0.033					0	0.064
Oral	9	1.18 (1.06 to 1.32) **	0.003	48.3			9	1.03 (0.64 to 1.64)	0.917	0.0		
Topical	3	0.77 (0.49 to 1.20)	0.255	25.2			5	0.26 (0.07 to 1.02)	0.054	0.0		
Severity of atopic dermatitis					0.012	0.021					0	0.036
Mild to moderate	2	0.73 (0.47 to 1.13)	0.163	33.1			3	0.16 (0.03 to 0.84) *	0.031	0.0		
Moderate to severe	10	1.18 (1.06 to 1.31) **	0.002	43.7			11	1.01 (0.64 to 1.60)	0.929	0.0		
Age of participants					0.019	0.483					0	0.200
Adults only	10	1.12 (0.99 to 1.26)	0.068	55.3			9	1.10 (0.63 to 1.93)	0.728	0.0		
Contain children or adolescents	2	1.41 (1.06 to 1.88) *	0.019	0.0			5	0.60 (0.29 to 1.26)	0.193	0.0		
Mechanism of action					0.012	0.062					0	0.750
Selective for JAK1 inhibition	3	1.29 (1.11 to 1.50) *	0.001	0.0			3	0.77 (0.39 to 1.52)	0.456	0.0		
Selective for JAK1/JAK2 inhibition	6	1.14 (0.98 to 1.31)	0.082	59.4			6	1.22 (0.60 to 2.51)	0.582	13.3		
Selective for JAK1/JAK3 inhibition	1	0.56 (0.32 to 1.00) *	0.049	NA			1	0.14 (0.01 to 2.59)	0.186	NA		
Pan-JAK inhibition	2	0.99 (0.66 to 1.48)	0.917	0.0			4	0.55 (0.11 to 2.63)	0.504	0.0		
Treatment duration					0.013	0.026					0	0.134
<12 weeks	4	0.84 (0.63 to 1.11)	0.223	8.2			6	0.37 (0.11 to 1.26)	0.120	0.0		
≥12 weeks	8	1.20 (1.07 to 1.34) **	0.002	52.5			8	1.01 (0.63 to 1.63)	0.965	0.0		

* $p < 0.05$; ** $p < 0.01$; CI, confidence interval; RR, risk ratio.

Table 3. Treatment-emergent adverse events reported in the studies included in the meta-analysis.

JAK Inhibitors by Mechanism	No. of Patients	No. (%) of Patients with Common TEAEs							
		Nasopharyngitis	URTI	Headache	Nausea	Diarrhea	Blood CPK Increase	Acne	Herpes Viral Infection
Selective for JAK1 inhibition									
Abrocitinib	834	73 (8.8)	85 (10.2)	64 (7.7)	94 (11.3)	10 (1.2)	8 (1.0)	11 (1.3)	10 (1.2)
Upadacitinib	126	9 (7.1)	17 (13.5)	10 (7.9)	7 (5.6)	4 (3.2)	7 (5.6)	12 (9.5)	0
Selective for JAK1/JAK2 inhibition									
Baricitinib	1318	118 (9.0)	36 (2.7)	64 (4.9)	2 (0.2)	25 (1.9)	27 (2.0)	5 (0.4)	74 (5.6)
Ruxolitinib	204	10 (4.9)	5 (2.5)	4 (2.0)	0	0	0	0	0
Selective for JAK1/JAK3 inhibition									
Tofacitinib	35	2 (5.7)	1 (2.9)	1 (2.9)	1 (2.9)	0	0	0	0
Pan-JAK inhibition									
Gusacitinib	27	3 (11.1)	0	7 (25.9)	5 (18.5)	3 (11.1)	0	0	0
Delgocitinib	439	28 (6.4)	0	0	0	0	0	4 (0.9)	0

AD, atopic dermatitis; AE, adverse event; NA, not applicable; RR, relative risk; SAE, serious adverse event; TEAE, treatment-emergent adverse event; URTI, upper respiratory tract infection.

Table 4. Certainty of evidence based on GRADE (Janus kinase inhibitors vs. placebo in atopic dermatitis).

Participants (Studies) Follow Up	Certainty Assessment						Summary of Findings	
	Risk of Bias	Inconsistency	Indirectness	Imprecision	Publication Bias	Overall Certainty of Evidence	Relative Effect (95% CI)	NNTs or NNHs
EASI-75 response								
3498 (12 RCTs)	Not serious	Not serious	Not serious	Not serious	Likely [a]	⊕⊕⊕⊖ MODERATE	2.84 (2.20 to 3.67)	3.97
IGA response								
2417 (11 RCTs)	Not serious	Not serious	Not serious	Not serious	Likely [a]	⊕⊕⊕⊖ MODERATE	2.99 (2.26 to 3.95)	5.72
Pruritus-NRS response								
3036 (8 RCTs)	Not serious	Not serious	Not serious	Not serious	Likely [a]	⊕⊕⊕⊖ MODERATE	2.52 (1.90 to 3.35)	4.91
TEAEs								
3402 (12 RCTs)	Serious [b]	Not serious	Not serious	Not serious	Likely [a]	⊕⊕⊖⊖ LOW	1.14 (1.02 to 1.28)	14.80
AEs leading to drug discontinuation								
3926 (14 RCTs)	Serious [b]	Not serious	Not serious	Not serious	Likely [a]	⊕⊕⊖⊖ LOW	0.89 (0.57 to 1.38)	NR

AEs, Adverse Events; CI, confidence interval; GRADE, Grading of Recommendations Assessment, Development and Evaluation; IGA, Investigator's Global Assessment; NNTs/NNHs, number-needed-to-treats/number-needed-to-harms; NR: not reasonable (no statistical significance in meta-analysis; therefore, calculation of this value is not reasonable); NRS, Numerical Rating Scale; RCT, randomized controlled trial; TEAEs, treatment emergent AEs. [a] Potential conflict of interest was indicated. [b] One study was judged as "high" bias risk.

4. Discussion

Our study provides evidence that JAK inhibitors are more effective in achieving EASI-75, IGA, and pruritus-NRS responses than placebo in patients with AD. AD patients treated with JAK inhibitors had relatively higher risks of developing TEAEs, but no higher risks were observed regarding AEs leading to drug discontinuation. From the viewpoint of evidence-based medicine based on the GRADE approach, the overall CoE of the efficacy outcomes was "moderate," while that of the safety outcomes was considered "low".

A previous meta-analysis of five RCTs demonstrated that JAK inhibitors lowered EASI and pruritus scores [20], which is consistent with the findings of this study. However, in contrast to the former study with a small sample size that represented only four countries, we included 15 multi-center RCTs in more than 10 countries and performed subgroup analyses and meta-regressions to identify potential effect modifiers of the efficacy and safety outcomes. Additionally, sensitivity analyses confirmed the robustness of our results. We also applied a GRADE assessment and furnished the NNT and NNH results to facilitate evidence-based decisions in the treatment of AD in clinical practice. Hence, our updated meta-analysis is robust and provides more evidence than a previously published meta-analysis [20].

Given that different kinds of JAK inhibitors seemed to have different effects in AD patients, there were no head-to-head comparisons between JAK inhibitors. According to our subgroup analyses of different JAK inhibitors at different time points, gusacitinib was unlikely to achieve EASI-75 and IGA responses. In the original article, gusacitinib showed benefits in achieving EASI-50 but not EASI-75 [47]. This may also be subject to the lack of statistical power due to an insufficient number of participants. Additionally, topical delgocitinib had higher rates of achieving EASI-75 response than placebo but not IGA response. Other topical agents such as tofacitinib or ruxolitinib demonstrated better response than placebos regarding IGA and pruritus-NRS responses. As seen in Table 3, ruxolitinib and delgocitinib seemed to have fewer TEAEs than other JAK inhibitors. This discovery is important to clinicians because these topical agents may serve as better options than oral forms for their effectiveness and fewer side effects.

We selected EASI as an efficacy outcome because it is adequately validated and recommended for the evaluation of the clinical signs of AD in RCTs [50,51]. However, an EASI assessment is not always feasible in routine practice as it is complex and time-consuming [50,51]. IGA is a rapid and easily interpreted alternative to EASI, and it should be included in the measurement outcomes for clinical trial approval under US drug regulations [52]. Despite the lack of standardization and validation, our meta-analysis of the IGA responses indicated less heterogeneity. Moreover, because EASI and IGA were evaluated by medical professionals, a patient-oriented scale is also critical for the assessment of drug efficacy. Consequently, considering chronic and intense pruritus is the major symptom observed in AD patients, we analyzed the previously validated pruritus-NRS as an efficacy outcome [53].

We performed several subgroup analyses and observed that children and adolescents had a higher RR of attaining an EASI-75 response. Only one RCT exclusively assessed pediatric patients. Therefore, no conclusions could be drawn regarding the efficacy of JAK inhibitors in this population.

The administration of JAK inhibitors was associated with an elevated risk of TEAEs. Nevertheless, most TEAEs were mild and tolerable. Nasopharyngitis, headache, and upper respiratory tract infection were the most common TEAEs observed in the enrolled RCTs, consistent with the findings of other systemic immunomodulators in AD management [54,55]. Recently, the warning black box issued by the Food and Drug Administration (FDA) reported an increased risk of serious cardiovascular problems with an oral form of tofacitinib, a JAK inhibitor in treating rheumatoid arthritis (RA) and ulcerative colitis [56]. Among the management of RA patients, JAK inhibitors (baricitinib, filgotinib, and tofacitinib) have also received warnings from the FDA about the increased risk of thromboembolic events and the higher rates of all-cause mortality. Even though the pharmacological features of the topical tofacitinib in AD may differ from that of oral usage in the above circumstances, these safety issues should not be ignored.

Recent studies have reported that AD exhibits complex dysregulations and multiple clinical phenotypes [57–59]. By contrast, between-study heterogeneity with seven distinct JAK inhibitors was observed to be unremarkable in most analyses. We hypothesized that the intracellular blockade by JAK inhibitors results in relatively less interference with the extracellular environment [60,61] and is indicated by the marked homogeneity among various types of JAK inhibitors in clinical settings. Furthermore, we identified administration route, severity, and treatment duration as potential effect modifiers for TEAE outcomes (Table 2). Systemic drug absorption via oral administration, severe inflammatory reactions in patients with moderate to severe AD, and longer treatment durations over 12 weeks could explain the results we obtained from the meta-regression analyses.

NNT/NNH is the average number of patients undergoing treatment with a particular therapy to achieve one additional positive/negative outcome compared with the placebo [62]. NNT < 10 and NNH $\geq$ 10 indicate "clinically desirable" benefit or harm of a particular therapeutic intervention [63]. In this study, the NNT was <10 for all efficacy outcomes, representing desirable effects compared with placebos. Despite the NNH for TEAEs being 14.80, the AEs were relatively innocuous. We believe that our findings could be helpful for clinical dermatologists in treating patients with AD.

A key strength of our study is the updated literature review and meta-analysis via an evidence-based approach. We provide CoE based on the GRADE system and calculate the NNTs/NNHs, which could guide clinicians in decision-making for AD treatment. However, the findings of this study must be considered with certain limitations in mind. First, we only compared the effects of JAK inhibitors against placebos. Comparisons of different types of JAK inhibitors were not performed in this study. Accordingly, we assume rigorous head-to-head RCTs to be beneficial in the comparison of the efficacy and safety outcomes of various JAK inhibitors. Second, we could not draw a firm conclusion concerning the efficacy of JAK inhibitors for the treatment of pediatric patients with AD because only one RCT that assessed patients aged less than 18 years was enrolled in this study. Given that pediatric AD is common, additional trials to clarify the effectiveness and safe dosage of JAK inhibitors in children and adolescents with AD are required. Third, it has only been five years since JAK inhibitors were approved for the treatment of AD; consequently, only a few RCTs with long-term follow-ups are available at present. Because we could only elucidate the short-term effects of JAK inhibitors, the results of this meta-analysis do not guarantee the long-term safety of JAK inhibitors. Hence, the evidence-based results presented herein must be interpreted with caution.

5. Conclusions

This systematic review and meta-analysis provide updated evidence for current AD guidelines. The findings demonstrate that JAK inhibitors have favorable efficacy (overall CoE: "moderate") in the treatment of AD with tolerable safety issues (overall CoE: "low"). However, planned prospective studies involving long-term follow-up of AEs and cost-effective analyses could aid clinical decisions in the application of JAK inhibitors for the treatment of AD.

Supplementary Materials: The following are available online at https://www.mdpi.com/article/10.3390/jpm11040279/s1, Figure S1: Flowchart of the Material and Methods: PRISMA flow diagram of the study. RCT, randomized controlled trial, Figure S2: Summary of Risk of Bias Assessment, Figure S3: Funnel Plot of Pruritus-NRS Response. Table S1: Search strategies modified in MEDLINE (a), Embase (b), Cochrane CENTRAL (c), and Web of Science (d), Table S2: Subgroup analyses and meta-regressions of efficacy outcomes, Table S3: Subgroup analyses of efficacy outcomes for various Janus kinase inhibitors at different time points, Table S4: Sensitivity analysis of overall effects of each outcome before and after modified Hartung–Knapp–Sidik–Jonkman (HKSJ) adjustment.

Author Contributions: H.-R.T., J.-W.L., L.-Y.C., and T.-L.C. had access to all the study data and take responsibility for the integrity of the data and the accuracy of data analysis. T.-L.C. conceptualized, designed, and supervised the study. H.-R.T., J.-W.L., and T.-L.C. performed data acquisition, analysis, or interpretation. All the authors contributed in drafting the manuscript and provided administrative, technical, or material support. T.-L.C. performed critical revision of the manuscript for important intellectual content. H.-R.T., J.-W.L., and T.-L.C. performed the statistical analysis. All authors have read and agreed to the published version of the manuscript.

Funding: This research received no external funding.

Institutional Review Board Statement: Ethical review and approval were waived for this study because the data were retrieved from published clinical trials in the public databases.

Informed Consent Statement: Patient consent was waived due to because the data were retrieved from published clinical trials, in which informed consent was obtained by the primary investigators.

Data Availability Statement: The data in this study were collated from published clinical trials, which could be accessed by the public.

Acknowledgments: We thank Ching-Ju Fang (Medical Library, National Cheng Kung University, Tainan, Taiwan) for her assistance and helpful comments that substantially improved the quality of our literature search. We also thank the Department of Medical Research of Hualien Tzu Chi Hospital and the Buddhist Tzu Chi Medical Foundation for their invaluable contributions to the methodology used in this systematic review and meta-analysis.

Conflicts of Interest: The authors declare no conflict of interest.

References

1. Silverberg, J.I.; Hanifin, J.M. Adult eczema prevalence and associations with asthma and other health and demographic factors: A US population-based study. *J. Allergy Clin. Immunol.* **2013**, *132*, 1132–1138. [CrossRef]
2. Bylund, S.; von Kobyletzki, L.B.; Svalstedt, M.; Svensson, Å. Prevalence and incidence of atopic dermatitis: A systematic review. *Acta Derm. Venereol.* **2020**, *100*, adv00160. [CrossRef] [PubMed]
3. Langan, S.M.; Irvine, A.D.; Weidinger, S. Atopic dermatitis. *Lancet* **2020**, *396*, 345–360. [CrossRef]
4. Kaufman, B.P.; Guttman-Yassky, E.; Alexis, A.F. Atopic dermatitis in diverse racial and ethnic groups-Variations in epidemiology, genetics, clinical presentation and treatment. *Exp. Dermatol.* **2018**, *27*, 340–357. [CrossRef]
5. Nettis, E.; Ortoncelli, M.; Pellacani, G.; Foti, C.; Di Leo, E.; Patruno, C.; Rongioletti, F.; Argenziano, G.; Ferrucci, S.M.; Macchia, L.; et al. A multicenter study on the prevalence of clinical patterns and clinical phenotypes in adult atopic dermatitis. *J. Investig. Allergol. Clin. Immunol.* **2020**, *30*, 448–450. [CrossRef] [PubMed]
6. Laughter, M.R.; Maymone, M.B.; Mashayekhi, S.; Arents, B.W.; Karimkhani, C.; Langan, S.M.; Dellavalle, R.P.; Flohr, C. The global burden of atopic dermatitis: Lessons from the global burden of disease study 1990–2017. *Br. J. Dermatol.* **2021**, *184*, 304–309. [CrossRef] [PubMed]
7. Eichenfield, L.F.; Tom, W.L.; Berger, T.G.; Krol, A.; Paller, A.S.; Schwarzenberger, K.; Bergman, J.N.; Chamlin, S.L.; Cohen, D.E.; Cooper, K.D.; et al. Guidelines of care for the management of atopic dermatitis, Section 2: Management and treatment of atopic dermatitis with topical therapies. *J. Am. Acad. Dermatol.* **2014**, *71*, 116–132. [CrossRef]
8. Ring, J.; Alomar, A.; Bieber, T.; Deleuran, M.; Fink-Wagner, A.; Gelmetti, C.; Gieler, U.; Lipozencic, J.; Luger, T.; Oranje, A.P.; et al. Guidelines for treatment of atopic eczema (atopic dermatitis) part I. *J. Eur. Acad. Dermatol. Venereol.* **2012**, *26*, 1045–1060. [CrossRef] [PubMed]
9. Katayama, I.; Aihara, M.; Ohya, Y.; Saeki, H.; Shimojo, N.; Shoji, S.; Taniguchi, M.; Yamada, H. Japanese guidelines for atopic dermatitis 2017. *Allergol. Int.* **2017**, *66*, 230–247. [CrossRef]
10. Worm, M.; Francuzik, W.; Kraft, M.; Alexiou, A. Modern therapies in atopic dermatitis: Biologics and small molecule drugs. *J. Dtsch. Dermatol. Ges.* **2020**, *18*, 1085–1092. [CrossRef]
11. Dattola, A.; Bennardo, L.; Silvestri, M.; Nisticò, S.P. What's new in the treatment of atopic dermatitis? *Dermatol. Ther.* **2019**, *32*, e12787. [CrossRef] [PubMed]
12. Yasuda, T.; Fukada, T.; Nishida, K.; Nakayama, M.; Matsuda, M.; Miura, I.; Dainichi, T.; Fukuda, S.; Kabashima, K.; Nakaoka, S.; et al. Hyperactivation of JAK1 tyrosine kinase induces stepwise, progressive pruritic dermatitis. *J. Clin. Invest.* **2016**, *126*, 2064–2076. [CrossRef] [PubMed]
13. Amano, W.; Nakajima, S.; Kunugi, H.; Numata, Y.; Kitoh, A.; Egawa, G.; Dainichi, T.; Honda, T.; Otsuka, A.; Kimoto, Y.; et al. The Janus kinase inhibitor JTE-052 improves skin barrier function through suppressing signal transducer and activator of transcription 3 signaling. *J. Allergy Clin. Immunol.* **2015**, *136*, 667–677. [CrossRef] [PubMed]
14. Fridman, J.S.; Scherle, P.A.; Collins, R.; Burn, T.; Neilan, C.L.; Hertel, D.; Contel, N.; Haley, P.; Thomas, B.; Shi, J.; et al. Preclinical evaluation of local JAK1 and JAK2 inhibition in cutaneous inflammation. *J. Invest. Dermatol.* **2011**, *131*, 1838–1844. [CrossRef]

15. Jin, W.; Huang, W.; Chen, L.; Jin, M.; Wang, Q.; Gao, Z.; Jin, Z. Topical application of JAK1/JAK2 inhibitor momelotinib exhibits significant anti-inflammatory responses in DNCB-induced atopic dermatitis model mice. *Int. J. Mol. Sci.* **2018**, *19*, 3973. [CrossRef]
16. Schwartz, D.M.; Kanno, Y.; Villarino, A.; Ward, M.; Gadina, M.; O'Shea, J.J. JAK inhibition as a therapeutic strategy for immune and inflammatory diseases. *Nat. Rev. Drug Discov.* **2017**, *17*, 78. [CrossRef]
17. Honstein, T.; Werfel, T. The show must go on: An update on clinical experiences and clinical studies on novel pharmaceutical developments for the treatment of atopic dermatitis. *Curr. Opin. Allergy Clin. Immunol.* **2020**, *20*, 386–394. [CrossRef]
18. Gadina, M.; Le, M.T.; Schwartz, D.M.; Silvennoinen, O.; Nakayamada, S.; Yamaoka, K.; O'Shea, J.J. Janus kinases to jakinibs: From basic insights to clinical practice. *Rheumatology* **2019**, *58*, i4–i16. [CrossRef]
19. Bieber, T.; Thyssen, J.P.; Reich, K.; Simpson, E.L.; Katoh, N.; Torrelo, A.; De Bruin-Weller, M.; Thaci, D.; Bissonnette, R.; Gooderham, M.; et al. Pooled safety analysis of baricitinib in adult patients with atopic dermatitis from 8 randomized clinical trials. *J. Eur. Acad. Dermatol. Venereol.* **2020**, *35*, 476–485. [CrossRef]
20. Arora, C.J.; Khattak, F.A.; Yousafzai, M.T.; Ibitoye, B.M.; Shumack, S. The effectiveness of Janus kinase inhibitors in treating atopic dermatitis: A systematic review and meta-analysis. *Dermatol. Ther.* **2020**, *33*, e13685. [CrossRef]
21. Higgins, J.P.T.; Thomas, J.; Chandler, J.; Cumpston, M.; Li, T.; Page, M.J.; Welch, V.A. Cochrane Handbook for Systematic Reviews of Interventions Version 6.2. Available online: www.training.cochrane.org/handbook (accessed on 25 January 2021).
22. Moher, D.; Liberati, A.; Tetzlaff, J.; Altman, D.G.; the PRISMA Group. Preferred reporting items for systematic reviews and meta-analyses: The PRISMA statement. *Ann. Intern. Med.* **2009**, *151*, 264–269. [CrossRef]
23. Sarri, G.; Patorno, E.; Yuan, H.; Guo, J.J.; Bennett, D.; Wen, X.; Zullo, A.R.; Largent, J.; Panaccio, M.; Gokhale, M.; et al. Framework for the synthesis of non-randomised studies and randomised controlled trials: A guidance on conducting a systematic review and meta-analysis for healthcare decision making. *BMJ Evid. Based Med.* **2020**, *9*. [CrossRef]
24. Sterne, J.A.; Savović, J.; Page, M.J.; Elbers, R.G.; Blencowe, N.S.; Boutron, I.; Cates, C.J.; Cheng, H.Y.; Corbett, M.S.; Eldridge, S.M.; et al. RoB 2: A revised tool for assessing risk of bias in randomised trials. *BMJ* **2019**, *366*, l4898. [CrossRef] [PubMed]
25. Page, M.J.; McKenzie, J.E.; Chau, M.; Green, S.E.; Forbes, A. Methods to select results to include in meta-analyses deserve more consideration in systematic reviews. *J. Clin. Epidemiol.* **2015**, *68*, 1282–1291. [CrossRef] [PubMed]
26. Cadham, C.J.; Jayasekera, J.C.; Advani, S.M.; Fallon, S.J.; Stephens, J.L.; Braithwaite, D.; Jeon, J.; Cao, P.; Levy, D.T.; Meza, R.; et al. Smoking cessation interventions for potential use in the lung cancer screening setting: A systematic review and meta-analysis. *Lung Cancer* **2019**, *135*, 205–216. [CrossRef]
27. Ueta, T.; Noda, Y.; Toyama, T.; Yamaguchi, T.; Amano, S. Systemic vascular safety of ranibizumab for age-related macular degeneration: Systematic review and meta-analysis of randomized trials. *Ophthalmology* **2014**, *121*, 2193–2203. [CrossRef]
28. Higgins, J.P.; Thompson, S.G.; Deeks, J.J.; Altman, D.G. Measuring inconsistency in meta-analyses. *BMJ* **2003**, *327*, 557–560. [CrossRef]
29. IntHout, J.; Ioannidis, J.P.; Borm, G.F. The Hartung-Knapp-Sidik-Jonkman method for random effects meta-analysis is straightforward and considerably outperforms the standard DerSimonian-Laird method. *BMC Med. Res. Methodol.* **2014**, *18*, 25. [CrossRef]
30. Hartung, J.; Knapp, G. On tests of the overall treatment effect in meta-analysis with normally distributed responses. *Stat. Med.* **2001**, *20*, 1771–1782. [CrossRef]
31. Saueressig, T.; Owen, P.J.; Zebisch, J.; Herbst, M.; Belavy, D.L. Evaluation of exercise interventions and outcomes after hip arthroplasty: A systematic review and meta-analysis. *JAMA Netw. Open* **2021**, *4*, e210254. [CrossRef]
32. Mc Cord, K.A.; Ewald, H.; Agarwal, A.; Glinz, D.; Aghlmandi, S.; Ioannidis, J.P.; Hemkens, L.G. Treatment effects in randomised trials using routinely collected data for outcome assessment versus traditional trials: Meta-research study. *BMJ* **2021**, *372*, n450. [CrossRef]
33. Janiaud, P.; Axfors, C.; Schmitt, A.M.; Gloy, V.; Ebrahimi, F.; Hepprich, M.; Smith, E.R.; Haber, N.A.; Khanna, N.; Moher, D.; et al. Association of convalescent plasma treatment with clinical outcomes in patients with COVID-19: A systematic review and meta-analysis. *JAMA* **2021**, *325*, 1185–1195. [CrossRef]
34. Guyatt, G.H.; Oxman, A.D.; Vist, G.E.; Kunz, R.; Falck-Ytter, Y.; Alonso-Coello, P.; Schünemann, H.J. GRADE: An emerging consensus on rating quality of evidence and strength of recommendations. *BMJ* **2008**, *336*, 924–926. [CrossRef]
35. Nakagawa, H.; Nemoto, O.; Igarashi, A.; Saeki, H.; Kaino, H.; Nagata, T. Delgocitinib ointment, a topical Janus kinase inhibitor, in adult patients with moderate to severe atopic dermatitis: A phase 3, randomized, double-blind, vehicle-controlled study and an open-label, long-term extension study. *J. Am. Acad. Dermatol.* **2020**, *82*, 823–831. [CrossRef]
36. Reich, K.; Kabashima, K.; Peris, K.; Silverberg, J.I.; Eichenfield, L.F.; Bieber, T.; Kaszuba, A.; Kolodsick, J.; Yang, F.E.; Gamalo, M.; et al. Efficacy and safety of baricitinib combined with topical corticosteroids for treatment of moderate to severe atopic dermatitis: A randomized clinical trial. *JAMA Dermatol.* **2020**, *156*, 1333–1343. [CrossRef]
37. Silverberg, J.I.; Simpson, E.L.; Thyssen, J.P.; Gooderham, M.; Chan, G.; Feeney, C.; Biswas, P.; Valdez, H.; DiBonaventura, M.; Nduaka, C.; et al. Efficacy and safety of abrocitinib in patients with moderate-to-severe atopic dermatitis: A randomized clinical trial. *JAMA Dermatol.* **2020**, *156*, 863–873. [CrossRef] [PubMed]
38. Simpson, E.L.; Lacour, J.P.; Spelman, L.; Galimberti, R.; Eichenfield, L.; Bissonnette, R.; King, B.; Thyssen, J.; Silverberg, J.; Bieber, T.; et al. Baricitinib in patients with moderate-to-severe atopic dermatitis and inadequate response to topical corticosteroids: Results from two randomized monotherapy phase III trials. *Br. J. Dermatol.* **2020**, *183*, 242–255. [CrossRef] [PubMed]

39. Simpson, E.L.; Sinclair, R.; Forman, S.; Wollenberg, A.; Aschoff, R.; Cork, M.; Bieber, T.; Thyssen, J.P.; Yosipovitch, G.; Flohr, C.; et al. Efficacy and safety of abrocitinib in adults and adolescents with moderate-to-severe atopic dermatitis (JADE MONO-1): A multicentre, double-blind, randomised, placebo-controlled, phase 3 trial. *Lancet* **2020**, *396*, 255–266. [CrossRef]
40. Bissonnette, R.; Papp, K.A.; Poulin, Y.; Gooderham, M.; Gooderham, M.; Raman, M.; Mallbris, L.; Wang, C.; Purohit, V.; Mamolo, C.; et al. Topical tofacitinib for atopic dermatitis: A phase IIa randomized trial. *Br. J. Dermatol.* **2016**, *175*, 902–911. [CrossRef] [PubMed]
41. Gooderham, M.J.; Forman, S.B.; Bissonnette, R.; Beebe, J.S.; Zhang, W.; Banfield, C.; Zhu, L.; Papacharalambous, J.; Vincent, M.S.; Peeva, E. Efficacy and safety of oral Janus kinase 1 inhibitor abrocitinib for patients with atopic dermatitis: A phase 2 randomized clinical trial. *JAMA Dermatol.* **2019**, *155*, 1371–1379. [CrossRef] [PubMed]
42. Guttman-Yassky, E.; Silverberg, J.I.; Nemoto, O.; Forman, S.B.; Wilke, A.; Prescilla, R.; de la Peña, A.; Nunes, F.P.; Janes, J.; Gamalo, M.; et al. Baricitinib in adult patients with moderate-to-severe atopic dermatitis: A phase 2 parallel, double-blinded, randomized placebo-controlled multiple-dose study. *J. Am. Acad. Dermatol.* **2019**, *80*, 913–921.e9. [CrossRef]
43. Guttman-Yassky, E.; Thaçi, D.; Pangan, A.L.; Hong, H.C.; Papp, K.A.; Reich, K.; Beck, L.A.; Mohamed, M.F.; Othman, A.A.; Anderson, J.K.; et al. Upadacitinib in adults with moderate to severe atopic dermatitis: 16-week results from a randomized, placebo-controlled trial. *J. Allergy Clin. Immunol.* **2020**, *145*, 877–884. [CrossRef]
44. Kim, B.S.; Howell, M.D.; Sun, K.; Papp, K.; Papp, K.; Nasir, A.; Kuligowski, M.E.; INCB 18424-206 Study Investigators. Treatment of atopic dermatitis with ruxolitinib cream (JAK1/JAK2 inhibitor) or triamcinolone cream. *J. Allergy Clin. Immunol.* **2020**, *145*, 572–582. [CrossRef]
45. Nakagawa, H.; Nemoto, O.; Igarashi, A.; Nagata, T. Efficacy and safety of topical JTE-052, a Janus kinase inhibitor, in Japanese adult patients with moderate-to-severe atopic dermatitis: A phase II, multicentre, randomized, vehicle-controlled clinical study. *Br. J. Dermatol.* **2018**, *178*, 424–432. [CrossRef] [PubMed]
46. Nakagawa, H.; Nemoto, O.; Igarashi, A.; Saeki, H.; Oda, M.; Kabashima, K.; Nagata, T. Phase 2 clinical study of delgocitinib ointment in pediatric patients with atopic dermatitis. *J. Allergy Clin. Immunol.* **2019**, *144*, 1575–1583. [CrossRef]
47. Bissonnette, R.; Maari, C.; Forman, S.; Bhatia, N.; Lee, M.; Fowler, J.; Tyring, S.; Pariser, D.; Sofen, H.; Dhawan, S.; et al. The oral Janus kinase/spleen tyrosine kinase inhibitor ASN002 demonstrates efficacy and improves associated systemic inflammation in patients with moderate-to-severe atopic dermatitis: Results from a randomized double-blind placebo-controlled study. *Br. J. Dermatol.* **2019**, *181*, 733–742. [CrossRef] [PubMed]
48. McGuinness, L.A.; Higgins, J.P.T. Risk-of-bias VISualization (robvis): An R package and Shiny web app for visualizing risk-of-bias assessments. *Res. Syn. Methods* **2021**, *12*, 55–61. [CrossRef] [PubMed]
49. Guyatt, G.H.; Oxman, A.D.; Montori, V.; Vist, G.; Kunz, R.; Brozek, J.; Alonso-Coello, P.; Djulbegovic, B.; Atkins, D.; Falck-Ytter, Y.; et al. GRADE guidelines: 5. Rating the quality of evidence–publication bias. *J. Clin. Epidemiol.* **2011**, *64*, 1277–1282. [CrossRef]
50. Schmitt, J.; Langan, S.; Deckert, S.; Svensson, A.; von Kobyletzki, L.; Thomas, K.; Spuls, P. Assessment of clinical signs of atopic dermatitis: A systematic review and recommendation. *J. Allergy Clin. Immunol.* **2013**, *132*, 1337–1347. [CrossRef]
51. Fishbein, A.B.; Silverberg, J.I.; Wilson, E.J.; Ong, P.Y. Update on atopic dermatitis: Diagnosis, severity assessment, and treatment selection. *J. Allergy Clin. Immunol. Pract.* **2020**, *8*, 91–101. [CrossRef] [PubMed]
52. Futamura, M.; Leshem, Y.A.; Thomas, K.S.; Nankervis, H.; Williams, H.C.; Simpson, E.; Information, P.E.K.F.C. A systematic review of Investigator Global Assessment (IGA) in atopic dermatitis (AD) trials: Many options, no standards. *J. Am. Acad. Dermatol.* **2016**, *74*, 288–294. [CrossRef]
53. Silverberg, J.I.; Margolis, D.J.; Boguniewicz, M.; Fonacier, L.; Grayson, M.H.; Ong, P.Y.; Fuxench, Z.C.; Simpson, E.L. Validation of five patient-reported outcomes for atopic dermatitis severity in adults. *Br. J. Dermatol.* **2020**, *182*, 104–111. [CrossRef] [PubMed]
54. Silverberg, J.I.; Pinter, A.; Pulka, G.; Poulin, Y.; Bouaziz, J.D.; Wollenberg, A.; Murrell, D.F.; Alexis, A.; Lindsey, L.; Ahmad, F.; et al. Phase 2B randomized study of nemolizumab in adults with moderate-to-severe atopic dermatitis and severe pruritus. *J. Allergy Clin. Immunol.* **2020**, *145*, 173–182. [CrossRef]
55. Guttman-Yassky, E.; Blauvelt, A.; Eichenfield, L.F.; Paller, A.S.; Armstrong, A.W.; Drew, J.; Gopalan, R.; Simpson, E.L. Efficacy and safety of lebrikizumab, a high-affinity interleukin 13 inhibitor, in adults with moderate to severe atopic dermatitis: A phase 2b randomized clinical trial. *JAMA Dermatol.* **2020**, *156*, 411–420. [CrossRef] [PubMed]
56. U.S. Food and Drug Administration. FDA Drug Safety Communication: FDA Approves Boxed Warning about Increased Risk of Blood Clots and Death with Higher Dose of Arthritis and Ulcerative Colitis Medicine Tofacitinib (Xeljanz, Xeljanz XR). 2019. Available online: https://www.fda.gov/drugs/drug-safety-and-availability/fda-approves-boxed-warning-about-increased-risk-blood-clots-and-death-higher-dose-arthritis-and (accessed on 2 April 2021).
57. Brunner, P.M.; Guttman-Yassky, E. Racial differences in atopic dermatitis. *Ann. Allergy Asthma Immunol.* **2019**, *122*, 449–455. [CrossRef] [PubMed]
58. Zhou, L.; Leonard, A.; Pavel, A.B.; Malik, K.; Raja, A.; Glickman, J.; Estrada, Y.D.; Peng, X.; Del Duca, E.; Sanz-Cabanillas, J.; et al. Age-specific changes in the molecular phenotype of patients with moderate-to-severe atopic dermatitis. *J. Allergy Clin. Immunol.* **2019**, *144*, 144–156. [CrossRef]
59. Løset, M.; Brown, S.J.; Saunes, M.; Hveem, K. Genetics of atopic dermatitis: From DNA sequence to clinical relevance. *Dermatology* **2019**, *235*, 355–364. [CrossRef]
60. Renert-Yuval, Y.; Guttman-Yassky, E. New treatments for atopic dermatitis targeting beyond IL-4/IL-13 cytokines. *Ann. Allergy Asthma Immunol.* **2020**, *124*, 28–35. [CrossRef]

61. Bieber, T. Interleukin-13: Targeting an underestimated cytokine in atopic dermatitis. *Allergy* **2020**, *75*, 54–62. [CrossRef] [PubMed]
62. Mendes, D.; Alves, C.; Batel-Marques, F. Number needed to treat (NNT) in clinical literature: An appraisal. *BMC Med.* **2017**, *15*, 112. [CrossRef]
63. Citrome, L. Quantifying clinical relevance. *Innov. Clin. Neurosci.* **2014**, *11*, 26–30. [PubMed]

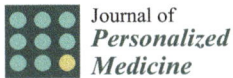

Article

Differential Expression of Estrogen-Responsive Genes in Women with Psoriasis

Vladimir Sobolev [1,*], Anna Soboleva [1,2], Elena Denisova [1,3], Malika Denieva [4], Eugenia Dvoryankova [1], Elkhan Suleymanov [5], Olga V. Zhukova [3], Nikolay Potekaev [3], Irina Korsunskaya [1] and Alexandre Mezentsev [1]

1. Centre of Theoretical Problems of Physico-Chemical Pharmacology, Russian Academy of Sciences, Russian Academy of Sciences, 119334 Moscow, Russia; annasobo@mail.ru (A.S.); evdenisova@rambler.ru (E.D.); edvoriankova@gmail.com (E.D.); marykor@bk.ru (I.K.); mesentsev@yahoo.com (A.M.)
2. Scientific Research Institute of Human Morphology, 3 Tsurupa Street, 117418 Moscow, Russia
3. Moscow Scientific and Practical Center of Dermatovenereology and Cosmetology, 119071 Moscow, Russia; klinderma@inbox.ru (O.V.Z.); klinderma@mail.ru (N.P.)
4. Department of Polyclinic Therapy, Chechen State University, 366007 Grozny, Russia; denieva54@mail.ru
5. P. Hertsen Moscow Oncology Research Institute, National Medical Research Radiological Centre of the Ministry of Health of the Russian Federation, 3, 2 Botkinskiy Proezd, 125284 Moscow, Russia; Docseasur@mail.ru
* Correspondence: vlsobolew@gmail.com

Abstract: In women, the flow of psoriasis is influenced by each phase of a woman's life cycle. According to previous findings, significant changes in the levels of sex hormones affect the severity of the disease. **Aim:** The aim of this study was to identify the estrogen-responsive genes that could be responsible for the exacerbation of psoriasis in menopausal women. **Methods:** Skin samples of lesional skin donated by psoriasis patients (n = 5) were compared with skin samples of healthy volunteers (n = 5) using liquid chromatography–tandem mass spectrometry (LC–MS/MS). The set of differentially expressed proteins was subjected to protein ontology analysis to identify differentially expressed estrogen-responsive proteins. The expression of discovered proteins was validated by qPCR and ELISA on four groups of female participants. The first group included ten psoriasis patients without menopause; the second included eleven postmenopausal patients; the third included five healthy volunteers without menopause; and the fourth included six postmenopausal volunteers. Moreover, the participants' blood samples were used to assess the levels of estradiol, progesterone, and testosterone. **Results:** We found that the levels of estradiol and progesterone were significantly lower and the levels of testosterone were significantly higher in the blood of patients compared to the control. The protein ontology analysis of LC–MS/MS data identified six proteins, namely HMOX1, KRT19, LDHA, HSPD1, MAPK1, and CA2, differentially expressed in the lesional skin of female patients compared to male patients. ELISA and qPCR experiments confirmed differential expression of the named proteins and their mRNA. The genes encoding the named proteins were differentially expressed in patients compared to volunteers. However, *KRT19* and *LDHA* were not differentially expressed when we compared patients with and without menopause. All genes, except *MAPK1*, were differentially expressed in patients with menopause compared to the volunteers with menopause. *HMOX1*, *KRT19*, *HSPD1*, and *LDHA* were differentially expressed in patients without menopause compared to the volunteers without menopause. However, no significant changes were found when we compared healthy volunteers with and without menopause. **Conclusion:** Our experiments discovered a differential expression of six estrogen-controlled genes in the skin of female patients. Identification of these genes and assessment of the changes in their expression provide insight into the biological effects of estrogen in lesional skin. The results of proteomic analysis are available via ProteomeXchange with identifier PXD021673.

Keywords: psoriasis; proteome analysis; estrogen; menopause

Citation: Sobolev, V.; Soboleva, A.; Denisova, E.; Denieva, M.; Dvoryankova, E.; Suleymanov, E.; Zhukova, O.V.; Potekaev, N.; Korsunskaya, I.; Mezentsev, A. Differential Expression of Estrogen-Responsive Genes in Women with Psoriasis. *J. Pers. Med.* **2021**, *11*, 925. https://doi.org/10.3390/jpm11090925

Academic Editors: Mircea Tampa, Monica Neagu, Constantin Caruntu and Simona Roxana Georgescu

Received: 14 June 2021
Accepted: 14 September 2021
Published: 17 September 2021

Publisher's Note: MDPI stays neutral with regard to jurisdictional claims in published maps and institutional affiliations.

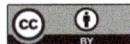

Copyright: © 2021 by the authors. Licensee MDPI, Basel, Switzerland. This article is an open access article distributed under the terms and conditions of the Creative Commons Attribution (CC BY) license (https://creativecommons.org/licenses/by/4.0/).

1. Introduction

Psoriasis is an immune-mediated disease that is driven by T_{h1} and T_{h17} cells [1]. The incidence of psoriasis is similar in men and women. The mean age at onset of psoriasis presentation ranges between 15 and 20 years of age and the second peak occurs at the ages of 55–60 [2]. It is well-documented that the endogenous factors such as hormonal changes may trigger psoriasis [3]. In women, the severity of psoriasis is influenced by each phase of a woman's life cycle and the disease frequency tends to peak during puberty, postpartum, and menopause. In contrast, the patients' condition often improves during pregnancy [4].

Although puberty is the period of life when the first signs of psoriasis often appear, there is a lack of evidence that female sex hormones trigger the disease. In fact, an increased production of estradiol (E2) and progesterone (PG) during the menstrual cycle has anti-inflammatory effects [5]. Moreover, PG shifts the balance between Th_1 and Th_2 responses toward Th_2 [6]. In pregnancy, an increased production of estriol and PG often results in an improvement of symptoms in a majority of psoriasis patients.

However, psoriasis exacerbates in the first months of the postpartum period and the body surface area covered by psoriasis (BSA) significantly increases [7]. There is also a negative correlation between the levels of estrogen (ES) and BSA [4]. Moreover, prolactin (PRL) released by the pituitary gland of the brain stimulates immunity [8]. Respectively, patients with hyperprolactinemia present with many different clinical manifestations, including psoriasis [9]. In addition, there is a correlation of the PRL level and disease severity [9].

In perimenopause, the remaining aging follicles produce less inhibin and ES [10]. Since they are suppressed, the synthesis and secretion of the follicle-stimulating hormone (FSH) and luteinizing hormone (LH) gradually increase and a higher production of FSH stabilizes the level of ES. For this reason, ES can be slightly elevated for a limited period of time. Then, ES drops because there are less ES-producing cells in the ovary and they require more FSH to produce the same amount of ES. Consequently, the level of FSH continues to increase due to an existence of the negative feedback between the synthesis of ES and production of FSH [11], and it is often accompanied by an exacerbation of psoriasis [8].

Our own observations suggest that young women diagnosed with psoriasis have lower ES levels compared to healthy controls [12,13]. In this paper, we aim to identity the genes that could be targeted by ES in the lesional and uninvolved skin of female patients.

2. Materials and Methods

2.1. Ethics Statement

All samples were obtained with informed written consent from healthy volunteers and psoriasis patients in accordance with Declaration of Helsinki principles. All protocols were approved by an institutional review board (I.I. Mechnikov Institute of Vaccines and Sera, Moscow, Russia).

2.2. Clinical Samples

Skin biopsies for LC–MS/MS study were obtained from 5 healthy volunteers (MS volunteers), namely 2 males and 3 females between the ages of 39 and 79 years (mean age: 61.6 years), and from an equal number of psoriasis patients (MS patients), namely 3 males and 2 females between the ages of 30 and 68 years (mean age: 49.2 years). Skin biopsies for qPCR and ELISA assays were obtained from female participants: 20 psoriasis patients and 11 healthy volunteers that we identified as qPCR/ELISA participants. To distinguish the changes in gene expression caused by the disease from ones caused by menopause, the participants were divided in four groups. The first group included 10 patients without menopause between the ages of 19 and 43 years (mean age: 31.5 years). The second group included 10 patients with menopause between the ages of 46 and 54 years (mean age: 50.2 years). The third group included 6 healthy volunteers without menopause between the ages of 26 and 38 years (mean age: 31 years). The fourth group included 5 healthy volunteers with menopause between the ages of 43 and 57 (mean age: 50.8 years). The additional details on participants of this study can be found in Table 1.

Table 1. Clinical characteristics of psoriasis patients and volunteers that participated in the LC–MS/MS, qPCR, and ELISA studies.

ID	Age	Medical History	ID	Age	Medical History
		LC-MS male patients			*qPCR/ELISA patients with menopause*
1	30	not reported			
2	40	stage 1 arterial hypertension, hyperuricemia, obesity,	1	46	gastritis, cholecystitis, pancreatitis, hypertension, coronary artery disease, angina pectoris, urolithiasis
3	68	psoriatic arthritis, hypertension, stage 2, bronchitis, dyscirculatory encephalopathy, hyperuricemia, obesity 1st degree	2	46	hypertension, stage 2, kidney cyst
			3	47	cholecystitis, cholelithiasis
			4	48	type II diabetes, obesity stage 3, arterial hypertension, nodular Hashimoto's thyroiditis, uterine fibroids, cerebrovascular disease, discirculatory encephalopathy arterial hypertension tachycardia
		LC-MS female patients			
1	48	stage 2 hypertension			
2	60	stage 2 hypertension			
		LC-MS male volunteers			
1	53	phlebeurysm			
2	77	arthrosclerosis			
		LC-MS female volunteers	5	51	
1	39	white line hernia			nodular Hashimoto's thyroiditis, osteochondrosis dorsopathy
2	60	incisional ventral hernia			
3	79	arthrosclerosis, abdominal aortic aneurysm, chronic pyelonephritis, dyslipidemia, hypertension			
			6	51	hypertension, stage 2;
			7	53	hypertension, stage 2; depression;
		qPCR/ELISA patients, without menopause	8	53	nodular goiter;
			9	53	hypertension, stage 2 type 2 diabetes, osteoarthritis; dorsopathy;
1	19	not reported			
2	21	erysipelas, obesity stage 4, cholecystitis, uterine fibroids	10	54	not reported
					qPCR/ELISA volunteers without menopause
3	28	not reported	1	26	not reported
4	30	goiter, euthyroid sick syndrome,	2	28	not reported
			3	29	not reported
5	32	bilateral otitis media, cholecystitis	4	32	not reported
			5	33	not reported
		vaginal yeast infection	6	38	not reported
6	32	not reported			
7	32	diffuse goiter, grade 2;			*qPCR/ELISA volunteers with menopause*
8	36	depression			
9	42	gastritis, pyelonephritis; insulin resistance, hypertension, stage 2, cerebrovascular disease, cholecystitis	1	43	not reported
			2	49	not reported
			3	50	not reported
			4	55	not reported
10	43	not reported	5	57	not reported

The patients that participated in our study discontinued topical treatment for 1 week prior to the biopsy collection (2 week in the case of systemic therapies). Each patient donated two 4 mm punch biopsies of lesional and uninvolved skin following a local anesthesia. Biopsies of uninvolved skin were taken at least 6 cm away from the nearest skin lesion. The collected biopsies were flash frozen in liquid nitrogen and stored at −80 °C until processing. Blood (3 mL) was withdrawn by venipuncture without anticoagulant at day 3 or 4 of the menstrual cycle. Serum was separated, divided into aliquots, and stored frozen at −20 °C until needed.

2.3. Preparation of Skin Samples for LC–MS/MS Experiments

Each sample was washed twice with 0.5 mL of phosphate-buffered saline. The samples were homogenized by mechanical disruption in liquid nitrogen. To prepare the protein samples, sodium deoxycholate (SDS) lysis as well as reduction and alkylation buffer pH 8.5, which contained 100 mM TRIS, 1% (w/v) SDS, 40 mM 2-chloroacetamide, and 10 mM TCEP, were added to the homogenized samples. The samples were sonicated and boiled for 10 min. Then, the protein concentration was determined by Bradford assay and the equal volumes of 1% trypsin solution (w/v) prepared in 100 mM TRIS pH 8.5 were added.

After overnight digestion at 37 °C, peptides were acidified with 1% trifluoroacetic acid (TFA). The samples (2 × 20 µg) were loaded on 14-gauge StageTips containing 2 layers of SDB-RPS discs. Respectively, 2 tips per a sample were used. The tips were consequently washed with equal volumes of ethyl acetate, 100 µL of 1% TFA prepared in ethyl acetate, and 100 µL of 0.2% TFA. After each washing, the excess of liquid was removed by centrifugation (300 g; 1.5 min.) Then, the peptides were eluted with 60 µL of 5% NH_4OH prepared in 80% acetonitrile. The eluates were vacuum-dried and stored at −80 °C. Prior to the experiment, the vacuum-dried samples were dissolved in 2% acetonitrile/0.1% TFA buffer and sonicated for 2 min.

2.4. LC-MS/MS Analysis

The reverse-phase chromatography was performed on the Ultimate 3000 Nano LC System (Thermo Fisher Scientific, Waltham, MA, USA) coupled to the Q Exactive Plus benchtop Orbitrap mass spectrometer (Thermo Fisher Scientific, Waltham, USA) using a chip-based nanoelectrospray source (Thermo Fisher Scientific, Waltham, USA). Samples prepared in the loading buffer (0.1% TFA and 2% acetonitrile in water) were loaded on the Inertsil ODS3 (GLSciences, Torrance, USA) trap column (0.1 × 20 mm, 3 µm) at 10 µL/min and separated on the Reprosil PUR C18AQ (Dr. Maisch, Germany) fused-silica column (0.1 × 500 mm, 1,9 µm) with a linear gradient of 3–35% buffer B (0.1% formic acid, 80% acetonitrile in water) for 55 min; 35–55% B for 5 min; and 55–100% B for 1 min at a flow rate of 440 nL/min. Prior to injection of the next sample, the column was washed with buffer B for 5 min and re-equilibrated with buffer A (0.1% formic acid and 3% acetonitrile in water) for 5 min.

Peptides were analyzed on the mass spectrometer with one full scan (350–2000 m/z, R = 70,000 at 200 m/z) at a target of 3 × 10^6 ions and a maximum ion fill-time of 50 ms, followed by up to 10 data-dependent MS/MS scans with higher-energy collisional dissociation (HCD) (target 1 × 10^5 ions, max ion fill time 45 ms, isolation window 1.4 m/z, normalized collision energy (NCE) 27%) detected in the Orbitrap (R = 17,500 at fixed first mass 100 m/z). Other settings included: charge exclusion: unassigned, 1, and more than 6; peptide match–preferred; excluded isotopes–on; and the dynamic exclusion of 40 s was enabled.

2.5. Analysis of LC–MS/MS Data

Label-free protein quantification was performed using MaxQuant software version 1.5.6.5 (Max Plank Institute of Biochemistry, Planegg, Germany) and a common contaminants database by the Andromeda search engine [14] with cysteine carbamidomethylation as a fixed modification was used. Oxidation of methionine and protein N-terminal acetylation were used as variable modifications. Peak lists were searched against the human protein sequences extracted from the Uniprot (28.06.19) database. The false discovery rate (FDR) was set to 0.01 for both proteins and peptides with a minimum length of seven amino acids. Peptide identification was performed with an allowed initial precursor mass deviation of up to 20 ppm and an allowed fragment mass deviation of 20 ppm. Downstream bioinformatics analysis was performed using Perseus software, version 1.5.5.1 (Max Plank Institute of Biochemistry, Planegg, Germany). Protein groups only identified by site, only from peptides identified also in the reverse database, or those belonging to the common contaminants database were excluded from the analyses. For Student's *t*-test, missing values were imputed with a width of 0.3 and a downshift of 1.8 over the total matrix. Two sample tests were performed in Perseus with s0 set to 0. Label-free quantification was performed using a minimum ratio count of 1. The protein levels were assessed by the iBAQ (intensity-based absolute quantification) method using MaxQuant software. To determine the relative abundance of identified proteins in the samples (riBAQ), we divided the obtained iBAQ values by the sum of all iBAQ values and expressed this ratio as percentage. The results were analyzed using Venn diagrams. Protein ontology analysis of the differentially expressed proteins (PO) was performed on gene ontology terms to catalog the biological processes using DAVID Bioinformatics resources, 6.7 (Frederick National Laboratory for Cancer Research, Frederick, MD, USA). The mass spectrometry proteomics data were deposited to the ProteomeXchange Consortium via the PRIDE [15] partner repository with the dataset identifier PXD021673.

2.6. Quantitative PCR

The gene expression analysis of *HMOX1*, *KRT19*, *LDHA*, *HSPD1*, *MAPK1*, and *CA2* in lesional and healthy skin was performed using the method of quantitative PCR (qPCR). The Qiagen RNeasy Mini Kit with spin columns was used to isolate the total RNA from the skin. The isolated total RNA was treated with DNase (Qiagen, Hilden, Germany) to remove the traces of genomic DNA. RNA concentration was measured with NanoDrop 1000 (Thermo Fisher Scientific, Waltham, USA). The M-MLV kit (Promega, Madison, WI, USA) was used for the reverse transcription with oligo-dT (DNA-Synthes, Moscow, Russia) primers according to the manufacturer's protocol.

The primers used in the qPCR experiments (Table 2) were designed in Primer blast (NCBI, USA), checked with the Multiple primer analyzer (Thermo Fisher Scientific, Waltham, USA) for the formation of potential secondary structures and dimers, and synthesized by DNA-Synthes (Moscow, Russia). The experiments were performed in the CFX96 Touch real-time DNA detection system (Bio-Rad, Hercules, CA, USA) using the SYBR-Green master mix supplied by Evrogen (Moscow, Russia) according to the manufacturer's instructions. The following conditions were used to amplify the DNA: 4 min at 95 °C, followed by 40 cycles of consequent incubations at 94 °C for 15 s and 60 °C for 30 s. Each reaction was run in triplicates. 18S RNA was used as a housekeeping gene to normalize the expression levels of the target genes.

Table 2. Gene-specific primers used in the qPCR experiments.

Gene	Reference Sequence	Primer Name	Primer Sequence	Product Size, bp
CA2	NM_000067.3	CA2 forward	GGCTGGTTGGTGCTTTGTTT	118
		CA2 re-verse	TTGTGAGTGCTCATCACCCT	
HMOX1	NM_002133.3	HMOX1 forward	GGCCTAAACTTCAGAGGGGG	99
		HMOX1 reverse	AGACAGCTGCCACATTAGGG	
HSPD1	NM_002156.5	HSPD1 forward	CTGGCACGCTCTATAGCCAA	142
		HSPD1 reverse	CAGGGGTGGTCACAGGTTTA	
KRT19	NM_002276.5	KRT19 forward	CCACTACTACACGACCATCCA	89
		KRT19 reverse	GTCGATCTGCAGGACAATCC	
LDHA	NM_005566.4	LDHA forward	TAAGCTGTCATGGGTGGGTC	100
		LDHA reverse	GGGTGCAGAGTCTTCAGAGAG	
MAPK1	NM_002745.5	MAPK1 forward	CAGTTCTTGACCCCTGGTCC	186
		MAPK1 reverse	TACATACTGCCGCAGGTCAC	
18S RNA	NR_003286.2	18S RNA forward	CTACCACATCCAAGGAAGCA	103
		18S RNA reverse	TTTTTCGTCACTACCTCCCCG	

The results were analyzed using the standard $2^{-\Delta\Delta CT}$ method [16] to compare the levels of expressed genes. Each ΔCt value was calculated as $\Delta Ct = Ct$ (tested gene) $- Ct$ (housekeeping gene). $\Delta\Delta Ct$ was calculated as $\Delta\Delta Ct = \Delta Ct$ (sample of psoriatic patient) $- \Delta Ct$ (sample of healthy individual). The experiments were repeated three times for each sample.

2.7. ELISA

The protein expression of KRT19 and HSPD1 in lesional and healthy skin was evaluated using ELISA kits (MyBiosource, Inc., San Diego, CA, USA, MBS2703060 and MBS450548, respectively) according to the manufacturer's protocol. Briefly, tissue samples were prepared in lysis buffer (25 mg per 1 mL), homogenized, centrifuged (10,000 g; 5 min; 4 °C), aliquoted, and stored at -80 °C. Before the experiment, samples, blanks, and standards were loaded on 96-well plates and incubated for 1 h at 37 °C. Then, the solutions were replaced by detection reagent A and incubation continued for the same period of time. After washing with wash solution (3 × 2 min) detection reagent B was added and incubation continued for another 20 min. Then, the wells were washed again (5 × 2 min). The presence of antigen was visualized with the chromogenic substrate 3,3′,5,5′-tetramethylbenzidine (TMB) and assayed using a microplate reader (Bio-Rad, Hercules, USA) at the wavelength 450 nm. The antigen was quantified with a standard curve generated with standards of known concentrations.

The blood levels of E2, PG, and TS were analyzed using ELISA kits (Diagnostics Biochem Canada, Inc., London, ON, Canada CAN-F-430, CAN-PRE-4500, and CAN-TE-250) according to the instructions provided by the manufacturer. To perform an assay, the calibrator, control, and specimen samples were loaded on 96-well plates and mixed with aliquots of horse radish peroxidase (HRP) conjugated to a tested hormone. The plate was incubated for 1 h at room temperature on a shaker (200 rpm). After washing 3 times with provided washing buffer, TMB was added and the incubation continued for another 10–15 min. Then, the presence of a tested hormone was revealed by measuring the absorbance using a microplate reader (Bio-Rad, Hercules, CA, USA) at the wavelength 450 nm. The antigen was quantified with a standard curve generated with standards of known concentrations.

2.8. Statistical Analysis

Due to small sample size, the data of LC–MS/MS were analyzed with non-parametric statistics using the Mann–Whitney U test. The Mann–Whitney U test was also used to evaluate gender-related differences in protein expression. Data variability was analyzed in R using the "prcomp" function. Two-sided unpaired Student's *t*-test was used to analyze the data of the qPCR and ELISA studies that were performed on larger groups of participants. In all cases, differences were considered statistically significant when $p < 0.05$.

3. Results

3.1. The Blood of Female Psoriasis Patients Contains Less Estradiol and Progesterone, and More Testosterone Compared to the Healthy Volunteers

The analysis of blood samples (Figure 1) revealed significant differences in the levels of sex hormones between qPCR/ELISA psoriasis patients (n = 20) and qPCR/ELISA healthy volunteers (n = 11). The levels of E2 and PG were significantly higher in healthy volunteers ($p = 0.042$ and 0.001, respectively). In contrast, the level of TS was significantly higher in patients ($p = 2 \times 10^{-4}$). In turn, the blood of participants with menopause, being either healthy volunteers or patients, contained less E2 and PG but more TS compared to their normally menstruating counterparts (Table 3).

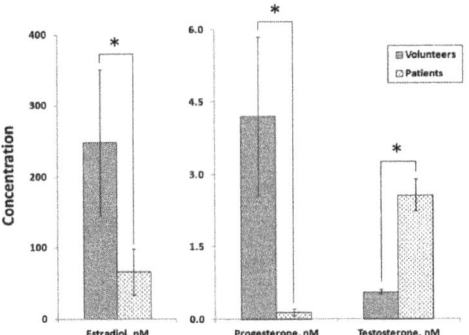

Figure 1. The levels of sex hormones in the blood of psoriasis patients and healthy volunteers that participated in the qPCR and ELISA experiments. The following individuals participated in these experiments: psoriasis patients without menopause (n = 10); psoriasis patients with menopause (n = 10); healthy volunteers without menopause (n = 6); and healthy volunteers with menopause (n = 5). * $p < 0.05$ when patients compared to healthy volunteers.

Table 3. The levels of sex hormones in blood samples of qPCR/ELISA participants with and without menopause. pM and nM are concentrations (pmol/L and nmol/L, respectively).

Group of Participants	N	Estradiol, pM	Progesterone, nM	Testosterone, nM
Volunteers without menopause	6	480.63 ± 157.43	8.18 ± 2.47	0.406 ± 0.078
Volunteers with menopause	5	53.8 ± 15.91	0.973 ± 0.206	0.733 ± 0.061
p-value		0.026	0.018	0.018
Patients without menopause	10	116.32 ± 45.85	0.159 ± 0.013	1.708 ± 0.362
Patients with menopause	10	14.51 ± 0.44	0.110 ± 0.011	3.428 ± 0.368
p-value		0.0495	0.011	0.005

3.2. LC–MS/MS Study Identifies Six Estrogen-Responsive Proteins That Are Differentially Expressed in Male and Female Psoriatic Skin

To identify a possible gender-specific response to the disease, we analyzed skin samples donated by MS psoriasis patients (n = 5) and MS healthy volunteers (n = 5) of both genders using LC/MS–MS. The analysis demonstrated that 756 proteins were differentially expressed in patients' lesional and uninvolved skin. The distribution of DEPs between the groups of samples is shown on a Venn diagram (Figure 2a). Samples of male lesional and uninvolved skin (n = 3) contained 479 and 128 DEPs (Figure 2b) compared to the skin of healthy volunteers (n = 5). Samples of female lesional and uninvolved skin (n = 2) contained 419 and 111 DEPs (Figure 2b) compared to the skin of healthy volunteers. Their paired comparison revealed 123 proteins that were differentially expressed in female skin and were not present in male skin (Supplementary Table S1). Particularly, 26 and 86 proteins were differentially expressed in female uninvolved and lesional skin. Moreover, 11 proteins were differentially expressed in both groups of samples (Figure 2b).

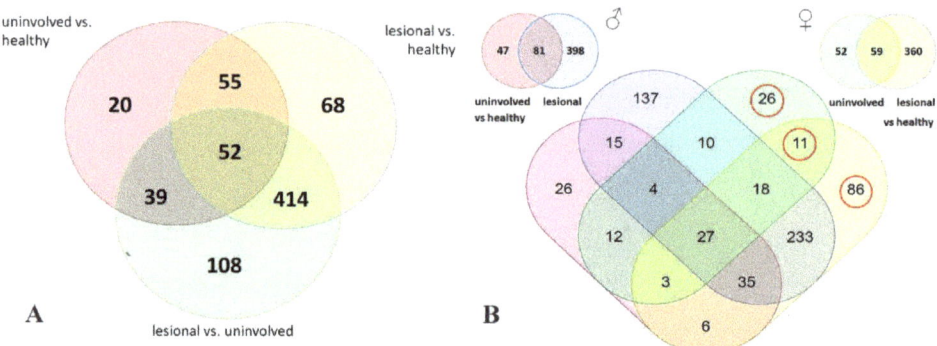

Figure 2. Venn diagram comparing DEPs in the donated skin samples as assessed by LC/MS–MS analysis. (**A**) Paired comparison of the samples obtained from lesional and uninvolved skin of the same psoriasis patients (n = 5) and skin of healthy volunteers (n = 5). (**B**) Analysis of gender-specific changes in protein expression. Samples of male (n = 3) and female (n = 2) psoriatic skin were compared to the skin of healthy volunteers (n = 5). The numbers indicated in the diagram are the numbers of DEPs in the compared groups of samples ($p < 0.05$). DEPs chosen for PO analysis are encircled. The data were compared using the Mann–Whitney U test.

The following protein ontology analysis of 123 proteins differentially expressed in female lesional and uninvolved skin performed on GO terms revealed 14 overrepresented biological processes (Table 4) including GO:0043627, which is the response to estrogen enriched by six DEPs, namely HMOX1, KRT19, LDHA, HSPD1, MAPK1, and CA2 ($p = 0.005$; FDR = 0.005). Four identified proteins, namely HMOX1, KRT19, LDHA, and MAPK1, were differentially expressed in female lesional skin, whereas HSPD1 and CA2 were also differentially expressed in female uninvolved skin. Among the mentioned six DEPs, CA2 was the only less abundant protein in patients' samples, whereas the others were more abundant in patients' skin samples compared to healthy skin. A similar analysis of the proteins differentially expressed in male lesional and uninvolved skin and were not differentially expressed in lesional and uninvolved female skin (Supplementary Table S1) revealed 11 overrepresented biological processes (Table 5).

Table 4. The ontology analysis of proteins differentially expressed in female lesional and uninvolved skin. The analyzed proteins were differentially expressed in female lesional and uninvolved skin and were not differentially expressed in male lesional and uninvolved skincompared to the skin of healthy volunteers.

Term	Genes	p-Value	FDR
Translational initiation	RPL30, RPL10, RPS7, RPS8, RPL11, RPL13A, RPL23A, RPS15, RPS27, RPS19, RPL14, EIF3C, RPL28, EIF3D, EIF4G1, RPS12	8.59×10^{-15}	6.62×10^{-12}
Nuclear-transcribed mRNA catabolic process, nonsense- mediated decay	RPL30, RPL10, RPS7, RPS8, RPL11, RPL13A, RPL23A, RPS15, RPS27, RPS19, RPL14, RPL28, EIF4G1, RPS12	6.03×10^{-13}	1.89×10^{-10}
SRP-dependent cotranslational protein targeting to membrane	RPL30, RPL10, RPS7, RPS8, RPL11, RPL13A, RPL23A, RPS15, RPS27, RPS19, RPL14, RPL28, RPS12	7.37×10^{-13}	1.89×10^{-10}
Viral transcription	RPL30, RPL10, RPS7, RPS8, RPL11, RPL13A, RPL23A, RPS15, RPS27, RPS19, RPL14, RPL28, RPS12	6.20×10^{-12}	1.19×10^{-9}
Translation	RPL30, RPL10, RPS7, RPS8, RPL11, RPL13A, SARS, RPL23A, RPS15, RPS27, RPS19, RPL14, RPL28, EIF4G1, RPS12	7.59×10^{-10}	1.17×10^{-7}
rRNA processing	RPL30, RPL10, RPS7, RPS8, RPL11, RPL13A, DDX21, RPL23A, RPS15, RPS27, RPS19, RPL14, RPL28, RPS12	1.03×10^{-9}	1.32×10^{-7}

Table 4. Cont.

Term	Genes	p-Value	FDR
Cell-cell adhesion	LDHA, AHNAK, HSPA5, RPL14, TACSTD2, EFHD2, RPL23A, TAGLN2, ENO1, ALDOA, SPTBN2, EIF4G1	1.24×10^{-6}	1.37×10^{-4}
Regulation of mRNA stability	PSMD6, PSMD7, PSMD13, PSMC1, PSMD3, HSPB1, HSPA1B, EIF4G1	4.20×10^{-6}	4.04×10^{-4}
Response to estrogen	LDHA, KRT19, CA2, HMOX1, MAPK1, HSPD1	5.83×10^{-5}	4.81×10^{-3}
Glycolytic process	GPI, LDHA, PGAM1, ENO1, ALDOA	6.24×10^{-5}	4.81×10^{-3}
Regulation of cellular amino acid metabolic process	PSMD6, PSMD7, PSMD13, PSMC1, PSMD3	3.09×10^{-4}	0.022
Canonical glycolysis	GPI, PGAM1, ENO1, ALDOA	5.88×10^{-4}	0.038
Antigen processing and presentation of exogenous peptide antigen via MHC class I, TAP-dependent	PSMD6, PSMD7, PSMD13, PSMC1, PSMD3	6.95×10^{-4}	0.041
NIK/NF-κB signaling	PSMD6, PSMD7, PSMD13, PSMC1, PSMD3	8.29×10^{-4}	0.046

Table 5. The ontology analysis of proteins differentially expressed in male lesional and uninvolved skin. The analyzed proteins were differentially expressed in male lesional and uninvolved skin and were not differentially expressed in female lesional and uninvolved skin compared to the skin of healthy volunteers.

Term	Genes	p-Value	FDR
SRP-dependent cotranslational protein targeting to membrane	RPS28, RPS16, RPL32, RPL23, RPL37A, RPL35A, FAU, RPL8, SRP14, RPL17, RPL19	4.74×10^{-9}	4.95×10^{-6}
Translational initiation	RPS28, RPS16, RPL32, EIF6, RPL23, RPL37A, RPL35A, FAU, RPL8, RPL17, RPL19	1.79×10^{-7}	9.32×10^{-5}
Viral transcription	RPS28, RPS16, RPL32, RPL23, RPL37A, RPL35A, FAU, RPL8, RPL17, RPL19	3.32×10^{-7}	1.16×10^{-4}
Nuclear-transcribed mRNA catabolic process, nonsense-mediated decay	RPS28, RPS16, RPL32, RPL23, RPL37A, RPL35A, FAU, RPL8, RPL17, RPL19	5.57×10^{-7}	1.45×10^{-4}
Translation	RPS28, RPS16, RPL32, RPL23, RPL37A, RPL35A, FAU, RPL8, RPL17, SLC25A6, RPL19	4.33×10^{-5}	0.009
Negative regulation of endopeptidase activity	CSTB, CSTA, ITIH2, SERPIND1, SERPINF1, SERPINH1, SERPING1, COL6A3	6.01×10^{-5}	0.010
rRNA processing	RPS28, RPS16, RPL32, RPL23, RPL37A, RPL35A, FAU, RPL8, RPL17, RPL19	6.56×10^{-5}	0.010
Regulation of complement activation	CFH, C9, C8B, PHB2, C8A	9.86×10^{-5}	0.013
Complement activation alternative pathway	CFH, C9, C8B, C8A	1.43×10^{-4}	0.017
Cell-cell adhesion	CNN2, PDLIM1, LAD1, DDX3X, ATIC, CTTN, RUVBL1, CHMP4B, PARK7, CNN3	3.86×10^{-4}	0.040
DNA duplex unwinding	DDX3X, XRCC5, DDX1, RUVBL2, RUVBL1	4.47×10^{-4}	0.042

3.3. The Identified Estrogen-Responsive Genes Were Differentially Expressed in Menopausal and Non-Menopausal Patients, and Their Expression Was Influenced by the Disease

Due to the small sample size of the performed LC–MS/MS study, we confirmed the differential expression of the identified estrogen-responsive proteins (ERPs) in women using qPCR and ELISA. The analysis of gene expression in skin samples by qPCR revealed that the genes encoding the identified ERPs were differentially expressed in lesional skin of qPCR/ELISA patients (n = 20) compared to the skin of qPCR/ELISA healthy volunteers (n = 11). Five identified genes, namely HMOX1 (38.97 ± 4.91; $p = 1.30 \times 10^{-7}$), KRT19 (45.90 ± 5.86; $p = 1.52 \times 10^{-7}$), LDHA (7.30 ± 2.55; $p = 0.01$), HSPD1 (17.32 ± 3.57; $p = 1.07 \times 10^{-4}$), and MAPK1 (3.20 ± 0.77; $p = 0.01$), were induced, whereas CA2 (0.43 ± 0.13; $p = 0.01$) was suppressed in lesional skin (Figure 3).

The expression profiles in qPCR/ELISA patients with and without menopause (Figure 3) were the same, i.e., the genes upregulated in patients without menopause (n = 10) were also upregulated in patients with menopause (n = 10) and vice versa, compared to qPCR/ELISA healthy volunteers (n = 11). All six identified ERGs had higher expression in patients without menopause compared to patients with menopause. Moreover, when patients with and without menopause were compared to each other, the changes in the expression of four genes, namely HMOX1 ($p = 0.001$), HSPD1 ($p = 0.008$), CA2 ($p = 0.006$), and MAPK1 ($p = 0.012$), were significant. In contrast, we did not see significant changes in gene expression (Figure 3) when we compared qPCR/ELISA healthy volunteers with and without menopause (n = 6 and 5, respectively).

The comparison of gene expression in qPCR/ELISA patients and healthy volunteers without menopause (n = 10 and 6, respectively) revealed a differential expression of five genes, namely HMOX1 ($p = 1.13 \times 10^{-6}$), KRT19 ($p = 1.81 \times 10^{-4}$), HSPD1 ($p = 9.00 \times 10^{-4}$), LDHA ($p = 0.047$), and MAPK1 ($p = 0.004$), as depicted in Figure 3. HMOX1, KRT19, HSPD1, and MAPK1 were upregulated in patients compared to healthy volunteers, whereas CA2 was downregulated. Considering the fact that the compared samples belonged to the individuals without menopause, we suggested that the observed changes in gene expression were caused by the disease. Similar results were obtained when we compared qPCR/ELISA patients and healthy volunteers with menopause (n = 10 and 5, respectively). In patients, changes in the expression of HMOX1, KRT19, LDHA, HSPD1, and CA2 were significant ($p < 0.05$). HMOX1, KRT19, LDHA, and HSPD1 were upregulated. The expression level of MAPK1 did not change ($p < 0.45$) and CA2 was downregulated.

In turn, the principle component analysis (PCA) of qPCR data revealed that a single factor (PC1) was responsible for 53% of the variability between the skin samples (Figure 3b). The K-mean clustering (Figure 3c) identified two clusters that contained samples of qPCR/ELISA psoriasis patients (n = 20) and healthy volunteers (n = 11). However, we could not completely separate patients with and without menopause, as well as similar groups of healthy volunteers.

A comparative analysis of gene expression in the PBMC obtained from the individuals that participated in the qPCR/ELISA experiments revealed significant changes in the expression of four genes, namely HMOX1, HSPD1, LDHA, and KRT19, whereas the expression MAPK1 and CA2 was not detected (Figure 3d). Similarly to skin cells, the expression levels of HMOX1, HSPD1, LDHA, and KRT19 were higher in non-menopausal patients compared to menopausal patients. However, the changes in gene expression were statistically insignificant, except for LDHA ($p = 0.047$). Moreover, we did not see any significant changes in gene expression when we compared non-menopausal and menopausal volunteers.

In non-menopausal patients, the expression levels of HMOX1, HSPD1, LDHA, and KRT19 were higher compared to non-menopausal volunteers (Figure 3d). In particular, we found that changes in the expression levels of KRT19 and HMOX1 were significant ($p = 0.022$ and 0.019, respectively), whereas changes in the expression levels of HSPD1 and LDHA were statistically insignificant ($p = 0.079$ and 0.072, respectively). Similarly, the expression levels of HMOX1, HSPD1, LDHA, and KRT19 were higher in menopausal patients compared to menopausal volunteers (Figure 3d). However, the changes in their expression levels were statistically insignificant ($p = 0.0503$ for HMOX1, $p = 0.053$ for HSPD1, $p = 0.102$ for LDHA, and $p = 0.080$ for KRT19).

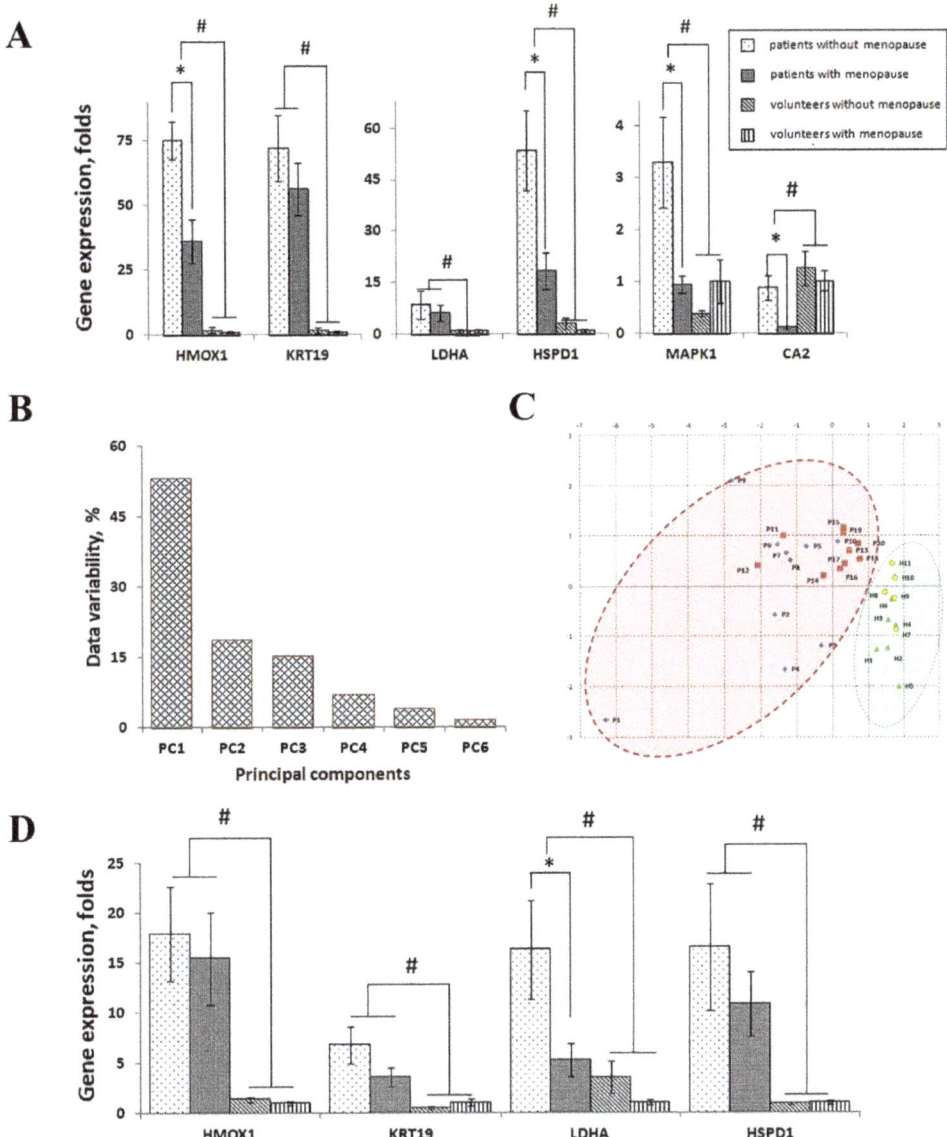

Figure 3. The expression of identified estrogen-responsive genes in clinical samples of psoriasis patients and healthy volunteers assessed by qPCR. (**A**). The levels of gene expression in the samples of patients' lesional skin and in the skin of healthy volunteers. (**B**). Assessment of a variation in gene expression in the lesional skin of psoriasis patients and healthy volunteers by principle component analysis. (**C**). The plot of two first principal components (PC1 and PC2). Different groups are indicated by data points of different colors and shapes: group 1 is represented by blue diamonds; group 2 is represented by red squares; group 3 is represented by green triangles; and group 4 is represented by yellow circles. (**D**). The expression of identified estrogen-responsive genes in the PBMC obtained from the blood of patients and healthy volunteers. The following individuals participated in these experiments: psoriasis patients without menopause (n = 10); psoriasis patients with menopause (n = 10); healthy volunteers without menopause (n = 6); and healthy volunteers with menopause (n = 5). * $p < 0.05$ when women without menopause compared to women with menopause. # $p < 0.05$ when patients compared to healthy volunteers. Gene expression in menopausal patients was set equal to 1.

3.4. Assessment of Protein Expression by ELISA Confirms a Differential Expression of KRT19 and HSPD1 in the Lesional Skin of Female Psoriasis Patients

Using ELISA, we analyzed the expression of KRT19 and HSPD1 in lesional skin as well as the PBMC of qPCR/ELISA psoriasis patients and healthy volunteers (Table 1). The performed analysis of skin samples revealed that the expression levels of both proteins were significantly higher in the lesional skin of patients compared to healthy volunteers (Figure 4a). Moreover, the expression levels of both proteins were significantly different ($p < 0.05$) in patients without menopause compared to patients with menopause. In contrast, we did not see significant differences in the expression of KRT19 and HSPD1 when we compared skin samples of non-menopausal and menopausal volunteers.

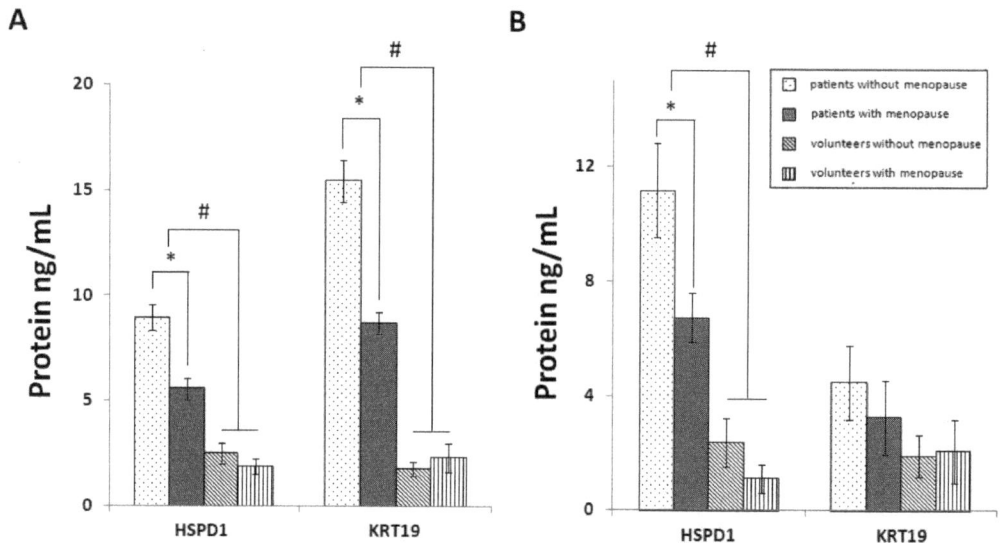

Figure 4. The levels of the expression of estrogen-responsive proteins in clinical samples of psoriasis patients and healthy volunteers, assessed by ELISA. (**A**). The levels of gene expression in the samples of patients' lesional skin and in the skin of healthy volunteers. (**B**). The levels of gene expression in the PBMC obtained from the patients' blood and from the blood of healthy volunteers. The following individuals participated in these experiments: psoriasis patients without menopause (n = 10); psoriasis patients with menopause (n = 10); healthy volunteers without menopause (n = 6); and healthy volunteers with menopause (n = 5). * $p < 0.05$ when women without menopause compared to women with menopause. # $p < 0.05$ when patients compared to healthy volunteers. Protein concentrations were measured in ng/mL.

A similar analysis of the PBMC also revealed a significantly higher expression of HSPD1 in the lesional skin of patients compared to that of the healthy volunteers (Figure 4b). In contrast, changes in the expression of KRT19 were statistically insignificant although the expression level of KRT19 in patients' PBMC was elevated compared to the PBMC of healthy volunteers. In a similar manner, the expression level of HSPD1 in the PBMC of the patients without menopause was significantly higher compared to the patients with menopause, although we did not see significant differences when we analyzed changes in the expression of KRT19. In addition, there were no significant differences in the expression of both proteins between non-menopausal and menopausal healthy volunteers.

4. Discussion

In this study, we analyzed skin samples of psoriasis patients using the LC–MS/MS method and reported of six ERPs, namely HMOX1, KRT19, LDHA, HSPD1, MAPK1, and CA2, that were differentially expressed in the lesional and uninvolved skin of female MS participants (Table 4) and were not present in the skin of their male counterparts

(Table 5), suggesting an existence of a gender-dependent response to the disease. Using independent methods of analysis, namely qPCR and ELISA (Figures 3 and 4), we examined their expression in menopausal and non-menopausal female patients and the respective groups of healthy volunteers (Figure 3a,d). We also assessed the levels of sex hormones, namely ES, PG, and TS, in their blood (Figure 1).

In performing qPCR and ELISA experiments on a larger cohort of women, we confirmed that the identified ERGs and their encoding proteins were differentially expressed in female lesional skin compared to healthy skin (Figures 3a and 4a). In comparing non-menopausal and menopausal patients, we found significant changes in the expression of *HMOX1*, *HSPD1*, *CA2*, and *MAPK1*. In contrast, the changes in their expression were insignificant when we compared non-menopausal and menopausal healthy volunteers. The results of the ELISA experiments were similar to the results of the qPCR analysis (Figure 4). Thus, the obtained data suggested that the observed changes in gene expression were caused by the differences in the levels of sex hormones and were associated with the disease because healthy volunteers did not have them. As we believe, the sex hormones, primarily E2, acted as modulators, altering the expression of ERGs and interfering with the disease.

This hypothesis is in agreement with our next finding. In performing the PCA of qPCR data, we found that a single factor was responsible for 53% of the variability between the samples (Figure 3a). Using K-mean clustering, we separated the samples in two groups that contained samples of qPCR/ELISA patients and samples of qPCR/ELISA volunteers. However, we could not achieve complete separation of individuals with and without menopause within those groups. Based on this finding, we proposed that in some women, changes in the expression of ERGs might not coincide with menopause. As we believe, deviations of this kind could be caused by a crosstalk of ES-activated signaling mechanisms and other signaling pathways (e.g., the pathways activated by proinflammatory cytokines).

In assessing the levels of sex hormones in the blood of qPCR/ELISA participants, we showed (Figure 1) that the blood of patients contained significantly less E2 and PG, and more TS compared to that of the healthy control. Moreover, menopausal patients and healthy volunteers contained less E2 and PG, and more TS compared to their non-menopausal counterparts (Table 3). These results suggested that sex hormones influenced the gene expression in psoriatic skin. They also confirmed the previous findings [4,6,8] regarding that the fluctuations in the levels of E2, PG, and TS could potentially modulate the course of the disease.

In comparing gene expression profiles in lesional skin (Figure 3a) and the patterns of sex hormones in patients' blood (Table 3), we discovered significant changes between menopausal and non-menopausal patients, as well as between healthy volunteers and any group of patients. The expression levels of *HMOX1*, *KRT19*, *LDHA*, *HSPD1*, and *MAPK1* were higher in patients with menopause compared to patients without menopause. Moreover, same individuals had higher blood levels of E2 and PG (Table 3). In addition, the expression levels of *CA2* and blood levels of TS were higher in patients with menopause compared to patients without menopause.

Furthermore, when we combined two groups of healthy volunteers with and without menopause (Figure 3a) and considered them as one group, we saw differences between the expression profiles of ERGs in lesional skin (Figure 3a) and in the patterns of sex hormones in their blood (Table 3). The expression levels of *HMOX1*, *KRT19*, *LDHA*, *HSPD1*, and *MAPK1* were lower in healthy volunteers compared to any group of patients. In contrast, their blood levels of E2 and PG were higher compared to the same groups. In contrast, the expression levels of *CA2* and blood levels of TS in both groups of patients were lower compared to that of healthy volunteers.

Based on these findings, we concluded that sex hormones differentially contributed to the expression of individual ERGs. Presumably, E2 and PG made a greater contribution to the regulation of *HMOX1*, *KRT19*, *LDHA*, *HSPD1*, and *MAPK1*, whereas TS made a greater contribution to the regulation of *CA2*. However, additional experimental studies on cultured cells are needed to clarify the role of particular sex hormones in the regulation of individual ERGs primarily in the skin because the biological effects of sex hormones are tissue-specific and their regulation of gene expression is often presented as a cross-talk of several signaling pathways.

In comparing the expression of the identified ERGs in the skin (Figure 3a) and of the PBMC (Figure 3d), we found similarities in their expression profiles. In particular, the expression levels of *HMOX1*, *KRT19*, *LDHA*, and *HSPD1* were significantly higher in the PBMC of patients compared to healthy volunteers, in non-menopausal patients compared to non-menopausal volunteers, and in menopausal patients compared to menopausal volunteers. However, most of these changes were statistically insignificant. Based on these findings, we concluded that sex hormones, primarily E2, influenced gene expression in both types of samples in a similar way. This result was anticipated since psoriasis is a systemic disorder that targets various tissues and is associated with multiple comorbidities. Expectedly, the same mechanism was activated in response to the disease in both the skin and PBMC.

The previous studies showed that female sex hormones have significant immunomodulatory effects. In particular, ES reduces the production of macrophage-attracting cytokines (CXCL8, CXCL10, CCL2, -5, and -8) and the production of IL12 in keratinocytes. These cytokines, namely CXCL10, CCL5, and -8, recruit activated T cells [17], macrophages [18], and neutrophils [19], respectively. E2 inhibits the production of IL12 and TNF by dendritic cells. Moreover, it decreases the blood level of neutrophils. Based on these findings, we may consider low E2 level in the blood of our patients (Figure 1) as a potential risk for exacerbation of the disease.

PG stimulates the production of the Th_2 cytokines, namely IL4 and IL5, by T cells without altering the production of Th_1 cytokines [20]. Moreover, PG blocks androgen receptors (AR) and, in inhibiting the release of LH, reduces the level of circulating androgens (AG) in the blood. In fibroblasts, PG suppresses the transcription of *CXCL8* [21]. In contrast, when the PG level is low, TS activates ARs, contributing to the development of an inflammatory response [22]. These data suggest that the reduction in the PG level in the patients' blood that we observed in our study (Figure 1) could also contribute to the pathogenesis of the disease.

To our knowledge, this is the first study focused on gender-specific differences in gene and protein expression in psoriatic skin. Three of the six identified genes, namely *KRT19*, *LDHA*, and *HSPD1* were not previously associated with psoriasis. Depending on the role of the particular ERG in the pathogenesis of psoriasis, its differential expression may either promote or limit the growth of psoriatic plaques in a disease-affected area. Hemoxygenase 1 (HMOX1) is a stress protein. The expression of *HMOX1* can be induced by a variety of stimuli, including the proinflammatory cytokines TNF and IL17, which are abundant in the lesional skin of psoriasis patients [23]. The anti-inflammatory and anti-oxidant activities of HMOX1 are well-documented and can be considered as a part of a protective mechanism that contains (controls) the inflammatory response in lesional skin. The others already showed that inducers of *HMOX1* attenuate the inflammatory response in lesional skin [24]. Moreover, a proteolytic cleavage of HMOX1 generates several biologically active metabolites. One of them, the N-terminal peptide, binds to the promoter of *IL23A*, interfering with biological activities of proinflammatory cytokines IL12 and IL23 [25]. The others, bilirubin and CO, produce potent antioxidant and anti-inflammatory effects [26,27].

MAPK1 is one of two known extracellular signal-regulated kinases (ERKs). Although the role of MAPK1 in the inflammatory response, primarily for the induction of TNF [28], is well-documented, in a general sense, it is a signaling molecule that can be activated by multiple stimuli, including ES [29]. Due to the high sequence homology of ERKs and its similar role in the cell, two proteins, namely MAPK1/ERK2 and MAPK3/ERK1, are considered as two isoforms of the same enzyme. However, their expression patterns in lesional skin are different. MAPK3/ERK1 is strongly increased, whereas the expression of MAPK1/ERK2 is slightly affected by the disease [30]. The cited paper also suggests that, similarly to HMOX1, ES is likely to contribute to the regulation of MAPK1 in lesional skin. Particularly, the involvement of ES would explain the strong induction of *MAPK1* in our female patients and answer the question concerning why the expression of *MAPK1* significantly decreases after menopause in patients (Figure 3a).

We also discovered that *LDHA*, which encodes LDH-M, the subunit of lactate dehydrogenase (LDH), was upregulated in lesional skin (Figure 3a). Compared to the other LDH subunits, LDH-M has a higher affinity to pyruvate. In other words, if lactate and pyruvate are equally available, LDH-M preferentially binds to pyruvate and converts pyruvate to lactate. It also oxidizes NADH, which is a coenzyme in this reaction, to NAD$^+$ [31]. According to the previously published data, *LDHA* is involved in several immunomodulatory processes that could potentially influence the flow of psoriasis. First, it decreases the proliferation of cytotoxic and other effector T cells and their production of cytokines because these cells become inactive at low glucose and high lactate concentrations in the medium [32]. Second, lactate activates a mechanism that stops the migration of T-cells, entrapping them in the inflamed area [33]. Third, a suppression of *LDHA* in macrophages reduces the phosphorylation of mitogen-activated protein kinase MAPK14/p38 [34]. At the same time, the accumulation of lactate in the inflamed tissue increases the production of IL17 by T cells [35]. In addition, *LDHA* is overexpressed in cancer cells that rely on aerobic glycolysis to maintain their higher proliferation and faster metabolic rates. For this reason, a higher expression of *LDHA* in lesional epidermis is also necessary due to hyperproliferation and acceleration of the metabolism in epidermal keratinocytes of psoriasis patients.

HSPD1 encodes the mitochondrial chaperonin HSP60 that provides a favorable environment for the correct folding of unfolded and misfolded proteins. Similarly to *HMOX1*, *MAPK1*, and *LDHA*, *HSPD1* is induced in stress conditions. In cancer cells, a higher expression of *HSPD1* is needed due to their faster metabolic and proliferation rates, and more intensive protein trafficking between the cytoplasm and mitochondria [36]. Moreover, a higher expression of *HSPD1* in lesional skin, as we observed (Figure 3a), would help to maintain a faster turnover of the epidermal keratinocytes.

KRT19 improves the rigidity of intermediate filaments [37]. Moreover, KRT19 activates NOTCH signaling pathways promoting nuclear translocation of β-catenin [38] and AKT [39]. The expression of *KRT19* in cancer cells increases their cell proliferation rate due to its ability to stabilize cyclin D3 [38]. A similar effect is observed in HaCaT cells that stop expressing *KRT19* before reaching the confluence [40]. We presume the upregulation of KRT19 in lesional skin helps epidermal keratinocytes to adapt to higher proliferation and metabolic rates in the areas affected by the disease.

CA2, which we also identified in our study, exhibits a higher catalytic rate for the conversion of bicarbonate to carbon dioxide compared to the other carbonic anhydrases. This prevents acidification of the cytoplasm. In the opposite direction, CA2 facilitates the diffusion of carbon dioxide through the cytoplasm, converting carbon dioxide to bicarbonate. According to our observations (Figure 3a), *CA2* levels were decreased in patients with menopause compared to either of the three groups, namely patients without menopause, healthy volunteers without menopause and healthy volunteers with menopause, suggesting that the downregulation of *CA2* in menopausal qPCR/ELISA patients (Figure 3a) could be caused by an action of an unidentified factor, such as TS which is capable of interfering with ES [41] and can be suppressed by PG [22].

The differential expression of the identified ERGs can be part of an adaptive mechanism (Figure 5) that protects the skin cells from chronic inflammatory responses. Presumably, this mechanism is more efficient in female patients without menopause since they have higher levels of female sex hormones. Cooperating with several transcription factors, ES modulates the responses to various stimuli such as oxidative stress [42] and hypoxia [43]. For instance, there is an abundance of evidence regarding synergism between ES and hypoxia-induced factor 1α (HIF1α), which is highly unstable under normoxic conditions [44]. However, HIF1α becomes more stable in lesional skin [45] because lactate, the preferential product of LDH-M, stabilizes HIF1α by inhibiting prolyl hydroxylase (PHD2). It also triggers the nuclear translocation of HIF1α and the following induction of hypoxia responsive genes [46]. In contrast, the inhibition of LDHA causes a rapid degradation of HIF1α in proteasomes [47]. Many genes, including ones that we mentioned above, are common targets of ES and HIF1α [44,48]. Respectively, their expression (Figure 5) also depends on both ES and HIF1α [49]. It can be suppressed by either ERα antagonists [44] or inhibitors of ERα or HIF1α, as well as by HIF1α destabilizing factors.

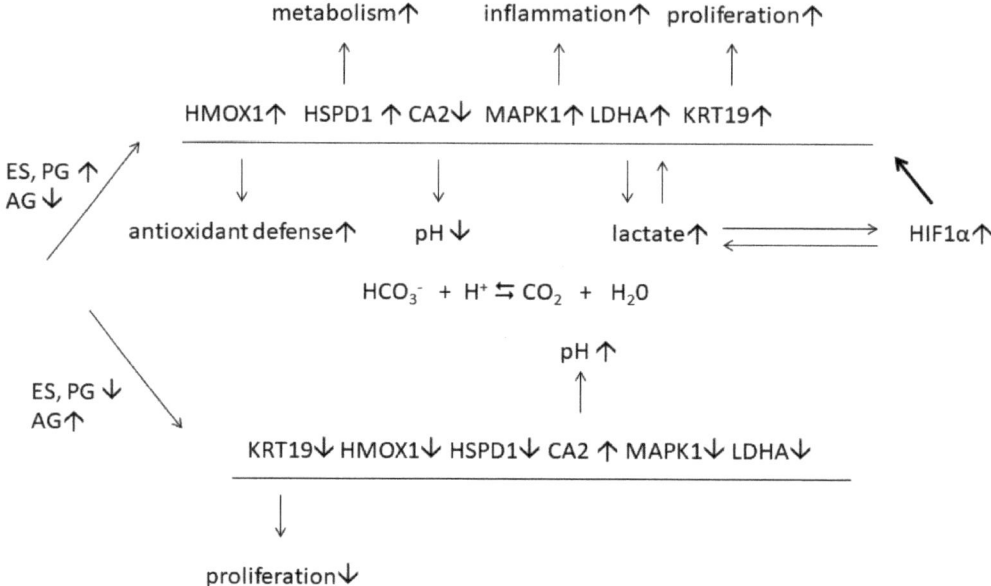

Figure 5. Regulation of estrogen-responsive proteins in lesional skin of female psoriasis patients with and without menopause: the proposed model. The signs ↑ and ↓ indicate that the protein expression is increased and decreased, respectively. The sign ⇌ indicates that chemical reaction between HCO_3^- and can be reversed.

The observed changes in the levels of sex hormones (Table 3) are of high clinical value. According to us (Figure 1) and others [22], low levels of sex hormones in the blood of women with psoriasis have a significant impact on the disease. Pregnant patients with moderate or severe forms of psoriasis have a higher risk of abortion, eclampsia, premature rupture of membranes, and macrosomia [50]. Another serious problem associated with psoriasis is female infertility [51]. However, it is still hard to say whether these complications are caused by psoriasis or comorbidities associated with the disease. For this reason, we explored the molecular basis of ES action in psoriatic skin and identified that there are six differentially expressed ERGs.

A medical correction of sex hormones may have a significant impact on the disease. The previously published data suggest that ES containing oral contraceptives [8] and hormone replacement therapy [52] may improve psoriasis. Conversely, it is well-documented that synthetic ES, if it is used as a therapeutic agent, can cause serious side effects such as cardiovascular events, thromboembolic disease, and breast cancer [53,54]. In this regard, knowledge of ERGs controlled by sex hormones in lesional skin suggests new hormone-free options to stabilize their expression in lesional skin, such as inducers of gene expression, biologically active peptides, and allosteric activators of their enzyme activity. Presumably, these potential treatment options may also help to avoid serious adverse effects.

In conclusion, a deficiency of female sex hormones seems to be among the risk factors that influence the flow of psoriasis in women. Respectively, the maintenance of their normal (physiological) levels may potentially prevent or suppress the disease. A detailed analysis of the proteins identified in the LC–MS/MS study, namely HMOX1, KRT19, LDHA, HSPD1, MAPK1, and CA2, revealed that they were differentially expressed in female lesional skin and were not present in male lesional skin. Using qPCR and ELISA, we found that the levels of their expression were higher in younger participants that were not in menopause. According to us and others, these proteins can be part of an adaptive mechanism that protects skin cells from the developing inflammatory response. In providing new insight on the molecular basis of ES signaling in female patients, we propose that ES mediates its anti-inflammatory effects in lesional skin, synergistically interacting with hormones/transcription factors that contribute to the stress response.

Supplementary Materials: The following are available online at https://www.mdpi.com/article/10.3390/jpm11090925/s1, Table S1: Excel-file with heat map that describes changes in protein expression in the skin of the male and female individuals that participated in the LC–MS/MS study and the results of the statistical analysis in male (n = 3) and female psoriasis patients (n = 2) compared to healthy volunteers (n = 5). The differences in protein expression were analyzed using the Mann–Whitney U test.

Author Contributions: Conceptualization, V.S.; Data curation, A.M.; Investigation, V.S. and A.S.; Project administration, V.S. and I.K.; Resources, E.D. (Elena Denisova), M.D., E.D. (Eugenia Dvoryankova), O.V.Z., E.S. and N.P.; Supervision, V.S.; Validation, A.M.; Visualization, A.M.; Writing—original draft, A.M. All authors have read and agreed to the published version of the manuscript.

Funding: This research received no external funding.

Institutional Review Board Statement: The study was conducted according to the guidelines of the Declaration of Helsinki and approved by the Institutional Review Board (Research Ethics Committees of Western Norway HR 2020-0870). The participants were informed of the nature of the study, gave their informed consent, and were told they could voluntary withdraw during the interviews at any time.

Informed Consent Statement: Written informed consent was obtained from all subjects involved in the study. Written informed consent has been obtained from the patient(s) to publish this paper.

Data Availability Statement: The mass spectrometry proteomics data were deposited to the ProteomeXchange Consortium via the PRIDE partner repository [15] with the dataset identifier PXD021673.

Conflicts of Interest: The authors declare no conflict of interest.

References

1. Deng, Y.; Chang, C.; Lu, Q. The Inflammatory Response in Psoriasis: A Comprehensive Review. *Clin. Rev. Allergy Immunol.* **2016**, *50*, 377–389. [CrossRef]
2. Queiro, R.; Tejón, P.; Alonso, S.; Coto, P. Age at disease onset: A key factor for understanding psoriatic disease. *Rheumatology* **2014**, *53*, 1178–1185. [CrossRef]
3. Naldi, L. Epidemiology of psoriasis. *Curr. Drug Targets. Inflamm. Allergy* **2004**, *3*, 121–128. [CrossRef] [PubMed]
4. Murase, J.E.; Chan, K.K.; Garite, T.J.; Cooper, D.M.; Weinstein, G.D. Hormonal effect on psoriasis in pregnancy and post partum. *Arch. Dermatol.* **2005**, *141*, 601–606. [CrossRef] [PubMed]
5. Straub, R.H. The complex role of estrogens in inflammation. *Endocr. Rev.* **2007**, *28*, 521–574. [CrossRef]
6. Shah, N.M.; Lai, P.F.; Imami, N.; Johnson, M.R. Progesterone-Related Immune Modulation of Pregnancy and Labor. *Front. Endocrinol.* **2019**, *10*, 198. [CrossRef]
7. Kurizky, P.S.; Ferreira Cde, C.; Nogueira, L.S.; Mota, L.M. Treatment of psoriasis and psoriatic arthritis during pregnancy and breastfeeding. *An. Bras. Dermatol.* **2015**, *90*, 367–375. [CrossRef] [PubMed]
8. Ceovic, R.; Mance, M.; Bukvic Mokos, Z.; Svetec, M.; Kostovic, K.; Stulhofer Buzina, D. Psoriasis: Female skin changes in various hormonal stages throughout life—Puberty, pregnancy, and menopause. *BioMed Res. Int.* **2013**, *2013*, 571912. [CrossRef]
9. Lee, Y.H.; Song, G.G. Association between circulating prolactin levels and psoriasis and its correlation with disease severity: A meta-analysis. *Clin. Exp. Dermatol.* **2018**, *43*, 27–35. [CrossRef]
10. Allshouse, A.; Pavlovic, J.; Santoro, N. Menstrual Cycle Hormone Changes Associated with Reproductive Aging and How They May Relate to Symptoms. *Obstet. Gynecol. Clin. N. Am.* **2018**, *45*, 613–628. [CrossRef]
11. Zhang, C.; Zhao, M.; Li, Z.; Song, Y. Follicle-Stimulating Hormone Positively Associates with Metabolic Factors in Perimenopausal Women. *Int. J. Endocrinol.* **2020**, *2020*, 7024321. [CrossRef] [PubMed]

12. Dobrohotova, J.E.; Zelenskaia, E.M.; Korsunskaia, I.M. Livial and some aspects of its infuentce on the skin of postmenopausal women. *Russ. Bull. Obstet. Gynecol.* **2007**, *7*, 72–76.
13. Morgulis, J.V.; Potekaev, N.N.; Korsunskaia, I.M. Non-invasive mechods to study the skin of menopausal females and clinical potential of hormone replacing therapy. *Russ. J. Clin. Dermatol. Venereol.* **2009**, *7*, 13–18.
14. Cox, J.; Hein, M.Y.; Luber, C.A.; Paron, I.; Nagaraj, N.; Mann, M. Accurate proteome-wide label-free quantification by delayed normalization and maximal peptide ratio extraction, termed MaxLFQ. *Mol. Cell. Proteom. MCP* **2014**, *13*, 2513–2526. [CrossRef] [PubMed]
15. Perez-Riverol, Y.; Csordas, A.; Bai, J.; Bernal-Llinares, M.; Hewapathirana, S.; Kundu, D.J.; Inuganti, A.; Griss, J.; Mayer, G.; Eisenacher, M.; et al. The PRIDE database and related tools and resources in 2019: Improving support for quantification data. *Nucleic Acids Res.* **2019**, *47*, D442–D450. [CrossRef]
16. Livak, K.J.; Schmittgen, T.D. Analysis of relative gene expression data using real-time quantitative PCR and the 2(-Delta Delta C(T)) Method. *Methods* **2001**, *25*, 402–408. [CrossRef] [PubMed]
17. Singh, K.P.; Zerbato, J.M.; Zhao, W.; Braat, S.; Deleage, C.; Tennakoon, G.S.; Mason, H.; Dantanarayana, A.; Rhodes, A.; Rhodes, J.W.; et al. Intrahepatic CXCL10 is strongly associated with liver fibrosis in HIV-Hepatitis B co-infection. *PLoS Pathog.* **2020**, *16*, e1008744. [CrossRef] [PubMed]
18. Mi, S.; Qu, Y.; Chen, X.; Wen, Z.; Chen, P.; Cheng, Y. Radiotherapy Increases 12-LOX and CCL5 Levels in Esophageal Cancer Cells and Promotes Cancer Metastasis via THP-1-Derived Macrophages. *Onco Targets Ther.* **2020**, *13*, 7719–7733. [CrossRef]
19. Edwards, C.K., 3rd; Green, J.S.; Volk, H.D.; Schiff, M.; Kotzin, B.L.; Mitsuya, H.; Kawaguchi, T.; Sakata, K.M.; Cheronis, J.; Trollinger, D.; et al. Combined anti-tumor necrosis factor-α therapy and DMARD therapy in rheumatoid arthritis patients reduces inflammatory gene expression in whole blood compared to DMARD therapy alone. *Front. Immunol.* **2012**, *3*, 366. [CrossRef]
20. Piccinni, M.P.; Scaletti, C.; Maggi, E.; Romagnani, S. Role of hormone-controlled Th1- and Th2-type cytokines in successful pregnancy. *J. Neuroimmunol.* **2000**, *109*, 30–33. [CrossRef]
21. Kanda, N.; Watanabe, S. Regulatory roles of sex hormones in cutaneous biology and immunology. *J. Dermatol. Sci.* **2005**, *38*, 1–7. [CrossRef] [PubMed]
22. Raghunath, R.S.; Venables, Z.C.; Millington, G.W. The menstrual cycle and the skin. *Clin. Exp. Dermatol.* **2015**, *40*, 111–115. [CrossRef]
23. Numata, I.; Okuyama, R.; Memezawa, A.; Ito, Y.; Takeda, K.; Furuyama, K.; Shibahara, S.; Aiba, S. Functional expression of heme oxygenase-1 in human differentiated epidermis and its regulation by cytokines. *J. Investig. Dermatol.* **2009**, *129*, 2594–2603. [CrossRef] [PubMed]
24. Campbell, N.K.; Fitzgerald, H.K.; Malara, A.; Hambly, R.; Sweeney, C.M.; Kirby, B.; Fletcher, J.M.; Dunne, A. Naturally derived Heme-Oxygenase 1 inducers attenuate inflammatory responses in human dendritic cells and T cells: Relevance for psoriasis treatment. *Sci. Rep.* **2018**, *8*, 10287. [CrossRef] [PubMed]
25. Ghoreschi, K.; Brück, J.; Kellerer, C.; Deng, C.; Peng, H.; Rothfuss, O.; Hussain, R.Z.; Gocke, A.R.; Respa, A.; Glocova, I.; et al. Fumarates improve psoriasis and multiple sclerosis by inducing type II dendritic cells. *J. Exp. Med.* **2011**, *208*, 2291–2303. [CrossRef] [PubMed]
26. Keum, H.; Kim, T.W.; Kim, Y.; Seo, C.; Son, Y.; Kim, J.; Kim, D.; Jung, W.; Whang, C.H.; Jon, S. Bilirubin nanomedicine alleviates psoriatic skin inflammation by reducing oxidative stress and suppressing pathogenic signaling. *J. Control. Release* **2020**, *325*, 359–369. [CrossRef]
27. Campbell, N.K.; Fitzgerald, H.K.; Dunne, A. Regulation of inflammation by the antioxidant haem oxygenase 1. *Nat. Rev. Immunol.* **2021**, *21*, 411–425. [CrossRef]
28. Sabio, G.; Davis, R.J. TNF and MAP kinase signalling pathways. *Semin. Immunol.* **2014**, *26*, 237–245. [CrossRef]
29. Madak-Erdogan, Z.; Lupien, M.; Stossi, F.; Brown, M.; Katzenellenbogen, B.S. Genomic collaboration of estrogen receptor alpha and extracellular signal-regulated kinase 2 in regulating gene and proliferation programs. *Mol. Cell. Biol.* **2011**, *31*, 226–236. [CrossRef]
30. Yu, X.J.; Li, C.Y.; Dai, H.Y.; Cai, D.X.; Wang, K.Y.; Xu, Y.H.; Chen, L.M.; Zhou, C.L. Expression and localization of the activated mitogen-activated protein kinase in lesional psoriatic skin. *Exp. Mol. Pathol.* **2007**, *83*, 413–418. [CrossRef]
31. Urbańska, K.; Orzechowski, A. Unappreciated Role of LDHA and LDHB to Control Apoptosis and Autophagy in Tumor Cells. *Int. J. Mol. Sci.* **2019**, *20*, 85. [CrossRef]
32. Macintyre, A.N.; Gerriets, V.A.; Nichols, A.G.; Michalek, R.D.; Rudolph, M.C.; Deoliveira, D.; Anderson, S.M.; Abel, E.D.; Chen, B.J.; Hale, L.P.; et al. The glucose transporter Glut1 is selectively essential for CD4 T cell activation and effector function. *Cell Metab.* **2014**, *20*, 61–72. [CrossRef] [PubMed]
33. Haas, R.; Smith, J.; Rocher-Ros, V.; Nadkarni, S.; Montero-Melendez, T.; D'Acquisto, F.; Bland, E.J.; Bombardieri, M.; Pitzalis, C.; Perretti, M.; et al. Lactate Regulates Metabolic and Pro-inflammatory Circuits in Control of T Cell Migration and Effector Functions. *PLoS Biol.* **2015**, *13*, e1002202. [CrossRef] [PubMed]
34. Song, Y.J.; Kim, A.; Kim, G.T.; Yu, H.Y.; Lee, E.S.; Park, M.J.; Kim, Y.J.; Shim, S.M.; Park, T.S. Inhibition of lactate dehydrogenase A suppresses inflammatory response in RAW 264.7 macrophages. *Mol. Med. Rep.* **2019**, *19*, 629–637. [CrossRef] [PubMed]
35. Pucino, V.; Certo, M.; Bulusu, V.; Cucchi, D.; Goldmann, K.; Pontarini, E.; Haas, R.; Smith, J.; Headland, S.E.; Blighe, K.; et al. Lactate Buildup at the Site of Chronic Inflammation Promotes Disease by Inducing CD4(+) T Cell Metabolic Rewiring. *Cell Metab.* **2019**, *30*, 1055–1074.e1058. [CrossRef]

36. Zhang, K.; Jiang, K.; Hong, R.; Xu, F.; Xia, W.; Qin, G.; Lee, K.; Zheng, Q.; Lu, Q.; Zhai, Q.; et al. Identification and characterization of critical genes associated with tamoxifen resistance in breast cancer. *PeerJ* **2020**, *8*, e10468. [CrossRef]
37. Saha, S.K.; Kim, K.; Yang, G.M.; Choi, H.Y.; Cho, S.G. Cytokeratin 19 (KRT19) has a Role in the Reprogramming of Cancer Stem Cell-Like Cells to Less Aggressive and More Drug-Sensitive Cells. *Int. J. Mol. Sci.* **2018**, *19*, 1423. [CrossRef]
38. Saha, S.K.; Choi, H.Y.; Kim, B.W.; Dayem, A.A.; Yang, G.M.; Kim, K.S.; Yin, Y.F.; Cho, S.G. KRT19 directly interacts with β-catenin/RAC1 complex to regulate NUMB-dependent NOTCH signaling pathway and breast cancer properties. *Oncogene* **2017**, *36*, 332–349. [CrossRef]
39. Ju, J.H.; Yang, W.; Lee, K.M.; Oh, S.; Nam, K.; Shim, S.; Shin, S.Y.; Gye, M.C.; Chu, I.S.; Shin, I. Regulation of cell proliferation and migration by keratin19-induced nuclear import of early growth response-1 in breast cancer cells. *Clin. Cancer Res.* **2013**, *19*, 4335–4346. [CrossRef]
40. Boukamp, P.; Petrussevska, R.T.; Breitkreutz, D.; Hornung, J.; Markham, A.; Fusenig, N.E. Normal keratinization in a spontaneously immortalized aneuploid human keratinocyte cell line. *J. Cell Biol.* **1988**, *106*, 761–771. [CrossRef]
41. Pennell, L.M.; Galligan, C.L.; Fish, E.N. Sex affects immunity. *J. Autoimmun.* **2012**, *38*, J282–J291. [CrossRef]
42. Fuentes, N.; Silveyra, P. Estrogen receptor signaling mechanisms. *Adv. Protein Chem. Struct. Biol.* **2019**, *116*, 135–170. [CrossRef]
43. Yi, J.M.; Kwon, H.Y.; Cho, J.Y.; Lee, Y.J. Estrogen and hypoxia regulate estrogen receptor alpha in a synergistic manner. *Biochem. Biophys. Res. Commun.* **2009**, *378*, 842–846. [CrossRef] [PubMed]
44. Yang, J.; AlTahan, A.; Jones, D.T.; Buffa, F.M.; Bridges, E.; Interiano, R.B.; Qu, C.; Vogt, N.; Li, J.L.; Baban, D.; et al. Estrogen receptor-α directly regulates the hypoxia-inducible factor 1 pathway associated with antiestrogen response in breast cancer. *Proc. Natl. Acad. Sci. USA* **2015**, *112*, 15172–15177. [CrossRef] [PubMed]
45. Ioannou, M.; Sourli, F.; Mylonis, I.; Barbanis, S.; Papamichali, R.; Kouvaras, E.; Zafiriou, E.; Siomou, P.; Klimi, E.; Simos, G.; et al. Increased HIF-1 alpha immunostaining in psoriasis compared to psoriasiform dermatitides. *J. Cutan. Pathol.* **2009**, *36*, 1255–1261. [CrossRef] [PubMed]
46. De Saedeleer, C.J.; Copetti, T.; Porporato, P.E.; Verrax, J.; Feron, O.; Sonveaux, P. Lactate activates HIF-1 in oxidative but not in Warburg-phenotype human tumor cells. *PLoS ONE* **2012**, *7*, e46571. [CrossRef]
47. Wang, Z.; Wang, D.; Han, S.; Wang, N.; Mo, F.; Loo, T.Y.; Shen, J.; Huang, H.; Chen, J. Bioactivity-guided identification and cell signaling technology to delineate the lactate dehydrogenase A inhibition effects of Spatholobus suberectus on breast cancer. *PLoS ONE* **2013**, *8*, e56631. [CrossRef]
48. Ma, L.; Li, G.; Zhu, H.; Dong, X.; Zhao, D.; Jiang, X.; Li, J.; Qiao, H.; Ni, S.; Sun, X. 2-Methoxyestradiol synergizes with sorafenib to suppress hepatocellular carcinoma by simultaneously dysregulating hypoxia-inducible factor-1 and -2. *Cancer Lett.* **2014**, *355*, 96–105. [CrossRef]
49. Wairagu, P.M.; Phan, A.N.; Kim, M.K.; Han, J.; Kim, H.W.; Choi, J.W.; Kim, K.W.; Cha, S.K.; Park, K.H.; Jeong, Y. Insulin priming effect on estradiol-induced breast cancer metabolism and growth. *Cancer Biol. Ther.* **2015**, *16*, 484–492. [CrossRef]
50. Ferreira, C.; Azevedo, A.; Nogueira, M.; Torres, T. Management of psoriasis in pregnancy—A review of the evidence to date. *Drugs Context* **2020**, *9*. [CrossRef]
51. De Simone, C.; Caldarola, G.; Moretta, G.; Piscitelli, L.; Ricceri, F.; Prignano, F. Moderate-to-severe psoriasis and pregnancy: Impact on fertility, pregnancy outcome and treatment perspectives. *G. Ital. Dermatol. Venereol.* **2019**, *154*, 305–314. [CrossRef] [PubMed]
52. Hall, G.; Phillips, T.J. Estrogen and skin: The effects of estrogen, menopause, and hormone replacement therapy on the skin. *J. Am. Acad. Dermatol.* **2005**, *53*, 555–568, quiz 569–572. [CrossRef]
53. Rozenberg, S.; Al-Daghri, N.; Aubertin-Leheudre, M.; Brandi, M.L.; Cano, A.; Collins, P.; Cooper, C.; Genazzani, A.R.; Hillard, T.; Kanis, J.A.; et al. Is there a role for menopausal hormone therapy in the management of postmenopausal osteoporosis? *Osteoporos. Int.* **2020**, *31*, 2271–2286. [CrossRef] [PubMed]
54. Sridevi, V.; Naveen, P.; Karnam, V.S.; Reddy, P.R.; Arifullah, M. Beneficiary and Adverse Effects of Phytoestrogens: A Potential Constituent of Plant-based Diet. *Curr. Pharm. Des.* **2021**, *27*, 802–815. [CrossRef] [PubMed]

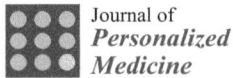 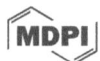

Article

S100A6, Calumenin and Cytohesin 2 as Biomarkers for Cutaneous Involvement in Systemic Sclerosis Patients: A Case Control Study

Paul Balanescu [1,2,3,*], Eugenia Balanescu [2], Cristian Baicus [1,2,3] and Anca Balanescu [4]

[1] Internal Medicine Chair, University of Medicine and Pharmacy Carol Davila, 020021 Bucharest, Romania; cristian.baicus@umfcd.ro
[2] Clinical Immunology Laboratory CDPC, Colentina Clinical Hospital, 020125 Bucharest, Romania; dzum_dzum@yahoo.com
[3] Clinical Research Unit RECIF (Reseau d'Epidemiologie Clinique International Francophone), 020125 Bucharest, Romania
[4] Pediatrics Chair, University of Medicine and Pharmacy Carol Davila, 020021 Bucharest, Romania; anca.balanescu@umfcd.ro
* Correspondence: paul.balanescu@umfcd.ro

Citation: Balanescu, P.; Balanescu, E.; Baicus, C.; Balanescu, A. S100A6, Calumenin and Cytohesin 2 as Biomarkers for Cutaneous Involvement in Systemic Sclerosis Patients: A Case Control Study. *J. Pers. Med.* **2021**, *11*, 368. https://doi.org/10.3390/jpm11050368

Academic Editor: Mircea Tampa

Received: 11 April 2021
Accepted: 30 April 2021
Published: 2 May 2021

Publisher's Note: MDPI stays neutral with regard to jurisdictional claims in published maps and institutional affiliations.

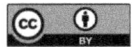

Copyright: © 2021 by the authors. Licensee MDPI, Basel, Switzerland. This article is an open access article distributed under the terms and conditions of the Creative Commons Attribution (CC BY) license (https://creativecommons.org/licenses/by/4.0/).

Abstract: Background: Systemic sclerosis (Ssc) is an autoimmune disease with incomplete known physiopathology. There is a high number of candidate proteomic biomarkers for Ssc that have not yet been confirmed on independent Ssc cohorts. The aim of the study was to confirm circulating S100A6, calumenin, and cytohesin 2 as biomarkers for Ssc. Methods: 53 Ssc patients and 26 age- and gender-matched controls were included. Serum S100A6, calumenin, and cytohesin 2 were evaluated with commercial ELISA kits. Associations between serum expression and clinical Ssc characteristics were evaluated. Results: Serum calumenin, S100A6, and cytohesin 2 were higher in Ssc patients compared to controls. Calumenin associated with extensive cutaneous fibrosis, frequency of Raynaud phenomenon, and low complement level, and had a tendency to be higher in Ssc patients with pulmonary fibrosis. S100A6 correlated with the number of active digital ulcers. Serum cytohesin 2 levels were higher in patients with teleangiectasia and associated with pulmonary artery pressure. Conclusions: Serum calumenin, S100A6, and cytohesin 2 were confirmed as biomarkers on an independent group of Ssc patients. Calumenin had the best predictive capacity for cutaneous Ssc manifestations. Future studies are needed to evaluate the prognostic value of these biomarkers and evaluate them as possible therapeutic targets.

Keywords: systemic sclerosis; biomarker; calumenin; S100A6; cytohesin 2

1. Introduction

Systemic sclerosis (Ssc) is a systemic autoimmune disease with incomplete known physiopathology. Its hallmark is represented by collagen deposition in various tissues that are accompanied by vascular injury [1]. As the clinical course of the disease can be severe in later Ssc stages, predictive biomarkers for severity and Ssc disease activity are necessary for better management of these patients [2]. Proteomic biomarkers are relatively easy to determine in the clinical laboratory setting using usual medical laboratory equipment. As such, there is an increased interest in research for proteomic biomarkers in Ssc patients. Previous mass spectrometry study pinpointed a relatively large number of candidate biomarkers for Ssc patients [3,4]. Nevertheless, the number of confirmed biomarkers on independent Ssc cohorts using specific assays (based on specific antibody-antigen reaction) is small. As such, studies are needed in order to confirm and evaluate the predictive value of candidate biomarkers on independent Ssc patient groups.

The study aimed to confirm circulating S100A6, calumenin, and cytohesin 2 as biomarkers for Ssc. These molecules were previously identified from various biological Ssc samples as candidate biomarkers. To the best of our knowledge, this is the first confirmatory study for these molecules as circulatory biomarkers in Ssc patients.

2. Materials and Methods

2.1. Patient Evaluation

Fifty-three consecutive Ssc patients that attended Colentina Clinical Hospital between January 2013 and January 2018 were included in the analysis (4 males and 49 females, median age 56 years). Patients were clinically evaluated and their cutaneous and visceral disease involvement was assessed.

Interstitial lung disease (ILD) was determined using X-ray imaging and high resolution CT. Flow spirometry and diffusing capacity for carbon monoxide-DLCO was determined in these patients (QUARK PFT station, Cosmed, Rome, Italy).

Pulmonary hypertension was indirectly determined by transthoracic echocardiography (Hitachi Aloka SSD 4000 ultrasound machine, Hitachi, Japan). Possible pulmonary hypertension was considered when the patients had at least 35 mm Hg at rest in pulmonary artery [5]. Cardiac involvement was determined using cardiac ultrasonography and EKG (Cardiocontrol, MDIMedical, Belfast, UK).

Frequency of Raynaud was interpreted as daily or less frequent. Presence of telangiectasias, ischemic digital ulcers, and calcinosis were recorded as previously defined in the literature [6]. Severity of skin involvement was evaluated using modified Rodnan skin score [7].

Disease activity score was evaluated with EUSTAR criteria [8]. Gastrointestinal involvement was evaluated using upper gastrointestinal endoscopy and radiographic examinations including barium swallow for esophageal motility. Inflammatory markers were also recorded in Ssc patients (erythrocyte sedimentation rate (ESR) and serum C reactive protein (CRP) concentration). Patient medication at the time of enrollment was also recorded.

Twenty-six age- and gender-matched controls were recruited in this study (2 males, 24 females, median age 51.5 years) from patients referred to Colentina Clinical Hospital. Controls had no previous record of Raynaud's phenomenon and no active inflammation.

Patients and controls signed the informed consent. The study was conducted according to the Declaration of Helsinki and was approved by the local ethics committee (decision No. 10/11 September 2020).

2.2. Sample Evaluation

Serum was separated and stored in an ultrafreezer at −80 °C. Indirect immunofluorescence was used for antinuclear antibodies analysis (ANA). Commercial enzyme linked immunosorbent assay (ELISA) kits were used to determine anti-Scl70 and anti-centromere antibodies (Euro Diagnostica, Malmo, Sweden).

2.2.1. S100A6 Assay

Serum S100A6 levels were determined using commercial sandwich ELISA kit (ELH-S-100A6-1 Raybiotech, Peachtree Corners, GA, USA) according to the manufacturer's instructions. The intra-assay and inter-assay coefficient of variation were 10% and 12%. The minimum detectable concentration of S100A6 was 0.06 ng/mL.

2.2.2. Calumenin Assay

Serum calumenin was determined using commercial sandwich ELISA kit (ELH-CALU-1 Raybiotech, Peachtree Corners, GA, USA) according to the manufacturer's instructions. The intra-assay and inter-assay coefficient of variation were 10% and 12%. The minimum detectable concentration of calumenin was 0.55 ng/mL.

2.2.3. Cytohesin 2 Assay

Serum cytohesin 2 levels were assayed using commercial competitive ELISA kit (ABIN857811, MyBiosource, San Diego, CA, USA). The intra-assay and inter-assay coefficient of variation were 10% and 10%. The minimum detectable concentration of cytohesin 2 was 0.1 ng/mL.

All samples were analyzed in duplicate, with optical densities evaluated at 450 nm using a microplate reader (Dynex, Buštěhrad, Czech Republic). In order to evaluate the standard curve and estimate the concentration of the samples, a four-parameter logistic regression curve was used (Aladyn software, Prague, Czech Republic). Results were presented as nanograms per milliliter (ng/mL).

2.3. Statistical Analysis

Continuous variables were presented as median and interquartile range (IQR) value if a non-normal distribution was found. Normality of distribution was tested with Kolmogorov-Smirnov tests. Fisher's exact tests were used to evaluate association between categorical variables. Differences between continuous variables were evaluated with Mann-Whitney U test. Spearman rho coefficient was used in order to assess correlations in continuous variables. A threshold for p-value ≤ 0.05 was considered significant. Statistical Software for Social Sciences (SPSS), Version 16 for Windows (Chicago, IL, USA) was used.

3. Results

Descriptive data of patients included in Ssc group and healthy controls are presented in Table 1.

Table 1. Characteristics of included Ssc patients and healthy controls.

Ssc Patient Characteristics	All Ssc Patients (n = 53)	Healthy Controls (n = 26)	Diffuse Ssc (n = 33)	Localized Ssc (n = 20)	p-Value (between Diffuse SSc and Localized SSc)
Age (median (IQR), years)	56 (15.75)	51.5 (12.50)	54 (14.25)	60.5 (20.25)	0.71 (NS)
Male/Female (n° of patients)	4/49	2/24	3/30	1/19	1 (NS)
Ssc disease duration (median (IQR), months)	84 (94.50)	N/A	102 (95)	77 (96)	0.22 (NS)
Interstitial lung disease (n° of patients)	28 (52.8%)	N/A	21 (63.6%)	7 (35%)	0.04
% DLCO (median (IQR)	78 (22)	N/A	77 (24)	85.5 (15.5)	0.10 (NS)
Pulmonary hypertension (n° of patients)	7 (13.2%)	N/A	3 (9.1%)	4 (20%)	0.26 (NS)
% predicted FVC (median (IQR))	97 (19.5)	N/A	98 (18)	96 (26.75)	0.83 (NS)
Presence of Raynaud phenomenon (n° of patients)	53 (100%)	N/A	33 (100%)	20 (100%)	1 (NS)
Digital ulcers (n° of patients)	12 (22.6%)	N/A	12 (36.4%)	0 (0%)	0.03
No of digital ulcers (median (IQR))	0 (2)	N/A	0 (2)	0 (0)	0.001
Presence of telangiectasia (no of patients)	27 (51%)	N/A	16 (48.5%)	11 (55%)	0.64 (NS)
Palpable friction rubs (n° of patients)	18 (34%)	N/A	14 (42.4%)	4 (20%)	0.10
PAP (median (IQR) mm Hg)	25 (4)	N/A	25 (4)	25 (8)	0.72 (NS)
ANA (n° of patients)	53 (100%)	N/A	33 (100%)	20 (100%)	1 (NS)
Presence of anti-centromere antibodies (n° of patients)	20 (37.7%)	N/A	0 (0%)	20 (100%)	< 0.001
Presence of anti Scl-70 antibodies (n° of positive patients)	23 (43.4%)	N/A	23 (70%)	0 (0%)	0.002
CRP (median (IQR) mg/L)	3.53 (7.28)	N/A	3.98 (11.24)	3.34 (6.44)	0.45 (NS)
ESR (median (IQR) mm/1 h)	16 (16.5)	N/A	16.5 (15.5)	14 (18.50)	0.38 (NS)
Hypocomplementemia (n° of patients)	6 (11.3%)	N/A	4 (12.1%)	2 (10%)	0.81 (NS)
EUSTAR score (median (IQR))	3 (2.50)	N/A	3.50 (2.75)	1.75 (2)	0.001
Steroid therapy (n° of patients)	30 (56.6%)	N/A	18 (54.4%)	12 (60%)	0.69 (NS)
Calcium blockers (n° of patients)	16 (30.2%)	N/A	10 (30.3%)	6 (30%)	0.98 (NS)
ACE inhibitors (n° of patients)	11 (20.7%)	N/A	8 (24.3%)	3 (15%)	0.42 (NS)

NS—not significant, PAP—pulmonary artery pressure, DLCO—diffuse lung capacity for carbon monoxide, ANA—antinuclear antibody, ESR—erythrocyte sedimentation rate; CRP—C-reactive protein; ACE—angiotensin-converting enzyme. n°—number; N/A—not applicable.

3.1. Serum Calumenin in Ssc Patients

Serum calumenin levels were higher in Ssc patients compared to controls (median 26.14 ng/mL (interquartile range—IQR 27.22) versus median 17.97 ng/mL (13.82), Mann Whitney U test, $p = 0.002$, Figure 1). Ssc patients with a modified Rodnan score ≥ 14 (thus with diffuse cutaneous fibrosis) had higher circulatory calumenin levels. Median calumenin levels in Ssc patients with diffuse cutaneous fibrosis were 30.55 ng/mL (30.12) versus 20.08 ng/mL (16.57), Mann Whitney U test, $p = 0.015$

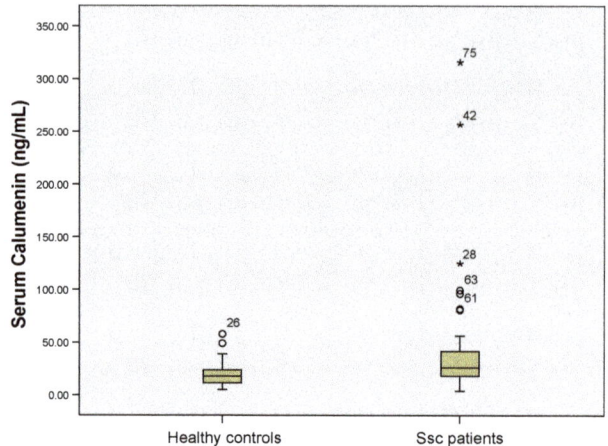

Figure 1. Serum calumenin levels were higher in Ssc (systemic sclerosis) patients compared to healthy controls ($p = 0.002$, Mann Whitney U test). The circles, stars and numbers in figure represent the patient ID in the database that are considered outliers by the statistical software used.

When used as a diagnostic test for diffuse cutaneous fibrosis, calumenin had a relatively good diagnostic capacity AUROC = 0.70 (95% confidence interval (0.56–0.86)), Figure 2.

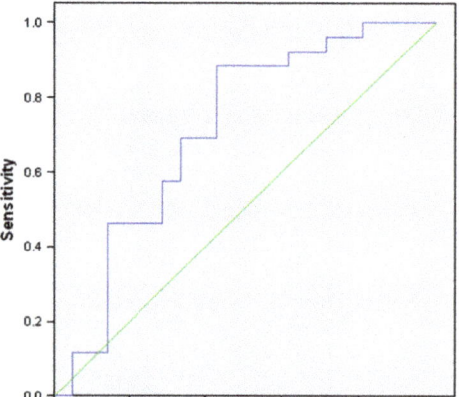

Figure 2. ROC curve for calumenin as diagnostic test for diffuse cutaneous fibrosis. AUROC = 0.70, 95% confidence interval 0.56–0.86.

In addition, patients with daily or higher frequency of Raynaud phenomenon had higher calumenin levels (30.36 ng/mL (35.11) versus 17.84 ng/mL (12.24), Mann Whitney U test, $p = 0.006$).

Patients with low C3 or C4 levels also had significantly higher calumenin levels (median 54.34 ng/mL (116.04) versus 23.71 ng/mL (15.19), Mann Whitney U test, $p = 0.03$). Circulating calumenin levels were positively correlated with modified Rodnan scores ($r = 0.40$, $p = 0.004$) with CRP levels ($r = 0.343$, $p = 0.02$) and with ESR ($r = 0.372$, $p = 0.01$).

Interestingly, patients with pulmonary fibrosis had a tendency for higher circulatory calumenin levels (30.22 ng/mL (34.62) versus 21.5 ng/mL (12.70) $p = 0.087$, Mann Whitney U test). Nevertheless, no significant differences between serum calumenin levels in diffuse versus localized Ssc patients were found.

3.2. Serum S100A6 in Ssc Patients

Serum S100A6 levels were statistically significant higher in the Ssc group compared to controls (median 81.06 ng/mL (18.80) versus median 13.24 ng/mL (4.85), Mann Whitney U test, $p < 0.001$, Figure 3).

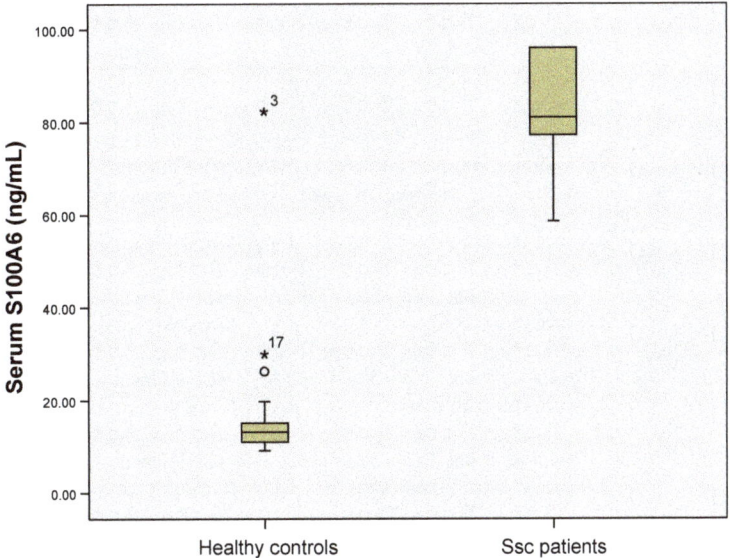

Figure 3. Serum S100A6 levels were higher in Ssc (systemic sclerosis) patients compared to healthy controls ($p < 0.001$, Mann Whitney U test). The circle, stars and numbers in figure represent the patient ID in the database that are considered outliers by the statistical software used.

Higher circulatory S100A6 levels were associated with digital ulcer presence (median 91.83 ng/mL in Ssc patients with digital ulcers (17.79) versus median 79.28 ng/mL in Ssc patients without digital ulcers (10.77), Mann Whitney U test, $p = 0.002$). Also, S100A6 levels were positively correlated with the number of active digital ulcers ($r = 0.33$, $p = 0.02$)

There were no significant differences between serum S100A6 levels in diffuse versus localized Ssc patients, nor with current Ssc medication.

3.3. Serum Cytohesin 2 in Ssc Patients

Serum cytohesin 2 levels were statistically significant higher in Ssc patients compared to controls (median 45.02 ng/mL (17.07) versus median 37.02 ng/mL (7.15), Mann Whitney U test, $p = 0.003$, Figure 4).

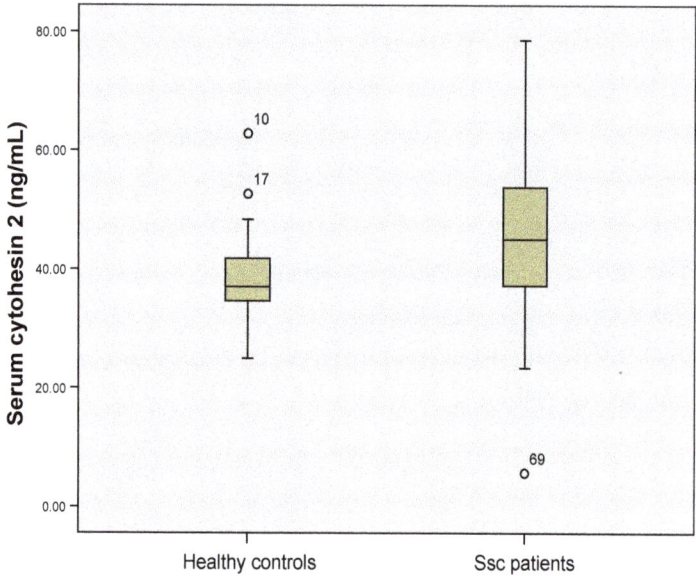

Figure 4. Serum cytohesin 2 levels were higher in Ssc (systemic sclerosis) patients compared to healthy controls ($p < 0.001$, Mann Whitney U test). The circle and numbers in figure represent the patient ID in the database that are considered outliers by the statistical software used.

Higher serum cytohesin 2 levels were observed in patients with telangiectasia presence (median 45.11 ng/mL (19.53) versus 40.46 ng/mL (11.68), Mann Whitney U test, $p = 0.025$).

Palpable tendon friction rubs were associated with lower circulating levels of cytohesin 2 (median 38.63 ng/mL (19.64) versus 46.06 (16.26), Mann Whitney U test, $p = 0.021$). Serum cytohesin 2 levels were positively correlated with inflammatory markers (ESR $r = 0.324$, $p = 0.024$, CRP $r = 0.486$, $p = 0.001$). There was a tendency for higher cytohesin 2 levels in patients with active disease, but without statistical significance ($p = 0.22$).

A cut-off value (53.97 ng/mL) defined as mean + two standard deviations of cytohesin 2 value of healthy controls was used to divide Ssc patients into two groups: high cytohesin 2 level and normal cytohesin 2 level. A total number of 13 Ssc patients (24.5%) had high cytohesin 2 levels. These patients had statistically significant higher PAP (pulmonary artery pressure) compared with patients with normal cytohesin 2 levels (median 28 mm Hg (20) versus median 25 mm Hg (2), Mann Whitney U test, $p = 0.03$). There were no significant differences between serum cytohesin 2 levels in diffuse versus localized Ssc patients, nor with current Ssc medication.

3.4. Correlations between Calumenin, S100A6 and Cytohesin 2

Calumenin levels were positively correlated with S100A6 levels ($r = 0.400$, $p < 0.001$), while a positive correlation was observed between S100A6 levels and cytohesin 2 levels ($r = 0.262$, $p = 0.02$).

4. Discussion

The results of the current study confirmed circulatory calumenin, S100A6 and cytohesin 2 as biomarkers for SSc patients. To the best of our knowledge, this is the first study that has evaluated circulatory levels of calumenin, S100A6, and cytohesin 2 on an independent cohort of Ssc patients.

Calumenin is a protein that binds calcium being localized in the endoplasmic reticulum. It belongs to a CREC chaperone alongside with Reticulocalbin 1, Cab45, and ERC-55, being involved in protein folding and the secretory pathway. Calumenin was described to be secreted in the surrounding medium [9]. It has been widely evaluated in various cancers by influencing tumorigenesis and therapeutic response [10]. Increased expression of calumenin was associated with poorer outcome in gliomas [11]. As such, this molecule could play a prognostic role for survival and for the therapeutic response in cancer. Secreted calumenin proved to have autocrine and paracrine effects, being linked to thrombosis and wound healing by modifying the fibroblast phenotype. [12]. Previous data suggest that calumenin is also secreted by activated thrombocytes and is localized in atherosclerotic lesion [13]. Having such an influence upon wound healing via fibroblast activity modulation calumenin could be an interesting and promising biomarker for Ssc patients as it has been previously isolated from biological samples from Ssc patients using mass spectrometry [14]. In this study, calumenin was confirmed as a circulatory biomarker and was associated with diffuse cutaneous fibrosis, inflammation, and low complement level. These data suggests that patients with higher inflammatory activity (that is continuously sustained by complement consumption) associate higher circulatory calumenin levels. However, no association was found between Ssc disease activity score and serum levels of calumenin and between patients with diffuse and localized Ssc. There was also a tendency for higher calumenin levels in patients with pulmonary fibrosis. Although the results did not reach statistical significance, this was most probably due to the relatively small sample size. The regulatory function of calumenin in tissues that are affected by the processes of cytoskeleton rearrangement points out calumenin as a candidate prognostic biomarker in Ssc patients, like has been previously suggested for another member of the CREC family (reticulocalbin 1) [15]. Future prospective studies including early Ssc patients should evaluate the prognostic capacity of circulatory calumenin in Ssc patients.

S100A6 (calcyclin) was extensively evaluated as a biomarker for digestive cancers. Serum S100A6 has a relatively good diagnostic capacity for cholangiocarcinoma [16]. Significant expression of S100A6 was observed also in placenta of women diagnosed with preeclampsia, and its expression is increased in oxidative stress response. [17]. S100A6 was much higher in Ssc patients compared to healthy controls. There were no associations with clinical Ssc features except for higher S100A6 levels in patients with active digital ulcers. Also, serum S100A6 positively correlated with the number of active digital ulcers. These data suggest that S100A6 could be a biomarker associated with more aggressive Ssc pattern. Another striking observation is the fact that S100A6 expression was a few folds higher in Ssc patients compared to controls. S100A6 is linked to the RAGE (Receptor for Advanced Glycation Endproducts) family by interacting with these molecules and acting as cytokines. It seems that S100A6 binding activates the NF-kB pathway and leads to apoptosis [18]. RAGE are known to be associated with various inflammatory cutaneous diseases (both autoimmune and infectious) [19]. RAGE pathway was reported to be involved in Ssc ulcerations development [20]. As a promotor for RAGE pathway, S100A6 could initiate and sustain the inflammatory process that is associated with digital ulceration. Also, very high levels of S100A6 were found in Ssc patients, which points out the fact that this specific molecule could be a potential future therapeutic target at least for prevention of digital ulcer development/aggravation. This hypothesis needs further testing in specific clinical settings on independent Ssc cohorts.

Cytohesin 2 is a guanine-nucleotide exchange factor (GEF) for ARF6 (ADP-ribosylation factor 6). It was previously showed that cytohesin 2 is localized on the plasma membrane and endosome [21]. It is involved in a multitude of signaling and trafficking pathways as it plays a major role in granule secretion in thrombocytes, chromaffin, and pancreatic β-cells [22]. Cytohesin 2 is an activator of both EGF and IGF-1 signaling pathways by direct interaction with the cytoplasmic domains of the activated EGF-R. In vitro studies on colorectal cells pointed out that cytohesin 2 blockade associated with a decreased cell proliferation, migration, and invasion of tumor cells, indicating cytohesin 2 as a potential therapeutic target in colorectal cancer [23]. A recent report also showed that inhibition of cytohesin 2 prevented the morphological changes in vascular smooth muscle cells due to resistin. Cytohesin 2 blockade modified the secretome of the vascular smooth muscle by decreasing matrix metalloproteinase expression [24].

IGF-1 and vascular smooth muscle cells are important pathogenic factors in Ssc, as they also seem to be involved in the progression from preclinical stages of Ssc to early stages [25]. Serum cytohesin 2 levels were increased in Ssc patients, but the prognostic value of these observed changes is not clear. Associations with some cutaneous features of Ssc were pointed out in this study (telangiectasia) alongside with positive correlations with inflammatory markers (especially CRP). Higher cytohesin 2 levels were associated with higher PAP but otherwise no associations with pulmonary Ssc involvement were found, although previous proteomic studies identified cytohesin 2 as a proteomic biomarker from BALF and suggested it as a candidate biomarker for pulmonary involvement in Ssc [14]. This is probably due to the fact the significant changes of cytohesin 2 levels are local rather than systemic. Confirmation studies for cytohesin 2, as a biomarker for IPF from BALF, are needed.

As previous findings pointed out that cytohesin 2 blockade is associated with a more quiescent cellular phenotype, it suggests that cytohesin 2 overexpression could also have a pathogenic effect in Ssc patients. Cytohesin 2 is localized at the crossroad of multiple pathogenic pathways in Ssc patients, and future in vitro studies on fibroblasts derived from Ssc samples are needed in order to evaluate cytohesin 2 blockade effects in Ssc derived cells and define cytohesin 2 as a potential Ssc therapeutic target.

The present study has important limitations. Firstly, the sample size is relatively small, especially for associations between serum levels of the biomarkers and all clinical characteristics of Ssc patients. This was due to the fact that the study was unicentric and Ssc is a rare disease. Secondly, this was only a confirmatory study of the proposed candidate biomarkers, without follow-up and dynamic evaluation of patients in order to validate them as biomarkers in Ssc patients. Thirdly, nailfold capillaroscopy data were not collected for these patients. As such, associations between nailfold capillaroscopy features and biomarkers were not evaluated. Future prospective validation studies on larger Ssc cohorts that also include nailfold capillaroscopy analysis are needed. Prospective studies evaluating the prognostic value of these biomarkers that include Ssc patients with early disease are of great interest.

5. Conclusions

In conclusion, this study confirmed circulatory cytohesin 2, calumenin and S100A6 as biomarkers in Ssc patients and found associations between the serum levels of these biomarkers and clinical characteristics, especially with severe cutaneous involvement (necrosis and diffuse sclerosis). Among all these biomarkers, calumenin had the best predictive capacity for cutaneous diffuse manifestation, while S100A6 was associated with digital ulcers. Independent confirmation of candidate biomarkers is the first essential step, and once the biomarkers are validated, it will eventually lead to a personalized approach of Ssc patients.

Author Contributions: Conceptualization, P.B., C.B. and A.B.; methodology, P.B.; formal analysis, P.B.; investigation, P.B. and E.B. writing—original draft preparation, P.B., A.B. and E.B.; writing—review and editing, P.B. and C.B.; supervision, C.B.; project administration, P.B. All authors have read and agreed to the published version of the manuscript.

Funding: This work was supported by a grant of theMinistry of Research, Innovation and Digitization, CNCS/CCCDI–UEFISCDI, project number PN-III-P1-1.1-PD-2019-0118, within PNCDI III.

Institutional Review Board Statement: The study was conducted according to the guidelines of the Declaration of Helsinki, and approved by the Ethics Committee of Colentina Clinical Hospital (decision No. 10/11 September 2020).

Informed Consent Statement: Informed consent was obtained from all subjects involved in the study.

Data Availability Statement: The data presented in this study are available upon reasonable request from the corresponding author.

Acknowledgments: This work was supported by a grant of the Ministry of Research, Innovation and Digitization, CNCS/CCCDI–UEFISCDI, project number PN-III-P1-1.1-PD-2019-0118, within PNCDI III.

Conflicts of Interest: The authors declare no conflict of interest.

References

1. Bhattacharyya, S.; Wei, J.; Varga, J. Understanding fibrosis in systemic sclerosis: Shifting paradigms, emerging opportunities. *Nat. Rev. Rheumatol.* **2012**, *8*, 42–54. [CrossRef]
2. Hasegawa, M. Biomarkers in systemic sclerosis: Their potential to predict clinical courses. *J. Dermatol.* **2016**, *43*, 29–38. [CrossRef]
3. Bălănescu, P.; Bălănescu, A.; Bălănescu, E.; Băicuş, C. Candidate proteomic biomarkers in systemic sclerosis discovered using mass-spectrometry: An update of a systematic review (2014–2020). *Rom. J. Intern. Med.* **2020**. [CrossRef]
4. Balanescu, P.; Ladaru, A.; Balanescu, E.; Baicus, C.; Dan, G.A. Systemic sclerosis biomarkers discovered using mass-spectrometry-based proteomics: A systematic review. *Biomark. Biochem. Indic. Expo. Responseand Susceptibility Chem.* **2014**, *19*, 345–355. [CrossRef] [PubMed]
5. Galie, N.; Humbert, M.; Vachiery, J.L.; Gibbs, S.; Lang, I.; Torbicki, A.; Simonneau, G.; Peacock, A.; Noordegraaf, A.V.; Beghetti, M.; et al. 2015 ESC/ERS Guidelines for the diagnosis and treatment of pulmonary hypertension The Joint Task Force for the Diagnosis and Treatment of Pulmonary Hypertension of the European Society of Cardiology (ESC) and the European Respiratory Society (ERS) Endorsed by: Association for European Paediatric and Congenital Cardiology (AEPC), International Society for Heart and Lung Transplantation (ISHLT). *Eur. Heart J.* **2016**, *37*, 67–119. [CrossRef] [PubMed]
6. Amanzi, L.; Braschi, F.; Fiori, G.; Galluccio, F.; Miniati, I.; Guiducci, S.; Conforti, M.L.; Kaloudi, O.; Nacci, F.; Sacu, O.; et al. Digital ulcers in scleroderma: Staging, characteristics and sub-setting through observation of 1614 digital lesions. *Rheumatology* **2010**, *49*, 1374–1382. [CrossRef] [PubMed]
7. Clements, P.; Lachenbruch, P.; Siebold, J.; White, B.; Weiner, S.; Martin, R.; Weinstein, A.; Weisman, M.; Mayes, M.; Collier, D.; et al. Inter and Intraobserver Variability of Total Skin Thickness Score (Modified Rodnan TSS) in Systemic-Sclerosis. *J. Rheumatol.* **1995**, *22*, 1281–1285.
8. Valentini, G.; D'Angelo, S.; Della Rossa, A.; Bencivelli, W.; Bombardieri, S. European Scleroderma Study Group to define disease activity criteria for systemic sclerosis. IV. Assessment of skin thickening by modified Rodnan skin score. *Ann. Rheum. Dis.* **2003**, *62*, 904–905. [CrossRef]
9. Vorum, H.; Hager, H.; Christensen, B.M.; Nielsen, S.; Honore, B. Human calumenin localizes to the secretory pathway and is secreted to the medium. *Exp. Cell Res.* **1999**, *248*, 473–481. [CrossRef]
10. Wang, Y.; Cui, X.X.; Wang, Y.L.; Fu, Y.; Guo, X.; Long, J.; Wei, C.X.; Zhao, M. Protective effect of miR378*on doxorubicin-induced cardiomyocyte injury via calumenin. *J. Cell. Physiol.* **2018**, *233*, 6344–6351. [CrossRef]
11. Yang, Y.; Wang, J.; Xu, S.H.; Shi, F.; Shan, A.J. Calumenin contributes to epithelial-mesenchymal transition and predicts poor survival in glioma. *Transl. Neurosci.* **2021**, *12*, 67–75. [CrossRef] [PubMed]
12. Ostergaard, M.; Hansen, G.A.W.; Vorum, H.; Honore, B. Proteomic profiling of fibroblasts reveals a modulating effect of extracellular calumenin on the organization of the actin cytoskeleton. *Proteomics* **2006**, *6*, 3509–3519. [CrossRef] [PubMed]
13. Coppinger, J.A.; Cagney, G.; Toomey, S.; Kislinger, T.; Belton, O.; McRedmond, J.P.; Cahill, D.J.; Emili, A.; Fitzgerald, D.J.; Maguire, P.B. Characterization of the proteins released from activated platelets leads to localization of novel platelet proteins in human atherosclerotic lesions. *Blood* **2004**, *103*, 2096–2104. [CrossRef] [PubMed]
14. Fietta, A.M.; Bardoni, A.M.; Salvini, R.; Passadore, I.; Morosini, M.; Cavagna, L.; Codullo, V.; Pozzi, E.; Meloni, F.; Montecucco, C. Analysis of bronchoalveolar lavage fluid proteome from systemic sclerosis patients with or without functional, clinical and radiological signs of lung fibrosis. *Arthritis Res. Ther.* **2006**, *8*. [CrossRef]
15. Balanescu, P.; Ladaru, A.; Balanescu, E.; Pompilian, V.; Gologanu, D.; Caraiola, S.; Baicus, C.; Dan, G.A. Circulating Reticulocalbin 1 and Reticulocalbin 3 in Systemic Sclerosis Patients: Results of a Case Control Study. *Clin. Lab.* **2016**, *62*, 1109–1116. [CrossRef] [PubMed]
16. Onsurathum, S.; Haonon, O.; Pinlaor, P.; Pairojkul, C.; Khuntikeo, N.; Thanan, R.; Roytrakul, S.; Pinlaor, S. Proteomics detection of S100A6 in tumor tissue interstitial fluid and evaluation of its potential as a biomarker of cholangiocarcinoma. *Tumour Biol.* **2018**, *40*, 1010428318767195. [CrossRef] [PubMed]
17. Guzel, C.; van den Berg, C.B.; Duvekot, J.J.; Stingl, C.; van den Bosch, T.P.P.; van der Weiden, M.; Steegers, E.A.P.; Steegers-Theunissen, R.P.M.; Luider, T.M. Quantification of Calcyclin and Heat Shock Protein 90 in Sera from Women with and without Preeclampsia by Mass Spectrometry. *Proteom. Clin. Appl.* **2019**, *13*. [CrossRef] [PubMed]
18. Leclerc, E.; Fritz, G.; Vetter, S.W.; Heizmann, C.W. Binding of S100 proteins to RAGE: An update. *Biochim. Biophys. Acta-Mol. Cell Res.* **2009**, *1793*, 993–1007. [CrossRef]
19. Guarneri, F.; Custurone, P.; Papaianni, V.; Gangemi, S. Involvement of RAGE and Oxidative Stress in Inflammatory and Infectious Skin Diseases. *Antioxidants* **2021**, *10*, 82. [CrossRef]

20. Yoshizaki, A.; Komura, K.; Iwata, Y.; Ogawa, F.; Hara, T.; Muroi, E.; Takenaka, M.; Shimizu, K.; Hasegawa, M.; Fujimoto, M.; et al. Clinical Significance of Serum HMGB-1 and sRAGE Levels in Systemic Sclerosis: Association with Disease Severity. *J. Clin. Immunol.* **2009**, *29*, 180–189. [CrossRef]
21. Donaldson, J.G.; Jackson, C.L. ARF family G proteins and their regulators: Roles in membrane transport, development and disease. *Nat. Rev. Mol. Cell Biol.* **2011**, *12*, 362–375. [CrossRef] [PubMed]
22. van den Bosch, M.T.J.; Poole, A.W.; Hers, I. Cytohesin-2 phosphorylation by protein kinase C relieves the constitutive suppression of platelet dense granule secretion by ADP-ribosylation factor 6. *J. Thromb. Haemost.* **2014**, *12*, 726–735. [CrossRef] [PubMed]
23. Pan, T.; Sun, J.F.; Hu, J.Y.; Hu, Y.W.; Zhou, J.; Chen, Z.G.; Xu, D.; Xu, W.H.; Zheng, S.; Zhang, S.Z. Cytohesins/ARNO: The Function in Colorectal Cancer Cells. *PLoS ONE* **2014**, *9*, e90997. [CrossRef] [PubMed]
24. Heun, Y.; Graff, P.; Lagara, A.; Schelhorn, R.; Mettler, R.; Pohl, U.; Mannell, H. IS The GEF Cytohesin-2/ARNO Mediates Resistin induced Phenotypic Switching in Vascular Smooth Muscle Cells. *Sci. Rep.* **2020**, *10*. [CrossRef]
25. Tabata, K.; Mikita, N.; Yasutake, M.; Matsumiya, R.; Tanaka, K.; Tani, S.; Okuhira, H.; Jinnin, M.; Fujii, T. Up-regulation of IGF-1, RANTES and VEGF in patients with anti-centromere antibody-positive early/mild systemic sclerosis. *Mod. Rheumatol.* **2021**, *31*, 171–176. [CrossRef]

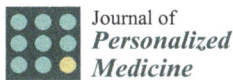

Article

Effectiveness of Platelet-Rich Plasma Therapy in Androgenic Alopecia—A Meta-Analysis

Simona Roxana Georgescu [1,2], Andreea Amuzescu [2,*], Cristina Iulia Mitran [3], Madalina Irina Mitran [3], Clara Matei [1], Carolina Constantin [4,5], Mircea Tampa [1,*] and Monica Neagu [4,5,6]

1 Department of Dermatology, "Carol Davila" University of Medicine and Pharmacy, 020021 Bucharest, Romania; simonaroxanageorgescu@yahoo.com (S.R.G.); matei_clara@yahoo.com (C.M.)
2 Department of Dermatology, "Victor Babes" Clinical Hospital for Infectious Diseases, 030303 Bucharest, Romania
3 Department of Microbiology, "Carol Davila" University of Medicine and Pharmacy, 020021 Bucharest, Romania; cristina.iulia.mitran@gmail.com (C.I.M.); madalina.irina.mitran@gmail.com (M.I.M.)
4 Immunology Department, "Victor Babes" National Institute of Pathology, 050096 Bucharest, Romania; caroconstantin@gmail.com (C.C.); neagu.monica@gmail.com (M.N.)
5 Colentina Clinical Hospital, 020125 Bucharest, Romania
6 Faculty of Biology, University of Bucharest, 76201 Bucharest, Romania
* Correspondence: amuzescuandreea@gmail.com (A.A.); dermatology.mt@gmail.com (M.T.)

Abstract: Platelet-rich plasma (PRP) represents a novel therapy tested and is used more and more frequently in dermatology and cosmetic surgery for a variety of conditions, including androgenic alopecia (AGA), a common condition with a complex pathogenesis involving genetic factors, hormonal status and inflammation. We performed an extensive literature search which retrieved 15 clinical trials concerning the use in AGA of PRP therapy, alone or in combination, in male, female or mixed patient groups. A quantitative statistical meta-analysis of $n = 17$ trial groups proved significant increases in hair density from 141.9 ± 108.2 to 177.5 ± 129.7 hairs/cm^2 (mean $\pm$ SD) following PRP ($p = 0.0004$). To the best of our knowledge, this is the first meta-analysis that proved a statistically significant correlation between the number of PRP treatments per month and the percentage change in hair density ($r = 0.5$, $p = 0.03$), as well as a negative correlation between the mean age of treatment group and the percentage change in hair density ($r = -0.56$, $p = 0.016$). Other factors considered for analysis were the PRP preparation method, amount used per treatment, hair diameter, terminal hairs and pull test. We conclude that PRP represents a valuable and effective therapy for AGA in both males and females if patients are rigorously selected.

Keywords: androgenic alopecia; clinical trial; hair density; inflammation; meta-analysis; platelet-rich plasma

Citation: Georgescu, S.R.; Amuzescu, A.; Mitran, C.I.; Mitran, M.I.; Matei, C.; Constantin, C.; Tampa, M.; Neagu, M. Effectiveness of Platelet-Rich Plasma Therapy in Androgenic Alopecia—A Meta-Analysis. *J. Pers. Med.* **2022**, *12*, 342. https://doi.org/10.3390/jpm12030342

Academic Editor: David S. Gibson

Received: 2 February 2022
Accepted: 22 February 2022
Published: 24 February 2022

Publisher's Note: MDPI stays neutral with regard to jurisdictional claims in published maps and institutional affiliations.

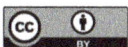

Copyright: © 2022 by the authors. Licensee MDPI, Basel, Switzerland. This article is an open access article distributed under the terms and conditions of the Creative Commons Attribution (CC BY) license (https://creativecommons.org/licenses/by/4.0/).

1. Introduction

Alopecia is a common condition that affects a large part of the population, particularly Caucasian males, the most common type being androgenic alopecia (AGA), a progressive disorder with significant psychosocial effects that can lead to depression. There are several theories trying to explain the complex multifactorial pathogeny of this condition. One of them postulates that chronic perifollicular microinflammation amplifies the expression of pro-inflammatory cytokines, leading to oxidative stress. The oxidative profile acts in combination with high levels of androgens, genetic predisposition and environmental factors such as stress, affecting the corticotropin-releasing hormone pathway and cortisol levels, hence generating the condition [1]. Gene variants that lead to increased activity of 5-α-reductase or increased sensitivity of androgen receptors are deemed to play an important role [2]. There is no single key mechanism involved in the disease, but a plethora of interconnected mechanisms that need to be treated simultaneously for a successful result. The reestablishment of healthy hair cell follicles can be influenced by certain growth factors that can stimulate the anagen phase of hair cycle, favoring cell proliferation, improvement of extracellular matrix and neoangiogenesis [3,4]. Recent studies have evidenced inflammatory infiltrates located in perifollicular/perivascular areas with histiocytes and lymphocytes. These findings, together with the implication of certain inflammatory genes (e.g., CASP7, TNF), strongly suggest a relationship between AGA and inflammatory pathways [1].

The close relationship between chronic inflammation and oxidative stress is well known [5–8]. There are many studies that show the involvement of oxidative stress in alopecia areata [9–12]. Recent research indicates an imbalance between oxidants and antioxidants in AGA [13,14]. The skin appendages, especially the hair follicle, can be exposed to elevated levels of oxidative stress. Reactive oxygen species (ROS) accumulate in the hair follicle and the antioxidant defense capacity is exceeded, resulting in premature aging of dermal papilla cells and eventually to the loss of their function [13,15]. Furthermore, it has been hypothesized that ROS may mediate the response of cells to growth factors [13]. In the light of oxidative stress involvement in AGA, Kaya Erdogan et al. consider that antioxidant therapies may be useful in the treatment of these patients [14].

Beyond classical AGA therapies such as minoxidil or finasteride, several new strategies have been proposed in recent years, each of them claiming long-term beneficial effects on hair follicle homeostasis [1,16], and offering multiple choices for personalized treatments. Among these new therapies, platelet-rich plasma (PRP) has been tested in several randomized case-control clinical trials [17,18]. The procedure involves collecting autologous blood from the patient under sterile conditions, on anticoagulant, and separating a platelet-rich plasma fraction by centrifugation. After a first spin, the second intermediate layer of plasma can be collected with a sterile syringe, dropping out the first layer of PPP (Platelet-Poor Plasma or buffy coat) and the red blood cells at the bottom of the tube. Some practitioners use a second spin to concentrate the PRP, as well as an activator of platelet α-granules release such as calcium or thrombin before injection into the scalp. There is a wide variation of protocols for preparation of PRP [3].

PRP therapy is already extensively used in dermatology and plastic surgery [19], being successfully applied for facial rejuvenation, treatment of wrinkles, scars, striae distensae, atrophic acne, vitiligo, facelift surgery, periorbital rejuvenation, dermal augmentation, as well as in other medical specialties such as orthopedic and trauma surgery, ocular surgery, stomatology, wound healing, urology, etc. [20,21]. Due to the important effects of growth factors present in PRP on skin rejuvenation, fibroblast and macrophage chemotaxis, fibroblast proliferation and extracellular matrix synthesis [22], this treatment is expected to exert beneficial effects on hair follicle degeneration, particularly in AGA. Autologous platelet rich fibrin (PRF), another related therapy, has been successfully used in both solid and liquid form administered intralesionally to accelerate healing in a case of facial pyoderma gangrenosum, due to its capacity to promote the prolonged release of multiple growth factors including TGF, EGF, FGF, KGF, CTGF, TNF-α [23], as well as in oral and maxillofacial surgery to cure medication-related osteonecrosis [24,25].

Until now, the only two effective treatments of AGA approved by the FDA are minoxidil for both men and women and finasteride for men [26–28]. Other treatment options are low-level laser therapy or hair transplant surgery, both with limited effectiveness, as well as synthetic PRP analogues such as growth factors biomimetic cocktails [16] or hair follicle dermal papilla stem cell cloning [29]. Considering their potential adverse reactions and other limiting factors, published results of clinical trials have to be carefully assessed via meta-analyses like the present one, which can be expanded for finding new possible therapy targets.

2. Materials and Methods

2.1. Literature Search and Selection of Studies

A search of the literature was performed by interrogating the PubMed database (on 27 July 2021) with the keyword combination "PRP AND alopecia AND clinical trial", a sufficiently specific search string that avoids sampling biases. We selected for meta-analysis the clinical trials that included treatment groups, using as therapy PRP alone, combined with or compared to other procedures. The exclusion criteria comprised clinical trials including patients with other types of alopecia (e.g., alopecia areata, seborrheic dermatitis, iatrogenic alopecia, *a.s.o.*). The stepwise procedure for selecting clinical trials included in the meta-analysis observed the methods, stages, as well as selected checklist items of the PRISMA (Preferred Reporting Items for Systematic Reviews and Meta-Analyses) guidelines and its subsequent updates [30,31].

2.2. Data Analysis

A number of qualitative or quantitative assessment variables (e.g., hair density, diameter, results of pull test, total number and frequency of PRP treatments, total amount of PRP per treatment, mean age of each group) were retrieved from each published clinical trial included in this meta-analysis. Data are expressed as means ± SD. The normality of the data samples was verified with the Kolmogorov-Smirnov, D'Agostino-Person and Shapiro-Wilk tests; normally distributed data were compared with Student's *t* test, and data sets that did not pass normality tests with its non-parametric versions: Mann-Whitney for independent data sets and Wilcoxon signed rank test for paired data. Most variables included in analysis were normally distributed, therefore we used directly Student's *t* test for independent samples (two-tailed), except for the absolute change in hair density, where we used its non-parametric variant, the non-directional Mann-Whitney test. We also performed linear correlation and regression analysis, indicating the values of Pearson's product-momentum correlation coefficient *r*, its statistical significance *p*, and the linear regression function. Statistical significance was assessed using a critical level $p = 0.05$. Forrest plots were generated with the clinical trials meta-analysis software Review Manager (RevMan) Version 5.4.1 The Cochrane Collaboration, 2020 [32].

3. Results

The literature search performed according to the criteria described within the Methods section resulted in the identification of 15 clinical trials, including studies on the effects of PRP treatment of AGA suitable for inclusion in our meta-analysis. The PRISMA flowchart describing the successive steps of the selection procedure is shown in Figure 1, while Table 1 presents the main features of the selected clinical trials. Most of them (86.7%) were randomized, 46.7% were double-blind, and 26.7% were single-blind. We found marked differences regarding the study design: 2 studies applied PRP/placebo on half-scalp and 3 studies on individual areas of the scalp in same patients, resulting in better case-control matching. Two studies included separate PRP and negative control (placebo) groups, while two other studies comprised two groups with different PRP administration protocols, differing in timing or preparation quality; three studies compared effects of PRP alone with those of PRP combined with minoxidil, or different PRP/minoxidil combinations, or other combinations of synthetic growth factors similar to those retrieved in PRP [16].

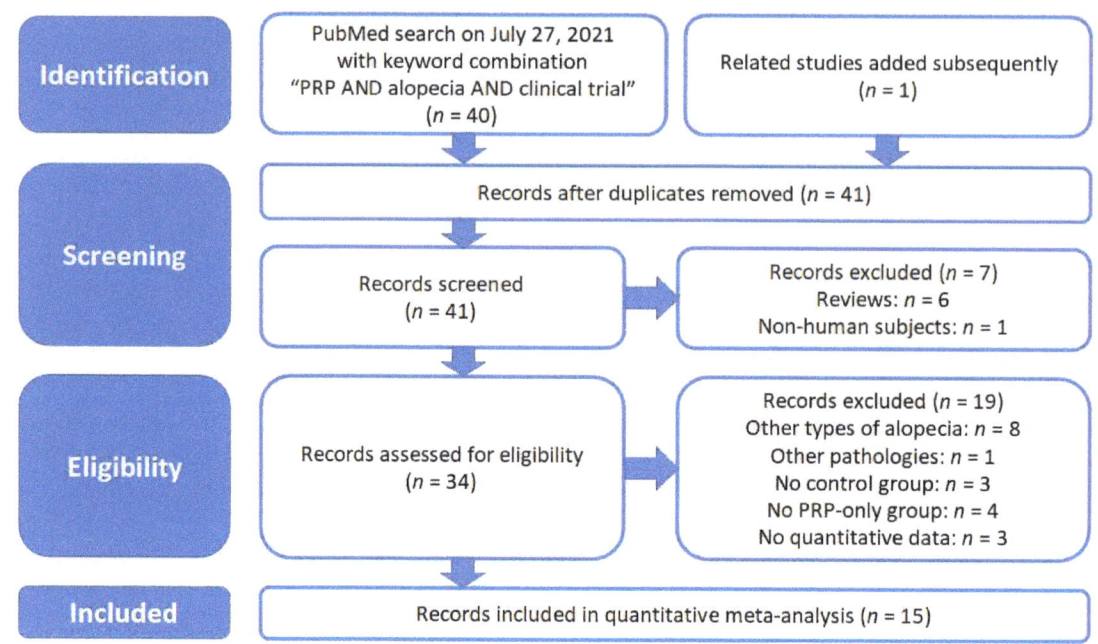

Figure 1. PRISMA flowchart showing the algorithm used for selection of the studies included in the current meta-analysis.

Table 1. Features of the clinical trials selected and included in the meta-analysis (in alphabetical order).

Study	Rando-Mized	Double-Blind	Groups	Mean Age &/Age Interval	Sex	mL PRP/ Treatment	Change in Hair Density (Hairs/cm^2) Initial–Final
Alves & Grimalt 2016 [26]	Y	Y	$n = 22$, PRP/placebo on half-scalp 3 PRP treatments (1/month)	39 (21–62)	M/F	3	165.7–179.9
Bayat et al. 2019 [33]	N	N	$n = 19$, 3 PRP treatments (0, 4, 8 weeks)	36.26 (28–40)	M	5	30.11–38.58
Bruce et al. 2020 [34]	Y	N	arm A–PRP then minoxidil ($n = 19$) 3 PRP treatments over 4 weeks 8 weeks wash-out then minoxidil 12 weeks	56 (20–79)	F	5	134–145
			arm B–minoxidil then PRP ($n = 18$) minoxidil 12 weeks, 8 weeks wash-out then 3 PRP treatments over 4 weeks	56 (20–79)	F	5	139–153
Butt et al. 2018 [35]	N	N	$n = 30$, 2 PRP treatments (1/month)	28.7 (19–47)	M/F	4	34.18–50.2
Butt et al. 2019 [36]	Y	N	PRP group ($n = 11$) 2 PRP treatments at 4 weeks	26.45	M/F	5	52.64–63.72
			stromal vascular fraction-PRP group ($n = 11$), same treatment timing	33.27	M/F	5	37.66–57.11
Gentile et al. 2015 [37]	Y	Y	$n = 23$, PRP/placebo on half-scalp 3 PRP treatments (1/month)	34.74 (19–63)	M	9	161.2–207.1
Hausauer & Jones 2018 [38]	Y	single-blind	PRP group 1 ($n = 20$) 3 PRP treatments (1/month) + 1 booster treatment after 3 months	40.1 (18–60)	M/F	5	160.4–207.1
			PRP group 2 ($n = 19$) 2 PRP treatments at 3 months	46.85 (18–60)	M/F	5	177.6–190.6

Table 1. Cont.

Study	Rando-Mized	Double-Blind	Groups	Mean Age &/Age Interval	Sex	mL PRP/ Treatment	Change in Hair Density (Hairs/cm^2) Initial–Final
Kapoor et al. 2020 [16]	Y	single-blind	group B (PRP) (n = 25) 8 PRP treatments at 3 weeks	25–50	M	1.5	167.2–176.1
Mapar et al. 2016 [39]	Y	single-blind	n = 17, PRP/placebo on squares 2 PRP treatments (1/month)	37.2 (25–45)	M	1.5	87.29–85.06
Pakhomova & Smirnova 2020 [40]	Y	single-blind	group I (PRP) (n = 25) 4 PRP treatments (1/month)	29.7 (18–53)	M	4	381.5–426.1
			group II (PRP + minoxidil) (n = 22) 4 PRP treatments (1/month)		M	4	408.4–539.6
Puig et al. 2016 [41]	Y	Y	PRP group (n = 15) 1 treatment placebo group (n = 11) 1 treatment	>18	F	10	no signifcant differences
Rodrigues et al. 2020 [42]	Y	Y	PRP group (n = 15) 4 treatments at 15 days intervals placebo group (n = 11) 4 treatments at 15 days intervals	32 (18–50)	M	2	140–180
Shapiro et al. 2020 [43]	Y	Y	n = 35, PRP/placebo on squares 3 PRP treatments (1/month)	36.5 (18–58)	M/F	5	151–170.96
Singh et al. 2020 [44]	Y	Y	PRP group (n = 20) 3 treatments (1/month)	26.5	M	3–3.5	93.73–143.2
			PRP+minoxidil group (n = 20) 3 treatments (1/month)	25.6	M	3–3.5	90.05–150.45
Tawfick & Osman 2017 [45]	Y	Y	n = 30, PRP/placebo on areas 4 PRP treatments (1/week)	29.3 (20–45)	F	0.9	73.66–150.94

The inclusion and exclusion criteria used within the clinical trials selected for analysis are listed in Table S1. Most studies used the Norwood-Hamilton scale for assessment of male patients with AGA and the Ludwig scale for female patients. Exclusion criteria were also largely similar among studies, including the use of other topical or systemic hair growth medications, other causes of alopecia, other general diseases (endocrine, inflammatory, autoimmune, neoplasia, platelet and other bleeding disorders), and risk factors such as alcohol use or smoking.

There were also important differences in the PRP preparation methods, as shown in Table S2. The amount of peripheral blood used for one PRP treatment ranged between 9 and 60 mL, centrifugation was done as a single-step or two-steps, and calcium chloride was the most frequently used agent for α-granule release by platelet fractions. The most widely used monitoring methods were digital photography and phototrichogram analysis using the standard TrichoScan method.

Figure 2 presents the absolute and relative changes in average hair density for n = 17 study groups included in this meta-analysis. The mean hair density within these groups varied from an initial value of 141.9 ± 108.2 hairs/cm^2 (mean ± SD) to 177.5 ± 129.7 hairs/cm^2 at the last evaluation, a statistically significant increase as proved by a two-tailed Wilcoxon signed rank test (p = 0.0004). The same study groups were analyzed for effects on hair density using a Forrest plot shown in Figure 3; the main difference between baseline and post-therapy levels was 36.84 hairs/cm^2 (95% confidence interval 22.63–51.06).

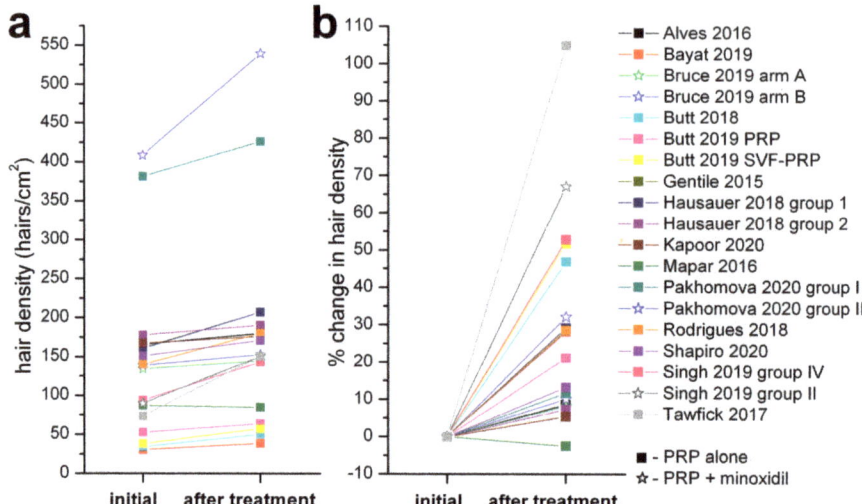

Figure 2. Effects of PRP treatments on absolute and percentage change in hair density within the clinical trials selected for meta-analysis. (**a**) absolute changes in hair density (hairs/cm^2) at the end of evaluation period. (**b**) percentage changes in hair density relative to initial values. The legend is the same for both graphs. Data for experimental groups where only PRP treatment was applied are marked with squares, those where minoxidil treatment was added are marked with hollow star symbols.

Study or Subgroup	After therapy Mean	SD	Total	Baseline Mean	SD	Total	Weight	Mean Difference IV, Random, 95% CI	Mean Difference IV, Random, 95% CI
Alves 2016 PRP	179.9	62.7	22	167.1	55.6	22	5.3%	12.80 [−22.22, 47.82]	
Bayat 2019 PRP	38.58	7.574	19	30.11	7.055	19	7.7%	8.47 [3.82, 13.12]	
Butt 2018 PRP	50.2	15.91	30	34.18	14.36	30	7.6%	16.02 [8.35, 23.69]	
Butt 2019 PRP	63.72	11.68	11	52.44	9.66	11	7.5%	11.28 [2.32, 20.24]	
Butt 2019 SVF-PRP	57.11	7.73	11	37.66	7.43	11	7.6%	19.45 [13.11, 25.79]	
Gentile 2015 PRP	207.1	56.3	23	161.2	41.9	23	5.9%	45.90 [17.22, 74.58]	
Hausauer 2018 PRP group 1	207.1	49.5	20	160.4	36.9	20	6.1%	46.70 [19.64, 73.76]	
Hausauer 2018 PRP group 2	190.6	66.9	19	177.6	62	19	4.7%	13.00 [−28.01, 54.01]	
Kapoor 2020 PRP	176.1	11.6	25	167.2	14.4	25	7.6%	8.90 [1.65, 16.15]	
Pakhomova 2020 PRP	426.1	50.1	25	381.5	45.4	25	6.1%	44.60 [18.10, 71.10]	
Pakhomova 2020 PRP+minoxidil	539.6	52.1	22	408.4	43.6	22	5.9%	131.20 [102.81, 159.59]	
Shapiro 2020 PRP	170.96	37.14	35	151	39.82	35	6.9%	19.96 [1.92, 38.00]	
Singh 2019 PRP	143.2	33.35	20	93.75	32.49	20	6.7%	49.45 [29.04, 69.86]	
Singh 2019 PRP+minoxidil	150.45	28.27	20	90.05	35.09	20	6.8%	60.40 [40.65, 80.15]	
Tawfik 2017 PRP	150.94	19.17	30	73.66	9.42	30	7.6%	77.28 [69.64, 84.92]	
Total (95% CI)			**332**			**332**	**100.0%**	**36.84 [22.63, 51.06]**	

Heterogeneity: Tau^2 = 677.62; Chi^2 = 341.33, df = 14 (P < 0.00001); I^2 = 96%
Test for overall effect: Z = 5.08 (P < 0.00001)

Figure 3. Forrest plot showing the effects of PRP treatment on hair density in selected study groups.

We have also assessed the correlations between the total number of PRP treatments and the absolute or relative change in hair density: both were statistically non-significant (r = 0.176, p = 0.47 for absolute and r = −0.115, p = 0.64 for relative changes, Figure 4). However, the percentage change in hair density was significantly correlated with the frequency of PRP treatments (r = 0.50, p = 0.03), but the absolute change in hair density was not (r = 0.135, p = 0.58) (Figure 5). We also found no significant correlation between the amount of PRP administered per treatment and the absolute (r = −0.069, p = 0.78) or relative change in hair density (r = −0.215, p = 0.38), while the mean ages of the treatment groups were significantly correlated with the absolute (r = −0.44, p = 0.07) and relative (r = −0.56, p = 0.016) change in hair density (Figure 6).

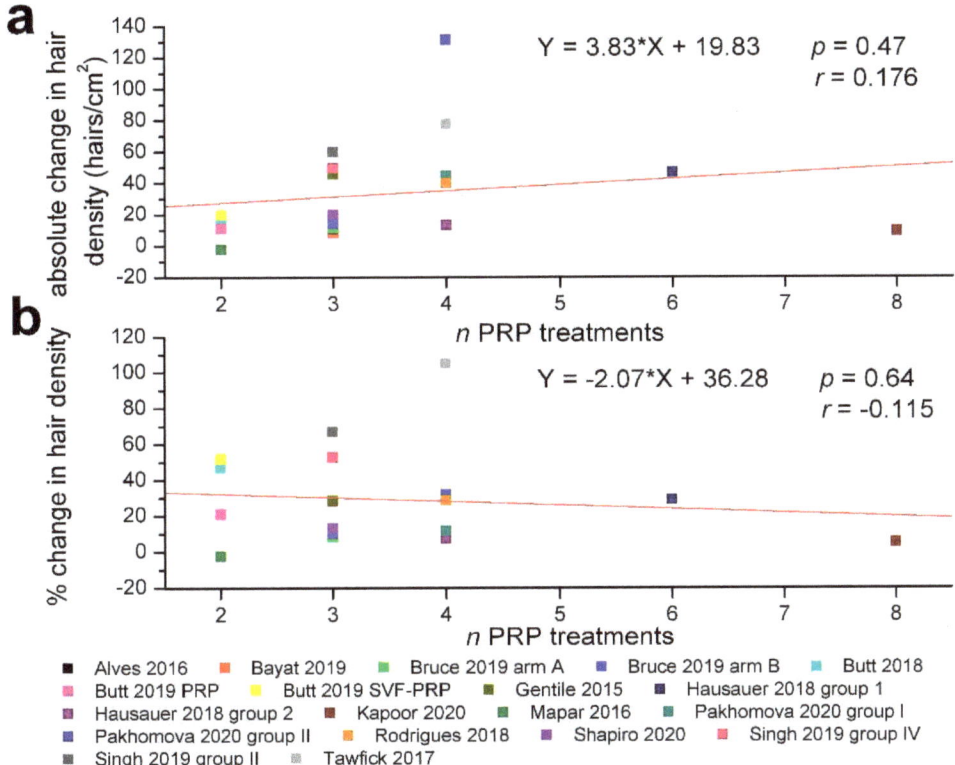

Figure 4. Absence of significant correlations between the number of PRP treatments and absolute or percentage change in hair density within the clinical trials selected for meta-analysis. (**a**) absolute changes in hair density (hairs/cm^2) at the end of evaluation period. (**b**) percentage changes in hair density relative to initial values (same legend for both graphs). The regression lines are plotted in red, and the corresponding equations, values of correlation coefficients r and their probabilities p are marked on each graph.

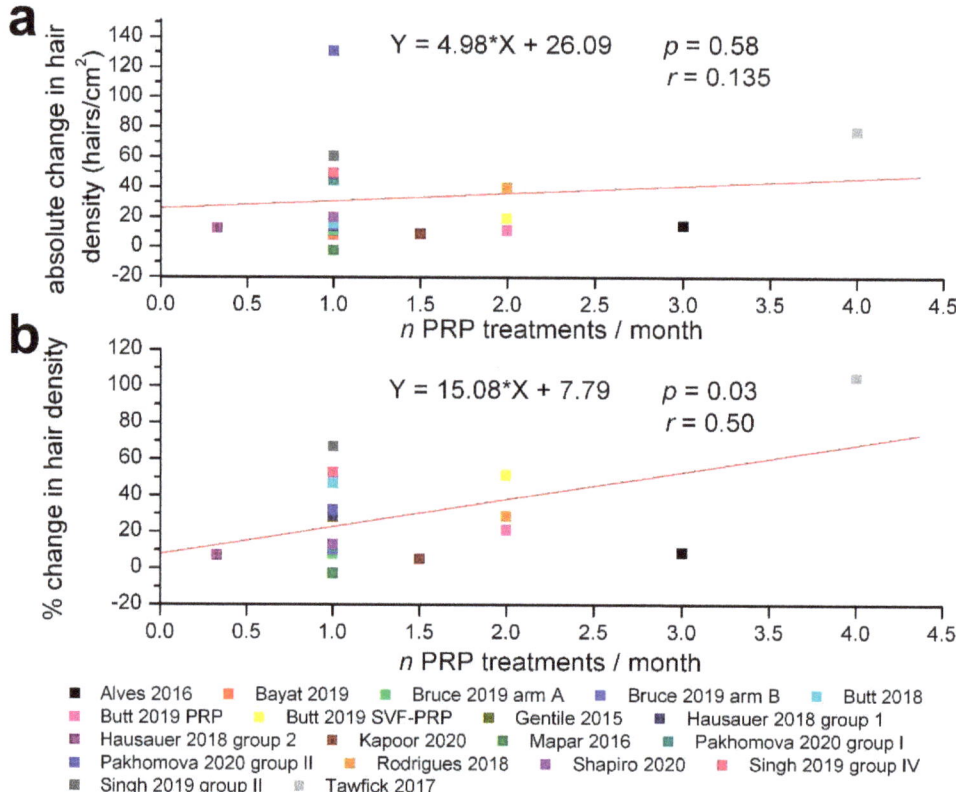

Figure 5. Correlations between the frequency of PRP treatments and absolute or percentage change in hair density within the clinical trials selected for meta-analysis. (**a**) lack of significant correlation of absolute changes in hair density (hairs/cm^2) at the end of evaluation period. (**b**) significant correlation with percentage changes in hair density relative to initial values (same legend for both graphs). The regression lines are plotted in red, and the corresponding equations, values of correlation coefficients r and their probabilities p are marked on each graph.

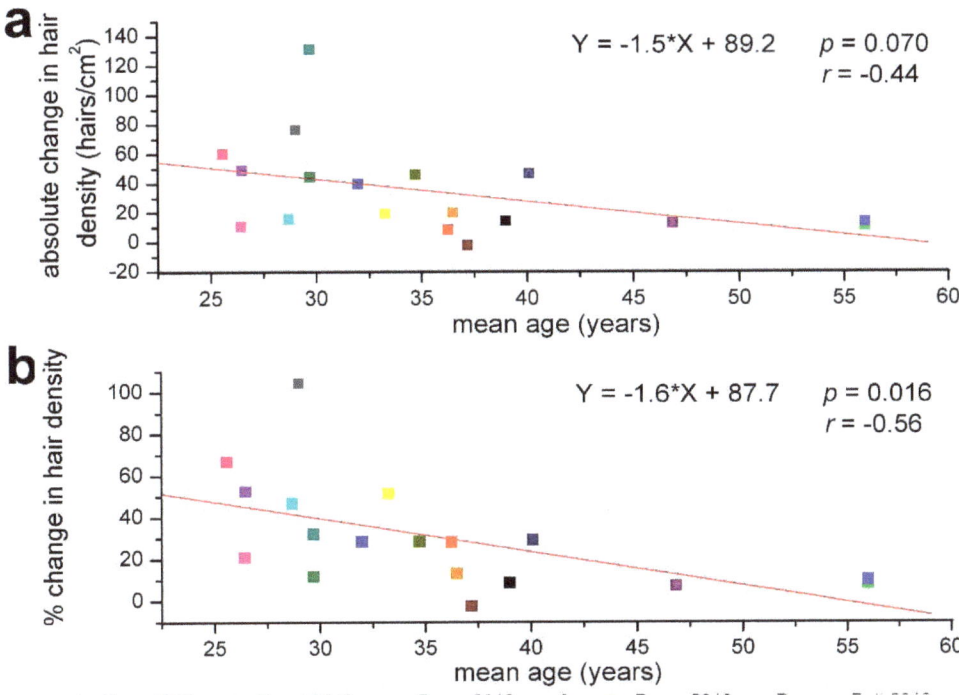

Figure 6. Correlations between the mean age of experimental groups and absolute or percentage change in hair density within the clinical trials selected for meta-analysis. (**a**) almost significant correlation with the absolute changes in hair density (hairs/cm^2) at the end of evaluation period. (**b**) significant correlation with percentage changes in hair density relative to initial values (same legend for both graphs). The regression lines are plotted in red, and the corresponding equations, the values of the correlation coefficients *r*, and their probabilities *p* are marked on each graph.

We verified if the sex composition of study groups exerted an effect on initial values, absolute and relative changes in hair density, using data exposed in Supplementary Table S3. Thus, the initial hair density, the absolute and the relative (%) change in hair density did not show significant differences between study groups formed exclusively from males vs. groups of females or with mixed gender composition.

Although relatively few studies of those included in the meta-analysis provided relevant data, we assessed the effects of PRP therapy on the mean hair diameter and the results of the pull test. Therefore, for n = 8 study groups the mean hair diameter increased by 15.67 μm after therapy (95% confidence interval 9.77–21.57) (Figure 7), while the results of the pull test decreased on average by 5.32 (95% confidence interval 2.84–7.80) for n = 5 study groups (Figure 8).

8 of the 15 studies included in the analysis (53.3%) reported use of patient self-assessment questionnaires, and 5 of them (33.3%) used physician assessments. Patient self-assessment comprised most often the degree of satisfaction following PRP therapy, usually at several time points, and divided on four levels (e.g., highly satisfied, satisfied, dissatisfied, highly dissatisfied). One study reported the percentage improvement after therapy on a 5-level scale [44], and another one on a 1-10 scale [45]. One self-assessment questionnaire included supplementary items such as evaluation of results (Yes, No, Unsure/maybe), recommendation to other patients (Yes, No, Maybe), and motivation to continue (Yes, No, Maybe) [38]. Physician assessments were based on analysis of global photographs of the scalp or four-level satisfaction questionnaires.

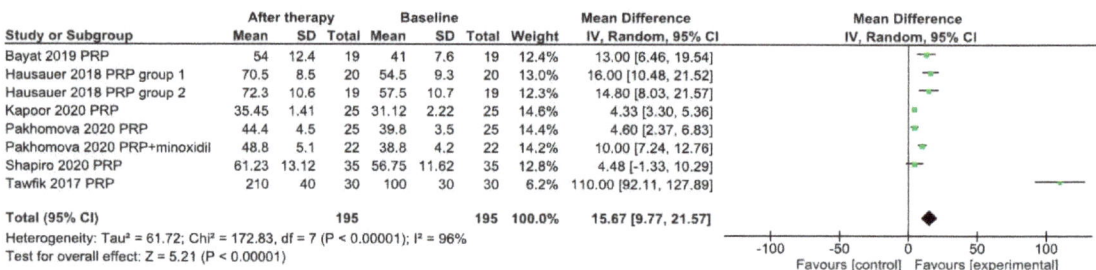

Figure 7. Forrest plot showing the effects of PRP treatment on mean hair diameter in selected study groups.

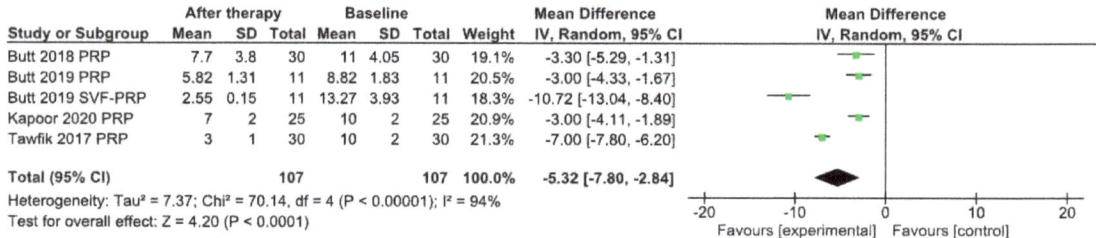

Figure 8. Forrest plot showing effects of PRP treatment on results of pull test in selected study groups.

4. Discussion

AGA is a challenging disorder for both healthcare providers and patients. Current therapeutic options for AGA may generate biochemical abnormalities and clinical adverse effects. Therefore, new personalized therapies are necessary according to the characteristics of the patients, with fewer side effects and satisfactory results [46–49]. An increasing body of evidence emphasizes an important dermal and follicular response to certain growth factors such as platelet-derived growth factor, transforming growth factor beta, etc. [17,50,51]. In line with this, recent research has focused on evaluating the effectiveness of PRP in AGA.

The present meta-analysis succeeded in retrieving a sufficiently large number of clinical trials including PRP treatments for AGA in male, female, or mixed gender groups to allow pertinent quantitative analysis of results. By comparison, a relatively recent similar meta-analysis, Giordano, Romeo and Lankinen (2017) [3], found only 6 out of 16 clinical trials of PRP in AGA accurately reporting changes in hair density following treatment. A similar attempt of meta-analysis, Kramer & Keaney (2018) [52], focusing on technical details of PRP preparation, concluded that only 21% of the 19 studies selected for analysis provided complete quantitative assessment of initial and final cellular composition of PRP preparations. Data reporting seems to have improved in recent clinical trials [17,53], so we were able to retrieve accurate quantitative estimates of changes in hair density obtained with reliable standardized methods in 14 out of 15 studies (Table 1), as well as sufficient details concerning PRP preparation or delivery protocols.

The amount of PRP administered per treatment varied between 0.9 and 10 mL (Tables 1 and S2), and it was distributed at multiple subcutaneous injection points, each receiving 100–150 µL. Interestingly, some studies reported significant increases in hair density even for the placebo treatment (e.g., from 151.04 ± 41.99 to 166.72 ± 37.13 hairs/cm^2, mean $\pm$ SD [43]). Although the authors explained such effects as resulting from a possible diffusion of the growth factors from the PRP-injected to the placebo-injected area, it is also plausible that microstimulation by needle puncture itself exerts beneficial effects on hair growth; this principle is currently applied in microneedling, another novel therapy used for AGA [54,55].

Among the 15 clinical trials selected for this meta-analysis, only two included histopathological and/or immunohistochemical assessment of PRP treatment effects. Gentile et al. (2015) showed significant increases in epidermal thickness and number of hair follicles after PRP injection on hematoxylin-eosin-stained scalp biopsies; they also assessed Ki67 proliferation index of hair follicle bulge cells and basal cells of epidermis [37]. Pakhomova and Smirnova (2020) proved by immunohistochemistry post-PRP treatment increases in areas of CD34 and β-catenin reactivity, as well as almost doubling of Ki67 proliferative index [40]. Rodrigues et al. (2018) used the multiplex method (Luminex®) to assess VEGF, PDGF and EGF concentrations in PRP preparations and correlate with their platelet counts, but also showed a lack of correlation with clinical effects on hair density [42].

Although there is no consensus concerning the molecular mechanisms and signaling pathways involved in PRP therapy, histological examination of biopsy samples from treated vs. control areas and immunohistochemical markers suggest multiple changes such as increased epidermal cell proliferation, particularly at hair follicles dermal papillae, augmentation of blood capillary network, and strengthening of the basal dermal extracellular matrix [43]. Platelet-secreted factors present in PRP preparations seem to enhance hair growth by stimulating multiple signaling pathways involved in the hair follicle cell cycle, such as the protein kinase B (Akt) pathway [18]. Upon Akt phosphorylation, subsequent Wnt/β-catenin transcription upregulation induces stem cell differentiation into hair follicle cells [56]. In vitro studies also showed that PRP causes papillary cells of the skin to grow by activating the extracellular signal-regulated kinases (ERK) [49]. Another important effect of PRP is reduction of hair follicle microinflammation associated with hair loss during AGA [1,57]. PRP growth and transcription factors signal the follicle to enter the anagen versus catagen phase, playing a role in regeneration and renewal; these effects partly overlap those of other effective AGA therapies such as minoxidil [58] or finasteride [59], justifying combined therapy approaches [44].

Due to these remarkable properties and activation of multiple signaling pathways by platelet-secreted factors, PRP raised a lot of interest as a potentially beneficial therapy in various medical fields, such as dermatology and cosmetology, ophthalmology, neurology, sports medicine, stomatology, gynaecology and reproductive medicine. A similar remedy is PRF, which is even easier to prepare in either leukocyte-rich or leukocyte-poor varieties, and includes cytokines and growth factors that are released for up to several weeks, resulting in enhanced wound healing [60,61].

Our study presents a number of limitations, such as those related to the extent of literature search, as well as the lack of accurate reporting of quantitative assessment variables and details concerning parameters of study groups, particularly in earlier published clinical trials. There is also a high degree of variability concerning PRP preparation and administration protocols, selection of experimental groups and general design of the trials, objective assessment methods. Possibly standardization requirements and larger patient samples will facilitate comparisons between objective outcomes of future studies.

5. Conclusions

PRP represents a relatively new therapeutic approach widely used in different areas of dermatology and plastic surgery [19,21,22], although its underlying mechanisms of action are not completely understood. The present meta-analysis proves the valuable role of PRP therapy in AGA for patients of both sexes, but also points to the need for personalized therapeutic indications and approaches. Although the total number of PRP treatments and the amount of PRP injected per treatment do not appear to influence the outcome, an increased frequency of application (number of treatments per month) results in larger increases in hair density. Other important factors are the age of patients and implicitly duration since alopecia onset. For best results it is advisable to apply a complex combined therapy protocol as early as possible.

Supplementary Materials: The following are available online at https://www.mdpi.com/article/10.3390/jpm12030342/s1, Table S1: Inclusion and exclusion criteria for the clinical trials included in the meta-analysis, Table S2: Methods of PRP preparation, injection and of patient monitoring for the clinical trials included in the meta-analysis, Table S3: Influence of sex composition of study groups on hair density (initial and after PRP treatment).

Author Contributions: All authors have equally contributed to this paper. Conceptualization, S.R.G., A.A. and M.T.; methodology, S.R.G., A.A. and C.M.; validation, C.I.M., M.I.M., C.C. and M.N.; formal analysis, A.A., M.T. and C.M.; investigation, A.A., C.I.M. and M.I.M.; resources, C.M.; data curation, C.C. and C.M.; writing—original draft preparation, A.A. and M.T.; writing—review and editing, M.T., C.I.M., M.I.M., C.C. and M.N.; visualization, S.R.G., C.M. and C.C.; supervision, S.R.G., M.N. and M.T.; project administration, S.R.G. and M.N. All authors have read and agreed to the published version of the manuscript.

Funding: The article processing charges are funded by Carol Davila University of Medicine and Pharmacy within the project Publish not perish.

Institutional Review Board Statement: Not applicable.

Informed Consent Statement: Not applicable.

Data Availability Statement: Not applicable.

Conflicts of Interest: The authors declare no conflict of interest.

Abbreviations

AGA	androgenic alopecia
CASP7	caspase 7
CD	cluster of differentiation
CTGF	connective tissue growth factor
EGF	epidermal growth factor
ERK	extracellular signal-regulated kinases
FDA	United States Food and Drug Administration
FGF	fibroblast growth factor
KGF	keratinocyte growth factor
PDGF	platelet-derived growth factor
PPP	platelet-poor plasma
PRF	platelet-rich fibrin
PRISMA	Preferred Reporting Items for Systematic Reviews and Meta-Analyses
PRP	platelet-rich plasma
ROS	reactive oxygen species
TGF	transforming growth factor
TNF-α	tumor necrosis factor α
VEGF	vascular endothelial growth factor

References

1. Sadick, N.S.; Callender, V.D.; Kircik, L.H.; Kogan, S. New Insight into the Pathophysiology of Hair Loss Trigger a Paradigm Shift in the Treatment Approach. *J. Drugs Dermatol.* **2017**, *16*, s135–s140.
2. Gupta, A.K.; Mays, R.R.; Dotzert, M.S.; Versteeg, S.G.; Shear, N.H.; Piguet, V. Efficacy of non-surgical treatments for androgenetic alopecia: A systematic review and network meta-analysis. *J. Eur. Acad. Dermatol. Venereol.* **2018**, *32*, 2112–2125. [CrossRef] [PubMed]
3. Giordano, S.; Romeo, M.; Lankinen, P. Platelet-rich plasma for androgenetic alopecia: Does it work? Evidence from meta analysis. *J. Cosmet. Dermatol.* **2017**, *16*, 374–381. [CrossRef]
4. Gupta, A.K.; Carviel, J.L. Meta-analysis of efficacy of platelet-rich plasma therapy for androgenetic alopecia. *J. Dermatolog. Treat.* **2017**, *28*, 55–58. [CrossRef] [PubMed]
5. Dandekar, A.; Mendez, R.; Zhang, K. Cross talk between ER stress, oxidative stress, and inflammation in health and disease. *Methods Mol. Biol.* **2015**, *1292*, 205–214.
6. Georgescu, S.R.; Tampa, M.; Mitran, C.I.; Mitran, M.I.; Caruntu, C.; Caruntu, A.; Lupu, M.; Matei, C.; Constantin, C.; Neagu, M. Tumour Microenvironment in Skin Carcinogenesis. *Adv. Exp. Med. Biol.* **2020**, *1226*, 123–142. [PubMed]

7. Hussain, T.; Tan, B.; Yin, Y.; Blachier, F.; Tossou, M.C.; Rahu, N. Oxidative Stress and Inflammation: What Polyphenols Can Do for Us? *Oxid. Med. Cell. Longev.* **2016**, *2016*, 7432797. [CrossRef]
8. Spychalowicz, A.; Wilk, G.; Śliwa, T.; Ludew, D.; Guzik, T.J. Novel therapeutic approaches in limiting oxidative stress and inflammation. *Curr. Pharm. Biotechnol.* **2012**, *13*, 2456–2466. [CrossRef]
9. Acharya, P.; Mathur, M.C. Oxidative stress in alopecia areata: A systematic review and meta-analysis. *Int. J. Dermatol.* **2020**, *59*, 434–440. [CrossRef]
10. Dizen-Namdar, N.; Emel Kocak, F.; Kidir, M.; Sarici, G.; Tak, H.; Altuntas, I. Evaluation of Serum Paraoxonase, Arylesterase, Prolidase Activities and Oxidative Stress in Patients with Alopecia Areata. *Skin Pharmacol. Physiol.* **2019**, *32*, 59–64. [CrossRef]
11. Georgescu, S.R.; Ene, C.D.; Tampa, M.; Matei, C.; Benea, V.; Nicolae, I. Oxidative stress-related markers and alopecia areata through latex turbidimetric immunoassay method. *Mater. Plast.* **2016**, *53*, 522–526.
12. Mustafa, A.I.; Khashaba, R.A.; Fawzy, E.; Baghdady, S.M.A.; Rezk, S.M. Cross talk between oxidative stress and inflammation in alopecia areata. *J. Cosmet. Dermatol.* **2021**, *20*, 2305–2310. [CrossRef] [PubMed]
13. Cwynar, A.; Olszewska-Słonina, D.M.; Czajkowski, R. The impact of oxidative stress in androgenic alopecia in women. *Postepy Dermatol. Alergol.* **2020**, *37*, 119–120. [CrossRef] [PubMed]
14. Kaya Erdogan, H.; Bulur, I.; Kocaturk, E.; Yildiz, B.; Saracoglu, Z.N.; Alatas, O. The role of oxidative stress in early-onset androgenetic alopecia. *J. Cosmet. Dermatol.* **2017**, *16*, 527–530. [CrossRef] [PubMed]
15. Jadkauskaite, L.; Coulombe, P.A.; Schäfer, M.; Dinkova-Kostova, A.T.; Paus, R.; Haslam, I.S. Oxidative stress management in the hair follicle: Could targeting NRF2 counter age-related hair disorders and beyond? *Bioessays* **2017**, *39*, 1700029. [CrossRef]
16. Kapoor, R.; Shome, D.; Vadera, S.; Ram, M.S. QR 678 & QR678 Neo Vs PRP-A randomised, comparative, prospective study. *J. Cosmet. Dermatol.* **2020**, *19*, 2877–2885. [PubMed]
17. Gentile, P.; Garcovich, S. Systematic Review of Platelet-Rich Plasma Use in Androgenetic Alopecia Compared with Minoxidil®, Finasteride®, and Adult Stem Cell-Based Therapy. *Int. J. Mol. Sci.* **2020**, *21*, 2702. [CrossRef] [PubMed]
18. Gupta, A.K.; Versteeg, S.G.; Rapaport, J.; Hausauer, A.K.; Shear, N.H.; Piguet, V. The Efficacy of Platelet-Rich Plasma in the Field of Hair Restoration and Facial Aesthetics-A Systematic Review and Meta-analysis. *J. Cutan. Med. Surg.* **2019**, *23*, 185–203. [CrossRef]
19. Leo, M.S.; Kumar, A.S.; Kirit, R.; Konathan, R.; Sivamani, R.K. Systematic review of the use of platelet-rich plasma in aesthetic dermatology. *J. Cosmet. Dermatol.* **2015**, *14*, 315–323. [CrossRef]
20. Bucur, M.; Constantin, C.; Neagu, M.; Zurac, S.; Dinca, O.; Vladan, C.; Cioplea, M.; Popp, C.; Nichita, L.; Ionescu, E. Alveolar blood clots and platelet-rich fibrin induce in vitro fibroblast proliferation and migration. *Exp. Ther. Med.* **2019**, *17*, 982–989. [CrossRef]
21. Elghblawi, E. Platelet-rich plasma, the ultimate secret for youthful skin elixir and hair growth triggering. *J. Cosmet. Dermatol.* **2017**, *17*, 423–430. [CrossRef] [PubMed]
22. Zhang, M.; Park, G.; Zhou, B.; Luo, D. Applications and efficacy of platelet-rich plasma in dermatology: A clinical review. *J. Cosmet. Dermatol.* **2018**, *17*, 660–665. [CrossRef] [PubMed]
23. Fortunato, L.; Barone, S.; Bennardo, F.; Giudice, A. Management of Facial Pyoderma Gangrenosum Using Platelet-Rich Fibrin: A Technical Report. *J. Oral Maxillofac. Surg.* **2018**, *76*, 1460–1463. [CrossRef] [PubMed]
24. Maluf, G.; Caldas, R.J.; Silva Santos, P.S. Use of Leukocyte- and Platelet-Rich Fibrin in the Treatment of Medication-Related Osteonecrosis of the Jaws. *J. Oral Maxillofac. Surg.* **2018**, *76*, 88–96. [CrossRef]
25. Soydan, S.S.; Uckan, S. Management of bisphosphonate-related osteonecrosis of the jaw with a platelet-rich fibrin membrane: Technical report. *J. Oral Maxillofac. Surg.* **2014**, *72*, 322–326. [CrossRef]
26. Alves, R.; Grimalt, R. Randomized Placebo-Controlled, Double-Blind, Half-Head Study to Assess the Efficacy of Platelet-Rich Plasma on the Treatment of Androgenetic Alopecia. *Dermatol. Surg.* **2016**, *42*, 491–497. [CrossRef]
27. Varothai, S.; Bergfeld, W.F. Androgenetic alopecia: An evidence-based treatment update. *Am. J. Clin. Dermatol.* **2014**, *15*, 217–230. [CrossRef]
28. Motofei, I.G.; Rowland, D.L.; Baconi, D.L.; Tampa, M.; Sârbu, M.I.; Păunică, S.; Constantin, V.D.; Bălălău, C.; Păunică, I.; Georgescu, S.R. Androgenetic alopecia; drug safety and therapeutic strategies. *Expert Opin. Drug Saf.* **2018**, *17*, 407–412. [CrossRef]
29. Talavera-Adame, D.; Newman, D.; Newman, N. Conventional and novel stem cell based therapies for androgenic alopecia. *Stem Cells Cloning* **2017**, *10*, 11–19. [CrossRef]
30. Moher, D.; Liberati, A.; Tetzlaff, J.; Altman, D.G. Preferred reporting items for systematic reviews and meta-analyses: The PRISMA statement. *J. Clin. Epidemiol.* **2009**, *62*, 1006–1012. [CrossRef]
31. Page, M.J.; McKenzie, J.E.; Bossuyt, P.M.; Boutron, I.; Hoffmann, T.C.; Mulrow, C.D.; Shamseer, L.; Tetzlaff, J.M.; Akl, E.A.; Brennan, S.E.; et al. The PRISMA 2020 statement: An updated guideline for reporting systematic reviews. *J. Clin. Epidemiol.* **2021**, *134*, 178–189. [CrossRef] [PubMed]
32. The Cochrane Collaboration. *Review Manager (RevMan)*; Vesion 5.3; The Nordic Cochrane Centre: Copenhagen, Denmark, 2014.
33. Bayat, M.; Yazdanpanah, M.J.; Hamidi Alamdari, D.; Banihashemi, M.; Salehi, M. The effect of platelet-rich plasma injection in the treatment of androgenetic alopecia. *J. Cosmet. Dermatol.* **2019**, *18*, 1624–1628. [CrossRef] [PubMed]
34. Bruce, A.J.; Pincelli, T.P.; Heckman, M.G.; Desmond, C.M.; Arthurs, J.R.; Diehl, N.N.; Douglass, E.J.; Bruce, C.J.; Shapiro, S.A. A Randomized, Controlled Pilot Trial Comparing Platelet-Rich Plasma to Topical Minoxidil Foam for Treatment of Androgenic Alopecia in Women. *Dermatol. Surg.* **2020**, *46*, 826–832. [CrossRef] [PubMed]

35. Butt, G.; Hussain, I.; Ahmed, F.J.; Choudhery, M.S. Efficacy of platelet-rich plasma in androgenetic alopecia patients. *J. Cosmet. Dermatol.* **2018**, *18*, 996–1001. [CrossRef] [PubMed]
36. Butt, G.; Hussain, I.; Ahmad, F.J.; Choudhery, M.S. Stromal vascular fraction-enriched platelet-rich plasma therapy reverses the effects of androgenetic alopecia. *J. Cosmet. Dermatol.* **2019**, *19*, 1078–1085. [CrossRef]
37. Gentile, P.; Garcovich, S.; Bielli, A.; Scioli, M.G.; Orlandi, A.; Cervelli, V. The Effect of Platelet-Rich Plasma in Hair Regrowth: A Randomized Placebo-Controlled Trial. *Stem Cells Transl. Med.* **2015**, *4*, 1317–1323. [CrossRef]
38. Hausauer, A.K.; Jones, D.H. Evaluating the Efficacy of Different Platelet-Rich Plasma Regimens for Management of Androgenetic Alopecia: A Single-Center, Blinded, Randomized Clinical Trial. *Dermatol. Surg.* **2018**, *44*, 1191–1200. [CrossRef]
39. Mapar, M.A.; Shahriari, S.; Haghighizadeh, M.H. Efficacy of platelet-rich plasma in the treatment of androgenetic (male-patterned) alopecia: A pilot randomized controlled trial. *J. Cosmet. Laser Ther.* **2016**, *18*, 452–455. [CrossRef]
40. Pakhomova, E.E.; Smirnova, I.O. Comparative Evaluation of the Clinical Efficacy of PRP-Therapy, Minoxidil, and Their Combination with Immunohistochemical Study of the Dynamics of Cell Proliferation in the Treatment of Men with Androgenetic Alopecia. *Int. J. Mol. Sci.* **2020**, *21*, 6516. [CrossRef]
41. Puig, C.J.; Reese, R.; Peters, M. Double-Blind, Placebo-Controlled Pilot Study on the Use of Platelet-Rich Plasma in Women With Female Androgenetic Alopecia. *Dermatol. Surg.* **2016**, *42*, 1243–1247. [CrossRef]
42. Rodrigues, B.L.; Montalvão, S.A.L.; Cancela, R.B.B.; Silva, F.A.R.; Urban, A.; Huber, S.C.; Júnior, J.; Lana, J.; Annichinno-Bizzacchi, J.M. Treatment of male pattern alopecia with platelet-rich plasma: A double-blind controlled study with analysis of platelet number and growth factor levels. *J. Am. Acad. Dermatol.* **2018**, *80*, 694–700. [CrossRef]
43. Shapiro, J.; Ho, A.; Sukhdeo, K.; Yin, L.; Lo Sicco, K. Evaluation of platelet-rich plasma as a treatment for androgenetic alopecia: A randomized controlled trial. *J. Am. Acad. Dermatol.* **2020**, *83*, 1298–1303. [CrossRef]
44. Singh, S.K.; Kumar, V.; Rai, T. Comparison of efficacy of platelet-rich plasma therapy with or without topical 5% minoxidil in male-type baldness: A randomized, double-blind placebo control trial. *Indian J. Dermatol. Venereol. Leprol.* **2020**, *86*, 150–157. [CrossRef]
45. Tawfik, A.A.; Osman, M.A.R. The effect of autologous activated platelet-rich plasma injection on female pattern hair loss: A randomized placebo-controlled study. *J. Cosmet. Dermatol.* **2017**, *17*, 47–53. [CrossRef]
46. Motofei, I.G.; Rowland, D.L.; Georgescu, S.R.; Tampa, M.; Baconi, D.; Stefanescu, E.; Baleanu, B.C.; Balalau, C.; Constantin, V.; Paunica, S. Finasteride adverse effects in subjects with androgenic alopecia: A possible therapeutic approach according to the lateralization process of the brain. *J. Dermatolog. Treat.* **2016**, *27*, 495–497. [CrossRef]
47. Motofei, I.G.; Rowland, D.L.; Georgescu, S.R.; Tampa, M.; Paunica, S.; Constantin, V.D.; Balalau, C.; Manea, M.; Baleanu, B.C.; Sinescu, I. Post-Finasteride Adverse Effects in Male Androgenic Alopecia: A Case Report of Vitiligo. *Skin Pharmacol. Physiol.* **2017**, *30*, 42–45. [CrossRef]
48. Pereira, A.F.J.R.; Coelho, T.O.A. Post-finasteride syndrome. *An. Bras. Dermatol.* **2020**, *95*, 271–277. [CrossRef]
49. Vasserot, A.P.; Geyfman, M.; Poloso, N.J. Androgenetic alopecia: Combing the hair follicle signaling pathways for new therapeutic targets and more effective treatment options. *Expert Opin. Ther. Targets* **2019**, *23*, 755–771. [CrossRef]
50. Emer, J. Platelet-Rich Plasma (PRP): Current Applications in Dermatology. *Skin Ther. Lett.* **2019**, *24*, 1–6.
51. Gupta, A.K.; Cole, J.; Deutsch, D.P.; Everts, P.A.; Niedbalski, R.P.; Panchaprateep, R.; Rinaldi, F.; Rose, P.T.; Sinclair, R.; Vogel, J.E.; et al. Platelet-Rich Plasma as a Treatment for Androgenetic Alopecia. *Dermatol. Surg.* **2019**, *45*, 1262–1273. [CrossRef]
52. Kramer, M.E.; Keaney, T.C. Systematic review of platelet-rich plasma (PRP) preparation and composition for the treatment of androgenetic alopecia. *J. Cosmet. Dermatol.* **2018**, *17*, 666–671. [CrossRef] [PubMed]
53. Zhou, S.; Qi, F.; Gong, Y.; Zhang, C.; Zhao, S.; Yang, X.; He, Y. Platelet-Rich Plasma in Female Androgenic Alopecia: A Comprehensive Systematic Review and Meta-Analysis. *Front. Pharmacol.* **2021**, *12*, 642980. [CrossRef]
54. Litchman, G.; Nair, P.A.; Badri, T.; Kelly, S.E. *Microneedling*; StatPearls Publishing LLC: Treasure Island, FL, USA, 2020.
55. Ocampo-Garza, S.S.; Fabbrocini, G.; Ocampo-Candiani, J.; Cinelli, E.; Villani, A. Micro needling: A novel therapeutic approach for androgenetic alopecia, A Review of Literature. *Dermatol. Ther.* **2020**, *33*, e14267. [CrossRef] [PubMed]
56. Gupta, A.K.; Carviel, J. A Mechanistic Model of Platelet-Rich Plasma Treatment for Androgenetic Alopecia. *Dermatol. Surg.* **2016**, *42*, 1335–1339. [CrossRef] [PubMed]
57. Mahé, Y.F.; Michelet, J.F.; Billoni, N.; Jarrousse, F.; Buan, B.; Commo, S.; Saint-Léger, D.; Bernard, B.A. Androgenetic alopecia and microinflammation. *Int. J. Dermatol.* **2000**, *39*, 576–584. [CrossRef]
58. Han, J.H.; Kwon, O.S.; Chung, J.H.; Cho, K.H.; Eun, H.C.; Kim, K.H. Effect of minoxidil on proliferation and apoptosis in dermal papilla cells of human hair follicle. *J. Dermatol. Sci.* **2004**, *34*, 91–98. [CrossRef]
59. Tosti, A.; Piraccini, B.M. Finasteride and the hair cycle. *J. Am. Acad. Dermatol.* **2000**, *42*, 848–849. [CrossRef]
60. Cecerska-Heryć, E.; Goszka, M.; Serwin, N.; Roszak, M.; Grygorcewicz, B.; Heryć, R.; Dołęgowska, B. Applications of the regenerative capacity of platelets in modern medicine. *Cytokine Growth Factor Rev.* **2021**, *6101*, 00090–00093. [CrossRef]
61. Inbarajan, A.; Veeravalli, P.T.; Seenivasan, M.K.; Natarajan, S.; Sathiamurthy, A.; Ahmed, S.R.; Vaidyanathan, A.K. Platelet-Rich Plasma and Platelet-Rich Fibrin as a Regenerative Tool. *J. Pharm. Bioallied Sci.* **2021**, *13*, S1266–S1267.

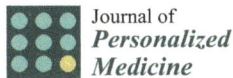

Review

Interrogating Epigenome toward Personalized Approach in Cutaneous Melanoma

Elena-Georgiana Dobre [1,*], Carolina Constantin [2,3], Marieta Costache [1] and Monica Neagu [1,2,3]

1. Faculty of Biology, University of Bucharest, Splaiul Independentei 91–95, 050095 Bucharest, Romania; marieta.costache@bio.unibuc.ro (M.C.); neagu.monica@gmail.com (M.N.)
2. Immunology Department, "Victor Babes" National Institute of Pathology, 050096 Bucharest, Romania; caroconstantin@gmail.com
3. Pathology Department, Colentina Clinical Hospital, 020125 Bucharest, Romania
* Correspondence: dobregeorgiana_95@yahoo.com

Abstract: Epigenetic alterations have emerged as essential contributors in the pathogenesis of various human diseases, including cutaneous melanoma (CM). Unlike genetic changes, epigenetic modifications are highly dynamic and reversible and thus easy to regulate. Here, we present a comprehensive review of the latest research findings on the role of genetic and epigenetic alterations in CM initiation and development. We believe that a better understanding of how aberrant DNA methylation and histone modifications, along with other molecular processes, affect the genesis and clinical behavior of CM can provide the clinical management of this disease a wide range of diagnostic and prognostic biomarkers, as well as potential therapeutic targets that can be used to prevent or abrogate drug resistance. We will also approach the modalities by which these epigenetic alterations can be used to customize the therapeutic algorithms in CM, the current status of epi-therapies, and the preliminary results of epigenetic and traditional combinatorial pharmacological approaches in this fatal disease.

Keywords: cutaneous melanoma; epigenetic regulation; inflammation; drug resistance; biomarkers; therapeutic targets; epigenetic therapy; immune response

Citation: Dobre, E.-G.; Constantin, C.; Costache, M.; Neagu, M. Interrogating Epigenome toward Personalized Approach in Cutaneous Melanoma. *J. Pers. Med.* **2021**, *11*, 901. https://doi.org/10.3390/jpm11090901

Academic Editor: Jun Fang

Received: 11 August 2021
Accepted: 6 September 2021
Published: 9 September 2021

Publisher's Note: MDPI stays neutral with regard to jurisdictional claims in published maps and institutional affiliations.

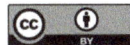

Copyright: © 2021 by the authors. Licensee MDPI, Basel, Switzerland. This article is an open access article distributed under the terms and conditions of the Creative Commons Attribution (CC BY) license (https://creativecommons.org/licenses/by/4.0/).

1. Introduction

Cutaneous melanoma (CM) is an aggressive neoplasm that evolves from the malignant transformation of neural crest stem cell-derived melanocytes [1]. The etiology of melanoma is multifactorial, and the most prominent factors include genetic predisposition, light skin color, multiple naevi, and excessive exposure to UV [2]. Although less prevalent than other skin malignancies, CM accounts for more than 70% of skin cancer-related deaths. Its incidence, however, is steadily increasing in fair-skinned populations worldwide [3]. Detected in the early stages, CM is generally curable, with a 5-year overall survival (OS) rate for the localized disease of 95%. In contrast, stage IV patients carry a grim prognosis, and the 5-year OS rate drops to 25%. CM mortality is usually related to delayed diagnosis or tumor refractoriness to conventional therapies, all of which contribute to metastatic disease [4]. The remarkable progress made in recent years in deciphering CM biology has resulted in the development of several targeted therapies and immune-checkpoint inhibitors (ICIs), such as anti-programmed death (PD-1) and anti-cytotoxic T lymphocyte antigen (CTLA-4), that have truly revolutionized metastatic CM treatment. For instance, therapies targeting critical nodes in the mitogen-activated protein kinase (MAPK) pathway have significantly improved patient OS [5,6]. Furthermore, immune therapies with ICIs led to more durable results and even pathological complete response (pCR) in several patients [7,8]. However, a significant proportion of CM patients fail to respond to these therapies due to the quick emergence of resistance, suggesting that it is critical to gain a deeper understanding of this disease's biology in order to improve its clinical management [9]. At present, CM diagnosis and prognosis rely on assessing clinicopathological variables that do not consider CM genomic and immune heterogeneity [10,11]. In CM, blood biomarkers are very few; S100 and melanoma inhibitory activity (MIA) are the only generally accepted biomarkers that can predict CM evolution and that can indicate therapy efficacy [12] Nevertheless, in tumor-free patients these biomarkers lack utility and additional biomarkers like those related to immune response can be used to monitor the disease dynamics [13]. Although still used in oncology as a general biomarker, serum lactate dehydrogenase (LDH) lacks specificity. An increase in serum LDH would indicate in late stages a high tumor burden, without providing any information on how to guide metastatic patient treatment [14]. Given the poor prognosis of advanced-stage CM, novel biomarkers are needed to assist in early diagnosis and prognosis and stratifying patients into different risk groups to optimize their therapeutic protocols [15].

The idealized model for CM development and progression is the Clark model. This model progressively describes the histopathological changes accompanying normal melanocytes' linear progression to metastatic melanoma via a benign naevus [16] (Figure 1). Nevi are growth-arrested, clonal neoplasms of melanocytes, triggered by certain specific mutations in the MAPK pathway, usually BRAF V600E mutations [17]. Subsequently, the benign nevus evolves into a dysplastic nevus, which progresses through the primary tumor's radial and vertical growth phases (RGP and VGP) and ultimately invades the dermis and regional lymph nodes, from which it metastasizes to distal sites [18]. However, current literature highlights that more than two-thirds of melanomas arise de novo in normal skin without requiring a nevus precursor [19,20]. Given that the annual risk of an individual nevus progressing into melanoma is estimated to be far less than one in 33,000 and the majority of CM patients lack atypical nevi, de novo genesis may be the main route of CM development [21,22]. Although nevus-associated melanomas correlate with favorable prognostic factors, the assessment of nevus as a biomarker in melanoma is still controversial due to certain unconventional models suggested for CM progression [21,23]. Finally, there is also an epigenetic progenitor model, which suggests that a polyclonal epigenetic disruption of tissue-specific (non-cancerous) stem/progenitor cells might act as a driving force of carcinogenesis. The subsequent accumulation of genetic and epigenetic alterations further enhances the tumorigenesis process [24,25] (Figure 1). Regardless of the controversy posed by CM progression, melanomagenesis is fueled by a pro-inflammatory environment. Multiple environmental agents can induce inflammation; however, UV radiation remains the most prominent aggressor, resulting in significant DNA damage and reactive oxygen species (ROS) generation [26]. Inflammation has acute and chronic stages that can shift the physiological balance towards skin regeneration or tumorigenesis, depending on their intensities [18,27]. If the inflammation is persistent and acquires chronic attributes, it may lead to a pre-cancerous lesion in the form of a dysplastic nevus. If detected by a fully functional immune system, this pre-cancerous lesion subsides to healing, and the melanocyte regains its physiological functions. However, if the entire process develops as a sustained chronic inflammation, it triggers a plethora of molecular and cellular networks shaping an immunosuppressive milieu that sustains skin tumorigenesis and further metastasis [18,28] (Figure 1).

Epigenetic alterations have emerged as essential contributors in the pathogenesis of various human diseases, including CM. Epigenetics is another layer of instructions apart from the genetic code that controls how genes are read and expressed, involving a change in the cell phenotype without changes in the genotype [29]. Epigenetic regulation is an umbrella term that encompasses several mechanisms such as DNA methylation, histone post-translational modifications (PTMs), nucleosome remodeling, histone variants, and RNA-mediated post-transcriptional regulation [30]. Influenced by lifestyle and environmental factors, epigenetic changes are highly dynamic and reversible and thus easy to regulate [31]. Given that these epigenetic alterations occur before the clinical diagnosis of CM, these molecular defects may serve as a foundation for developing novel diagnostic tools for early detection [32]. Furthermore, the discovery that distinct epigenetic signatures may associate with different disease subtypes highlights that these changes may also have prognostic applications in CM management [33,34]. Additionally, the study of epigenetic enzymes facilitates the design of novel treatment strategies that may help in delaying or reversing drug resistance, either as monotherapy or in combinations [35,36]. Of particular importance, observations that epigenetic regulators are often mutated in CM [37] and that mutant genes differ significantly between patients [38] suggest not only that the signaling pathways in these tumors are induced in a patient-dependent manner but also the need to implement personalized medicine in the clinical management of CM. Accordingly, once a certain abnormality is identified, it must be targeted with a specific treatment to reduce the side effects and maximize the therapeutic benefit of the patients [39]. Therefore, a better understanding of CM epigenetics will guide the precision medicine initiative in the field towards the identification of more specific diagnostic, prognostic, and predictive biomarkers, as well as more potent epigenetic inhibitors for the treatment of specific subtypes of CM.

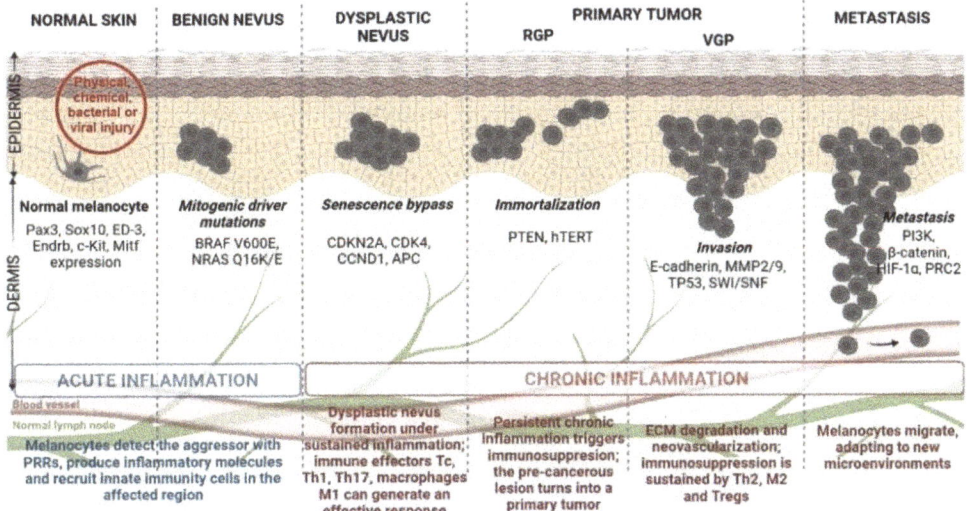

Figure 1. Schematic representation of CM development from healthy melanocyte to metastatic disease (the Clark model) under a pro-inflammatory milieu. Abbreviations: PRRs—pattern recognition receptors, Tc—cytotoxic T cells, Th1-T—helper type 1 cells, Tregs—regulatory T cells, Pax3—paired box gene 3, Sox10—SRY-box transcription factor 10, Endrb—endothelin receptor type B, c-Kit—human receptor tyrosine kinase c-kit, Mitf—microphthalmia-associated transcription factor, CDKN2A—cyclin dependent kinase inhibitor 2A, CDK4—cyclin dependent kinase 4, CCND1—cyclin D1, APC—adenomatous polyposis coli, PTEN—phosphatase and tensin homolog, hTERT—human telomerase reverse transcriptase, MMP2—matrix metalloproteinase 2, SWI/SNF—switch/sucrose non-fermentable chromatin remodeling complex, PI3K—phosphoinositide 3-kinase, HIF-1α—hypoxia-inducible factor-1α, PRC2—polycomb repressive complex 2.

We present herein both old and new evidence regarding the roles of DNA methylation and chromatin modifications in melanoma pathogenesis and discuss recent advances in investigating their translational potential as biomarkers and therapeutic targets.

2. Epigenetics: Another Layer of Information in Gene Expression Regulation

The epigenetics field focuses on the study of heritable alterations in gene expression with no underlying changes in the DNA sequence. Epigenetic regulation has been extensively reviewed in association with various human biological processes, such as embryogenesis, cell differentiation, X chromosome inactivation, and pathologies such as cancer [40,41]. The best-characterized epigenetic mechanisms are DNA methylation and histone modifications; however, the epigenetic scenario is much more complicated with new players and new mechanisms including non-coding RNA (ncRNA)-mediated regulation, histone variants, and ATP-dependent chromatin remodeling [42–44]. All these discrete but reversible modifications may orchestrate extensive changes in chromatin structure and conformation, interfering with the transcriptional machinery's ability to access its target genes and promoters [45,46].

The epigenetic machinery carefully modifies the homeostatic balance between euchromatin and heterochromatin, which is essential to genomic stability [31]. The epigenetic players involved are divided into three classes: writers (generally enzymes that induce chemical modifications in histones and DNA), erasers (entities that erase these chemical signatures), and readers (enzymes that recognize and interpret various chemical modifications) [47]. Within the review, we will focus mainly on DNA methylation and histone modifications. These two types of epigenetic changes appear to influence each other in the deposition during mammalian development and carcinogenesis; histone methylation appears to direct DNA methylation patterns, while DNA methylation may serve as a model for establishing certain histone changes [32]. Moreover, in CM, DNA methylation is gaining increased importance in PD-related immune therapy [48], while histone alterations are associated with BRAF-targeted therapy [49].

In mammals, DNA methylation is an epigenetic signature that occurs at the 5′ position of the cytosine preceding a guanine nucleotide (denoted CpG, where p implies the phosphodiester bond between the two nucleosides) [50]. CpG-enriched regions, called 'CpG islands', are found in about 40% of mammalian gene promoters, making these particular regions prone to methylation [51]. Interestingly, methylation's biological effects can vary widely depending on genomic location; thus, methylation in the promoter regions of genes is usually associated with transcriptional repression, while methylation in the gene body promotes transcription [31]. The enzymes that perform this modification are DNA methyltransferases (DNMTs), using S-adenosylmethionine (SAM) as a donor of methyl groups [52]. The human genome encodes at least four DNMTs: DNMT1, DNMT3A, DNMT3B, and DNMT3L [53]. DNMT1 is responsible for maintaining DNA methylation, while DNMT3A and DNMT3B catalyze the de novo synthesis of 5-mC [52,54]. Conversely, 5-mC methylation marks can be deleted by ten-eleven translocation (TET) proteins [55]. DNMTs may play critical roles in embryonic development and the intergenerational propagation of specific methylation patterns [56]; thus, any disorder in the functionality of these enzymes can have important physiological consequences [53]. DNMTs were recently shown to be involved in immune therapy resistance in CM, as further detailed in [57].

Histones, especially their N-terminal tails (containing an average of 15–30 residues), can undergo a plethora of PTMs, such as acetylation, methylation, phosphorylation, and more rarely, ubiquitination, sumoylation, and glycosylation [58]. The acetylation (ac) of histone lysines (K), is associated with the transition to an "open" conformation; this weakens DNA–histone interactions, increases DNA accessibility, and facilitates transcription. Acetylated lysine residues may also serve as binding platforms for transcription factors and other histone-modifying enzymes, such as bromodomains [59]. Another type of histone modification is methylation (me) of lysine and arginine (R) residues. Histone methylation can be present in several forms, so that the lysine residues may be mono-, di- or trimethylated, while the arginine residues may be mono- or di-methylated. Methylated histone residues are recognized by several protein domains such as plant homeodomain zinc fingers, Tudor domains, or WD40 repeats. While histone acetylation is usually associated with transcriptional activation, histone methylation has various functions, depending on the type of histone, the type of amino acid, the degree of modification, and another histone's PTMs in the vicinity [60,61]. For example, in the promoter region, di- or tri-methylation of histone H3 at lysine 4 (H3K4me2, H3K4me3) is associated with transcriptional activation; in contrast, H3K27me3 and H3K9me3 are transcriptionally repressive marks [62]. Combinations of H3K4me1, H3K27me3, and H3K27ac marks can be used to distinguish active enhancers (H3K4me1 and H3K27ac positive) from inactive (H3K4me1 positive and H3K27ac negative) or poised (H3K4me1 and H3K27me3 positive) gene enhancers [63]. Interestingly, promoters of lineage-controlling developmental genes display a particular epigenetic signature that combines the activating H3K4me3 and the repressive H3K27me3 mark; these bivalent domains, which have also been reported in cancers, allow for rapid activation of developmental genes during embryogenesis, while maintaining repression in the absence of differentiation signals [64,65]. However, the balance between histone methylation and acetylation is tightly controlled by histone methyltransferases (HMTs)/demethylases (HDMs) and histone acetyltransferases (HATs)/histone deacetylases (HDACs), respectively [66]. Alterations in histone "writers" or "erasers" have been associated with many pathologies, including cancer [31,45,67]. Histone modifications can be associated in CM with therapy resistance [68] and/or with epithelial–mesenchymal transition (EMT) and metastasis [69].

3. CM Epigenetics

Recent advancements in next-generation sequencing (NGS) technologies and their coupling with chromatin-immunoprecipitation (CHIP), altogether RNA interference (RNAi) screening methods, and matrix-assisted laser desorption/ionization time-of-flight (MALDI-TOF) proteomic tools have allowed the dissection of the epigenome for various cancers [70]. In particular, for CM, epigenomic interrogation revealed aberrant DNA methylation in gene promoters [71], histone PTMs [72], alteration of epigenetic regulators [73], and dysregulated ncRNAs [74] (Figure 2). It seems that in CM these epigenetic alterations may allow melanocytes to overcome senescence and metastasize at a distance [75,76], support the immune escape of CM [77], but also the transcriptomic reprogramming of cancer cells to overcome the cancer therapy-induced apoptosis [78].

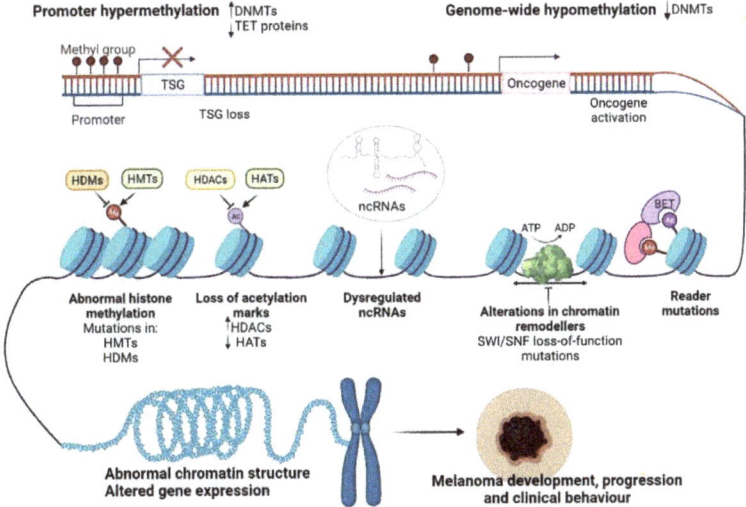

Figure 2. Epigenetic changes regulating CM progression and clinical behavior. Abbreviations: Me—methylation, Ac—acetylation, DNMTs—DNA methyltransferases, TET—ten-eleven-translocation enzyme, TSG—tumor suppressor gene, HDMs—histone demethylases, HMTs—histone methyltransferases, HDACs—histone deacetylases, HATs—histone acetyltransferases, SWI/SNF—switch/sucrose non-fermentable chromatin remodeling complex, BET—bromodomain and extra-terminal domain protein, ncRNAs—non-coding RNAs, ATP—adenosine triphosphate, ADP—adenosine diphosphate. Figure created with https://biorender.com/.

Inflammation and epigenetic alterations play pivotal roles in CM initiation and development. However, in recent years, considerable research efforts have been devoted to identifying a potential link between these processes in the context of cancer. Current literature confirms that these two phenomena are interconnected and mutually regulate each other [79,80]. Epigenetics can modulate tumor antigen presentation and immune cell functions, therefore impacting tumor development and clinical behavior [81]. Conversely, inflammation can induce epigenetic alterations in resident skin cells, promoting immune evasion and tumorigenesis [80]. We will focus herein mainly on inflammation-induced epigenetic changes in CM, as it is a less studied topic in the field. In the first instance, inflammation can disrupt epigenetic programs by altering the metabolic state of a cell [82]. Their activation determines alteration of immune cells' metabolism and activated immune cells further disrupt the metabolic processes in neighboring tissues. Since the activity of many epigenetic enzymes depends on cellular metabolism intermediates, a dysfunctional metabolism will significantly impact the molecular processes within the cell [82]. For example, DNMTs and HMTs use SAM as a cofactor, while HDMs and TET proteins require α-ketoglutarate produced in the tricarboxylic acid cycle for their activity [83]. Moreover, it has been reported that increased production of cytokines, chemokines, and ROS, including hydrogen peroxides, can orchestrate dramatic epigenetic changes in resident epithelial cells. For instance, DNA damage triggered by ROS exposure can interfere with the ability of certain epigenetic regulators to bind to DNA, leading to abnormal DNA methylation patterns and altered gene expression [84]. Additionally, long-term production and accumulation of cytokines and ROS/reactive nitrogen species (RNS) have been correlated with the activation of STAT3 and NF-κB oncogenic pathways in epithelial cells [27,85]. In parallel, antigen-presenting cells (APCs) and cytokines can activate T cells, involving transcription factors that participate in their transcriptomic reprogramming, which includes epigenetic changes, among others [80]. Epigenetic alterations are usually pro-tumorigenic, facilitating the suppression of tumor suppressor genes and the activation of oncogenes. These reversible changes may also help tumors escape the immune response by reducing the expression of genes involved in the antigen processing and presentation or viral defense pathways. In line with these observations, myeloid-derived suppressor cells (MDSCs) may differentiate into tumor-associated macrophages (TAMs) or interfere with T cell activity, promoting tumorigenesis as transcription factors induce alternative transcriptional programs resulting in epigenetic alterations [80]. Here, we will describe the current status of knowledge regarding the roles of DNA methylation and chromatin modifications in CM as a problematic inflammatory malignancy.

4. Epigenetic Alterations Driving CM initiation and Progression

4.1. DNA Methylation in CM Development

Disruption of DNA methylation is a common event in cancer. Both focal hypermethylation at CpG islands and global hypomethylation are constant hallmarks of the cancer genome and often coexist in tumor cells, impacting tumor biology and behavior. As with other cancers, CM initiation and progression have been associated with loss of tumor suppressors and oncogene activation (Figure 2) [86].

Inactivation of tumor suppressor genes (TSGs) due to specific DNA methylation in the promoter regions was the first epigenetic alteration studied in CM more than 10 years ago [87] (Figure 1). So far, dozens of genes are known to be regulated by this mechanism. These genes appear to be involved in various signaling pathways, usually disrupted in CM, such as the phosphatidylinositol 3-kinase/protein kinase B (PI3K/Akt) and MAPK pathways, cell cycle, DNA repair, retinoblastoma (RB) and Wnt signaling [86]. Furthermore, it was also observed that three TSGs are frequently inactivated by methylation: RASSF1A (55%), RAR-β2 (70%), and MGMT (34%) can also be identified in the circulating tumor DNA of CM patients, which makes them useful diagnostic and prognostic biomarkers in the clinical setting [88,89]. In several cancers, but also in a significant proportion of melanomas, a gradual increase in DNA hypermethylation was observed along with tumor aggressiveness; this phenomenon, called CpG methylator phenotype (CIMP), was reported for the first time in colorectal cancers, a finding that highlighted a tight correlation between altered DNA methylation patterns and the clinical outcome of the affected patients.

Tanemura at al. demonstrated that during tumor progression, several tumor-related genes and loci, including WIF1, SOCS1, RASSF1A, TFPI2, MINT17, and MINT31, gain methylation with advancing stages. These genes have been suggested to constitute CM's CIMP [90]; however, recent research highlights that CIMP is usually associated with an NRAS-mutant phenotype, which is more aggressive than a non-NRAS-mutant tumor [91]. Therefore, future approaches should correlate CIMP with CM patients' clinical outcomes and mutational profiles. This information would be essential for developing novel tools for prognosis and response to therapy in the clinical cohorts of melanoma patients.

Epigenetic silencing of tumor suppressor genes has been one of the best-studied phenomena in CM; however, although less studied, DNA hypomethylation is equally important in the initiation and development of CM. It was shown that in many cancers, hypomethylation contributes to tumor progression by inducing genome instability via the demethylation of transposons and pericentromeric repeats or the activation of certain oncogenes [92]. Figure 2 depicts hypomethylation mechanisms as a hallmark of melanomagenesis. LINE-1 elements are one of the most abundant classes of mobile DNAs within the human genome [93]. LINE-1 hypomethylation, detected in both tissues and plasma circulating DNA of melanoma patients seems to be a hallmark of the metastatic capacity of primary melanomas [94,95]. Other reports highlighted that LINE-1 hypomethylation may predict the OS in stage III CM patients [96,97]. In parallel, DNA hypomethylation has been described as one of the main mechanisms regulating the expression of cancer-testis-antigens (CTAs) in human melanomas [98]. CTAs are a specific group of tumor-associated antigens (TAAs) whose expression in normal tissues is generally restricted to the gametogenic tissues of the testis and fetal ovaries [99]; nonetheless, CTAs were found to be re-expressed via hypomethylation in CM, regulating vital cellular processes such as tumor cell division, differentiation, invasion and drug resistance [98,100–102].

Several studies have revealed that DNA methylome analysis may help discriminate between normal melanocytes, nevi, and melanomas. For instance, Fujiwara et al. identified several novel genes that were hypermethylated in melanomas compared to melanocytes, such as KRTCAP3, AGAP2, ZNF490, and TTC22, in addition to those previously documented, such as COL1A2, GPX3, and NPM2 [103]. Among those genes, they found that NPM2 showed distinct immunohistochemical (IHC) staining in normal melanocytes, whereas its expression was lost in CM samples [103]. Moreover, Gao et al. reported a diagnostic algorithm based on the methylation patterns of CLDN11, CDH11, and PPP1R3C genes that can differentiate between dysplastic nevi and primary melanomas with a specificity of 89% and a sensitivity of 67% [104]. Other reports highlighted that several methylation subgroups might be associated with different clinical characteristics of the disease, potentiating that the evaluation of DNA methylomes may have prognostic applications in CM. A study led by Lauss et al. revealed three methylation clusters: MS1, MS2, and MS3, which differ significantly in terms of promoter methylation, proliferation, and presence in immune cells [33]. The MS1 group has the highest methylation level, especially at CpG islands and poised promoters, enriched in polycomb repressive complex (PRC2) target genes. The MS1 subtype also showed an increased frequency of homologous deletions of CDKN2A and IDH1R132 hotspot mutations. The MS3 group had the lowest methylation levels, similar to peripheral blood leukocytes, and MS2 was intermediate. No correlations were identified between methylation clusters and clinicopathological variables or actionable mutations such as BRAF or NRAS. However, the tumors bearing MS1-signature were associated with the lower patient OS (20 months for MS1 vs. 60 months for MS3). Interestingly, genetic analysis revealed methylation clusters are associated with different biological and clinical behaviors. The MS1 subtype termed "proliferative" was associated with the upregulation of TP53, MDM2, CDK4, CDK6, CCND1, CCNE1, and E2F3, as well as epigenetic modifiers TET1, JARID1B, SWI/SNF chromatin remodelers, and DNMT3A; in contrast, the MS3 subtype harbored an "immune high" signature, possibly explaining the better survival of patients appending to the MS3 cluster [33]. Similarly, Yamamoto et al. stratified 51 CM into two risk groups based on the promoter region's methylation status.

The high-methylated subgroup was positively associated with a thicker tumor progression and hence a worse clinical prognosis. Among the 27 genes proposed to distinguish between the two subtypes, TFPI2 was the most frequently hypermethylated gene in the aggressive subtype [34]. In addition, altered methylation patterns of the homeobox D cluster were linked with melanoma metastasizing to the brain [105].

Further complicating this scenario, genome-wide mapping of CM revealed that 5 hmC levels are progressively lost during tumor progression from benign nevus to malignant melanoma, via IDH2 and TET family downregulation [106]. Elevated levels of 5 hmC were subsequently validated by IHC staining as predictors of metastasis-free survival and overall survival in CM patients [107]. Taken together, all this information supports the further development of 5-hmC IHC expression as a prognostic biomarker that can add some precision to the American Joint Committee on Cancer (AJCC) staging system [108].

4.2. Histone-Modifying Enzymes and PTMs in CM Development

In addition to the undeniable role of DNA methylation in melanomagenesis, histone PTMs mediated by several writers, readers and erasers may also alter some transcriptional processes closely associated with CM initiation and progression [109].

The involvement of histone modifications in CM development has been suggested since benign nevi, which usually carry the BRAF V600E oncogenic mutation, rarely become melanoma, as this conversion requires additional events. Yet, valuable insights on the importance of histone-modifying enzymes and PTMs in melanomagenesis were obtained using zebrafish melanoma models [110]. Patton et al. developed the first experimental model of BRAF V600E driven melanoma using a zebrafish model expressing BRAF V600E under the control of the mitfa promoter in a p53 loss-of-function background [111]. Only a fraction of zebrafish developed melanocytic tumors, highlighting the existence of additional molecular events operating in concert with genetic alterations in melanoma. To examine these processes in more detail, the researchers developed a triple transgenic zebrafish model (p53/BRAF/crestin: EGFP), in which the crestin/EGFP gene marks neural crest stem and progenitor cells, from which melanocytes originate [111]. Melanocytic tumors reported in zebrafish models re-expressed crestin-EGFP gene, suggesting that these cancer cells are maintaining their neural crest identity. Notably, they identified enrichment of H3K27ac marks in super-enhancers at the sox10 locus, a major regulator of neural crest formation and melanomagenesis, suggesting that epigenetic regulation of SOX10 is an important step in melanoma initiation [111]. Later on, Scahill at al. revealed that loss of kdm2aa, an orthologue of KDM2A, triggered the spontaneous formation of melanomas at a high frequency in zebrafish [112]. These tumors were generated independently of BRAF V600E and other melanoma-related mutations in oncogenes and tumor suppressors. Finally, gene expression analysis revealed altered levels of genes involved in DNA replication, translation, and chromatin regulation after kdm2aa silencing, confirming on an alternative pathway that histone methylation may have vital roles in melanomagenesis [112].

4.2.1. Histone Modifications "Writers"

H3K4 Methyltransferases (KMT2D)

One of the chromatin's writer enzymes that has been identified to function aberrantly in melanomas is the KMT2D, also known as MLL2. KMT2D is associated with gene promoter and enhancer regions and catalyzes H3K4 monomethylation [113–115]. Several recent in vitro genetic screen studies have revealed important details regarding the roles of KMT2D in CM tumorigenesis [38,73]. By performing the first in vivo genetic screen with shRNA libraries targeting fundamental epigenetic players in CM, Bossi et al. observed multiple genes involved in melanomagenesis [38]. Among them, KMT2D orchestrates a migratory transcriptional program in NRAS melanomas. The authors also reported some interpatient heterogeneity in their study [38]. Interestingly, KMT2D silencing resulted in the inactivation of a subset of KMT2D-bound enhancers (reduced H3K4me1 and H3K27ac) and downregulation of MFGE8 and RPL39L cell motility genes. Notably, the closest genes to these enhancers were the KMT2D target genes, suggesting that KMT2D can deregulate enhancer activity to promote tumorigenesis [38]. Therefore, a better understanding of the roles of KMT2D in CM may help expand the number of biomarkers and druggable genes in the clinical management of CM patients.

After the first published results in 2016, KMT2D was reported as frequently mutated in a variety of solid and hematologic tumors, including melanomas (15%) [73]. Recently, Maitituoheti at al. identified KMT2D serving tumor suppressor roles in CM. In addition to KMT2D, the authors identified seven more epigenetic regulators in CM cell lines (KDM1A, APOBEC2, HDAC6, KMT2F, SETD4, KAT4, and KDM5B) whose loss accelerates CM tumor progression. Among them, KMT2D, KDM5B, KMT2F and KDM1A were mainly associated with H3K4 methylation. However, the most potent phenotypes were linked with mutations in KMT2D. To investigate CM genesis in more detail, the authors developed a genetically engineered mouse model (GEMM) based on conditional and melanocyte-specific ablation of KMT2D [73]. It has been further observed that H3K4me1-marked enhancer reprogramming by KMT2D loss is associated with a drastic alteration of the central metabolic pathways in the tumor cells. Furthermore, the authors observed a preferential dependence of glycolysis in deficient KMT2D tumors compared to WT cells, most likely to provide cancerous tumors' energy and biomass needs. Interestingly, pharmacological inhibition of glycolysis and the IGF signaling pathway reduced the proliferation of KMT2D-deficient tumor cells in both murine models and human melanoma cell lines [73]. Thus, this study highlights exciting aspects of the biology of mutant KMT2D tumors and identifies new potential therapeutic vulnerabilities concerning them.

The Roles of H3K4 Methylation Marks

H3K4me1, H3K4me2 and H3K4me3 are generally associated with active gene transcription [116]. Although partially overlapping with H3K4me3 at the 5'-end level of transcribing genes, H3K4me2 decorates genomic regions independently of H3K4me3 [117]. H3Kme2's role as a biomarker in the diagnosis and prognosis of CM patients has been suggested by several studies. For example, Uzdensky at al. found elevated levels of H3K4me2 in tumor samples compared to paired normal skin [118]. Later on, Kampilafkos at al. observed that H3K4me2 and H3K27me3 levels were lower in metastatic compared to primary melanomas and that combined IHC analysis of H3K4me2, H3K27me3, and EZH2 may help identify cancer cells with stem cell-like behaviors, particularly at the invasion front of CM [72]. This study highlighted that the combination of several genetic alterations may be more relevant for characterizing and predicting complex events such as metastasis and that all these epigenetic changes can be integrated as a code that can provide valuable information about the biology of melanocytic tumors.

H3K4me3 is a chromatin landmark of promoters of transcriptionally active genes or genes poised for activation in mammalian cells [116]. In particular, for CM, Cheng at al. observed that human metastatic tissues are highly heterogeneous in terms of H3K4me3 levels [115]. Further analysis showed that metastatic lesions that displayed low levels of H3K4me3 were associated with repressed genes in embryonic stem cells (ESCs) and PRC2-target genes. In contrast, elevated H3K4me3 levels correlated with interferon and inflammatory response genes [115]. However, Terranova at al. found that metastatic melanomas harbor exceptionally wide H3K4me3 domains [119]. These domains can span tens of thousands of kilobases, and appear to be involved in the regulation of several EMT transcription factors (POU3F2, SOX9, and PDGFRA) as well as melanocyte-specific master regulators (MITF, ZEB2, and TFAP2A) [120]. Terranova et al. finally highlighted that particular events such as BRAF or NRAS mutations may employ specific chromatin states (bivalent states and broad H3K4me3 domains) to orchestrate transcriptional changes unique to a genotype, suggesting that epigenetic mechanisms play important roles in regulating CM behaviors [119].

H3K27 Methyltransferases (EZH2)

Histone lysine methyltransferase EZH2, responsible for H3K27 trimethylation, was also found to be dysregulated during the development of human melanomas. EZH2 is the catalytic subunit of the PRC2 complex and appears overexpressed in various tumors, including melanoma [121]. PRC2 trimethylates H3K27, orchestrating the repression of transcriptional programs [121]. Particularly for melanoma, PRC2 levels have been reported to increase gradually over the progression from benign nevi to malignant melanomas, suggesting that this protein plays a key role in CM initiation and progression [72]. Moreover, EZH2 and H3K27me3 are overexpressed in highly invasive melanoma cells and metastatic melanomas, leading to TSGs inactivation [72,76,121,122]. Finally, other studies have revealed that increased EZH2 levels are associated with poor prognosis in CM patients [123].

Regarding the roles played by EZH2 in the pathogenesis of CM, several mechanisms by which it supports tumor growth and metastasis have been proposed. Some authors have shown that EZH2 expression is associated with the suppression of senescence in human melanoma cells. For example, Fan at al. have shown that EZH2 can support unlimited melanocyte proliferation by repressing CDKN1A, which is not mediated by H3K27me3 deposition [124]. Conversely, EZH2 silencing inhibits cell proliferation, restoring senescent phenotype and p21/CDKN1A expression in a p53-independent manner. It was further observed that depletion of EZH2 removes HDAC1 from the transcriptional start site of CDKN1A, resulting in increased H3 acetylation and transcriptional activation. These observations confirm the existence of a synergistic relationship between EZH2, as part of PRC2 and HDAC, in mediating the suppression of certain senescence-related genes in melanoma cells [124]. In parallel, De Donatis at al. showed that EZH2 oncogenic activation is mediated by the non-canonical NF-kB signaling pathway; interestingly, NF-kB2 silencing was associated with reconversion to the senescent phenotype, suggesting the pivotal roles of the NF-kB2/EZH2 axis in CM initiation and development [125]. Other studies have shown that induction of EZH2 in benign BrafV600E- or NrasQ61K-expressing melanocytes facilitates tumor metastasis and invasiveness by silencing genes relevant for cell surface organelle primary cilium integrity and by activating Wnt/β-catenin oncogenic signaling [77]. Finally, it is also worth mentioning that EZH2 gain-of-function mutations usually co-occur with BRAF V600E mutations in CM, promote aggressive cell morphologies and enhance melanoma tumor growth in vitro [126].

H3K9 Methyltransferases

Another histone-modifying enzyme involved in CM pathogenesis is bifurcated domain SUV39/SET 1 (SETDB1), which belongs to the SUV39 family of histone lysine methyltransferases [127]. This enzyme is involved in the trimethylation of H3K9, which is a specific signature of transcriptionally repressive chromatin [128].

In human melanoma samples, SETB1 often appears amplified in association with another histone methyltransferase, EHMT1 [129]. Subsequently, a positive association between SETB1 expression and several prognostic factors such as increased mitotic index, advanced Clark levels, and epidermal involvement in tissue biopsies of CM patients was also described [130]. A recent study, led by Orouji at al., revealed that the expression and amplification rate of SETDB1 may serve as an individual prognostic biomarker in CM, with increased levels of SETB1 protein being associated with metastasis and lower patient survival rates [131]. Compared to normal melanocytes, melanoma cells showed 8–13.9 times higher levels of SETDB1. Interestingly, they found that all those SETDB1 highly amplified human cell lines were BRAF V600E mutants [131]. Functional studies have shown that SETDB1 exerts its oncogenic effects in CM by modulating the expression of thrombospondin 1, a molecule known for its involvement in cell migration and invasiveness [131]. Surprisingly, it was found that SETDB1 regulates not only H3K9 methylation patterns but also H3K4me1 deposition, emphasizing that SETDB1's involvement in tumorigenesis is much broader than previously thought. Furthermore, treatment with an H3K9me-specific histone methyltransferase inhibitor is highly effective in this context, leading to a considerable decrease in tumor cell viability. Interestingly, melanoma cells harboring low levels of SETDB1 were not affected by treatment with epigenetic inhibitors, underscoring SETDB1's role as a valuable therapeutic target in CM [131].

4.2.2. Histone Modifications "Readers"

Protein readers can recognize specific chromatin changes or combinations of PTMs and histone variants to further direct the transcriptional outcome [47]. Some of the best-studied families of chromatin readers are the bromodomain and extra-terminal domain (BET) family of adapter proteins (BRD2, BRD3, BRD4, and BRDT). BET proteins have an increased affinity for acetylated histone residues, enabling transcriptional activation by interaction with the transcriptional machinery [132]. Notably, the SWI/SNF complex, which uses energy from ATP hydrolysis to reshape the structure of chromatin, is also dependent on the presence of bromodomain-containing domains to be fully functional [133]. BET protein involvement in melanomagenesis was demonstrated by Segura at al. when it was shown that BRD2 and BRD4 are overexpressed in human melanoma cell lines and tissues, controlling the expression of certain genes involved in cell cycle progressions and survival [134]. Gene expression and IHC analysis of human tissue biopsies have confirmed higher levels of BRD2 and BRD4 in primary and metastatic tumors relative to melanocytes and nevi, suggesting that these BET proteins are involved in melanoma tumorigenesis [134]. Treatment with BET inhibitors (BETi) significantly reduced tumor growth and metastasis in both in vitro and in vivo models, and those effects were recapitulated by individual silencing of BRD4. Notably, the pharmacological capabilities of BETi have not been influenced by the mutational status of BRAF or NRAS, offering new promises for the treatment of patients that do not harbor actionable mutations [134]. Collectively, all these observations potentiate the pivotal role of the BRD4 protein in CM tumorigenesis, propelling it as a potential prognosis biomarker and therapeutic target in CM.

4.2.3. Histone Modifications "Erasers"

Histone Deacetylases (HDACs)

One of the most important classes of chromatin erasers associated with CM pathogenesis is HDACs, which catalyze the deletion of acetyl groups from histone tails [135]. At least 18 mammalian HDACs were identified and subdivided into four main classes, depending on their location and functional characteristics. Given the significant differences reported between the acetylation patterns of benign nevi and the malignant tissues of patients diagnosed with CM, it was thought that aberrant histone deacetylation could play important roles in the pathobiology of CM [136]. Subsequent studies with patient-derived cell cultures have indeed shown that there is a loss of acetylation marks (H3K27Ac, H2BK5Ac, and H4K5Ac) and H3K4me2/3 during the transition from premalignant to the malignant phenotype, resulting in alterations of some essential signaling pathways in CM formation, including PI3K, interferon (IFN) -γ, and TRAIL- and platelet-derived growth factor (PDGF) signaling [136].

Many other studies have shown that various HDACs are involved in skin tumorigenesis and can be exploited as biomarkers or therapeutic targets in melanomas. For instance, Wilmott et al. identified that increased expression of nuclear HDAC3 and cytoplasmic HDAC8 may serve as indicators of better prognosis in stage IV melanoma patients [35]. They also revealed an increase in HDAC8 levels in BRAF-mutant tumors [35]. Additionally, HDAC6 expression has recently been correlated with advanced stages and with an unfavorable prognosis [137]. In line with these observations, certain in vitro studies have shown that HDAC5 and HDAC6 are overexpressed in melanoma cell lines versus normal skin cells, being required for melanoma proliferation and metastasis through different signaling pathways [138]. Interestingly, HDAC6 inhibition inhibited tumor cell proliferation, and when knocked down cells were inoculated in animal models a decreased PD-L1 production and an augmented T-cell-mediated immune response was obtained [138].

Another epigenetic player investigated for its involvement in CM initiation is SIRT1 (class III HDAC proteins), which was found overexpressed in human melanoma cells and tissues in comparison to normal skin and melanocytes [139]. Further studies suggested that SIRT1 is upregulated in metastatic tumors compared to primary tumors, most likely due to its ability to support EMT programs via autophagic degradation of E-cadherin [140]. SIRT1, SIRT3 and SIRT6 were also proposed to support tumor growth in CM [141,142]. Interestingly, a recent study showed that dual inhibition of SIRT1 and SIRT3 mediated by 4′-bromo-resveratrol inhibits melanoma cell proliferation and growth [143]. Thus, all this information suggests that pro-tumorigenic sirtuins have not only the value of prognosis biomarkers but also of potential therapeutic targets in CM and that inhibition of multiple sirtuins may be a promising strategy for improving clinical management of CM.

Histone Demethylases (HDMs)

The scientific progress made in recent years in deciphering the cancer epigenome has revealed the critical roles of histone H3 lysine 4 (H3K4) JARID1B/KDM5B demethylase in the tumorigenesis of various human tumors, including melanoma [144]. One of the pioneering studies in the field revealed that H3K4 demethylase JARID1B is overexpressed in melanocyte nevi and almost absent in melanoma samples [145]. However, subsequent studies have revealed increased heterogeneity of KDM5B in CM, and its expression levels have been documented to define distinct cellular states, even with antithetical effects on cellular tumor fate depending on the biological and clinical context [146]. KDM5B was found to mark a slow-cycling subpopulation of tumor cells which is essential for continuous tumor growth and resistance to therapy [147]. This population displays similar behaviors to that of cancer stem cells and give rise to a heterogeneous population of melanoma cells, being a major contributor to the increased heterogeneity observed in CM tumors [129]. Therefore, the assessment of KDM5B expression and H3K4 deposition patterns can provide valuable information about the clinical behavior of these tumors and may lead to more personalized therapies for CM patients.

H3K9me3 is an epigenetic mark of heterochromatin, which is often present on distal regions of genes [129]. H3K9 methyl groups may be erased by members of the lysine-specific histone demethylase (LSD) family. LSD1, often referred to as KDM1A, has the ability to demethylate histone 3 on lysine residues at position 4 (H3K4- gene promoter) and 9 (H3K9- distal) [129]. Interestingly, Yu et al. reported that oncogene-induced senescence of melanocytes relies on the deposition of H3K9me3 at the promoters of proliferation-related genes [75]. This is in accordance with their findings highlighting that benign naevi displayed increased senescence-associated H3K9me3 levels, with almost no detectable activity of H3 lysine 9 demethylases LSD1 and Jumonji Domain-Containing Protein 2D (JMJD2C/KDM4C), whilst human melanoma tissues generally harbored increased expression of LSD1 and JMJD2C and reduced H3K9me3 reactivity [75]. To gain a broader understanding of the molecular mechanisms that are involved in this process, the authors induced the expression of LSD1 and JMJD2C in mouse and zebrafish models. It was further shown that these two enzymes cooperated to overcome the oncogenic Ras G12V/BRAF V600E-induced senescence by preventing H3K9me3 deposition at E2F target gene promoters, which further augmented melanomagenesis [75]. Of note, targeted inhibition of LSD1 and JMJD2C demethylases restored cellular senescence and growth arrest, potentiating LSD1 and JMJD2C regulation as a potential anti-cancer therapeutic strategy [75].

5. Epigenetic Alterations Involved in CM Drug Resistance

5.1. Resistance to MAPK Inhibitors (MAPKi)

Genomic profiling of CMs revealed several actionable mutations in tumors that may be matched with targeted therapies. Recurrent driver alterations such as BRAF V600, NRAS, and NF-1 facilitated the design of BRAF inhibitors (BRAFi: vemurafenib and dabrafenib) and MEKi (trametinib, cobimetinib, and binimetinib) that have significantly improved patient OS [5,6]. Although 60–80% of BRAF-mutated CM patients respond well to targeted therapy, a significant proportion of them develop resistance, which results in life-threatening metastases and death [109,148,149]. The phenomenon of MAPKi resistance is complex and multifactorial and involves, among others, alterations of the BRAF V600E gene (amplification, aberrant splicing) [150–152], which leads to MAPK pathway hyperactivation, mutations that activate alternative survival pathways [153], modifications in apoptotic machinery [154], RTK hyperactivation [155,156], and the presence of slow-cycling populations [147], to which are added other MITFs, c-AMP, and NF-kB related mechanisms [9]. In CM, tumor refractoriness has been extensively linked with genetic alterations in many cancer-related genes; however, in some cases, the cause of the resistance appears to be non-genetic in nature [157]. Peculiarities such as the rapid kinetics and the transient nature of refractory phenotypes suggest the existence of an epigenetic basis for drug resistance in CM, pointing out that epigenetic remodeling is a fundamental feature of tumor development and adaptation to therapy [157,158]. Therefore, new therapeutic targets and therapies are critically necessary to improve the therapeutic management of CM. In this section, epigenetic alterations associated with MAPKi resistance and how they can be exploited in the future to become therapeutic targets and biomarkers in CM will be highlighted.

5.1.1. DNA Methylation and MAPKi Resistance

Studies highlighting the involvement of DNA methylation in CM targeted therapy resistance are relatively few. Al Emran et al. reported DNMT3A, DNMT3B, and DNMT1 as differentially expressed in the BRAF V600E melanoma cells refractory to MAPKi, which resulted in low DNA methylation levels. However, genome-wide integrated epigenetic analyses revealed that altered histone methylation patterns, rather than DNA methylation, are involved in the transition from the normal state toward the resistant phenotype [159]. In parallel, Hugo at al. observed that drug resistance programs are associated with dramatic transcriptomic and methylomic alterations in MAPKi-treated CM patients. Transcriptomic analyses indicated dysregulated mRNA levels of LEF1, TAP1, CD8, and DUSP4 genes in MAPKi-resistant tumors, which correlated with differential methylation at CpG islands, suggesting the critical roles of DNA methylation in transcriptomic reprogramming of melanoma cells to support MAPKi resistance [160].

5.1.2. Histone-Modifying Enzymes and PTMs Involved in MAPKi Resistance

One of the clinical observations that have postulated the link between epigenetic regulation and resistance to cancer therapy is the so-called "drug holiday" concept, which refers to intermittent treatment programs or treatment breaks. This strategy is often applied to delay the onset of resistance to therapy but is not potent on a genetically resistant phenotype [59]. Particularly for CM, it was observed that rechallenging patients with BRAFi after a free period of treatment and tumor progression resulted in a significant clinical response upon BRAFi and BRAF + MEKi treatments [161]. Recently, several studies have shown that the administration of a third-line BRAF-targeted therapy following first-line targeted therapy and second-line immunotherapy may be an effective strategy in CM metastatic patients [162,163]. Targeted therapy rechallenge in subjects who previously progressed on targeted therapies and immunotherapy was associated with a 2.7–5.9 month median progression-free survival (PFS), 9.3–19 month median OS and a 34–35% disease control rate. Notably, the time between treatment initiation and rechallenge did not seem to impact treatment responses [162,163].

Another aspect that advocates for epigenetically mediated drug-resistance phenotypes is that of slow-cycling cell populations, which appear to be endowed with reversible drug tolerance. One of the most important observations in this regard is that a very small fraction of cells can survive following exposure to drug concentrations 100-fold higher than IC_{50} [164]. These cells were found in a quiescent state and G1 arrest and continued to be viable in the presence of the drug. The induction of a "drug holiday", however, resensitized these cells to initial therapy, potentiating the plasticity of the drug-tolerant phenotype of these cells. These refractory tumor populations showed an altered chromatin state, with elevated KDM5A expression levels and a dramatic depletion of H3K4me2/3 marks. Notably, RNA-mediated KDM5A silencing confirmed that this histone demethylase allows for the maintenance of a reversible drug-tolerant state in human melanoma cells [164]. The critical role of the KDM5B epigenetic regulator in the generation of cell subpopulations with distinct drug sensitivity profiles was recently confirmed in the study of Liu et al. [78]. They found in mouse melanomas two cell subpopulations, CD34+ and CD34−, endowed with the characteristics of stem and progenitor cells, which may differ considerably in their clinical behaviors. It was further observed that the CD34+ and CD34− subpopulations displaying the BRAFV600E mutation may respond differently to targeted BRAFi. Interestingly, KDM5B overexpression reprogrammed melanoma cells to a CD34−, more drug-tolerant, phenotype, while KDM5B loss shifted melanoma cells to a more BRAFi-responsive CD34+ state, potentiating the pivotal role of KDM5A in modulating intratumoral heterogeneity in CM [78]. Moreover, KDM5B, another H3K4 demethylase, has been observed to play similar roles in the responsiveness of CM tumors to targeted therapies [165].

Further complicating the drug-resistance scenario, several studies have highlighted those particularities of the tumor microenvironment such as hypoxia and nutrient starvation alongside genotoxic pressure exerted by drugs can give rise to induced drug-tolerant cells (IDTCs) rather than a selection of a pre-existing subpopulation. One of these studies revealed that continuous exposure of melanoma cells to sub-lethal BRAFi concentrations induced surviving cells to adopt a less differentiated state and become refractory to 20-fold higher BRAFi concentrations, as well as to other MEKi and platinum salts [166]. At the molecular level, it has been observed that IDTCs display exacerbated expression of drug efflux ATB-binding cassette transporters and melanoma stem cell markers and loss of differentiation markers such as melan-A and Tyrosinase, which are MITF-target genes. Depletion of histone marks H3K4me3, H3K27me3 alongside a remarkable increase in H3K9me3 was observed in IDTCs cells. The authors also reported an overexpression of several histone-modifying enzymes including the H3K27-specific demethylases, KDM6A, KDM6B, and the H3K4-specific demethylases, KDM1B, KDM5A, and KDM5B, in the IDTC states. Interestingly, as was observed for the KDM5A-enriched subpopulation, IDTCs regained their therapeutic sensitivity seven days after treatment interruption [166]. Hypoxic conditions and nutrient starvation were also associated with the transition to an H3K4me3low/H3K27me3low/H3K9me3high phenotype and the IDTCs generated in this manner exhibited increased refractoriness to BRAFi, suggesting an epigenetically regulated drug-independent stress response that allows cancer cells to cope with difficult environmental conditions [166]. All these observations enhance the role of tumor heterogeneity of CM as the main determinant of resistance to targeted therapies.

It is also well documented that epigenetic alterations can interfere with the MAPKi mechanism of action. MAPK inhibitors cause cellular apoptosis by adjusting the balance between members of the Bcl-2 family, more precisely, by inducing the pro-apoptotic factors Bim and Bmf and by reducing Mcl-1 expression [167,168]. In contrast, MAPKi-resistant melanoma cells showed overexpression of Mcl-1, concomitantly with Noxa downregulation, which counteracted the MAPKi-induced cell death [154,169]. Notably, inhibition of EZH2 expression has been associated with the release of apoptosis-inducing factor (AIFM1) from mitochondria and the induction of caspase-independent apoptosis in human melanoma cell lines [170]. Therefore, all this information suggests that using EZH2 inhibition in conjunction with MAPKi may be a promising strategy to combat the hurdle of drug resistance in CM. Moreover, it is well documented that the BET family of histone reader proteins also turns melanoma cells against apoptosis. There are at least two BET proteins in melanoma, in this case BRD2 and BRD4, that are documented to be overexpressed during melanoma progression. Interestingly, several studies have potentiated that inhibition of BET proteins is associated with an increase in BIM, which synergizes with the induction of BIM after MAPK inhibition, and that the combination of BETi and MAPKi may be an effective pharmacological approach in CM [134,171]. Equally exciting results were obtained by combining HDACi with BETi in CM cell lines, leading to deregulation of anti-apoptotic proteins and components of the AKT and Hippo/YAP signaling pathways [172].

Despite the remarkable progress made in understanding the biology of melanocytic tumors, drug resistance remains a major problem in CM therapeutic management. Epigenetic reprogramming has the potential to reshape the metabolic and signaling networks in cancers, facilitating the emergence of tumor cell subpopulations with distinct behavior and antigenic profile [173]. This intratumor heterogeneity drives new resistance mechanisms to escape the genotoxic pressure or the immune system, facilitating metastasis and disease relapse [109]. However, novel omics technologies such as single-cell analysis and clustered regularly interspaced short palindromic repeats (CRISPR)-associated protein 9 (Cas9) genome editing tool are expected to revolutionize CM research and partially solve the issue of intratumoral heterogeneity, either by screening for novel therapeutic targets or by functional genome/epigenome editing.

5.2. Resistance to Immunotherapy

The development of immunotherapy, which has transformed the management of metastatic tumors, has undoubtedly been fostered by a comprehensive understanding of the tumor microenvironment (TME) and its immunophenotype. Tumors can be reduced to two main compartments that are closely intertwined: the malignant cells and TME. TME is composed of a variety of stromal cells embedded in an extracellular matrix irrigated by a complex network of blood and lymphatic vessels [174]. The cells within the stromal compartment can include immune cells (macrophages, B lymphocytes and cytotoxic T lymphocytes (CTLs), natural killer cells (NKCs), neutrophils, and dendritic cells), mesenchymal cells (fibroblasts, myofibroblasts, cancer stem cells- CSCs, mesenchymal stem cells- MSCs, adipocytes, and endothelial cells), and MDSCs [175,176]. Moreover, in melanoma's TME, TAMs are abundant and due to their pro-tumoral M2 phenotype these "tumor hijacked" cells sustain therapy resistance [15]. Stromal cells are in close communication with tumor cells and help them adapt to a changing microenvironment, survive, and replicate. As melanomas have a clear immune fate since immunosurveillance favors efficient tumor elimination and immunotolerance promotes tumor survival [175], therapy resistance has a clear immunological background. Additionally, it is well known that melanomas have an increased mutational rate and express a plethora of antigens, for example CTAs, which attracts immune cells that can eradicate the tumor or can be diverted towards pro-tumoral activity [177].

Natural immunosuppression has emerged as a physiological mechanism, but in TME immunosuppression usually interferes with CTL activity and functions [178,179]. Tumor cells mediate immunosuppression taking over inhibitory checkpoint proteins such as PD-1, T cell immunoglobulin and mucin domain 3 (TIM-3), lymphocyte activation gene 3 (LAG-3), and CTLA-4 expressed on the surface of T lymphocytes [180,181]. PD-1 and CTLA-4 bind to specific ligands such as PD-L1 and PD-L2, or CD80 and CD86, respectively, to negatively regulate T cell activity, leading to immune cell escape [181]. Therefore, the task of immunotherapy is much more challenging than it seems, as its goal is not to induce apoptosis but to modulate TME to induce a state of immunosurveillance that destroys cancer cells [109]. Anti-CTLA-4 antibody (Ipilimumab/Tramelimumab), approved for clinical management of CM more than five years ago [182] and followed closely by the approval of anti-PD1 (Nivolumab) [183], is the main immune therapeutical player that changed the fate of melanoma patients. Recently published data regarding the long-term therapy with individual and/or combined therapies in melanoma patients has shown that complete response is witnessed in 28% of patients and that there is still a great percentage of patients with incomplete response, patients that gain resistance and/or patients that due to immune-related adverse effect have to cease their immune therapy [184].

To date, the proposed mechanisms for CM resistance to immunotherapy are downregulation of MHC molecules, loss of antigenic expression, T-cell exhaustion, aberrant expression of PD-L1 in response to IFN-γ production by T cells, along with the altered expression of chemokines such as CCL3, CXCL1, and CCL4 [9]. Although it is well known that epigenetic regulation has critical roles in shaping the identity and differentiation of immune cells, the administration of epigenetic therapy should be done with caution in immunotherapy-resistant CMs, as these agents can affect other cells within TME in addition to tumor cells [59].

5.2.1. DNA Methylation and Resistance to Immunotherapy

The discovery that the immune system can be harnessed to fight cancer and improve clinical outcomes in CM was recognized with a Nobel prize in 2018 [185]. Nevertheless, further studies drove research toward elucidating how DNA methylation can impact the function and activity of immune system components [57]. Earlier studies have shown that DNA methylation appears to be involved in regulating T cell differentiation and exhaustion [186,187], but also in modulating immune checkpoint genes [188], which are the main biomarkers for the response to immunotherapy.

Several authors have reported a mechanistic link between DNA methylation status and immune checkpoint gene expression that may have important predictive and monitoring implications for immunotherapy-treated CM patients. For instance, methylation of immune checkpoint CTLA4 has recently been associated with worse response and progression-free survival (PFS) in stage IV CM patients treated with ipilimumab [189]. The same study also highlighted an inverse correlation between CTLA4 promoter methylation and the presence of tumor-infiltrating lymphocytes (TILs), which play a critical role in tumor control and response to immunotherapy. Therefore, melanoma samples with a low level of methylation are likely to have an increased immune cell infiltration, and an increased number of TILs is an indicator of a good clinical response. However, no significant correlation was reported between CTLA4 promoter methylation and CTLA-4 protein expression, suggesting that the level of protein expression of CTLA4 cannot be used as a predictive biomarker in CM [189]. Other authors have shown that the pattern of PD-L1 methylation may also be suggestive of the response to immunotherapy. Briefly, it has been shown that the degree of DNA methylation of melanoma cells facilitates the stratification of CM patients into four subgroups based on the expression of PD-L1 and TILs and that this information may provide clues about the therapeutic response and survival rates of these CM patients [190,191]. Earlier studies have shown that highly responsive patients showed elevated levels of TILs and PD-L1, while the nonresponsive group displayed low levels of TILs and PD-L1 [190]. In the meantime, while clinical information has been gathered about this clear-cut PD-L1 high expression, efficient immune therapy has been shaken due to various newly discovered molecular mechanisms [192]. DNA methylome analysis of 52 stage III patients from TCGA revealed that low/absent PD-L1 expression is associated with high DNA methylation, differential expression of immune-related genes and worse survival [193]. In parallel, Micevic at al. confirmed that PD-L1 methylation regulates PD-L1 expression and identified for the first time the existence of methylated CpG loci at the PD-L1 promoter [194]. The authors further stratified melanomas into 2 groups based on PD-L1 status and observed that PD-L1 hypomethylation is associated with increased PD-L1 expression and superior OS in CM patients regardless of the diagnosed stages [194]. Moreover, studies on melanoma cells showed that treatment with the hypomethylating agent 5-azacytidine can orchestrate transcriptional derepression in hypermethylated PD-L1 tumors, leading to amplification of PD-L1 expression [194]. Finally, some other studies confirmed the epigenetic regulation of immune checkpoint gene LAG3 via DNA methylation in CM [195]. LAG3 is a molecule involved in blocking tumor cell proliferation and regulating the production of IFN-γ and TNFα cytokines. Interestingly, it has been shown that LAG3 promoter hypomethylation positively associates with increased levels of tumor-infiltrating immune cells and better PFS in CM patients [195].

Given that anti-PD-L1 and anti-PD-1 antibodies are the most extensively used immunotherapies in the clinical setting, and PD-L1 hypermethylation renders CM resistant to

ICIs, applying DNMTi treatments appears a tempting strategy to reverse CM immunotherapy resistance. Interestingly, it has been noted that DNMTi hs the ability to activate endogenous retroviruses (ERVs) and virus defense-related pathways in melanoma cells [196]. In the TCGA, the expression levels of viral defense genes may help in stratifying primary samples from multiple tumors, including CM, into two risk groups where a high defense signature positively associates with improved OS and more durable clinical response. Moreover, combining anti-CTLA-4 with low doses of DNMTi proved to be an effective strategy in augmenting the immunotherapy efficiency in a mouse melanoma model [196]. Therefore, the use of immune checkpoint inhibitors in conjunction with DNMTi may be a promising strategy for maximizing the therapeutic benefit in CM patients. Certainly, we will soon find out more about the efficacy and safety of combining DNMTi with immunotherapy, given that ongoing clinical trials are studying the oral use of azacitidine with pembrolizumab in patients with metastatic CM (NCT02816021).

5.2.2. Histone-Modifying Enzymes and PTMs Involved in Immunotherapy Resistance

To date, information on histone enzymes and PTMs involved in immunotherapy resistance are even vaguer than in the case of epigenetic regulation by DNA methylation. Several studies have suggested a mechanistic link between EZH2 activity and resistance to immunotherapy. For example, Zingg at al. observed that anti-CTLA-4 or IL-2 immunotherapy leads to TNFα amplification and T cell infiltration, resulting in EZH2 overexpression and loss of tumor control in melanoma mouse models [197]. Mechanistically, EZH2 catalyzes the deposition of H3K27me3 marks and the suppression of a plethora of immune-related genes. Notably, EZH2 inactivation reversed the drug-resistant phenotype and amplified the effects of anti-CTLA-4 and IL-2 immunotherapy in melanoma mouse models, thus blocking CM growth and dissemination [197]. Therefore, in this study, Zingg at al. have demonstrated not only that EZH2 expression is a valuable biomarker for monitoring the response to immunotherapy but can also be exploited as a therapeutic target to restore and enhance the effects of immunotherapy.

Additional studies have reinforced that the involvement of EZH2 in resistance to CM immunotherapy could be much broader. Tiffen at al. analyzed 471 cases of CM in the TCGA and found that 20% of patients displayed copy number amplifications and mRNA upregulation, along with activating mutations in EZH2 [198]. RNAseq analysis further showed that these alterations correlated with DNA hypermethylation and downregulation of certain genes involved in tumor suppression, antigen processing, and presentation pathways. Treatment with the EZH2 inhibitor GSK126 reversed the transcriptional silencing driven by EZH2 alterations in CM cells, suggesting that EZH2 inhibition is a promising pharmacological strategy for improving the therapeutic response in CM [198]. From these observations, it appears that there may be a close link between EZH2 and the activity of DNMTs in regulating tumor biological properties, including the response to immunotherapy in CM. It is well documented that the ATRX_DNMT3_DNMT3L (ADD) domain of DNMT3A may interact with several epigenetic players, such as SUV39H1 methyltransferases, HDAC1, and EZH2, among others [199]. Moreover, it was postulated that the activity of DNMTs is supported by EZH2, a well-known target of PI3K/Akt signaling, and that they cooperate in cancer pathogenesis [200]. In support of this idea is the observation that EZH2 and DNMTs are regulated by similar upstream signaling cascades, such as MEK/ERK and PI3K/Akt, and transcription factors such as NF-kB2 [57]. Last but not least, it appears that EZH2 can pre-mark genes for DNMTs methylation [201]. Therefore, although still in its infancy, the study of epigenetic mechanisms concerning the response to immunotherapy is expected to not only guide and revolutionize the treatment of refractory patients, but also to stratify them into risk groups to provide personalized therapeutic solutions.

6. Epigenetics-Based Therapies for CM

Given the critical roles of epigenetic alterations in CM development and its drug resistance, targeting or co-targeting these epigenetic events appears to be a promising strategy for improving the clinical condition of CM patients [109]. Although epigenetic biomarkers have not yet found their place in clinical practice, an impressive number of epigenetic drugs are constantly being developed and tested for their cytotoxicity and efficacy in clinical trials in various human cancers, including CM [89,202]. These epigenetic drugs include both general epigenetic inhibitors such as HDACi or DNMTi, but also more specific inhibitors targeting enhancer of zeste homolog 2 (EZH2i), bromodomain and extra-terminal domain proteins (BETi), or JMJD3 and JARID1B demethylases [203]. Table 1 summarizes the current status of those CM therapies (Table 1).

Table 1. Overview of the most common epigenetic inhibitors and their current status in CM [1].

Class	Agent	Mechanism of Action	Development Stage	Combination	References
DNMTi	Azacitidine (Vidaza©)		Phase I/II clinical trials	- (NCT02223052)	[204]
				Pembrolizumab (NCT02816021)	[205]
				Carboplatin + Avelumab (ACTRN12618000053224)	[206]
	Decitabine (Dacogen©)	Incorporation into DNA, covalently linking the DNMTs, leading to DNMTs exhaustion and DNA damage	Phase I/II clinical trials	- (NCT00002980)	[207]
				TCR-engineered T-cell immunotherapy (NCT02650986)	[208]
				Decitabine, Temozolomide and Panobinostat (NCT00925132)	[209]
				Temozolomide (NCT00715793)	[210]
				Vemurafenib (NCT01876641)	[211]
				Vemurafenib + Cobimetinib (NCT01876641)	[212]
	Guadecitabine (SGI-110)		Phase I/II clinical trials	Ipilimumab (NCT02608437)	[213,214]
				Nivolumab + ipilimumab (NCT04250246)	[215]
	Zebularine		Preclinical	-	[216]
	Disulfiram (Antabuse©)	Prevent the interaction of DNMTs with their target sequences either by binding to the catalytic site of DNMTs or by binding to CpG-enriched sequences	Phase I clinical trials	- (NCT00256230)	[217]
				Arsenic Trioxide (NCT00571116)	[218]
HDACi	Vorinostat/ Suberoylanilide hydroxamic acid (SAHA/Zolinza©)	Targeting class I, II and IV HDACs	Phase I/II clinical trials	- (NCT02836548)	[219]
	Domatinostat (4SC-202)	Targeting class I HDACs	Phase I clinical trials	Nivolumab + Ipilimumab (NCT04133948)	[220]

Table 1. Cont.

Class	Agent	Mechanism of Action	Development Stage	Combination	References
HDACi	Panobinostat (LBH589)	Inhibition of class I, II, and IV enzymes	Phase I clinical trials	- (NCT01065467)	[221]
				Ipilimumab (NCT02032810)	[222]
	Romidepsin (Despipeptide/ FR901228)	Targeting class I HDACs	Phase II clinical trials	- (NCT00104884)	[223]
	Entinostat (SNDX-275/ MS-275)	Inhibition of class I HDACs	Phase II clinical trials	Pembrolizumab (NCT02437136)	[224]
	Mocetinostat (DB11830)	Targeting class I HDACs	Phase I clinical trials	Ipilimumab (NCT03565406)	[225]
	Tinostamustine	Targeting all the classical HDACs	Phase I clinical trials	Nivolumab (NCT03903458)	[226]
	Valproic acid (Depakote©)	Inhibition of class I and II enzymes	Phase I clinical trials	Chemoimmunotherapy	[227]
	Sulforaphane	Regulation of inflammatory and cell survival pathways	Pilot clinical studies	- (NCT01568996)	[228]
	Trichostatin A (TSA)	Induction of cell cycle arrest and apoptotic pathways	Preclinical	-	[229]
	Dacinostat (LAQ824)	Regulation of cell cycle and apoptosis	Preclinical	-	[229]
	Suberic bishydroxamate (SBHA)	Induction of apoptosis	Preclinical	-	[229]
EZH2i	Tazemetostat	Targeting EZH2 activity	Phase I/II clinical studies	Dabrafenib trametinib (NCT04557956)	[230]
	CPI-1205	Targeting EZH2 activity	Phase I clinical studies	Ipilimumab (NCT03525795)	[231]
BETi	ODM-207	Preventing BETs-acetylated histones interaction	Phase I clinical studies	- (NCT03035591)	[232]
	NHWD-870	Preventing BETs-acetylated histones interaction	Preclinical	-	[233]
	PLX51107	Preventing BETs-acetylated histones interaction, regulation of TME	Preclinical	PLX3397	[234]

[1] (-) none; (+) combination therapy.

DNA methylation and histone acetylation were the first and most extensively studied epigenetic alterations in cancer. The progress made in understanding them led to the development of DNA methyltransferase inhibitors (DNMTIs) and histone deacetylase inhibitors (HDACi), which constitute the first generation of epigenetic inhibitors [39]. These first-generation epigenetic inhibitors were tested in clinical trials either alone or combined with other therapeutic agents; notably, these molecules showed limited selectivity and stability, increased cytotoxicity, and low efficiency in solid tumors especially when employed as a single therapy [235]. Their clinical use is currently restricted to hematological malignancies:

myelodysplastic syndromes and leukemias. The low efficacy of epi-therapies in solid tumors compared to blood cancers is still poorly understood. One possible explanation may be that these agents reach their therapeutic concentrations more efficiently in blood cancers so that their short life may not affect their activities as it may do in solid tumors [236]. Another explanation refers to the fact that solid and hematological tumors differ considerably in terms of cell differentiation and epigenetic plasticity, with solid tumors originating from a more terminally differentiated state that is much more difficult to be transcriptomically reprogrammed [39].

The introduction of the second-generation of epi-drugs, which included certain DNMTi (such as zebularine and guadecitabine) and HDACi (belinostat, panobinostat, hydroxamic acid, tucidinostat, and valproic acid) has brought considerable advantages over its predecessors. These compounds have improved pharmacological properties, fewer side effects, and amplified selectivity, their targets being key drivers or pivotal regulators of tumor growth [202]. Despite the scientific efforts devoted to its development, the second generation of epigenetic drugs also showed reduced efficacy when administered as monotherapy [237]. This called for the development of the third generation of epi-therapies, which include, among others, histone methyltransferase inhibitors (HMTi), histone demethylase inhibitors (HDMi), enhancer of zest homolog 2 inhibitors (EZH2i), and bromodomain and extra-terminal domain inhibitors (BETi) [39]. The development of the third generation of epi-drugs took into account the principles of precision medicine, in which the existence of a high degree of selectivity is a supreme desideratum [39]. The development of the third generation of epi-drugs revealed that epigenetic factors that can write, erase or read epigenetic marks are usually protein complexes, emphasizing that a better understanding of the epigenetic regulators' interactome may help to design more effective and selective epi-therapies [238]. In this section we will review the current status of epigenetic therapies used either as single agents or in combination with conventional approaches in CM.

6.1. Epigenetic Drugs as Monotherapies in CM

6.1.1. DNMTi

DNMTis are potent antineoplastic compounds able to reverse the DNA hypermethylation status of TSGs. Depending on their mode of action, DNMTIs can be divided into two classes: cytosine analogue inhibitors and non-nucleotide analogue inhibitors [239].

Cytosine analogues such as azacytidine, decitabine, zebularine, guadecitabine (SGI-110), fazarabine, and pseudois cytidine, may replace C-5 of cytosine with N-5 into the DNA or RNA backbone, leading to DNMTs degradation, DNA damage, and subsequently, apoptosis [239]. Although they gained FDA approval for the treatment of hematologic malignancies, azacitidine and decitabine showed disappointing results in CM and other cancer patients with solid tumors when employed as monotherapy in Phase I/II clinical trials [240]. The clinical benefits seen in patients with solid tumors exposed to high doses of azacytidine and decitabine are offset by severe adverse effects, such as hematological toxicity [203]. The lowest dose at which decitabine was shown to be effective in treating a solid tumor was 50 mg/m^2 but the reported side effects were severe [241]. Interestingly, the incidence of hematotoxicity may be reduced if these nucleoside analogues are administered by hepatic arterial infusion and not via the intravenous route [242]. Moreover, it seems that low doses of DNMTis (~20 mg/m^2) can minimize toxicity and side effects while making tumor cells more sensitive to immunotherapeutic or chemotherapeutic agents [242]. Further clinical research revealed that cytosine analogs can induce ERVs and CTA expression in cancer patients so that cancer cells end up expressing a plethora of neoantigens that can be targeted by immunotherapy [243]. Moreover, it has been reported that DNMTi exposure can induce the activation of transposable elements such as Alu or LINEs, leading to a state of viral mimicry in which treated tumor cells translate the induced expression as caused by an exogenous viral infection, ultimately triggering an innate immune response [203]. Combining DNMTi with chemotherapy is another intensively investigated strategy to improve the clinical management of CM patients. A Phase I/II study combining decitabine with temozolomide in patients with metastatic melanoma showed promising results in terms of efficiency and safety profile (NCT00715793) [244]. The study reported that administration of decitabine in combination with temozolomide re-sensitizes CM patients to temozolomide by dual modulation of DNA repair machinery due to depletion of DNA repair protein O6-methylguanine-DNA-methyltransferase (MGMT) and subsequent induction of DNA mismatch repair (MMR) pathway in temozolomide-refractory melanoma cells [244].

Other cytosine analogues that are gaining considerable research interest for clinical use in CM are guadecitabine and zebularine. Although these next-generation DNMTis act similarly with azacytidine and decitabine, they have a longer half-life and better bioavailability when compared to their predecessors [237,239]. Guadecitabine has been tested in over 30 clinical trials in cancers, including certain phase III trials (https://clinicaltrials.gov). In particular, for CM, there are no clinical trials in which guadecitabine is tested as monotherapy, there are only two ongoing clinical trials, but in which it is administered in conjunction with immunotherapy (NCT02608437, NCT04250246). Zebularine is another second-generation DNMTi that acts by sequestering DNMTs after incorporation into DNA, interfering with their catalytic activities [245]. Preclinical studies in CM highlighted that zebularine treatments can reverse the mechanisms developed by the tumor to get rid of anti-tumoral immunity, priming it for the action of immunotherapies. That is, zebularine allows for the re-expression of intercellular adhesion molecule-1 (ICAM-1) on tumor endothelial cells, which results in restored leukocyte-endothelial cell adhesion and enhanced leukocyte infiltration [216]. Zebularine remains to be further evaluated in clinical trials in CM.

Another class of DNMTi is the class of non-nucleotide analogue inhibitors. This class encompasses small molecules that block the interaction of DNMTs with target sequences either by binding to the catalytic site of DNMTs or by binding to CpG-enriched sequences; however, the antineoplastic effects of non-nucleotide analog inhibitors are inferior to those of cytosine analog inhibitors. They include several compounds such as hydralazine, epigallocatechin gallate (EGCG), and disulfiram [239]. Disulfiram is one of the best-studied non-nucleotide analog inhibitors in cancers, and implicitly in CM. In numerous in vitro experimental studies, disulfiram and its metabolites were extremely potent in blocking tumor growth and inducing apoptosis in tumor cells, but with the disadvantage of strong cytotoxic effects. However, no clinical reports attest to a measurable efficacy of disulfiram as a mono-therapeutic agent against solid tumors to date, most likely due to the low circulating bioavailability of this compound [246]. Due to the potent antiapoptotic activity of disulfiram in tumor cells, it remains a promising approach when administered in conjunction with other pharmacological approaches such as chemotherapy, targeted therapy, radiotherapy, or immunotherapy. However, to minimize the cytotoxic effects and increase the therapeutic benefit of cancer and CM patients, extensive testing of disulfiram is needed in experimental studies and clinical combinatorial trials [246].

6.1.2. HDACi

HDACis are a class of compounds capable of rectifying the aberrant acetylation status of histone and non-histone proteins in cancers to orchestrate TSG activation. In addition, cancer cells display an increased sensitivity to HDACi-induced apoptosis, making those epigenetic agents promising anti-cancer strategies [239]. The FDA has approved four HDACis for use in cancer patients. Three of these compounds are the hydroxamic acids vorinostat, belinostat, and panobinostat, which have been described as non-specific HDAC inhibitors targeting all classical HDACs (classes I, II, and IV). In contrast, the fourth HDACi that gained FDA approval, romidepsin, also known as FK228 or depsipeptide, has been reported to act specifically on Class I HDACs [247]. Other HDACis that have been tested in vitro or are in current clinical trials are well characterized by the scientific literature [203]. Proposed mechanisms of action for HDACis include cell cycle arrest by p53-dependent or -independent induction of the p21CIP/WAF1 axis, downregulation of oncogenes, enhanced

ROS production, autophagy induction, as well as suppression of genes involved in cell survival and EMT programs [245,248].

Several HDACis, including both specific (class I HDAC inhibitor entinostat) and non-specific agents (panobinostat), have recently been tested in phase I/II clinical trials in metastatic CM patients; yet, they have shown reduced efficacy and poor tolerability as monotherapies [249,250]. The most common side effects associated with HDAC inhibition are hematotoxicity, fatigue, nausea, and hyperglycemia [229]. Valproic acid (VA) administration also led to disappointing results in CM clinical cohorts [227]. This was mainly because valproic acid requires a long period, up to several weeks, to reach full dose in most patients, making it almost ineffective in the case of aggressive and rapidly dividing CM tumors. VA was linked to serious adverse effects, such as grade 3 neurological toxicity and intracerebral hemorrhage [227]. In a phase II clinical trial, vorinostat (suberoyl-anilide-hydroxamic acid: SAHA) demonstrated some early responses in patients with advanced CM; however, for the majority of these patients, the disease state was stable, and vorinostat did not meet its primary endpoint of response [251]. As expected, vorinostat therapy was associated with significant side effects, such as lymphopenia, fatigue, and nausea [251]. Surprisingly, quisinostat, an HDACi with increased affinity for class I and II HDACs, showed strong antineoplastic activities and an acceptable safety profile in phase I clinical study of metastatic melanoma patients, calling for further investigation of its clinical efficiency and tolerability in different doses and combinations [252].

In recent years, considerable attention has been paid to sulforaphane (SFN), a natural compound found in cruciferous vegetables, such as broccoli, cauliflower, cabbage, and Brussels sprouts. Being a natural compound, SFN brings with it the advantage of being well-tolerated in human subjects [245]. Additionally, in CM preclinical studies, SFN consumption was linked with the inhibition of UV-induced inflammation and tumorigenesis [253,254]. It was further reported that SFN, through its inhibition of HDACs properties, can regulate apoptotic programs and cell survival pathways to induce cell arrest and apoptosis in melanoma cells [255]. Other mechanisms by which SFN can control tumor growth and evolution in CM cells are by downregulating the metastasis-promoting enzymes MMP-9 and sulfatase-2 [256,257]. However, a pilot study with 17 patients with at least two atypical nevi and a prior history of melanoma revealed that SFN treatment is relevant for chemoprevention in this clinical condition [228]. SFN treatment at 200 μmol daily for 28 days resulted in a significant reduction of the proinflammatory cytokines IL-10 (CXCL10), MCP-1 (CCL-2), MIG (CXCL9), and MIP-1β, and overexpression of tumor suppressor decorin. These encouraging results support that further testing of SFN should be performed in phase II clinical trials at higher doses and over a longer period, ideally accompanied by morphological, histopathological, and molecular analyses of excised tumors [228]. Other HDACis such as trichostatin A (TSA) and suberic bishydroxamate (SBHA) are currently in the preclinical development phase for CM treatment [229].

6.1.3. Next-Generation Epigenetic Agents

Novel epigenetic targets identified in cancers have given rise to the next generation of epigenetic therapies that include enhancer of zest homolog 2 inhibitors (EZH2i), bromodomain, and extra-terminal domain inhibitors (BETi), inhibitors of the demethylases JMJD3 and JARID1B, as well as many other compounds [202]. The observation that EZH2 is often overexpressed in cancers led to the development of certain small molecule agents targeting this histone methyltransferase such as EPZ-6438 (tazemetostat), GSK2816126, and CPI-1205 [239,258]; these drugs are currently in early clinical studies reporting clinical responses with acceptable tolerability in many cancers [258,259]. EZH2 is also amplified in CM, and increased levels have been linked with aggressive disease and poor prognosis [77]. Notably, the use of EZH2i in the treatment of wild-type and mutant melanoma cell lines led to a reduction in cell proliferation and growth, legitimating EZH2 as a veritable target in melanoma cells [170]. Another study highlighted that EZH2 depletion may interfere with cancer cell proliferation both in vitro and in vivo via the induction of the p21/CDKN1A-mediated senescence [124]. Moreover, conditional ablation of EZH2 in a melanoma mouse model impaired tumor growth and attenuated metastasis without affecting the functionality of normal melanocytes [76]. These effects were recapitulated by pharmacological inhibition of EZH2, suggesting that EZH2 inhibitors are promising therapeutic approaches for the treatment of CM patients [76].

Another class of epi-therapies that is gaining considerable research interest in cancers is that of BET inhibitors (BETi). BETis exert their anti-neoplastic activities in tumor cells by preventing BETs-acetylated histones interaction [239]. So far, several BETis, such as thienodiazepine JQ1, I-BET151/GSK1210151A, I-BET762/GSK525762, ABBV-075, PLX51107, ODM-207, and ZEN003694 have shown encouraging clinical outcomes with tolerable toxicity and increased efficiency in various tumor types [260,261]. BRD4 is a notorious BET family member that is consistently reported to be amplified or overexpressed in human melanoma lines and primary tumors [262]. Notably, one study suggested that BETi treatments significantly affected melanoma cell proliferation in vitro and tumor growth and metastasis in vivo due to the downregulation of genes involved in cell cycle progression (SKP2, ERK1, and c-MYC) and concomitant accumulation of cyclin-dependent kinase inhibitors (p21 and p27). These effects were also reported upon individual silencing of BRD4. However, the efficiency of BETi was not affected by the BRAF or NRAS mutational status, suggesting that BRD4 inhibitors may be a promising approach for the treatment of CM patients that are not eligible for targeted therapy [134]. NHWD-870, a novel BRD4 inhibitor that suppresses the secretion of macrophage colony-stimulating factor (CSF)-1 by tumor cells and disrupts the BRD4/HIF-1α axis, is currently under preclinical investigation for the treatment of CM [233]. Another BETi, I-BET151, triggered the selective inhibition of the NF-κB signaling pathway in melanoma cells, regulating genes involved in inflammation (VEGF, CCL-20) and cell cycle progression (CDK6) and suppressing the production of IL-6 and IL-8 via BRD2 displacement [263]. PLX51107, a next-generation BETi, impaired tumor growth to differing degrees in BRAF V600E syngeneic mouse models, effects that were linked to the influx of TAMs. Tumors that were poorly responsive to BET inhibition displayed an increased influx of pro-tumoral macrophages and the addition of PLX3397 resulted in improved response rates to PLX51107, offering a novel combination therapy for metastatic CM patients [234]. In another study, PLX51107 slowed the growth of mouse BRAF V600E melanoma tumors by inducing the CD8$^+$ T cell-mediated anti-tumor effects; moreover, PLX51107 proved to be an effective second-line therapy for CM tumors that harbored resistance to PD1/PDL1 checkpoint inhibition [264]. While certain BETis have recently started to be evaluated in phase I clinical trials in CM patients [232], novel pharmacological inhibitors continue to be tailored to target other classes of epigenetic enzymes, such as JMJD3 and JARID1B histone demethylases [265,266]. Therefore, the continuous enrichment of the anti-cancer armamentarium with next-generation therapies and their exploration either alone or in conjunction with traditional therapies is expected to positively impact CM therapeutic management and open up new opportunities for precision medicine in those patients.

6.2. Combinatorial Therapies in CM

Several lines of evidence support that, in addition to their potential use as single agents, epigenetic drugs may be extremely potent in sensitizing tumor cells to other anti-cancer therapies or may help in circumventing the major hurdle of acquired drug resistance [68,203,267]. Chemotherapy, targeted therapy, and immunotherapy are the major pillars of the anti-cancer treatment arsenal in CM. In this section, we review the current literature by which epi-drugs may regulate the sensitivity of cancer cells to targeted therapies and immunotherapies, two of the most used therapies in CM clinical management.

6.2.1. Combinations with Targeted Therapy

Several research groups have shown that the administration of epigenetic inhibitors, such as HDACs, BETi, or DNMTi in combination with BRAFi and/or MEKi can reverse acquired resistance to targeted therapy. For instance, the use of BRAFi encorafenib in combination with HDACi panobinostat decreases PI3K oncogenic pathway activity and increases the expression levels of pro-apoptotic proteins BIM and NADPH oxidase activator (NOXA) in CM cell lines with acquired BRAFi resistance [268]. In parallel, it has been reported that BETi JQ1 treatment can sensitize vemurafenib-resistant melanoma cells to BRAFi by modulating the histone acetylation patterns of the P-gp gene in the promoter region to prevent drug efflux [267]. Additionally, combining BET and HDAC inhibitors has strong synergistic effects in the induction of apoptosis and suppression of Akt and Yap signaling in melanoma cells, even in those with acquired resistance to BRAFi [172]. In addition, the combination of vemurafenib and decitabine has shown increased efficacy and tolerability in BRAF V600E metastatic tumors in a Phase I clinical trial (NCT01876641) [212]. Although this study was prematurely terminated due to loss of funding, 3/14 patients achieved a complete response, 3/14 had a partial response, and 5/14 had stable disease. The highest response rate was reported in clinical cohorts that utilized low-dose, long-term decitabine, emphasizing that future studies should focus on long-term use of decitabine at the lowest dose of 0.1 mg/kg [212]. At the moment, a phase II clinical trial is testing the efficacy and safety of tazemetostat in combination with dual BRAF/MEK inhibition in patients with BRAF-mutated metastatic melanoma who progressed on prior BRAF/MEKi therapy (NCT04557956).

6.2.2. Combinations with Immunotherapy

Several other reports highlighted that combining epigenetic therapies with immunotherapeutics may result in considerable clinical benefits in cancer patients. This is possible due to the ability of epigenetic therapies to modulate the immune response in tumors [269]. The mechanisms by which these epi-therapies exert their activity are not fully elucidated, but it has been suggested that they may involve reactivation of ERVs, upregulation of tumor-surface antigens, stimulation of antigen-presenting mechanisms, activation of IFN response pathways, transcriptomic reprogramming of TME cells, or induction of immune checkpoint blockade targets such as PD-1/PD-L1 on both tumor cells and lymphocytes alongside reversal of T cell exhaustion [79]. The mechanisms underlying these actions are depicted in Figure 3.

A bourgeoning body of evidence suggests that despite their reduced anti-cancer activities, DNMTis have the potential to increase the immunogenicity and immune recognition of CM cells [270]. Pioneering studies in this field have highlighted that DNMTi hypomethylating agent decitabine may orchestrate re-expression of HLA class I antigens on melanoma cells, which enables tumor cell recognition by MAGE-specific cytotoxic T lymphocytes and their further elimination [271]. Since the studied melanoma cell line was obtained from a metastatic lesion of a nonresponding patient undergoing MAGE-3.A1 T-cell-based peptide immunotherapy, the authors postulated that hypermethylation-induced loss of HLA class I expression may be the cause of the impaired response to vaccination; however, this study highlights for the first time that DNMTis should be tested for their efficiency on reversing the acquired resistance to immunotherapy in CM [271]. Other preclinical studies have shown that DNMTi may trigger the activation of ERVs, which are normally transcriptionally silenced, leading to the activation of a type I IFN response and cytotoxic T cell recruitment into the TME [196,272]. DNMTi treatments were also linked with CTA induction in melanoma cells, with important pharmacological applications in CM management, as the homogeneous expression of a therapeutic target in neoplastic cells is a prerequisite to effectively target tumors by vaccination-induced CTA-directed immune response [273]. MAGE-A3 and NYESO-1-based vaccines are currently being tested in clinical trials for the regression of CM (Li at al. 2020). Therefore, epigenetic regulation may be harnessed to broaden the eligibility and benefits of vaccine-based therapies in CM patients, but also to tailor specific immunotherapies for each patient [273].

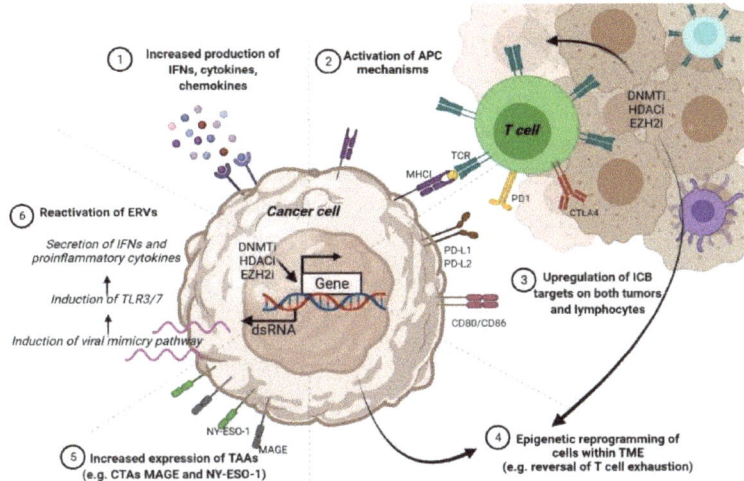

Figure 3. The proposed mechanisms by which epigenetic agents may regulate the immune response in cancers. Abbreviations: IFNs—interferons; APC—antigen-presenting cell; MHCI—major histocompatibility complex I; TCR—T-cell receptor; PD-1—programmed cell death protein 1; CTLA4—cytotoxic T-lymphocyte-associated protein 4; ICB—immune checkpoint blockade; PD-L1—programmed death-ligand 1; CD80—cluster of differentiation 80; TME—tumor microenvironment; TAAs—tumor-associated antigens; CTAs—cancer testis antigens; MAGE—human melanoma antigen; NY-ESO-1—New York esophageal squamous cell carcinoma 1; TLR3—Toll-like receptor; dsRNA—double-stranded RNA.

Currently, two clinical trials evaluating the safety and efficiency of DNMTi combined with immunotherapy are underway in CM. Preliminary results of a phase II study of azacitidine in combination with pembrolizumab in patients with metastatic melanoma (NCT02816021) revealed that although the combination is relatively well tolerated, it is potent only in PD-1-naïve patients (55% ORR) [274]. However, these observations remain to be further confirmed in larger clinical cohorts and correlated with the molecular characteristics of tumor biopsies. Another phase I clinical trial evaluating guadecitabine with anti-CTLA-4 showed promising tumor immunomodulatory and anti-cancer activities in CM metastatic patients; briefly, the use of DNMTi led to the induction of HLA class I molecules and IFNγ signaling pathways and increased tumor infiltration by CD8[+] T cells, rendering those tumors more sensitive to immunotherapy [214].

Recent studies have provided evidence that the efficiency of immunotherapy may also be potentiated in cancers when used in combination with HDACis. HDACis are known to increase MHC class I and II expression on the cell surface or regulate PD-L1 and PD-L2 expression on cancer cells, thereby rendering the tumor vulnerable to T-cell mediated immune responses [275,276]. Furthermore, it is well documented that HDACis may be involved in TME reprogramming to deactivate immunosuppressive cells such as MDSCs and increase cytotoxic T cell activity within the TME [277]. Interestingly, in a melanoma mouse model, HDAC6 inhibitor Nexturastat A given in conjunction with anti-PD-1 antibodies significantly impaired tumor growth by causing a decrease in the anti-inflammatory phenotype of macrophages and increased infiltration of CD8[+] T cells and NK cells into the TME [278]. Moreover, upon exposure to the HDACi entinostat in combination with azacytidine, the syngeneic mouse melanoma models displayed improved rates of response to both anti-PD-1 and anti-CTLA-4 immunotherapies, and the tumors were eradicated in 80% of the experimental animals [279]. Functional analysis revealed that the primary targets of the epigenetic drugs were the MDSCs, which exert immunosuppressive effects in tumors [279]. Similarly, mocetinostat decreases immunosuppressive immune cell phenotypes while augmenting anti-tumor phenotypes in both preclinical and clinical settings, providing a rationale for the use of these agents in conjunction with ICIs in CM [225]. The promising results of treatment regimens incorporating immunotherapy and HDACi have led to the recent initiation of several clinical trials in CM. Preliminary results from a phase I clinical trial evaluating the combination of pembrolizumab and HDACi entinostat demonstrated a favorable response in patients with immune checkpoint inhibitor-resistant CM and acceptable safety (NCT02437136) [224]. Notably, for one patient with a confirmed partial response, transition from a PD-L1 negative phenotype (pretreatment tumor biopsy) to a PD-L1 positive state (post-treatment biopsy) was reported, as a hallmark of increased sensitivity to immunotherapy [224]. In contrast, in another phase I clinical trial, panobinostat showed limited efficiency when added to standard ipilimumab therapy in CM metastatic patients (NCT02032810) [222]. Other drug combinations such as that of anti-PD-L1 antibody nivolumab with tinostamustine, an alkylating HDACi (NCT03903458) are now under clinical investigation in refractory, locally advanced, or metastatic CM patients (Table 1).

Finally, several studies that highlight the combination of EZH2i and MAPKi or immunotherapy show an enhanced apoptosis and increased tumor control in CM cell lines and mouse models [197,198]. There is also the possibility of using EZH2i in conjunction with DNMTi and/or HDAC inhibitors as these agents have demonstrated the ability to upregulate immune response pathways in many solid cancers, including CM [57,235].

7. Discussion

Notorious for its increased unpredictable behaviors, distant metastatic patterns, increased inflammatory status, and intrinsic resistance to therapy, CM is an unsolved clinical and social issue [280]. The remarkable progress made in recent years in deciphering CM biology has resulted in the development of several targeted therapies and immune checkpoint inhibitors that have truly revolutionized the treatment of metastatic CM. For instance, therapies targeting nodes in the MAPK pathway have greatly improved OS; furthermore, immune therapies with immune-checkpoint modulators have led to more durable results and even pCR in several patients [192]. Despite these promising results, targeted and immune therapies' effectiveness is often limited by the emergence of drug resistance. In CM, tumor refractoriness has been extensively linked with mutations in genes regulating drug efflux mechanisms, apoptotic machinery, DNA damage repair, cancer stemness, as well as many other biological processes [280–283]; however, for a significant proportion of CM, the cause of the resistance appears to be non-genetic. Peculiarities such as the rapid kinetics and the transient nature of refractory phenotypes suggest the existence of an epigenetic basis for drug resistance in CM, pointing out that epigenetic regulation is a fundamental feature of tumor development and adaptation to therapy [157]. Accordingly, epigenetic alterations are currently being investigated as potential biomarkers and are being envisioned as promising therapeutic targets for CM clinical management [284].

We revised how epigenetic mechanisms such as DNA methylation and histone modifications are fine-tuning gene expression programs in CM, thus influencing almost all the biological properties of these tumors. Distinct epigenetic signatures show promise for assisting in distinguishing between benign and malignant lesions, as well as between certain disease subtypes histologically classified or evaluated into blood circulation [34,103,285]. Moreover, altered epigenetic patterns have been shown to contribute to the acquisition of drug resistant phenotypes in CM and some of these modifications seem to have important prognostic and predictive applications [189,195]. Given the critical roles of epigenetic alterations in CM development and drug resistance, but also their reversible nature, targeting or co-targeting these epigenetic events appears to be a promising strategy for improving the clinical condition of CM patients. Although epigenetic biomarkers have not yet found their place in clinical practice, an impressive number of epigenetic drugs are constantly being developed and tested for their cytotoxicity and efficacy in clinical trials in CM [203].

There are several generations of epigenetic drugs. The first two generations of epi-therapies include DNMTis and HDACis, some of which have already gained FDA approval for the treatment of blood cancers [202]. Notably, these earliest generations of epigenome-targeted therapies were tailored according to the "one size fits all" principle, showing poor efficiency and selectivity and increased toxicity in CM patients [39]. However, clinical responses achieved with certain third-generation epigenetic agents designed according to precision medicine paradigms have provided new hope in the treatment of solid cancers [286,287]. Therefore, epi-drug development should follow a more personalized approach, with further identification of robust predictive biomarker selection and subsequent validation of this strategy in clinical studies [39]. Current literature highlights that, besides their use as monotherapy, epigenetic drugs may synergize with other anti-cancer compounds and reverse therapy resistance in both preclinical and clinical settings [236]. The administration of certain epigenetic drugs before chemotherapy or targeted therapy can be used for priming cancer cells to be more sensitive to these approaches, as epigenetic drugs can induce chromatin decompaction, making it more accessible to antineoplastic compounds [203]. A phase I clinical study (NCT01876641) has already shown that vemurafenib is more effective in CM patients when given in combination with decitabine in low doses. In line with these observations, the preclinical assessment reported activity of the combination and an increased potential in delaying the development of acquired resistance [212]. Moreover, co-administration of two epigenetic agents (such as DNMTi and HDACi) with different mechanisms of action may allow these compounds to increase each other's efficiency and overcome the issue of CM drug resistance [279]. Another rationale for using DNMTi in conjunction with HDACi is that such a combination may be extremely potent in stimulating the immune system to fight against tumors [39]. Finally, combinations of epigenetic agents with immunotherapy are currently tested in CM in clinical trials, holding promise to enhance antitumor immune responses or to reverse acquired resistance to ICIs. Even though most clinical studies have simple designs with both agents used simultaneously and continuously, epi-drugs and immunotherapy combinations are generally well tolerated in human subjects, in contrast to regimens incorporating targeted therapies and immunotherapies [39]. However, long-term use of certain epigenetic agents may have detrimental effects on antitumor immune response; for instance, prolonged use of BETi was linked with T cell depletion [288]. Therefore, to use these epigenetic drugs in immuno-oncology, more scientific effort is required to understand how the dose and scheduling of these therapies modulate the immune response and adverse effects in the clinical setting of melanoma management.

Author Contributions: Conceptualization, E.-G.D. and M.N.; writing—original draft preparation, E.-G.D.; writing—review and editing, M.N., C.C. and M.C.; supervision, M.N., C.C. and M.C.; funding acquisition, M.N. All authors have read and agreed to the published version of the manuscript.

Funding: This study was supported by the Core Program, implemented with the support of NASR, projects PN 19.29.01.01 grant PN-III-P1-1.2-PCCDI-2017-0341/2018. The authors also wish to acknowledge Horizon2020 funded projects COST 16120 (EPITRAN) and CA18127-International Nucleome Consortium (INC).

Institutional Review Board Statement: Not applicable.

Informed Consent Statement: Not applicable.

Data Availability Statement: Data sharing not applicable.

Acknowledgments: The present study will be integrated into the PhD thesis of the first author and PhD student Georgiana Dobre.

Conflicts of Interest: The authors declare no conflict of interest.

Abbreviations

MAPK—mitogen-activated protein kinase; OS—overall survival; ICIs—immune-checkpoint inhibitors; PD-1—anti-programmed death; CTLA-4—anti-cytotoxic T lymphocyte antigen; LDH—serum lactate dehydrogenase; S100—S-100 protein; MIA—melanoma inhibitory activity; PTMs—post-translational modifications; EZH2—enhancer of zeste 2 polycomb repressive complex 2 subunit; SWI/SNF—switch/sucrose non-fermentable chromatin remodeling complex; pCR—pathological complete response; CDKN2A—cyclin-dependent kinase inhibitor 2; CDK4—cyclin dependent kinase 4; RASSF1A—ras association domain family member; RAR-β2—retinoic acid receptor-beta; WIF-1—WNT inhibitory factor 1; Socs1—suppressor of cytokine signaling 1; TFPI2—tissue factor pathway inhibitor 2; KRTCAP3—keratinocyte associated protein 3; STAT3—signal transducer and activator of transcription 3; NF-κB—nuclear factor kappa B; AGAP2—Arf-GAP with GTPase, ANK repeat and PH domain-containing protein 2; ZNF490—zinc finger protein 490; TTC22—tetratricopeptide repeat protein 22; COL1A2—collagen type I alpha 2 chain; GPX3—glutathione peroxidase 3; CLDN11—claudin 11; CDH11—cadherin 11; PPP1R3C—protein phosphatase 1 regulatory subunit 3C; NPM2—nucleophosmin/nucleoplasmin 2; CCND1—cyclin D1; CCNE1—cyclin E1; E2F3—E2F transcription factor 3; JARID1B—jumonji AT-rich interactive domain 1B; TFPI2—tissue factor pathway inhibitor 2; IDH1/2—isocitrate dehydrogenase $\frac{1}{2}$; KDM1A—lysine demethylase 1A; APOBEC2—apolipoprotein B mRNA editing enzyme catalytic subunit 2; SETD4—SET domain containing 4; KDM5B—lysine demethylase 5B; POU3F2—POU class 3 homeobox 2; SOX9—SRY-box transcription factor 9; PDGFRA—Platelet derived growth factor receptor alpha; MITF—melanocyte inducing transcription factor; ZEB2—zinc finger E-box binding homeobox 2; TFAP2A—transcription factor AP-2 alpha; EHMT1—euchromatic histone lysine methyltransferase 1; RTKs—receptor tyrosine kinases; LEF1—lymphoid enhancer binding factor 1; TAP1—transporter associated with antigen processing 1; CD8—cluster of differentiation 8; DUSP4—dual specificity phosphatase 4; CCL3—chemokine (C-C motif) ligand 3; CXCL1—C-X-C motif chemokine ligand 1; TNFα—tumor necrosis factor alpha; p21CIP/WAF1—cyclin-dependent kinase inhibitor 1A.

References

1. Shain, A.H.; Bastian, B.C. From melanocytes to melanomas. *Nat. Rev. Cancer* **2016**, *16*, 345–358. [CrossRef] [PubMed]
2. Leonardi, G.C.; Falzone, L.; Salemi, R.; Zanghì, A.; Spandidos, D.A.; Mccubrey, J.A.; Candido, S.; Libra, M. Cutaneous melanoma: From pathogenesis to therapy (Review). *Int. J. Oncol.* **2018**, *52*, 1071–1080. [CrossRef] [PubMed]
3. Gershenwald, J.E.; Guy, G.P. Stemming the Rising Incidence of Melanoma: Calling Prevention to Action. *J. Natl. Cancer Inst.* **2016**, *108*, 381. [CrossRef]
4. Rebecca, V.W.; Somasundaram, R.; Herlyn, M. Pre-clinical modeling of cutaneous melanoma. *Nat. Commun.* **2020**, *11*, 2858. [CrossRef] [PubMed]
5. Chapman, P.B.; Hauschild, A.; Robert, C.; Haanen, J.B.; Ascierto, P.; Larkin, J.; Dummer, R.; Garbe, C.; Testori, A.; Maio, M.; et al. Improved survival with vemurafenib in melanoma with BRAF V600E mutation. *N. Engl. J. Med.* **2011**, *364*, 2507–2516. [CrossRef]
6. Long, G.V.; Weber, J.S.; Infante, J.R.; Kim, K.B.; Daud, A.; Gonzalez, R.; Sosman, J.A.; Hamid, O.; Schuchter, L.; Cebon, J.; et al. Overall Survival and Durable Responses in Patients With BRAF V600-Mutant Metastatic Melanoma Receiving Dabrafenib Combined With Trametinib. *J. Clin. Oncol. Off. J. Am. Soc. Clin. Oncol.* **2016**, *34*, 871–878. [CrossRef] [PubMed]
7. Long, G.V.; Schachter, J.; Ribas, A.; Arance, A.M.; Grob, J.-J.; Mortier, L.; Daud, A.; Carlino, M.S.; McNeil, C.M.; Lotem, M.; et al. 4-year survival and outcomes after cessation of pembrolizumab (pembro) after 2-years in patients (pts) with ipilimumab (ipi)-naive advanced melanoma in KEYNOTE-006. *J. Clin. Oncol.* **2018**, *36*, 9503. [CrossRef]
8. Hamid, O.; Robert, C.; Daud, A.; Hodi, F.S.; Hwu, W.J.; Kefford, R.; Wolchok, J.D.; Hersey, P.; Joseph, R.; Weber, J.S.; et al. Five-year survival outcomes for patients with advanced melanoma treated with pembrolizumab in KEYNOTE-001. *Ann. Oncol. Off. J. Eur. Soc. Med. Oncol.* **2019**, *30*, 582–588. [CrossRef]
9. Gallagher, S.J.; Tiffen, J.C.; Hersey, P. Histone Modifications, Modifiers and Readers in Melanoma Resistance to Targeted and Immune Therapy. *Cancers* **2015**, *7*, 1959–1982. [CrossRef]
10. Song, L.-B.; Zhang, Q.-J.; Hou, X.-Y.; Xiu, Y.-Y.; Chen, L.; Song, N.-H.; Lu, Y. A twelve-gene signature for survival prediction in malignant melanoma patients. *Ann. Transl. Med.* **2020**, *8*, 312. [CrossRef]
11. Reuben, A.; Spencer, C.N.; Prieto, P.A.; Gopalakrishnan, V.; Reddy, S.M.; Miller, J.P.; Mao, X.; De Macedo, M.P.; Chen, J.; Song, X.; et al. Genomic and immune heterogeneity are associated with differential responses to therapy in melanoma. *NPJ Genom. Med.* **2017**, *2*, 1–11. [CrossRef] [PubMed]

12. Uslu, U.; Schliep, S.; Schliep, K.; Erdmann, M.; Koch, H.-U.; Parsch, H.; Rosenheinrich, S.; Anzengruber, D.; Bosserhoff, A.K.; Schuler, G.; et al. Comparison of the Serum Tumor Markers S100 and Melanoma-inhibitory Activity (MIA) in the Monitoring of Patients with Metastatic Melanoma Receiving Vaccination Immunotherapy with Dendritic Cells. *Anticancer Res.* **2017**, *37*, 5033–5037. [CrossRef]
13. Neagu, M.; Constantin, C.; Zurac, S. Immune parameters in the prognosis and therapy monitoring of cutaneous melanoma patients: Experience, role, and limitations. *Biomed Res. Int.* **2013**, *2013*, 107940. [CrossRef] [PubMed]
14. Petrelli, F.; Ardito, R.; Merelli, B.; Lonati, V.; Cabiddu, M.; Seghezzi, S.; Barni, S.; Ghidini, A. Prognostic and predictive role of elevated lactate dehydrogenase in patients with melanoma treated with immunotherapy and BRAF inhibitors: A systematic review and meta-analysis. *Melanoma Res.* **2019**, *29*, 1–12. [CrossRef]
15. Georgescu, S.R.; Tampa, M.; Mitran, C.I.; Mitran, M.I.; Caruntu, C.; Caruntu, A.; Lupu, M.; Matei, C.; Constantin, C.; Neagu, M. Tumour Microenvironment in Skin Carcinogenesis. *Adv. Exp. Med. Biol.* **2020**, *1226*, 123–142. [CrossRef] [PubMed]
16. Clark, W.H.J.; Elder, D.E.; Guerry, D., 4th; Epstein, M.N.; Greene, M.H.; Van Horn, M. A study of tumor progression: The precursor lesions of superficial spreading and nodular melanoma. *Hum. Pathol.* **1984**, *15*, 1147–1165. [CrossRef]
17. Schiferle, E.B.; Cheon, S.Y.; Ham, S.; Son, H.G.; Messerschmidt, J.L.; Lawrence, D.P.; Cohen, J.V.; Flaherty, K.T.; Moon, J.J.; Lian, C.G.; et al. Rejection of benign melanocytic nevi by nevus-resident CD4(+) T cells. *Sci. Adv.* **2021**, *7*. [CrossRef] [PubMed]
18. Neagu, M.; Constantin, C.; Engin, A.B.; Popescu, I. Snapshot-changing melanocyte identity in melanoma developing route, 2020. *J. Cell Identity* **2020**, *1*, 33–47. [CrossRef]
19. Reiter, O.; Kurtansky, N.; Nanda, J.K.; Busam, K.J.; Scope, A.; Musthaq, S.; Marghoob, A.A. The differences in clinical and dermoscopic features between in situ and invasive nevus-associated melanomas and de novo melanomas. *J. Eur. Acad. Dermatol. Venereol.* **2021**, *35*, 1111–1118. [CrossRef]
20. Pampena, R.; Kyrgidis, A.; Lallas, A.; Moscarella, E.; Argenziano, G.; Longo, C. A meta-analysis of nevus-associated melanoma: Prevalence and practical implications. *J. Am. Acad. Dermatol.* **2017**, *77*, 938–945.e4. [CrossRef]
21. Vezzoni, R.; Conforti, C.; Vichi, S.; Giuffrida, R.; Retrosi, C.; Magaton-Rizzi, G.; Di Meo, N.; Pizzichetta, M.A.; Zalaudek, I. Is There More Than One Road to Nevus-Associated Melanoma? *Dermatol. Pract. Concept.* **2020**, *10*, e2020028. [CrossRef] [PubMed]
22. Cymerman, R.M.; Shao, Y.; Wang, K.; Zhang, Y.; Murzaku, E.C.; Penn, L.A.; Osman, I.; Polsky, D. De Novo vs. Nevus-Associated Melanomas: Differences in Associations With Prognostic Indicators and Survival. *J. Natl. Cancer Inst.* **2016**, *108*. [CrossRef] [PubMed]
23. de Souza, C.F.; Morais, A.S.; Jasiulionis, M.G. Biomarkers as Key Contributors in Treating Malignant Melanoma Metastases. *Dermatol. Res. Pract.* **2012**, *2012*, 156068. [CrossRef] [PubMed]
24. Feinberg, A.P.; Ohlsson, R.; Henikoff, S. The epigenetic progenitor origin of human cancer. *Nat. Rev. Genet.* **2006**, *7*, 21–33. [CrossRef]
25. Bruschi, M. The Epigenetic Progenitor Origin of Cancer Reassessed: DNA Methylation Brings Balance to the Stem Force. *Epigenomes* **2020**, *4*, 8. [CrossRef]
26. Voiculescu, V.M.; Lisievici, C.V.; Lupu, M.; Vajaitu, C.; Draghici, C.C.; Popa, A.V.; Solomon, I.; Sebe, T.I.; Constantin, M.M.; Caruntu, C. Mediators of Inflammation in Topical Therapy of Skin Cancers. *Mediat. Inflamm.* **2019**, *2019*, 8369690. [CrossRef] [PubMed]
27. Ciążyńska, M.; Olejniczak-Staruch, I.; Sobolewska-Sztychny, D.; Narbutt, J.; Skibińska, M.; Lesiak, A. Ultraviolet Radiation and Chronic Inflammation-Molecules and Mechanisms Involved in Skin Carcinogenesis: A Narrative Review. *Life* **2021**, *11*, 326. [CrossRef]
28. Neagu, M.; Constantin, C.; Caruntu, C.; Dumitru, C.; Surcel, M.; Zurac, S. Inflammation: A key process in skin tumorigenesis. *Oncol. Lett.* **2019**, *17*, 4068–4084. [CrossRef] [PubMed]
29. Sang, Y.; Deng, Y. Current insights into the epigenetic mechanisms of skin cancer. *Dermatol. Ther.* **2019**, *32*, e12964. [CrossRef] [PubMed]
30. Chen, W.; Cheng, P.; Jiang, J.; Ren, Y.; Wu, D.; Xue, D. Epigenomic and genomic analysis of transcriptome modulation in skin cutaneous melanoma. *Aging* **2020**, *12*, 12703–12725. [CrossRef]
31. Lee, J.J.; Murphy, G.F.; Lian, C.G. Melanoma epigenetics: Novel mechanisms, markers, and medicines. *Lab. Investig.* **2014**, *94*, 822–838. [CrossRef]
32. Besaratinia, A.; Tommasi, S. Epigenetics of human melanoma: Promises and challenges. *J. Mol. Cell Biol.* **2014**, *6*, 356–367. [CrossRef] [PubMed]
33. Lauss, M.; Ringnér, M.; Karlsson, A.; Harbst, K.; Busch, C.; Geisler, J.; Lønning, P.E.; Staaf, J.; Jönsson, G. DNA methylation subgroups in melanoma are associated with proliferative and immunological processes. *BMC Med. Genom.* **2015**, *8*, 73. [CrossRef] [PubMed]
34. Yamamoto, Y.; Matsusaka, K.; Fukuyo, M.; Rahmutulla, B.; Matsue, H.; Kaneda, A. Higher methylation subtype of malignant melanoma and its correlation with thicker progression and worse prognosis. *Cancer Med.* **2020**, *9*, 7194–7204. [CrossRef] [PubMed]
35. Wilmott, J.S.; Colebatch, A.J.; Kakavand, H.; Shang, P.; Carlino, M.S.; Thompson, J.F.; Long, G.V.; Scolyer, R.A.; Hersey, P. Expression of the class 1 histone deacetylases HDAC8 and 3 are associated with improved survival of patients with metastatic melanoma. *Mod. Pathol. Off. J. USA Can. Acad. Pathol. Inc.* **2015**, *28*, 884–894. [CrossRef] [PubMed]

36. Park, W.-Y.; Hong, B.-J.; Lee, J.; Choi, C.; Kim, M.-Y. H3K27 Demethylase JMJD3 Employs the NF-κB and BMP Signaling Pathways to Modulate the Tumor Microenvironment and Promote Melanoma Progression and Metastasis. *Cancer Res.* **2016**, *76*, 161–170. [CrossRef] [PubMed]
37. Lee, J.J.; Sholl, L.M.; Lindeman, N.I.; Granter, S.R.; Laga, A.C.; Shivdasani, P.; Chin, G.; Luke, J.J.; Ott, P.A.; Hodi, F.S.; et al. Targeted next-generation sequencing reveals high frequency of mutations in epigenetic regulators across treatment-naïve patient melanomas. *Clin. Epigenetics* **2015**, *7*, 59. [CrossRef] [PubMed]
38. Bossi, D.; Cicalese, A.; Dellino, G.I.; Luzi, L.; Riva, L.; D'Alesio, C.; Diaferia, G.R.; Carugo, A.; Cavallaro, E.; Piccioni, R.; et al. In Vivo Genetic Screens of Patient-Derived Tumors Revealed Unexpected Frailty of the Transformed Phenotype. *Cancer Discov.* **2016**, *6*, 650–663. [CrossRef] [PubMed]
39. Morel, D.; Jeffery, D.; Aspeslagh, S.; Almouzni, G.; Postel-Vinay, S. Combining epigenetic drugs with other therapies for solid tumours past lessons and future promise. *Nat. Rev. Clin. Oncol.* **2020**, *17*, 91–107. [CrossRef]
40. Sharma, S.; Kelly, T.K.; Jones, P.A. Epigenetics in cancer. *Carcinogenesis* **2010**, *31*, 27–36. [CrossRef] [PubMed]
41. Payer, B.; Lee, J.T.; Namekawa, S.H. X-inactivation and X-reactivation: Epigenetic hallmarks of mammalian reproduction and pluripotent stem cells. *Hum. Genet.* **2011**, *130*, 265–280. [CrossRef]
42. Dobre, E.-G.; Dinescu, S.; Costache, M. Connecting the missing dots: Ncrnas as critical regulators of therapeutic susceptibility in breast cancer. *Cancers* **2020**, *12*, 2698. [CrossRef] [PubMed]
43. Ferrand, J.; Rondinelli, B.; Polo, S.E. Histone Variants: Guardians of Genome Integrity. *Cells* **2020**, *9*, 2424. [CrossRef]
44. Hasan, N.; Ahuja, N. The Emerging Roles of ATP-Dependent Chromatin Remodeling Complexes in Pancreatic Cancer. *Cancers* **2019**, *11*, 1859. [CrossRef]
45. Dueñas-González, A.; Lizano, M.; Candelaria, M.; Cetina, L.; Arce, C.; Cervera, E. Epigenetics of cervical cancer. An overview and therapeutic perspectives. *Mol. Cancer* **2005**, *4*, 1–24. [CrossRef] [PubMed]
46. Mitsis, T.; Efthimiadou, A.; Bacopoulou, F.; Vlachakis, D.; Chrousos, G.; Eliopoulos, E. Transcription factors and evolution: An integral part of gene expression (Review). *World Acad. Sci. J.* **2020**, *2*, 3–8. [CrossRef]
47. Gillette, T.G.; Hill, J.A. Readers, writers, and erasers: Chromatin as the whiteboard of heart disease. *Circ. Res.* **2015**, *116*, 1245–1253. [CrossRef]
48. Hoffmann, F.; Zarbl, R.; Niebel, D.; Sirokay, J.; Fröhlich, A.; Posch, C.; Holderried, T.A.W.; Brossart, P.; Saavedra, G.; Kuster, P.; et al. Prognostic and predictive value of PD-L2 DNA methylation and mRNA expression in melanoma. *Clin. Epigenetics* **2020**, *12*, 94. [CrossRef] [PubMed]
49. Grigore, F.; Yang, H.; Hanson, N.D.; VanBrocklin, M.W.; Sarver, A.L.; Robinson, J.P. BRAF inhibition in melanoma is associated with the dysregulation of histone methylation and histone methyltransferases. *Neoplasia* **2020**, *22*, 376–389. [CrossRef] [PubMed]
50. Esteller, M. CpG island hypermethylation and tumor suppressor genes: A booming present, a brighter future. *Oncogene* **2002**, *21*, 5427–5440. [CrossRef]
51. Fatemi, M.; Pao, M.M.; Jeong, S.; Gal-Yam, E.N.; Egger, G.; Weisenberger, D.J.; Jones, P.A. Footprinting of mammalian promoters: Use of a CpG DNA methyltransferase revealing nucleosome positions at a single molecule level. *Nucleic Acids Res.* **2005**, *33*, e176. [CrossRef]
52. Shen, H.; Laird, P.W. Interplay between the cancer genome and epigenome. *Cell* **2013**, *153*, 38–55. [CrossRef]
53. Jin, B.; Robertson, K.D. DNA methyltransferases, DNA damage repair, and cancer. *Adv. Exp. Med. Biol.* **2013**, *754*, 3–29. [CrossRef] [PubMed]
54. Kulis, M.; Esteller, M. DNA methylation and cancer. *Adv. Genet.* **2010**, *70*, 27–56. [CrossRef]
55. Kohli, R.M.; Zhang, Y. TET enzymes, TDG and the dynamics of DNA demethylation. *Nature* **2013**, *502*, 472–479. [CrossRef]
56. Stenz, L.; Schechter, D.S.; Serpa, S.R.; Paoloni-Giacobino, A. Intergenerational Transmission of DNA Methylation Signatures Associated with Early Life Stress. *Curr. Genom.* **2018**, *19*, 665–675. [CrossRef]
57. Emran, A.A.; Chatterjee, A.; Rodger, E.J.; Tiffen, J.C.; Gallagher, S.J.; Eccles, M.R.; Hersey, P. Targeting DNA Methylation and EZH2 Activity to Overcome Melanoma Resistance to Immunotherapy. *Trends Immunol.* **2019**, *40*, 328–344. [CrossRef]
58. Gross, D.S.; Chowdhary, S.; Anandhakumar, J.; Kainth, A.S. Chromatin. *Curr. Biol.* **2015**, *25*, R1158–R1163. [CrossRef] [PubMed]
59. Hammerlindl, H.; Schaider, H. Epigenetics in Melanoma Development and Drug Resistance. In *Human Skin Cancers Pathways, Mechanisms, Targets and Treatments*; InTech: Tokyo, Japan, 2018.
60. Greer, E.L.; Shi, Y. Histone methylation: A dynamic mark in health, disease and inheritance. *Nat. Rev. Genet.* **2012**, *13*, 343–357. [CrossRef]
61. Aparicio Pelaz, D.; Yerkesh, Z.; Kirchgäßner, S.; Mahler, H.; Kharchenko, V.; Azhibek, D.; Jaremko, M.; Mootz, H.D.; Jaremko, Ł.; Schwarzer, D.; et al. Examining histone modification crosstalk using immobilized libraries established from ligation-ready nucleosomes. *Chem. Sci.* **2020**, *11*, 9218–9225. [CrossRef] [PubMed]
62. Zhao, Z.; Shilatifard, A. Epigenetic modifications of histones in cancer. *Genome Biol.* **2019**, *20*, 1–16. [CrossRef] [PubMed]
63. Pradeepa, M.M. Causal role of histone acetylations in enhancer function. *Transcription* **2017**, *8*, 40–47. [CrossRef]
64. Kumar, D.; Jothi, R. Bivalent chromatin protects reversibly repressed genes from irreversible silencing. *bioRxiv* **2020**. [CrossRef]
65. Dunican, D.S.; Mjoseng, H.K.; Duthie, L.; Flyamer, I.M.; Bickmore, W.A.; Meehan, R.R. Bivalent promoter hypermethylation in cancer is linked to the H327me3/H3K4me3 ratio in embryonic stem cells. *BMC Biol.* **2020**, *18*, 25. [CrossRef]
66. Ghosh, K.; O'Neil, K.; Capell, B.C. Histone modifiers: Dynamic regulators of the cutaneous transcriptome. *J. Dermatol. Sci.* **2018**, *89*, 226–232. [CrossRef]

67. Calcagno, D.Q.; Gigek, C.O.; Chen, E.S.; Burbano, R.R.; de Arruda Cardoso Smith, M. DNA and histone methylation in gastric carcinogenesis. *World J. Gastroenterol.* **2013**, *19*, 1182–1192. [CrossRef] [PubMed]
68. Yeon, M.; Kim, Y.; Jung, H.S.; Jeoung, D. Histone Deacetylase Inhibitors to Overcome Resistance to Targeted and Immuno Therapy in Metastatic Melanoma. *Front. Cell Dev. Biol.* **2020**, *8*, 486. [CrossRef] [PubMed]
69. Azevedo, H.; Pessoa, G.C.; De Luna Vitorino, F.N.; Nsengimana, J.; Newton-Bishop, J.; Reis, E.M.; Da Cunha, J.P.C.; Jasiulionis, M.G. Gene co-expression and histone modification signatures are associated with melanoma progression, epithelial-to-mesenchymal transition, and metastasis. *Clin. Epigenetics* **2020**, *12*, 127. [CrossRef] [PubMed]
70. Farooqi, A.A.; Fayyaz, S.; Poltronieri, P.; Calin, G.; Mallardo, M. Epigenetic deregulation in cancer: Enzyme players and non-coding RNAs. *Semin. Cancer Biol.* **2020**. [CrossRef]
71. de Unamuno Bustos, B.; Murria Estal, R.; Pérez Simó, G.; Simarro Farinos, J.; Pujol Marco, C.; Navarro Mira, M.; Alegre de Miquel, V.; Ballester Sánchez, R.; Sabater Marco, V.; Llavador Ros, M.; et al. Aberrant DNA methylation is associated with aggressive clinicopathological features and poor survival in cutaneous melanoma. *Br. J. Dermatol.* **2018**, *179*, 394–404. [CrossRef]
72. Kampilafkos, P.; Melachrinou, M.; Kefalopoulou, Z.; Lakoumentas, J.; Sotiropoulou-Bonikou, G. Epigenetic modifications in cutaneous malignant melanoma: EZH2, H3K4me2, and H3K27me3 immunohistochemical expression is enhanced at the invasion front of the tumor. *Am. J. Dermatopathol.* **2015**, *37*, 138–144. [CrossRef]
73. Maitituoheti, M.; Keung, E.Z.; Tang, M.; Yan, L.; Alam, H.; Han, G.; Singh, A.K.; Raman, A.T.; Terranova, C.; Sarkar, S.; et al. Enhancer Reprogramming Confers Dependence on Glycolysis and IGF Signaling in KMT2D Mutant Melanoma. *Cell Rep.* **2020**, *33*, 108293. [CrossRef] [PubMed]
74. Neagu, M.; Constantin, C.; Cretoiu, S.M.; Zurac, S. miRNAs in the Diagnosis and Prognosis of Skin Cancer. *Front. Cell Dev. Biol.* **2020**, *8*, 71. [CrossRef] [PubMed]
75. Yu, Y.; Schleich, K.; Yue, B.; Ji, S.; Lohneis, P.; Kemper, K.; Silvis, M.R.; Qutob, N.; van Rooijen, E.; Werner-Klein, M.; et al. Targeting the Senescence-Overriding Cooperative Activity of Structurally Unrelated H3K9 Demethylases in Melanoma. *Cancer Cell* **2018**, *33*, 322–336.e8. [CrossRef] [PubMed]
76. Zingg, D.; Debbache, J.; Schaefer, S.M.; Tuncer, E.; Frommel, S.C.; Cheng, P.; Arenas-Ramirez, N.; Haeusel, J.; Zhang, Y.; Bonalli, M.; et al. The epigenetic modifier EZH2 controls melanoma growth and metastasis through silencing of distinct tumour suppressors. *Nat. Commun.* **2015**, *6*, 6051. [CrossRef] [PubMed]
77. Zingg, D.; Debbache, J.; Peña-Hernández, R.; Antunes, A.T.; Schaefer, S.M.; Cheng, P.F.; Zimmerli, D.; Haeusel, J.; Calçada, R.R.; Tuncer, E.; et al. EZH2-Mediated Primary Cilium Deconstruction Drives Metastatic Melanoma Formation. *Cancer Cell* **2018**, *34*, 69–84.e14. [CrossRef]
78. Liu, X.; Zhang, S.-M.; McGeary, M.K.; Krykbaeva, I.; Lai, L.; Jansen, D.J.; Kales, S.C.; Simeonov, A.; Hall, M.D.; Kelly, D.P.; et al. KDM5B Promotes Drug Resistance by Regulating Melanoma-Propagating Cell Subpopulations. *Mol. Cancer Ther.* **2019**, *18*, 706–717. [CrossRef] [PubMed]
79. Licht, J.D.; Bennett, R.L. Leveraging epigenetics to enhance the efficacy of immunotherapy. *Clin. Epigenetics* **2021**, *13*, 115. [CrossRef]
80. Maiuri, A.R.; O'Hagan, H.M. Interplay Between Inflammation and Epigenetic Changes in Cancer. *Prog. Mol. Biol. Transl. Sci.* **2016**, *144*, 69–117. [CrossRef]
81. Maes, K.; Mondino, A.; Lasarte, J.J.; Agirre, X.; Vanderkerken, K.; Prosper, F.; Breckpot, K. Epigenetic Modifiers: Anti-Neoplastic Drugs With Immunomodulating Potential. *Front. Immunol.* **2021**, *12*, 652160. [CrossRef] [PubMed]
82. Kominsky, D.J.; Campbell, E.L.; Colgan, S.P. Metabolic shifts in immunity and inflammation. *J. Immunol.* **2010**, *184*, 4062–4068. [CrossRef]
83. Johnson, C.; Warmoes, M.O.; Shen, X.; Locasale, J.W. Epigenetics and cancer metabolism. *Cancer Lett.* **2015**, *356*, 309–314. [CrossRef] [PubMed]
84. Franco, R.; Schoneveld, O.; Georgakilas, A.G.; Panayiotidis, M.I. Oxidative stress, DNA methylation and carcinogenesis. *Cancer Lett.* **2008**, *266*, 6–11. [CrossRef]
85. Fan, Y.; Mao, R.; Yang, J. NF-κB and STAT3 signaling pathways collaboratively link inflammation to cancer. *Protein Cell* **2013**, *4*, 176–185. [CrossRef]
86. Micevic, G.; Theodosakis, N.; Bosenberg, M. Aberrant DNA methylation in melanoma: Biomarker and therapeutic opportunities. *Clin. Epigenetics* **2017**, *9*, 34. [CrossRef]
87. Howell, P.M.J.; Liu, S.; Ren, S.; Behlen, C.; Fodstad, O.; Riker, A.I. Epigenetics in human melanoma. *Cancer Control* **2009**, *16*, 200–218. [CrossRef] [PubMed]
88. Hoon, D.S.B.; Spugnardi, M.; Kuo, C.; Huang, S.K.; Morton, D.L.; Taback, B. Profiling epigenetic inactivation of tumor suppressor genes in tumors and plasma from cutaneous melanoma patients. *Oncogene* **2004**, *23*, 4014–4022. [CrossRef] [PubMed]
89. Palanca-Ballester, C.; Rodriguez-Casanova, A.; Torres, S.; Calabuig-Fariñas, S.; Exposito, F.; Serrano, D.; Redin, E.; Valencia, K.; Jantus-Lewintre, E.; Diaz-Lagares, A.; et al. Cancer Epigenetic Biomarkers in Liquid Biopsy for High Incidence Malignancies. *Cancers* **2021**, *13*, 3016. [CrossRef] [PubMed]
90. Tanemura, A.; Terando, A.M.; Sim, M.-S.; van Hoesel, A.Q.; de Maat, M.F.G.; Morton, D.L.; Hoon, D.S.B. CpG island methylator phenotype predicts progression of malignant melanoma. *Clin. cancer Res. an Off. J. Am. Assoc. Cancer Res.* **2009**, *15*, 1801–1807. [CrossRef]

91. Garcia-Alvarez, A.; Ortiz, C.; Muñoz-Couselo, E. Current Perspectives and Novel Strategies of NRAS-Mutant Melanoma. *Onco. Targets. Ther.* **2021**, *14*, 3709–3719. [CrossRef] [PubMed]
92. Ehrlich, M. DNA hypomethylation in cancer cells. *Epigenomics* **2009**, *1*, 239–259. [CrossRef]
93. Ponomaryova, A.A.; Rykova, E.Y.; Gervas, P.A.; Cherdyntseva, N.V.; Mamedov, I.Z.; Azhikina, T.L. Aberrant Methylation of LINE-1 Transposable Elements: A Search for Cancer Biomarkers. *Cells* **2020**, *9*, 2017. [CrossRef] [PubMed]
94. Ecsedi, S.I.; Hernandez-Vargas, H.; Lima, S.C.; Herceg, Z.; Adany, R.; Balazs, M. Transposable hypomethylation is associated with metastatic capacity of primary melanomas. *Int. J. Clin. Exp. Pathol.* **2013**, *6*, 2943–2948. [PubMed]
95. De Araújo, É.S.S.; Kashiwabara, A.Y.; Achatz, M.I.W.; Moredo, L.F.; De Sá, B.C.S.; Duprat, J.P.; Rosenberg, C.; Carraro, D.M.; Krepischi, A.C. V LINE-1 hypermethylation in peripheral blood of cutaneous melanoma patients is associated with metastasis. *Melanoma Res.* **2015**, *25*, 173–177. [CrossRef] [PubMed]
96. Sigalotti, L.; Fratta, E.; Bidoli, E.; Covre, A.; Parisi, G.; Colizzi, F.; Coral, S.; Massarut, S.; Kirkwood, J.M.; Maio, M. Methylation levels of the "long interspersed nucleotide element-1" repetitive sequences predict survival of melanoma patients. *J. Transl. Med.* **2011**, *9*, 78. [CrossRef] [PubMed]
97. Tonella, L.; Pala, V.; Ponti, R.; Rubatto, M.; Gallo, G.; Mastorino, L.; Avallone, G.; Merli, M.; Agostini, A.; Fava, P.; et al. Prognostic and Predictive Biomarkers in Stage III Melanoma: Current Insights and Clinical Implications. *Int. J. Mol. Sci.* **2021**, *22*, 4561. [CrossRef] [PubMed]
98. Colemon, A.; Harris, T.M.; Ramanathan, S. DNA hypomethylation drives changes in MAGE-A gene expression resulting in alteration of proliferative status of cells. *Genes Environ. Off. J. Japanese Environ. Mutagen Soc.* **2020**, *42*, 24. [CrossRef]
99. Faramarzi, S.; Ghafouri-Fard, S. Melanoma: A prototype of cancer-testis antigen-expressing malignancies. *Immunotherapy* **2017**, *9*, 1103–1113. [CrossRef]
100. Sigalotti, L.; Coral, S.; Nardi, G.; Spessotto, A.; Cortini, E.; Cattarossi, I.; Colizzi, F.; Altomonte, M.; Maio, M. Promoter methylation controls the expression of MAGE2, 3 and 4 genes in human cutaneous melanoma. *J. Immunother.* **2002**, *25*, 16–26. [CrossRef] [PubMed]
101. Sigalotti, L.; Covre, A.; Zabierowski, S.; Himes, B.; Colizzi, F.; Natali, P.G.; Herlyn, M.; Maio, M. Cancer testis antigens in human melanoma stem cells: Expression, distribution, and methylation status. *J. Cell. Physiol.* **2008**, *215*, 287–291. [CrossRef]
102. Danilova, A.; Misyurin, V.; Novik, A.; Girdyuk, D.; Avdonkina, N.; Nekhaeva, T.; Emelyanova, N.; Pipia, N.; Misyurin, A.; Baldueva, I. Cancer/testis antigens expression during cultivation of melanoma and soft tissue sarcoma cells. *Clin. Sarcoma Res.* **2020**, *10*, 3. [CrossRef] [PubMed]
103. Fujiwara, S.; Nagai, H.; Jimbo, H.; Jimbo, N.; Tanaka, T.; Inoie, M.; Nishigori, C. Gene Expression and Methylation Analysis in Melanomas and Melanocytes From the Same Patient: Loss of NPM2 Expression Is a Potential Immunohistochemical Marker for Melanoma. *Front. Oncol.* **2018**, *8*, 675. [CrossRef] [PubMed]
104. Gao, L.; van den Hurk, K.; Moerkerk, P.T.M.; Goeman, J.J.; Beck, S.; Gruis, N.A.; van den Oord, J.J.; Winnepenninckx, V.J.; van Engeland, M.; van Doorn, R. Promoter CpG island hypermethylation in dysplastic nevus and melanoma: CLDN11 as an epigenetic biomarker for malignancy. *J. Invest. Dermatol.* **2014**, *134*, 2957–2966. [CrossRef]
105. Marzese, D.M.; Scolyer, R.A.; Huynh, J.L.; Huang, S.K.; Hirose, H.; Chong, K.K.; Kiyohara, E.; Wang, J.; Kawas, N.P.; Donovan, N.C.; et al. Epigenome-wide DNA methylation landscape of melanoma progression to brain metastasis reveals aberrations on homeobox D cluster associated with prognosis. *Hum. Mol. Genet.* **2014**, *23*, 226–238. [CrossRef] [PubMed]
106. Lian, C.G.; Xu, Y.; Ceol, C.; Wu, F.; Larson, A.; Dresser, K.; Xu, W.; Tan, L.; Hu, Y.; Zhan, Q.; et al. Loss of 5-hydroxymethylcytosine is an epigenetic hallmark of melanoma. *Cell* **2012**, *150*, 1135–1146. [CrossRef] [PubMed]
107. Saldanha, G.; Joshi, K.; Lawes, K.; Bamford, M.; Moosa, F.; Teo, K.W.; Pringle, J.H. 5-Hydroxymethylcytosine is an independent predictor of survival in malignant melanoma. *Mod. Pathol. Off. J. United States Can. Acad. Pathol. Inc* **2017**, *30*, 60–68. [CrossRef] [PubMed]
108. Khaliq, M.; Fallahi-Sichani, M. Epigenetic Mechanisms of Escape from BRAF Oncogene Dependency. *Cancers* **2019**, *11*, 1480. [CrossRef] [PubMed]
109. Strub, T.; Ballotti, R.; Bertolotto, C. The "ART" of Epigenetics in Melanoma: From histone "Alterations, to Resistance and Therapies". *Theranostics* **2020**, *10*, 1777–1797. [CrossRef] [PubMed]
110. Frantz, W.T.; Ceol, C.J. From Tank to Treatment: Modeling Melanoma in Zebrafish. *Cells* **2020**, *9*, 1289. [CrossRef] [PubMed]
111. Patton, E.E.; Widlund, H.R.; Kutok, J.L.; Kopani, K.R.; Amatruda, J.F.; Murphey, R.D.; Berghmans, S.; Mayhall, E.A.; Traver, D.; Fletcher, C.D.M.; et al. BRAF mutations are sufficient to promote nevi formation and cooperate with p53 in the genesis of melanoma. *Curr. Biol.* **2005**, *15*, 249–254. [CrossRef]
112. Scahill, C.M.; Digby, Z.; Sealy, I.M.; Wojciechowska, S.; White, R.J.; Collins, J.E.; Stemple, D.L.; Bartke, T.; Mathers, M.E.; Patton, E.E.; et al. Loss of the chromatin modifier Kdm2aa causes BrafV600E-independent spontaneous melanoma in zebrafish. *PLoS Genet.* **2017**, *13*, e1006959. [CrossRef]
113. Herz, H.-M.; Mohan, M.; Garruss, A.S.; Liang, K.; Takahashi, Y.-H.; Mickey, K.; Voets, O.; Verrijzer, C.P.; Shilatifard, A. Enhancer-associated H3K4 monomethylation by Trithorax-related, the Drosophila homolog of mammalian Mll3/Mll4. *Genes Dev.* **2012**, *26*, 2604–2620. [CrossRef] [PubMed]
114. Wang, C.; Lee, J.-E.; Lai, B.; Macfarlan, T.S.; Xu, S.; Zhuang, L.; Liu, C.; Peng, W.; Ge, K. Enhancer priming by H3K4 methyltransferase MLL4 controls cell fate transition. *Proc. Natl. Acad. Sci. USA* **2016**, *113*, 11871–11876. [CrossRef] [PubMed]

115. Cheng, C.S.; Rai, K.; Garber, M.; Hollinger, A.; Robbins, D.; Anderson, S.; Macbeth, A.; Tzou, A.; Carneiro, M.O.; Raychowdhury, R.; et al. Semiconductor-based DNA sequencing of histone modification states. *Nat. Commun.* **2013**, *4*, 2672. [CrossRef] [PubMed]
116. Gu, B.; Lee, M.G. Histone H3 lysine 4 methyltransferases and demethylases in self-renewal and differentiation of stem cells. *Cell Biosci.* **2013**, *3*, 39. [CrossRef] [PubMed]
117. Bernstein, B.E.; Kamal, M.; Lindblad-Toh, K.; Bekiranov, S.; Bailey, D.K.; Huebert, D.J.; McMahon, S.; Karlsson, E.K.; Kulbokas, E.J., 3rd; Gingeras, T.R.; et al. Genomic maps and comparative analysis of histone modifications in human and mouse. *Cell* **2005**, *120*, 169–181. [CrossRef]
118. Uzdensky, A.; Demyanenko, S.; Bibov, M.; Sharifulina, S.; Kit, O.; Przhedetski, Y.; Pozdnyakova, V. Expression of proteins involved in epigenetic regulation in human cutaneous melanoma and peritumoral skin. *Tumour Biol. J. Int. Soc. Oncodevelopmental Biol. Med.* **2014**, *35*, 8225–8233. [CrossRef]
119. Terranova, C.; Tang, M.; Maitituoheti, M.; Raman, A.T.; Schulz, J.; Amin, S.B.; Orouji, E.; Tomczak, K.; Sarkar, S.; Oba, J.; et al. Bivalent and broad chromatin domains regulate pro-metastatic drivers in melanoma. *bioRxiv* **2019**, 721480. [CrossRef]
120. Neagu, M.; Constantin, C.; Bostan, M.; Caruntu, C.; Ignat, S.R.; Dinescu, S.; Costache, M. Proteomic Technology "Lens" for Epithelial-Mesenchymal Transition Process Identification in Oncology. *Anal. Cell. Pathol.* **2019**, *2019*, 3565970. [CrossRef]
121. Hoffmann, F.; Niebel, D.; Aymans, P.; Ferring-Schmitt, S.; Dietrich, D.; Landsberg, J. H3K27me3 and EZH2 expression in melanoma: Relevance for melanoma progression and response to immune checkpoint blockade. *Clin. Epigenetics* **2020**, *12*, 24. [CrossRef] [PubMed]
122. McHugh, J.B.; Fullen, D.R.; Ma, L.; Kleer, C.G.; Su, L.D. Expression of polycomb group protein EZH2 in nevi and melanoma. *J. Cutan. Pathol.* **2007**, *34*, 597–600. [CrossRef]
123. Bachmann, I.M.; Halvorsen, O.J.; Collett, K.; Stefansson, I.M.; Straume, O.; Haukaas, S.A.; Salvesen, H.B.; Otte, A.P.; Akslen, L.A. EZH2 expression is associated with high proliferation rate and aggressive tumor subgroups in cutaneous melanoma and cancers of the endometrium, prostate, and breast. *J. Clin. Oncol. Off. J. Am. Soc. Clin. Oncol.* **2006**, *24*, 268–273. [CrossRef] [PubMed]
124. Fan, T.; Jiang, S.; Chung, N.; Alikhan, A.; Ni, C.; Lee, C.-C.R.; Hornyak, T.J. EZH2-dependent suppression of a cellular senescence phenotype in melanoma cells by inhibition of p21/CDKN1A expression. *Mol. Cancer Res.* **2011**, *9*, 418–429. [CrossRef] [PubMed]
125. De Donatis, G.M.; Le Pape, E.; Pierron, A.; Cheli, Y.; Hofman, V.; Hofman, P.; Allegra, M.; Zahaf, K.; Bahadoran, P.; Rocchi, S.; et al. NF-kB2 induces senescence bypass in melanoma via a direct transcriptional activation of EZH2. *Oncogene* **2016**, *35*, 2735–2745. [CrossRef] [PubMed]
126. Barsotti, A.M.; Ryskin, M.; Zhong, W.; Zhang, W.-G.; Giannakou, A.; Loreth, C.; Diesl, V.; Follettie, M.; Golas, J.; Lee, M.; et al. Epigenetic reprogramming by tumor-derived EZH2 gain-of-function mutations promotes aggressive 3D cell morphologies and enhances melanoma tumor growth. *Oncotarget* **2015**, *6*, 2928–2938. [CrossRef] [PubMed]
127. Ceol, C.J.; Houvras, Y.; Jane-Valbuena, J.; Bilodeau, S.; Orlando, D.A.; Battisti, V.; Fritsch, L.; Lin, W.M.; Hollmann, T.J.; Ferré, F.; et al. The histone methyltransferase SETDB1 is recurrently amplified in melanoma and accelerates its onset. *Nature* **2011**, *471*, 513–517. [CrossRef] [PubMed]
128. Schultz, D.C.; Ayyanathan, K.; Negorev, D.; Maul, G.G.; Rauscher, F.J. 3rd SETDB1: A novel KAP-1-associated histone H3, lysine 9-specific methyltransferase that contributes to HP1-mediated silencing of euchromatic genes by KRAB zinc-finger proteins. *Genes Dev.* **2002**, *16*, 919–932. [CrossRef] [PubMed]
129. Orouji, E.; Utikal, J. Tackling malignant melanoma epigenetically: Histone lysine methylation. *Clin. Epigenetics* **2018**, *10*, 145. [CrossRef]
130. Kostaki, M.; Manona, A.D.; Stavraka, I.; Korkolopoulou, P.; Levidou, G.; Trigka, E.-A.; Christofidou, E.; Champsas, G.; Stratigos, A.J.; Katsambas, A.; et al. High-frequency p16(INK)(4A) promoter methylation is associated with histone methyltransferase SETDB1 expression in sporadic cutaneous melanoma. *Exp. Dermatol.* **2014**, *23*, 332–338. [CrossRef]
131. Orouji, E.; Federico, A.; Larribère, L.; Novak, D.; Lipka, D.B.; Assenov, Y.; Sachindra, S.; Hüser, L.; Granados, K.; Gebhardt, C.; et al. Histone methyltransferase SETDB1 contributes to melanoma tumorigenesis and serves as a new potential therapeutic target. *Int. J. Cancer* **2019**, *145*, 3462–3477. [CrossRef]
132. Trivedi, A.; Mehrotra, A.; Baum, C.E.; Lewis, B.; Basuroy, T.; Blomquist, T.; Trumbly, R.; Filipp, F.V.; Setaluri, V.; De La Serna, I.L. Bromodomain and extra-terminal domain (BET) proteins regulate melanocyte differentiation. *Epigenetics Chromatin* **2020**, *13*, 1–18. [CrossRef] [PubMed]
133. Denis, G.V.; McComb, M.E.; Faller, D.V.; Sinha, A.; Romesser, P.B.; Costello, C.E. Identification of transcription complexes that contain the double bromodomain protein Brd2 and chromatin remodeling machines. *J. Proteome Res.* **2006**, *5*, 502–511. [CrossRef] [PubMed]
134. Segura, M.F.; Fontanals-Cirera, B.; Gaziel-Sovran, A.; Guijarro, M.V.; Hanniford, D.; Zhang, G.; González-Gomez, P.; Morante, M.; Jubierre, L.; Zhang, W.; et al. BRD4 sustains melanoma proliferation and represents a new target for epigenetic therapy. *Cancer Res.* **2013**, *73*, 6264–6276. [CrossRef]
135. Li, Y.; Seto, E. HDACs and HDAC Inhibitors in Cancer Development and Therapy. *Cold Spring Harb. Perspect. Med.* **2016**, *6*. [CrossRef] [PubMed]
136. Fiziev, P.; Akdemir, K.C.; Miller, J.P.; Keung, E.Z.; Samant, N.S.; Sharma, S.; Natale, C.A.; Terranova, C.J.; Maitituoheti, M.; Amin, S.B.; et al. Systematic Epigenomic Analysis Reveals Chromatin States Associated with Melanoma Progression. *Cell Rep.* **2017**, *19*, 875–889. [CrossRef] [PubMed]

137. Hu, Z.; Rong, Y.; Li, S.; Qu, S.; Huang, S. Upregulated Histone Deacetylase 6 Associates with Malignant Progression of Melanoma and Predicts the Prognosis of Patients. *Cancer Manag. Res.* **2020**, *12*, 12993–13001. [CrossRef] [PubMed]
138. Liu, J.; Gu, J.; Feng, Z.; Yang, Y.; Zhu, N.; Lu, W.; Qi, F. Both HDAC5 and HDAC6 are required for the proliferation and metastasis of melanoma cells. *J. Transl. Med.* **2016**, *14*, 7. [CrossRef] [PubMed]
139. Wilking, M.J.; Singh, C.; Nihal, M.; Zhong, W.; Ahmad, N. SIRT1 deacetylase is overexpressed in human melanoma and its small molecule inhibition imparts anti-proliferative response via p53 activation. *Arch. Biochem. Biophys.* **2014**, *563*, 94–100. [CrossRef]
140. Sun, T.; Jiao, L.; Wang, Y.; Yu, Y.; Ming, L. SIRT1 induces epithelial-mesenchymal transition by promoting autophagic degradation of E-cadherin in melanoma cells article. *Cell Death Dis.* **2018**, *9*, 1–10. [CrossRef]
141. George, J.; Nihal, M.; Singh, C.K.; Zhong, W.; Liu, X.; Ahmad, N. Pro-Proliferative Function of Mitochondrial Sirtuin Deacetylase SIRT3 in Human Melanoma. *J. Invest. Dermatol.* **2016**, *136*, 809–818. [CrossRef] [PubMed]
142. Garcia-Peterson, L.M.; Ndiaye, M.A.; Singh, C.K.; Chhabra, G.; Huang, W.; Ahmad, N. SIRT6 histone deacetylase functions as a potential oncogene in human melanoma. *Genes Cancer* **2017**, *8*, 701–712. [CrossRef]
143. George, J.; Nihal, M.; Singh, C.K.; Ahmad, N. 4′-Bromo-resveratrol, a dual Sirtuin-1 and Sirtuin-3 inhibitor, inhibits melanoma cell growth through mitochondrial metabolic reprogramming. *Mol. Carcinog.* **2019**, *58*, 1876–1885. [CrossRef] [PubMed]
144. Kuźbicki, L.; Lange, D.; Strączyńska-Niemiec, A.; Chwirot, B.W. JARID1B expression in human melanoma and benign melanocytic skin lesions. *Melanoma Res.* **2013**, *23*, 8–12. [CrossRef] [PubMed]
145. Roesch, A.; Becker, B.; Meyer, S.; Wild, P.; Hafner, C.; Landthaler, M.; Vogt, T. Retinoblastoma-binding protein 2-homolog 1: A retinoblastoma-binding protein downregulated in malignant melanomas. *Mod. Pathol. Off. J. USA Can. Acad. Pathol. Inc* **2005**, *18*, 1249–1257. [CrossRef]
146. Chauvistré, H.; Daignault, S.; Shannan, B.; Ju, R.; Picard, D.; Vogel, F.; Egetemaier, S.; Krepler, C.; Rebecca, V.; Sechi, A.; et al. The Janus-faced role of KDM5B heterogeneity in melanoma: Differentiation as a situational driver of both growth arrest and drug-resistance. 2020; preprint. [CrossRef]
147. Roesch, A.; Fukunaga-Kalabis, M.; Schmidt, E.C.; Zabierowski, S.E.; Brafford, P.A.; Vultur, A.; Basu, D.; Gimotty, P.; Vogt, T.; Herlyn, M. A temporarily distinct subpopulation of slow-cycling melanoma cells is required for continuous tumor growth. *Cell* **2010**, *141*, 583–594. [CrossRef] [PubMed]
148. Flaherty, K.T.; Robert, C.; Hersey, P.; Nathan, P.; Garbe, C.; Milhem, M.; Demidov, L.V.; Hassel, J.C.; Rutkowski, P.; Mohr, P.; et al. Improved survival with MEK inhibition in BRAF-mutated melanoma. *N. Engl. J. Med.* **2012**, *367*, 107–114. [CrossRef] [PubMed]
149. Flaherty, K.T.; Infante, J.R.; Daud, A.; Gonzalez, R.; Kefford, R.F.; Sosman, J.; Hamid, O.; Schuchter, L.; Cebon, J.; Ibrahim, N.; et al. Combined BRAF and MEK inhibition in melanoma with BRAF V600 mutations. *N. Engl. J. Med.* **2012**, *367*, 1694–1703. [CrossRef]
150. Shi, H.; Hugo, W.; Kong, X.; Hong, A.; Koya, R.C.; Moriceau, G.; Chodon, T.; Guo, R.; Johnson, D.B.; Dahlman, K.B.; et al. Acquired resistance and clonal evolution in melanoma during BRAF inhibitor therapy. *Cancer Discov.* **2014**, *4*, 80–93. [CrossRef]
151. Clark, M.E.; Rizos, H.; Pereira, M.R.; McEvoy, A.C.; Marsavela, G.; Calapre, L.; Meehan, K.; Ruhen, O.; Khattak, M.A.; Meniawy, T.M.; et al. Detection of *BRAF* splicing variants in plasma-derived cell-free nucleic acids and extracellular vesicles of melanoma patients failing targeted therapy therapies. *Oncotarget* **2020**, *11*, 4016–4027. [CrossRef] [PubMed]
152. Shi, H.; Moriceau, G.; Kong, X.; Lee, M.-K.; Lee, H.; Koya, R.C.; Ng, C.; Chodon, T.; Scolyer, R.A.; Dahlman, K.B.; et al. Melanoma whole-exome sequencing identifies (V600E)B-RAF amplification-mediated acquired B-RAF inhibitor resistance. *Nat. Commun.* **2012**, *3*, 724. [CrossRef] [PubMed]
153. Perna, D.; Karreth, F.A.; Rust, A.G.; Perez-Mancera, P.A.; Rashid, M.; Iorio, F.; Alifrangis, C.; Arends, M.J.; Bosenberg, M.W.; Bollag, G.; et al. BRAF inhibitor resistance mediated by the AKT pathway in an oncogenic BRAF mouse melanoma model. *Proc. Natl. Acad. Sci. USA* **2015**, *112*, E536–E545. [CrossRef]
154. Basile, K.J.; Aplin, A.E. Downregulation of Noxa by RAF/MEK inhibition counteracts cell death response in mutant B-RAF melanoma cells. *Am. J. Cancer Res.* **2012**, *2*, 726–735. [PubMed]
155. Nazarian, R.; Shi, H.; Wang, Q.; Kong, X.; Koya, R.C.; Lee, H.; Chen, Z.; Lee, M.-K.; Attar, N.; Sazegar, H.; et al. Melanomas acquire resistance to B-RAF(V600E) inhibition by RTK or N-RAS upregulation. *Nature* **2010**, *468*, 973–977. [CrossRef]
156. Dugo, M.; Nicolini, G.; Tragni, G.; Bersani, I.; Tomassetti, A.; Colonna, V.; Del Vecchio, M.; De Braud, F.; Canevari, S.; Anichini, A.; et al. A melanoma subtype with intrinsic resistance to BRAF inhibition identified by receptor tyrosine kinases gene-driven classification. *Oncotarget* **2015**, *6*, 5118–5133. [CrossRef]
157. Su, Y.; Lu, X.; Li, G.; Liu, C.; Kong, Y.; Lee, J.W.; Ng, R.; Wong, S.; Robert, L.; Warden, C.; et al. Kinetic Inference Resolves Epigenetic Mechanism of Drug Resistance in Melanoma. *Cell* **2019**. preprint. [CrossRef]
158. Wilting, R.H.; Dannenberg, J.H. Epigenetic mechanisms in tumorigenesis, tumor cell heterogeneity and drug resistance. *Drug Resist. Updat.* **2012**, *15*, 21–38. [CrossRef] [PubMed]
159. Al Emran, A.; Marzese, D.M.; Menon, D.R.; Stark, M.S.; Torrano, J.; Hammerlindl, H.; Zhang, G.; Brafford, P.; Salomon, M.P.; Nelson, N.; et al. Distinct histone modifications denote early stress-induced drug tolerance in cancer. *Oncotarget* **2018**, *9*, 8206–8222. [CrossRef]
160. Hugo, W.; Shi, H.; Sun, L.; Piva, M.; Song, C.; Kong, X.; Moriceau, G.; Hong, A.; Dahlman, K.B.; Johnson, D.B.; et al. Non-genomic and Immune Evolution of Melanoma Acquiring MAPKi Resistance. *Cell* **2015**, *162*, 1271–1285. [CrossRef] [PubMed]
161. Seghers, A.C.; Wilgenhof, S.; Lebbé, C.; Neyns, B. Successful rechallenge in two patients with BRAF-V600-mutant melanoma who experienced previous progression during treatment with a selective BRAF inhibitor. *Melanoma Res.* **2012**, *22*, 466–472. [CrossRef]

162. Atkinson, V.; Batty, K.; Long, G.V.; Carlino, M.S.; Peters, G.D.; Bhave, P.; Moore, M.A.; Xu, W.; Brown, L.J.; Arneil, M.; et al. Activity and safety of third-line BRAF-targeted therapy (TT) following first-line TT and second-line immunotherapy (IT) in advanced melanoma. *J. Clin. Oncol.* **2020**, *38*, 10049. [CrossRef]
163. Cybulska-Stopa, B.; Rogala, P.; Czarnecka, A.M.; Galus, Ł.; Dziura, R.; Rajczykowski, M.; Kubiatowski, T.; Wiśniewska, M.; Gęga-Czarnota, A.; Teterycz, P.; et al. BRAF and MEK inhibitors rechallenge as effective treatment for patients with metastatic melanoma. *Melanoma Res.* **2020**, *30*, 465–471. [CrossRef]
164. Sharma, S.V.; Lee, D.Y.; Li, B.; Quinlan, M.P.; Takahashi, F.; Maheswaran, S.; McDermott, U.; Azizian, N.; Zou, L.; Fischbach, M.A.; et al. A chromatin-mediated reversible drug-tolerant state in cancer cell subpopulations. *Cell* **2010**, *141*, 69–80. [CrossRef]
165. Roesch, A.; Vultur, A.; Bogeski, I.; Wang, H.; Zimmermann, K.M.; Speicher, D.; Körbel, C.; Laschke, M.W.; Gimotty, P.A.; Philipp, S.E.; et al. Overcoming intrinsic multidrug resistance in melanoma by blocking the mitochondrial respiratory chain of slow-cycling JARID1B(high) cells. *Cancer Cell* **2013**, *23*, 811–825. [CrossRef]
166. Ravindran Menon, D.; Das, S.; Krepler, C.; Vultur, A.; Rinner, B.; Schauer, S.; Kashofer, K.; Wagner, K.; Zhang, G.; Bonyadi Rad, E.; et al. A stress-induced early innate response causes multidrug tolerance in melanoma. *Oncogene* **2015**, *34*, 4448–4459. [CrossRef] [PubMed]
167. Cartlidge, R.A.; Thomas, G.R.; Cagnol, S.; Jong, K.A.; Molton, S.A.; Finch, A.J.; McMahon, M. Oncogenic BRAF(V600E) inhibits BIM expression to promote melanoma cell survival. *Pigment Cell Melanoma Res.* **2008**, *21*, 534–544. [CrossRef] [PubMed]
168. Tsai, J.; Lee, J.T.; Wang, W.; Zhang, J.; Cho, H.; Mamo, S.; Bremer, R.; Gillette, S.; Kong, J.; Haass, N.K.; et al. Discovery of a selective inhibitor of oncogenic B-Raf kinase with potent antimelanoma activity. *Proc. Natl. Acad. Sci. USA* **2008**, *105*, 3041–3046. [CrossRef] [PubMed]
169. Mohana-Kumaran, N.; Hill, D.S.; Allen, J.D.; Haass, N.K. Targeting the intrinsic apoptosis pathway as a strategy for melanoma therapy. *Pigment Cell Melanoma Res.* **2014**, *27*, 525–539. [CrossRef]
170. Tiffen, J.C.; Gunatilake, D.; Gallagher, S.J.; Gowrishankar, K.; Heinemann, A.; Cullinane, C.; Dutton-Regester, K.; Pupo, G.M.; Strbenac, D.; Yang, J.Y.; et al. Targeting activating mutations of EZH2 leads to potent cell growth inhibition in human melanoma by derepression of tumor suppressor genes. *Oncotarget* **2015**, *6*, 27023–27036. [CrossRef]
171. Gallagher, S.J.; Mijatov, B.; Gunatilake, D.; Tiffen, J.C.; Gowrishankar, K.; Jin, L.; Pupo, G.M.; Cullinane, C.; Prinjha, R.K.; Smithers, N.; et al. The epigenetic regulator I-BET151 induces BIM-dependent apoptosis and cell cycle arrest of human melanoma cells. *J. Invest. Dermatol.* **2014**, *134*, 2795–2805. [CrossRef]
172. Heinemann, A.; Cullinane, C.; De Paoli-Iseppi, R.; Wilmott, J.S.; Gunatilake, D.; Madore, J.; Strbenac, D.; Yang, J.Y.; Gowrishankar, K.; Tiffen, J.C.; et al. Combining BET and HDAC inhibitors synergistically induces apoptosis of melanoma and suppresses AKT and YAP signaling. *Oncotarget* **2015**, *6*, 21507–21521. [CrossRef]
173. Neagu, M. Metabolic Traits in Cutaneous Melanoma. *Front. Oncol.* **2020**, *10*, 851. [CrossRef]
174. Witz, I.P. Tumor-microenvironment interactions: Dangerous liaisons. *Adv. Cancer Res.* **2008**, *100*, 203–229. [CrossRef] [PubMed]
175. Falcone, I.; Conciatori, F.; Bazzichetto, C.; Ferretti, G.; Cognetti, F.; Ciuffreda, L.; Milella, M. Tumor Microenvironment: Implications in Melanoma Resistance to Targeted Therapy and Immunotherapy. *Cancers* **2020**, *12*, 2870. [CrossRef] [PubMed]
176. Mazurkiewicz, J.; Simiczyjew, A.; Dratkiewicz, E.; Ziętek, M.; Matkowski, R.; Nowak, D. Stromal Cells Present in the Melanoma Niche Affect Tumor Invasiveness and Its Resistance to Therapy. *Int. J. Mol. Sci.* **2021**, *22*, 529. [CrossRef] [PubMed]
177. Passarelli, A.; Mannavola, F.; Stucci, L.S.; Tucci, M.; Silvestris, F. Immune system and melanoma biology: A balance between immunosurveillance and immune escape. *Oncotarget* **2017**, *8*, 106132–106142. [CrossRef]
178. Farhood, B.; Najafi, M.; Mortezaee, K. CD8(+) cytotoxic T lymphocytes in cancer immunotherapy: A review. *J. Cell. Physiol.* **2019**, *234*, 8509–8521. [CrossRef]
179. Liu, Y.; Guo, J.; Huang, L. Modulation of tumor microenvironment for immunotherapy: Focus on nanomaterial-based strategies. *Theranostics* **2020**, *10*, 3099–3117. [CrossRef] [PubMed]
180. Qin, S.; Xu, L.; Yi, M.; Yu, S.; Wu, K.; Luo, S. Novel immune checkpoint targets: Moving beyond PD-1 and CTLA-4. *Mol. Cancer* **2019**, *18*, 155. [CrossRef] [PubMed]
181. Turnis, M.E.; Andrews, L.P.; Vignali, D.A.A. Inhibitory receptors as targets for cancer immunotherapy. *Eur. J. Immunol.* **2015**, *45*, 1892–1905. [CrossRef]
182. Yervoy (ipilimumab) FDA Approval History Drugs.com. Available online: https://www.drugs.com/history/yervoy.html (accessed on 17 February 2021).
183. Opdivo (nivolumab) FDA Approval History Drugs.com. Available online: https://www.drugs.com/history/opdivo.html (accessed on 17 February 2021).
184. Asher, N.; Ben-Betzalel, G.; Lev-Ari, S.; Shapira-Frommer, R.; Steinberg-Silman, Y.; Gochman, N.; Schachter, J.; Meirson, T.; Markel, G. Real World Outcomes of Ipilimumab and Nivolumab in Patients with Metastatic Melanoma. *Cancers* **2020**, *12*, 2329. [CrossRef]
185. Nobel Prize Awarded to Cancer Immunotherapy Researchers. Available online: https://www.cancer.org/latest-news/nobel-prize-awarded-to-cancer-immunotherapy-researchers.html (accessed on 17 February 2021).
186. Lee, P.P.; Fitzpatrick, D.R.; Beard, C.; Jessup, H.K.; Lehar, S.; Makar, K.W.; Pérez-Melgosa, M.; Sweetser, M.T.; Schlissel, M.S.; Nguyen, S.; et al. A critical role for Dnmt1 and DNA methylation in T cell development, function, and survival. *Immunity* **2001**, *15*, 763–774. [CrossRef]
187. Scanlon, S. DNA methylation makes for tired T cells. *Science* **2017**, *357*, 367–368. [CrossRef]

188. Xiao, Q.; Nobre, A.; Piñeiro, P.; Berciano-Guerrero, M.-Á.; Alba, E.; Cobo, M.; Lauschke, V.M.; Barragán, I. Genetic and Epigenetic Biomarkers of Immune Checkpoint Blockade Response. *J. Clin. Med.* **2020**, *9*, 286. [CrossRef] [PubMed]
189. Fietz, S.; Zarbl, R.; Niebel, D.; Posch, C.; Brossart, P.; Gielen, G.H.; Strieth, S.; Pietsch, T.; Kristiansen, G.; Bootz, F.; et al. CTLA4 promoter methylation predicts response and progression-free survival in stage IV melanoma treated with anti-CTLA-4 immunotherapy (ipilimumab). *Cancer Immunol. Immunother.* **2020**. [CrossRef] [PubMed]
190. Madore, J.; Vilain, R.E.; Menzies, A.M.; Kakavand, H.; Wilmott, J.S.; Hyman, J.; Yearley, J.H.; Kefford, R.F.; Thompson, J.F.; Long, G.V.; et al. PD-L1 expression in melanoma shows marked heterogeneity within and between patients: Implications for anti-PD-1/PD-L1 clinical trials. *Pigment Cell Melanoma Res.* **2015**, *28*, 245–253. [CrossRef]
191. Sznol, M.; Chen, L. Antagonist antibodies to PD-1 and B7-H1 (PD-L1) in the treatment of advanced human cancer. *Clin. cancer Res. an Off. J. Am. Assoc. Cancer Res.* **2013**, *19*, 1021–1034. [CrossRef] [PubMed]
192. Eddy, K.; Chen, S. Overcoming Immune Evasion in Melanoma. *Int. J. Mol. Sci.* **2020**, *21*, 8984. [CrossRef] [PubMed]
193. Madore, J.; Strbenac, D.; Vilain, R.; Menzies, A.M.; Yang, J.Y.H.; Thompson, J.F.; Long, G.V.; Mann, G.J.; Scolyer, R.A.; Wilmott, J.S. PD-L1 Negative Status is Associated with Lower Mutation Burden, Differential Expression of Immune-Related Genes, and Worse Survival in Stage III Melanoma. *Clin. cancer Res. an Off. J. Am. Assoc. Cancer Res.* **2016**, *22*, 3915–3923. [CrossRef]
194. Micevic, G.; Thakral, D.; McGeary, M.; Bosenberg, M.W. PD-L1 methylation regulates PD-L1 expression and is associated with melanoma survival. *Pigment Cell Melanoma Res.* **2019**, *32*, 435–440. [CrossRef]
195. Fröhlich, A.; Sirokay, J.; Fietz, S.; Vogt, T.J.; Dietrich, J.; Zarbl, R.; Florin, M.; Kuster, P.; Saavedra, G.; Valladolid, S.R.; et al. Molecular, clinicopathological, and immune correlates of LAG3 promoter DNA methylation in melanoma. *EBioMedicine* **2020**, *59*, 102962. [CrossRef]
196. Chiappinelli, K.B.; Strissel, P.L.; Desrichard, A.; Li, H.; Henke, C.; Akman, B.; Hein, A.; Rote, N.S.; Cope, L.M.; Snyder, A.; et al. Inhibiting DNA Methylation Causes an Interferon Response in Cancer via dsRNA Including Endogenous Retroviruses. *Cell* **2015**, *162*, 974–986. [CrossRef]
197. Zingg, D.; Arenas-Ramirez, N.; Sahin, D.; Rosalia, R.A.; Antunes, A.T.; Haeusel, J.; Sommer, L.; Boyman, O. The Histone Methyltransferase Ezh2 Controls Mechanisms of Adaptive Resistance to Tumor Immunotherapy. *Cell Rep.* **2017**, *20*, 854–867. [CrossRef] [PubMed]
198. Tiffen, J.; Wilson, S.; Gallagher, S.J.; Hersey, P.; Filipp, F. V Somatic Copy Number Amplification and Hyperactivating Somatic Mutations of EZH2 Correlate With DNA Methylation and Drive Epigenetic Silencing of Genes Involved in Tumor Suppression and Immune Responses in Melanoma. *Neoplasia* **2016**, *18*, 121–132. [CrossRef]
199. Chen, B.-F.; Chan, W.-Y. The de novo DNA methyltransferase DNMT3A in development and cancer. *Epigenetics* **2014**, *9*, 669–677. [CrossRef]
200. Badeaux, A.I.; Shi, Y. Emerging roles for chromatin as a signal integration and storage platform. *Nat. Rev. Mol. Cell Biol.* **2013**, *14*, 211–224. [CrossRef] [PubMed]
201. Schlesinger, Y.; Straussman, R.; Keshet, I.; Farkash, S.; Hecht, M.; Zimmerman, J.; Eden, E.; Yakhini, Z.; Ben-Shushan, E.; Reubinoff, B.E.; et al. Polycomb-mediated methylation on Lys27 of histone H3 pre-marks genes for de novo methylation in cancer. *Nat. Genet.* **2007**, *39*, 232–236. [CrossRef] [PubMed]
202. Montalvo-Casimiro, M.; González-Barrios, R.; Meraz-Rodriguez, M.A.; Juárez-González, V.T.; Arriaga-Canon, C.; Herrera, L.A. Epidrug Repurposing: Discovering New Faces of Old Acquaintances in Cancer Therapy. *Front. Oncol.* **2020**, *10*, 605386. [CrossRef]
203. Majchrzak-Celińska, A.; Warych, A.; Szoszkiewicz, M. Novel Approaches to Epigenetic Therapies: From Drug Combinations to Epigenetic Editing. *Genes* **2021**, *12*.
204. Bioequivalence & Food Effect Study in Patients With Solid Tumor or Hematologic Malignancies Full Text View ClinicalTrials.gov. Available online: https://clinicaltrials.gov/ct2/show/NCT02223052?term=azacitidine&cond=Melanoma&draw=6&rank=6 (accessed on 9 August 2021).
205. Hussein Tawbi PHD, M.D. Study of Oral Azacitidine (CC-486) in Combination With Pembrolizumab (MK-3475) in Patients With Metastatic Melanoma. Available online: https://clinicaltrials.gov/ct2/show/NCT02816021?term=azacitidine&cond=Melanoma&draw=2&rank=1 (accessed on 9 August 2021).
206. Van Der Westhuizen, A.; Graves, M.; Levy, R.; Majid, A.; Vilain, R.; Bowden, N. PRIME002: Early phase II study of azacitidine and carboplatin priming for avelumab in patients with advanced melanoma who are resistant to immunotherapy. In *Abstracts B, Proceedings of the 44th ESMO Congress (ESMO 2019), Barcelona, Spain, 27 September—1 October 2019*; European Society for Medical Oncology: Lugano, Switzerland, 2019; Volume 561, p. 30. [CrossRef]
207. Decitabine in Treating Patients With Melanoma or Other Advanced Cancer Full Text View ClinicalTrials.gov. Available online: https://clinicaltrials.gov/ct2/show/NCT00002980?term=azacitidine&cond=Melanoma&draw=2&rank=9 (accessed on 9 August 2021).
208. Gene-Modified T Cells With or Without Decitabine in Treating Patients With Advanced Malignancies Expressing NY-ESO-1 Full Text View ClinicalTrials.gov. Available online: https://clinicaltrials.gov/ct2/show/NCT02650986?term=azacitidine&cond=Melanoma&draw=5&rank=11 (accessed on 9 August 2021).
209. Xia, C.; Leon-Ferre, R.; Laux, D.; Deutsch, J.; Smith, B.J.; Frees, M.; Milhem, M. Treatment of resistant metastatic melanoma using sequential epigenetic therapy (decitabine and panobinostat) combined with chemotherapy (temozolomide). *Cancer Chemother. Pharmacol.* **2014**, *74*, 691–697. [CrossRef] [PubMed]

210. Combination of Decitabine and Temozolomide in the Treatment of Patients With Metastatic Melanoma Full Text View ClinicalTrials.gov. Available online: https://clinicaltrials.gov/ct2/show/NCT00715793?term=decitabine&cond=Melanoma&draw=4&rank=3 (accessed on 9 August 2021).
211. Phadke, S.D.; Engelman, E.S.; Leon-Ferre, R.A.; Abushahin, L.I.; Mott, S.C.; Zakharia, Y.; Milhem, M.M. A phase I study of vemurafenib and decitabine in metastatic melanoma. *J. Clin. Oncol.* 2015, 33, 9056. [CrossRef]
212. Zakharia, Y.; Monga, V.; Swami, U.; Bossler, A.D.; Freesmeier, M.; Frees, M.; Khan, M.; Frydenlund, N.; Srikantha, R.; Vanneste, M.; et al. Targeting epigenetics for treatment of BRAF mutated metastatic melanoma with decitabine in combination with vemurafenib: A phase Ib study. *Oncotarget* 2017, 8, 89182–89193. [CrossRef]
213. A Study Investigating SGI-110 in Combination With Ipilimumab in Unresectable or Metastatic Melanoma Patients Full Text View ClinicalTrials.gov. Available online: https://clinicaltrials.gov/ct2/show/NCT02608437?term=Guadecitabine&cond=Melanoma&draw=2&rank=1 (accessed on 3 August 2021).
214. Giacomo, A.M.D.; Covre, A.; Finotello, F.; Rieder, D.; Danielli, R.; Sigalotti, L.; Giannarelli, D.; Petitprez, F.; Lacroix, L.; Valente, M.; et al. Guadecitabine Plus Ipilimumab in Unresectable Melanoma: The NIBIT-M4 Clinical Trial. *Clin. Cancer Res.* 2019, 25, 7351–7362. [CrossRef]
215. A Study of NIVO Plus IPI and Guadecitabine or NIVO Plus IPI in Melanoma and NSCLC Resistant to Anti-PD1/PDL1 Full Text View ClinicalTrials.gov. Available online: https://clinicaltrials.gov/ct2/show/NCT04250246?term=Guadecitabine&cond=Melanoma&draw=2&rank=2 (accessed on 3 August 2021).
216. Hellebrekers, D.M.E.I.; Castermans, K.; Viré, E.; Dings, R.P.M.; Hoebers, N.T.H.; Mayo, K.H.; Egbrink, M.G.A.; Molema, G.; Fuks, F.; Engeland, M.; et al. Epigenetic Regulation of Tumor Endothelial Cell Anergy: Silencing of Intercellular Adhesion Molecule-1 by Histone Modifications. *Cancer Res.* 2006, 66, 10770–10777. [CrossRef]
217. Disulfiram in Patients With Metastatic Melanoma Full Text View ClinicalTrials.gov. Available online: https://clinicaltrials.gov/ct2/show/NCT00256230?term=disulfiram&cond=Melanoma&draw=2&rank=2 (accessed on 9 August 2021).
218. Disulfiram Plus Arsenic Trioxide In Patients With Metastatic Melanoma and at Least One Prior Systemic Therapy Full Text View ClinicalTrials.gov. Available online: https://clinicaltrials.gov/ct2/show/NCT00571116?term=disulfiram&cond=Melanoma&draw=2&rank=1 (accessed on 9 August 2021).
219. Huijberts, S.; Wang, L.; de Oliveira, R.L.; Rosing, H.; Nuijen, B.; Beijnen, J.; Bernards, R.; Schellens, J.; Wilgenhof, S. Vorinostat in patients with resistant BRAF(V600E) mutated advanced melanoma: A proof of concept study. *Future Oncol.* 2020, 16, 619–629. [CrossRef] [PubMed]
220. Reijers, I.L.M.; Dimitriadis, P.; Rozeman, E.A.; Versluis, J.M.; Broeks, A.; Bosch, L.J.W.; Bouwman, J.; Cornelissen, S.; Krijgsman, O.; Gonzalez, M.; et al. Personalized combination of neoadjuvant domatinostat, nivolumab and ipilimumab in macroscopic stage III melanoma patients stratified according to the interferon-gamma signature: The DONIMI study. *J. Clin. Oncol.* 2020, 38, TPS10087. [CrossRef]
221. Panobinostat (LBH589) in Patients With Metastatic Melanoma Full Text View ClinicalTrials.gov. Available online: https://clinicaltrials.gov/ct2/show/NCT01065467 (accessed on 9 August 2021).
222. Khushalani, N.I.; Markowitz, J.; Eroglu, Z.; Giuroiu, I.; Ladanova, V.; Reiersen, P.; Rich, J.; Thapa, R.; Schell, M.J.; Sotomayor, E.M.; et al. A phase I trial of panobinostat with ipilimumab in advanced melanoma. *J. Clin. Oncol.* 2017, 35, 9547. [CrossRef]
223. FR901228 in Treating Patients With Unresectable Stage III or Stage IV Malignant Melanoma Full Text View ClinicalTrials.gov. Available online: https://clinicaltrials.gov/ct2/show/NCT00104884 (accessed on 9 August 2021).
224. Johnson, M.L.; Gonzalez, R.; Opyrchal, M.; Gabrilovich, D.; Ordentlich, P.; Brouwer, S.; Sankoh, S.; Schmidt, E.V.; Meyers, M.L.; Agarwala, S.S. ENCORE 601: A phase I study of entinostat (ENT) in combination with pembrolizumab (PEMBRO) in patients with melanoma. *J. Clin. Oncol.* 2017, 35, 9529. [CrossRef]
225. Woods, D.M.; Laino, A.S.; Vassallo, M.; Weber, J. Abstract PO-007: The Class I/IV HDAC Inhibitor Mocetinostat Augments Anti-Tumor Immune Responses in Melanoma Patients. *Cancer Res.* 2020, 80, PO-007. [CrossRef]
226. Tinostamustine and Nivolumab in Advanced Melanoma Full Text View ClinicalTrials.gov. Available online: https://clinicaltrials.gov/ct2/show/NCT03903458 (accessed on 9 August 2021).
227. Rocca, A.; Minucci, S.; Tosti, G.; Croci, D.; Contegno, F.; Ballarini, M.; Nolè, F.; Munzone, E.; Salmaggi, A.; Goldhirsch, A.; et al. A phase I–II study of the histone deacetylase inhibitor valproic acid plus chemoimmunotherapy in patients with advanced melanoma. *Br. J. Cancer* 2009, 100, 28–36. [CrossRef] [PubMed]
228. Tahata, S.; Singh, S.V.; Lin, Y.; Hahm, E.-R.; Beumer, J.H.; Christner, S.M.; Rao, U.N.; Sander, C.; Tarhini, A.A.; Tawbi, H.; et al. Evaluation of Biodistribution of Sulforaphane after Administration of Oral Broccoli Sprout Extract in Melanoma Patients with Multiple Atypical Nevi. *Cancer Prev. Res.* 2018, 11, 429–438. [CrossRef]
229. Garmpis, N.; Damaskos, C.; Garmpi, A.; Dimitroulis, D.; Spartalis, E.; Margonis, G.A.; Schizas, D.; Deskou, I.; Doula, C.; Magkouti, E.; et al. Targeting histone deacetylases in malignant melanoma: A future therapeutic agent or just great expectations? *Anticancer Res.* 2017, 37, 5355–5362. [PubMed]
230. Testing the Addition of the Anti-cancer Drug, Tazemetostat, to the Usual Treatment (Dabrafenib and Trametinib) for Metastatic Melanoma That Has Progressed on the Usual Treatment Full Text View ClinicalTrials.gov. Available online: https://clinicaltrials.gov/ct2/show/NCT04557956 (accessed on 9 August 2021).
231. ORIOn-E: A Study Evaluating CPI-1205 in Patients With Advanced Solid Tumors Full Text View ClinicalTrials.gov. Available online: https://clinicaltrials.gov/ct2/show/NCT03525795 (accessed on 9 August 2021).

232. Ameratunga, M.; Braña, I.; Bono, P.; Postel-Vinay, S.; Plummer, R.; Aspegren, J.; Korjamo, T.; Snapir, A.; de Bono, J.S. First-in-human Phase 1 open label study of the BET inhibitor ODM-207 in patients with selected solid tumours. *Br. J. Cancer* **2020**, *123*, 1730–1736. [CrossRef] [PubMed]
233. Yin, M.; Guo, Y.; Hu, R.; Cai, W.L.; Li, Y.; Pei, S.; Sun, H.; Peng, C.; Li, J.; Ye, R.; et al. Potent BRD4 inhibitor suppresses cancer cell-macrophage interaction. *Nat. Commun.* **2020**, *11*, 1833. [CrossRef] [PubMed]
234. Erkes, D.A.; Rosenbaum, S.R.; Field, C.O.; Chervoneva, I.; Villanueva, J.; Aplin, A.E. PLX3397 inhibits the accumulation of intra-tumoral macrophages and improves bromodomain and extra-terminal inhibitor efficacy in melanoma. *Pigment Cell Melanoma Res.* **2020**, *33*, 372–377. [CrossRef]
235. Rollins, R.A.; Kim, K.H.; Tsao, C.-C. *The Emerging Epigenetic Landscape in Melanoma. In Human Skin Cancer, Potential Biomarkers and Therapeutic Targets*; InTech: London, UK, 2016.
236. Jin, N.; George, T.L.; Otterson, G.A.; Verschraegen, C.; Wen, H.; Carbone, D.; Herman, J.; Bertino, E.M.; He, K. Advances in epigenetic therapeutics with focus on solid tumors. *Clin. Epigenetics* **2021**, *13*, 83. [CrossRef]
237. Ganesan, A.; Arimondo, P.B.; Rots, M.G.; Jeronimo, C.; Berdasco, M. The timeline of epigenetic drug discovery: From reality to dreams. *Clin. Epigenetics* **2019**, *11*, 1–17. [CrossRef] [PubMed]
238. Cartron, P.-F.; Cheray, M.; Bretaudeau, L. Epigenetic protein complexes: The adequate candidates for the use of a new generation of epidrugs in personalized and precision medicine in cancer. *Epigenomics* **2020**, *12*, 171–177. [CrossRef]
239. Lu, Y.; Chan, Y.-T.; Tan, H.-Y.; Li, S.; Wang, N.; Feng, Y. Epigenetic regulation in human cancer: The potential role of epi-drug in cancer therapy. *Mol. Cancer* **2020**, *19*, 79. [CrossRef]
240. Martinez-Useros, J.; Martin-Galan, M.; Florez-Cespedes, M.; Garcia-Foncillas, J. Epigenetics of Most Aggressive Solid Tumors: Pathways, Targets and Treatments. *Cancers* **2021**, *13*, 3209. [CrossRef]
241. Chu, B.F.; Karpenko, M.J.; Liu, Z.; Aimiuwu, J.; Villalona-Calero, M.A.; Chan, K.K.; Grever, M.R.; Otterson, G.A. Phase I study of 5-aza-2′-deoxycytidine in combination with valproic acid in non-small-cell lung cancer. *Cancer Chemother. Pharmacol.* **2013**, *71*, 115–121. [CrossRef]
242. Jansen, Y.J.L.; Verset, G.; Schats, K.; Van Dam, P.-J.; Seremet, T.; Kockx, M.; Van Laethem, J.-L.B.; Neyns, B. Phase I clinical trial of decitabine (5-aza-2′-deoxycytidine) administered by hepatic arterial infusion in patients with unresectable liver-predominant metastases. *ESMO Open* **2019**, *4*, e000464. [CrossRef]
243. Jones, P.A.; Ohtani, H.; Chakravarthy, A.; De Carvalho, D.D. Epigenetic therapy in immune-oncology. *Nat. Rev. Cancer* **2019**, *19*, 151–161. [CrossRef] [PubMed]
244. Tawbi, H.A.; Beumer, J.H.; Tarhini, A.A.; Moschos, S.J.; Egorin, M.J.; Buch, S.C.; Lin, Y.; Kirkwood, J.M. Phase I/II study of the combination of decitabine (DAC) and temozolomide (TMZ) in patients (pts) with metastatic melanoma (MM). *J. Clin. Oncol.* **2010**, *28*, 8533. [CrossRef]
245. Patnaik, S. Anupriya Drugs Targeting Epigenetic Modifications and Plausible Therapeutic Strategies Against Colorectal Cancer. *Front. Pharmacol.* **2019**, *10*, 588. [CrossRef] [PubMed]
246. Meraz-Torres, F.; Plöger, S.; Garbe, C.; Niessner, H.; Sinnberg, T. Disulfiram as a Therapeutic Agent for Metastatic Malignant Melanoma—Old Myth or New Logos? *Cancers* **2020**, *12*, 3538. [CrossRef]
247. Hull, E.E.; Montgomery, M.R.; Leyva, K.J. HDAC Inhibitors as Epigenetic Regulators of the Immune System: Impacts on Cancer Therapy and Inflammatory Diseases. *Biomed Res. Int.* **2016**, *2016*, 8797206. [CrossRef]
248. Mrakovcic, M.; Fröhlich, L.F. Molecular Determinants of Cancer Therapy Resistance to HDAC Inhibitor-Induced Autophagy. *Cancers* **2019**, *12*, 109. [CrossRef]
249. Ibrahim, N.; Buchbinder, E.I.; Granter, S.R.; Rodig, S.J.; Giobbie-Hurder, A.; Becerra, C.; Tsiaras, A.; Gjini, E.; Fisher, D.E.; Hodi, F.S. A phase I trial of panobinostat (LBH589) in patients with metastatic melanoma. *Cancer Med.* **2016**, *5*, 3041–3050. [CrossRef]
250. Hauschild, A.; Trefzer, U.; Garbe, C.; Kaehler, K.; Ugurel, S.; Kiecker, F.; Eigentler, T.; Krissel, H.; Schadendorf, D. A phase II multicenter study on the histone deacetylase (HDAC) inhibitor MS-275, comparing two dosage schedules in metastatic melanoma. *J. Clin. Oncol.* **2006**, *24*, 8044. [CrossRef]
251. Haas, N.B.; Quirt, I.; Hotte, S.; McWhirter, E.; Polintan, R.; Litwin, S.; Adams, P.D.; McBryan, T.; Wang, L.; Martin, L.P.; et al. Phase II trial of vorinostat in advanced melanoma. *Invest. New Drugs* **2014**, *32*, 526–534. [CrossRef]
252. Venugopal, B.; Baird, R.; Kristeleit, R.S.; Plummer, R.; Cowan, R.; Stewart, A.; Fourneau, N.; Hellemans, P.; Elsayed, Y.; McClue, S.; et al. A phase I study of quisinostat (JNJ-26481585), an oral hydroxamate histone deacetylase inhibitor with evidence of target modulation and antitumor activity, in patients with advanced solid tumors. *Clin. cancer Res. Off. J. Am. Assoc. Cancer Res.* **2013**, *19*, 4262–4272. [CrossRef] [PubMed]
253. Dinkova-Kostova, A.T.; Jenkins, S.N.; Fahey, J.W.; Ye, L.; Wehage, S.L.; Liby, K.T.; Stephenson, K.K.; Wade, K.L.; Talalay, P. Protection against UV-light-induced skin carcinogenesis in SKH-1 high-risk mice by sulforaphane-containing broccoli sprout extracts. *Cancer Lett.* **2006**, *240*, 243–252. [CrossRef] [PubMed]
254. Shibata, A.; Nakagawa, K.; Yamanoi, H.; Tsuduki, T.; Sookwong, P.; Higuchi, O.; Kimura, F.; Miyazawa, T. Sulforaphane suppresses ultraviolet B-induced inflammation in HaCaT keratinocytes and HR-1 hairless mice. *J. Nutr. Biochem.* **2010**, *21*, 702–709. [CrossRef] [PubMed]
255. Arcidiacono, P.; Ragonese, F.; Stabile, A.; Pistilli, A.; Kuligina, E.; Rende, M.; Bottoni, U.; Calvieri, S.; Crisanti, A.; Spaccapelo, R. Antitumor activity and expression profiles of genes induced by sulforaphane in human melanoma cells. *Eur. J. Nutr.* **2018**, *57*, 2547–2569. [CrossRef] [PubMed]

256. Pradhan, S.J.; Mishra, R.; Sharma, P.; Kundu, G.C. Quercetin and sulforaphane in combination suppress the progression of melanoma through the down-regulation of matrix metalloproteinase-9. *Exp. Ther. Med.* **2010**, *1*, 915–920. [CrossRef]
257. Alyoussef, A.; Taha, M. Antitumor activity of sulforaphane in mice model of skin cancer via blocking sulfatase-2. *Exp. Dermatol.* **2019**, *28*, 28–34. [CrossRef]
258. Duan, R.; Du, W.; Guo, W. EZH2: A novel target for cancer treatment. *J. Hematol. Oncol.* **2020**, *13*, 104. [CrossRef] [PubMed]
259. Yap, T.A.; Winter, J.N.; Giulino-Roth, L.; Longley, J.; Lopez, J.; Michot, J.-M.; Leonard, J.P.; Ribrag, V.; McCabe, M.T.; Creasy, C.L.; et al. Phase I Study of the Novel Enhancer of Zeste Homolog 2 (EZH2) Inhibitor GSK2816126 in Patients with Advanced Hematologic and Solid Tumors. *Clin. Cancer Res.* **2019**, *25*, 7331–7339. [CrossRef]
260. Doroshow, D.B.; Eder, J.P.; LoRusso, P.M. BET inhibitors: A novel epigenetic approach. *Ann. Oncol.* **2017**, *28*, 1776–1787. [CrossRef]
261. Shorstova, T.; Foulkes, W.D.; Witcher, M. Achieving clinical success with BET inhibitors as anti-cancer agents. *Br. J. Cancer* **2021**, *124*, 1478–1490. [CrossRef] [PubMed]
262. Deng, G.; Zeng, F.; Su, J.; Zhao, S.; Hu, R.; Zhu, W.; Hu, S.; Chen, X.; Yin, M. BET inhibitor suppresses melanoma progression via the noncanonical NF-κB/SPP1 pathway. *Theranostics* **2020**, *10*, 11428–11443. [CrossRef]
263. Gallagher, S.J.; Mijatov, B.; Gunatilake, D.; Gowrishankar, K.; Tiffen, J.; James, W.; Jin, L.; Pupo, G.; Cullinane, C.; McArthur, G.A.; et al. Control of NF-kB activity in human melanoma by bromodomain and extra-terminal protein inhibitor I-BET151. *Pigment Cell Melanoma Res.* **2014**, *27*, 1126–1137. [CrossRef]
264. Erkes, D.A.; Field, C.O.; Capparelli, C.; Tiago, M.; Purwin, T.J.; Chervoneva, I.; Berger, A.C.; Hartsough, E.J.; Villanueva, J.; Aplin, A.E. The next-generation BET inhibitor, PLX51107, delays melanoma growth in a CD8-mediated manner. *Pigment Cell Melanoma Res.* **2019**, *32*, 687–696. [CrossRef]
265. Punnia-Moorthy, G.; Hersey, P.; Emran, A.A.; Tiffen, J. Lysine Demethylases: Promising Drug Targets in Melanoma and Other Cancers. *Front. Genet.* **2021**, *12*, 680633. [CrossRef] [PubMed]
266. Vogel, F.C.E.; Bordag, N.; Zügner, E.; Trajkovic-Arsic, M.; Chauvistré, H.; Shannan, B.; Váraljai, R.; Horn, S.; Magnes, C.; Thomas Siveke, J.; et al. Targeting the H3K4 Demethylase KDM5B Reprograms the Metabolome and Phenotype of Melanoma Cells. *J. Invest. Dermatol.* **2019**, *139*, 2506–2516.e10. [CrossRef] [PubMed]
267. Zhao, B.; Cheng, X.; Zhou, X. The BET-bromodomain inhibitor JQ1 mitigates vemurafenib drug resistance in melanoma. *Melanoma Res.* **2018**, *28*, 521–526. [CrossRef]
268. Gallagher, S.J.; Gunatilake, D.; Beaumont, K.A.; Sharp, D.M.; Tiffen, J.C.; Heinemann, A.; Weninger, W.; Haass, N.K.; Wilmott, J.S.; Madore, J.; et al. HDAC inhibitors restore BRAF-inhibitor sensitivity by altering PI3K and survival signalling in a subset of melanoma. *Int. J. cancer* **2018**, *142*, 1926–1937. [CrossRef]
269. Héninger, E.; Krueger, T.E.G.; Lang, J.M. Augmenting antitumor immune responses with epigenetic modifying agents. *Front. Immunol.* **2015**, *6*, 29. [CrossRef] [PubMed]
270. Dan, H.; Zhang, S.; Zhou, Y.; Guan, Q. DNA Methyltransferase Inhibitors: Catalysts For Antitumour Immune Responses. *Onco. Targets. Ther.* **2019**, *12*, 10903–10916. [CrossRef]
271. Serrano, A.; Tanzarella, S.; Lionello, I.; Mendez, R.; Traversari, C.; Ruiz-Cabello, F.; Garrido, F. Rexpression of HLA class I antigens and restoration of antigen-specific CTL response in melanoma cells following 5-aza-2′-deoxycytidine treatment. *Int. J. Cancer* **2001**, *94*, 243–251. [CrossRef]
272. Jansz, N.; Faulkner, G.J. Endogenous retroviruses in the origins and treatment of cancer. *Genome Biol.* **2021**, *22*, 147. [CrossRef] [PubMed]
273. Li, X.-F.; Ren, P.; Shen, W.-Z.; Jin, X.; Zhang, J. The expression, modulation and use of cancer-testis antigens as potential biomarkers for cancer immunotherapy. *Am. J. Transl. Res.* **2020**, *12*, 7002–7019.
274. Burton, E.M.; Woody, T.; Glitza, I.C.; Amaria, R.N.; Keung, E.Z.-Y.; Diab, A.; Patel, S.P.; Wong, M.K.K.; Yee, C.; Hwu, P.; et al. A phase II study of oral azacitidine (CC-486) in combination with pembrolizumab (PEMBRO) in patients (pts) with metastatic melanoma (MM). *J. Clin. Oncol.* **2019**, *37*, 9560. [CrossRef]
275. Woods, D.M.; Sodré, A.L.; Villagra, A.; Sarnaik, A.; Sotomayor, E.M.; Weber, J. HDAC Inhibition Upregulates PD-1 Ligands in Melanoma and Augments Immunotherapy with PD-1 Blockade. *Cancer Immunol. Res.* **2015**, *3*, 1375–1385. [CrossRef] [PubMed]
276. Banik, D.; Moufarrij, S.; Villagra, A. Immunoepigenetics Combination Therapies: An Overview of the Role of HDACs in Cancer Immunotherapy. *Int. J. Mol. Sci.* **2019**, *20*, 2241. [CrossRef] [PubMed]
277. Wang, H.-F.; Ning, F.; Liu, Z.-C.; Wu, L.; Li, Z.-Q.; Qi, Y.-F.; Zhang, G.; Wang, H.-S.; Cai, S.-H.; Du, J. Histone deacetylase inhibitors deplete myeloid-derived suppressor cells induced by 4T1 mammary tumors in vivo and in vitro. *Cancer Immunol. Immunother.* **2017**, *66*, 355–366. [CrossRef] [PubMed]
278. Knox, T.; Sahakian, E.; Banik, D.; Hadley, M.; Palmer, E.; Noonepalle, S.; Kim, J.; Powers, J.; Gracia-Hernandez, M.; Oliveira, V.; et al. Selective HDAC6 inhibitors improve anti-PD-1 immune checkpoint blockade therapy by decreasing the anti-inflammatory phenotype of macrophages and down-regulation of immunosuppressive proteins in tumor cells. *Sci. Rep.* **2019**, *9*, 6136. [CrossRef] [PubMed]
279. Kim, K.; Skora, A.D.; Li, Z.; Liu, Q.; Tam, A.J.; Blosser, R.L.; Diaz, L.A.J.; Papadopoulos, N.; Kinzler, K.W.; Vogelstein, B.; et al. Eradication of metastatic mouse cancers resistant to immune checkpoint blockade by suppression of myeloid-derived cells. *Proc. Natl. Acad. Sci. USA* **2014**, *111*, 11774–11779. [CrossRef]
280. Winder, M.; Virós, A. Mechanisms of Drug Resistance in Melanoma. *Handb. Exp. Pharmacol.* **2018**, *249*, 91–108. [CrossRef]

281. Signetti, L.; Elizarov, N.; Simsir, M.; Paquet, A.; Douguet, D.; Labbal, F.; Debayle, D.; Di Giorgio, A.; Biou, V.; Girard, C.; et al. Inhibition of Patched Drug Efflux Increases Vemurafenib Effectiveness against Resistant Braf(V600E) Melanoma. *Cancers* **2020**, *12*, 1500. [CrossRef]
282. Zhang, J.; Shih, D.J.H.; Lin, S.-Y. Role of DNA repair defects in predicting immunotherapy response. *Biomark. Res.* **2020**, *8*, 23. [CrossRef] [PubMed]
283. Czerwinska, P.; Jaworska, A.M.; Wlodarczyk, N.A.; Mackiewicz, A.A. Melanoma Stem Cell-Like Phenotype and Significant Suppression of Immune Response within a Tumor Are Regulated by TRIM28 Protein. *Cancers* **2020**, *12*, 2998. [CrossRef]
284. Mancarella, D.; Plass, C. Epigenetic signatures in cancer: Proper controls, current challenges and the potential for clinical translation. *Genome Med.* **2021**, *13*, 23. [CrossRef] [PubMed]
285. Wouters, J.; Vizoso, M.; Martinez-Cardus, A.; Carmona, F.J.; Govaere, O.; Laguna, T.; Joseph, J.; Dynoodt, P.; Aura, C.; Foth, M.; et al. Comprehensive DNA methylation study identifies novel progression-related and prognostic markers for cutaneous melanoma. *BMC Med.* **2017**, *15*, 101. [CrossRef] [PubMed]
286. Stacchiotti, S.; Schoffski, P.; Jones, R.; Agulnik, M.; Villalobos, V.M.; Jahan, T.M.; Chen, T.W.-W.; Italiano, A.; Demetri, G.D.; Cote, G.M.; et al. Safety and efficacy of tazemetostat, a first-in-class EZH2 inhibitor, in patients (pts) with epithelioid sarcoma (ES) (NCT02601950). *J. Clin. Oncol.* **2019**, *37*, 11003. [CrossRef]
287. Lewin, J.; Soria, J.-C.; Stathis, A.; Delord, J.-P.; Peters, S.; Awada, A.; Aftimos, P.G.; Bekradda, M.; Rezai, K.; Zeng, Z.; et al. Phase Ib Trial With Birabresib, a Small-Molecule Inhibitor of Bromodomain and Extraterminal Proteins, in Patients With Selected Advanced Solid Tumors. *J. Clin. Oncol. Off. J. Am. Soc. Clin. Oncol.* **2018**, *36*, 3007–3014. [CrossRef] [PubMed]
288. Bolden, J.E.; Tasdemir, N.; Dow, L.E.; van Es, J.H.; Wilkinson, J.E.; Zhao, Z.; Clevers, H.; Lowe, S.W. Inducible in vivo silencing of Brd4 identifies potential toxicities of sustained BET protein inhibition. *Cell Rep.* **2014**, *8*, 1919–1929. [CrossRef]

Case Report

Dealing with Corticosteroid and High-Dose Cyclosporine Therapy in a Pyoderma Gangrenosum Patient Contracting a COVID-19 Infection

Marcella Ricardis May [1], Albert Rübben [1,2], Andrea Lennertz [3], Luk Vanstreels [2] and Marike Leijs [1,2,*]

1. Department of Dermatology and Allergology, University Hospital of the RWTH Aachen University, 52074 Aachen, Germany; marcella.may@rwth-aachen.de (M.R.M.); Albert.Ruebben@post.rwth-aachen.de (A.R.)
2. Department of Dermatology, St. Nikolaus Hospital, 4700 Eupen, Belgium; luk.vanstreels@hospital-eupen.be
3. Department of Internal Medicine, St. Nikolaus Hospital, 4700 Eupen, Belgium; andrea.lennertz@hospital-eupen.be
* Correspondence: mleijs@ukaachen.de or marike.leijs@hospital-eupen.be; Tel.: +32-87-599312; Fax: +32-87-599322

Abstract: Pyoderma gangrenosum (PG) is a rare and chronic neutrophil inflammation belonging to the spectrum of autoinflammatory disorders. Immunosuppressive therapy is the cornerstone of successful treatment. However, due to the global COVID-19 pandemic, physicians struggle with therapeutic strategies during infection. This paper describes the case of a 58-year-old patient with a very painful, rapidly increasing wound on his right foot, which was diagnosed as pyoderma gangrenosum. Five weeks after the initial treatment with high-dose immunosuppressives (combination therapy with cyclosporine A and systemic methylprednisolone), he became infected with COVID-19. Reduction in the immunosuppressive dosage proved effective, as the patient recovered from COVID-19 without any complication and showed rapid wound healing.

Keywords: COVID-19; pyoderma gangrenosum; immunosuppression; cyclosporine; corticosteroids; autoinflammatory disease

1. Introduction

Currently, we are facing a global pandemic with severe acute respiratory syndrome coronavirus 2 (SARS-CoV-2) infection. While vaccines diminished the number of new infections, hospital admissions, and deaths, the number of so-called breakthrough hospital admissions of fully vaccinated individuals is increasing. Vulnerable patients with immunosuppressive medication, in particular, are at high risk of suffering from severe symptoms during an infection. In addition, there is always a part of the population that is not vaccinated. This can be due to underlying medical conditions or because a few individuals refuse to be vaccinated. Studies reported that immunosuppressed and multimorbid patients have a poor immune response following the SARS-CoV-2 vaccination [1]. In addition, experiences with other coronaviruses showed that immunosuppression could lead to atypical presentations including prolonged incubation periods, a persistence in asymptomatic viral shedding, and atypical symptoms such as gastroenterological disease and encephalitis. Experience and research evidence on COVID-19 in such patients are still very limited [2–7]. The severity of the COVID-19 infection is correlated with age, as well as gender and comorbidities such as cardiovascular diseases, diabetes, chronic respiratory diseases, hypertension, and cancers. A measured high number of white blood cells and neutrophils, as well as elevated D-dimer levels, are observed in COVID-19 patients with severe outcomes [8,9].

Pyoderma gangrenosum (PG) is a rare and chronic neutrophil inflammation. It belongs to the spectrum of autoinflammatory diseases and is characterized by recurrent episodes of progressive and often painful sterile inflammation. PG can be found solitary and multiple. According to Frank C. Powell (1996), six forms can be classified [10]. The classic and most frequent form is the ulcerous form. It develops fast and is mostly laminar. PG is a rare disease, as the global incidence is estimated to be around three to ten cases per one million population per year [9]. Moreover, it is frequently associated with several comorbidities especially inflammatory intestinal diseases (IBDs) (25%) [11], autoimmune disease (14.1%), hematological disorder (6.2%), and others (17.2%) [9]. PG is more often present in women than in men and most prevalent in 50–70-year-old individuals. Diagnosing PG properly is indispensable since PG is linked with a major reduction in quality of life and even with death [8]. To avoid misdiagnosis the Delphi score (D), as well as the so-called PARACELSUS score (P), which is an acronym, considers the following criteria (Table 1) [12,13]:

Table 1. The Major and Minor Criteria of the Delphi and PARACELSUS score.

Major Criteria	Minor Criteria
Rapidly progressing course of disease (P)	Prompt alleviation of symptoms by immunosuppressants (P *)
Reddish-violaceous wound border (P)	Characteristically irregular shape of the ulcer (P)
Exclusion of relevant differential diagnoses (P)	Extreme pain (P)
Neutrophilic infiltrate found in the ulcer edge (D)	Lesion at site of trauma (P)
	Exclusion of infection (D)
	Pathergy (D)
	History of inflammatory bowel disease or inflammatory arthritis (D)
	History of papule, pustule, or vesicle ulcerating within 4 days of appearing (D)
	Peripheral erythema, undermining border, and tenderness at ulceration site; (D)
	multiple ulcerations, at least 1 on an anterior lower leg (D)
	Cribriform or "wrinkled paper" scar(s) at healed ulcer sites (D)
	Decreased ulcer size within 1 month of initiating immunosuppressive medication(s) (D)

* The Paracelsus score contains three additional criteria: suppurative inflammation in histopathology, undermined wound border, systemic disease associated.

The pathogenesis of this autoinflammatory disease is not just multifactorial but also still unknown. In addition, the different PG types are differing in pathogenesis according to their form. Abnormalities in the function of the immune system including inflammatory cytokines, neutrophilic dysfunction, and specific genetic mutations have been observed. Evaluation of 21 patients with PG demonstrated infiltrates of CD-31 T cells and CD-1631 macrophages with high levels of interleukin (IL)-8 in the lesion. As IL-8 is a potent chemotactic for neutrophils, this explains the typical neutrophilic infiltrates, which can be visible in histopathological examination [14]. Overexpression of interleukin (IL)-1β plays an important role in PG as well but is not specific [15]. It has been suggested that PG and rheumatic diseases share a commonality in T-cell abnormalities. It was proposed that autoreactive T cells, which destroy pilosebaceous units, contribute to the pathophysiology since complete hair loss is found after healing [16]. An elevation of several chemotactic cytokines and interleukins was found in another study: CXC motif chemokine ligand

(CXCL) 9, CXCL 10, CXCL 11, chemokine C-C ligand 3 (CCL-3) and CCL-5, interleukin (IL)-36G, IL-17A, IL-8 (a neutrophil chemokine), and interferon gamma have been identified in PG lesions. In addition, an upregulation of certain transcription factors (STAT 1 and STAT 4) responsible for promoting Th1 differentiation was found in another study [17]. Very rare PG can appear as a monogenetic disease such as the PAPA syndrome in which case it is accompanied by arthritis and cystic acne [18]. Early diagnosis of pyoderma gangrenosum is important in order to minimize the size and necrotic painful character of the ulcer, as well as the formation of disfiguring scars [16]. In addition, secondary bacterial infections can occur and should be prevented.

Immunocompromised patients, including those requiring immunosuppressive therapy following autoinflammatory skin disease, are at high risk for developing severe disease following SARS-CoV-2 infection [2]. Neither the data regarding the best medical management of immune-compromised patients testing positive for SARS-CoV-2 nor strategies for reducing or modifying immunosuppression are easy to standardize yet [2]. In this case, in this study, we describe a 58-year-old man who became infected with COVID-19 while being treated with (high-dose) corticosteroids and cyclosporine. As cases similar to this are not commonly discussed, the aim of this paper was to set an example for other clinicians of how an adjustment of immunosuppressive therapy in patients with a rare autoinflammatory disease such as PG contracting a COVID-19 infection could be successfully performed.

2. Case Report

We present a 58-year-old Caucasian European male with an extremely painful ulcer at his right lateral malleolus (see Figure 1a). Anamnesis revealed that the wound appeared after massage therapy that he received for Achilles tendinitis. Initially, he reported a painful bulla, which became ulcerative. Due to other physical problems (otitis media and necrosis of the temporomandibular joint) and the fact that he was taking antibiotics and analgesics, the patient did not seek medical treatment at an earlier stage of the disease. However, the wound expanded within two weeks rapidly and became very painful. Medical history revealed comorbidities of diverticulosis and hypercholesterolemia.

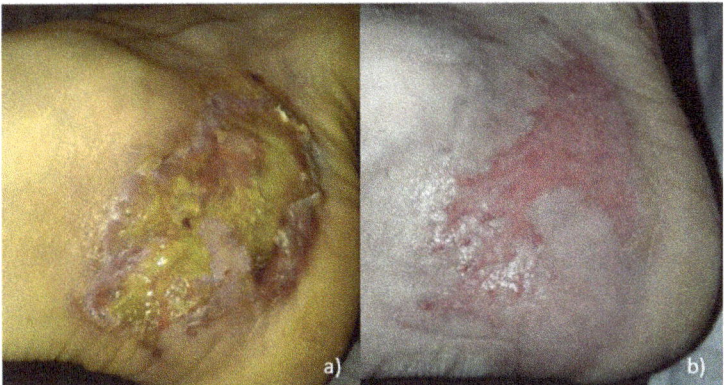

Figure 1. Pictures of the ulcer: (**a**) at the time of hospitalization; (**b**) healed ulcer 8.5 weeks after initial diagnosis.

Clinical evaluation revealed a 4 cm × 8 cm ulcer with tissue necrosis, as well as a very painful livid erythematous encircling undermined edge (Figure 1a). No signs of venous insufficiency were visible. Clinical assessment showed normal peripheral vascularization.

An infectious ulcer was excluded by a negative microbiological swab. Peripheral arterial occlusive disease and venous insufficiency could be excluded with duplex sonography. Computed tomography of the foot and ankle was used to exclude osteomyelitis.

Two skin biopsies were taken from the edge of the ulcus. As seen more often in PG, histopathological findings were not specific. However, the dermis showed fibrosis including mixed cellular inflammatory infiltrates. These were mainly perivascular lymphocytic but also mixed lymphohistiocytic infiltrates including some neutrophil granulocytes. Infiltrates contained mostly CD-3 positive T lymphocytes.

We diagnosed the ulcer as an ulcerating form of pyoderma gangrenosum due to its typical clinical presentation and as the minor criteria (Delphi) and major and minor criteria of the PARACELSUS score of pyoderma gangrenosum (which is discussed in detail in the Introduction Section) were fulfilled [12].

We decided to start directly a combination therapy with (2.5 mg/kg) cyclosporine A (CsA) twice a day and systemic methylprednisolone (1 mg/kg) per day because of severe pain and a rapidly increasing wound (despite premedication with 20 mg methylprednisolone from the patients' otorhinolaryngologist) and in order to avoid side effects of long-term steroid usage [8]. A local corticosteroid and a calcineurin inhibitor ointment were applied once a day, and an adsorbing dressing was added.

An improvement in pain and a decrease in ulcer size were observed. Moreover, the C-reactive protein (CRP) declined satisfactorily under this treatment. After 5 days of treatment, the CRP declined from 198.3 mg/L (see Table 2) to 37.7 mg/L (RV < 8.0).

Table 2. The laboratory parameters at the time of the patient's hospitalization.

Laboratory Parameter	Value	Reference
Hemoglobin	9.8 g/dL	13.3–17.7 g/dL
Hematocrite	30%	40–52%
Red Blood Cells	$3.67 \times 10^6/mm^3$	$4.40-5.90 \times 10^6/mm^3$
Blood Platelets (in Ethylenediaminetetraacetic Acid (EDTA))	544 million/μL	3.9–10.6 million/μL
Reticulocytes	2.05%	0.50–2.00%
Neutrophiles	70.7%	40.0–70.0%
Lymphocytes	14.3%	20.0–45.0%
Eosinohiles	0.7%	<4.0%
Basophiles	0.4%	<2.0%
Monocytes	13.9%	<12.0%
Creatinin	0.55 mg/dL	0.80–1.30 mg/dL
Uric Acid	4.5 mg/dL	2.6–7.2 mg/dL
Sodium	133 mmol/L	135–145 mmol/L
Potassium	4.6 mmol/L	3.5–5.1 mmol/L
Chloride	99 mmol/L	97–107 mmol/L
CRP (c-reactive proteine ultrasensitive)	**198.3 mg/L**	**<8.0 mg/L**
Protein total	60.3 g/L	58.0–83.0 g/L
AST (spartate aminotransferase)	31 U/L	<42 U/L
GPT (alanine transaminase)	33 U/L	<40 U/L
LDH (lactaatdehydrogenase)	125 U/L	<250 U/L
Alkaline Phosphatases	57 U/L	30–120 U/L
Gamma-GT (glutamyl transferase)	34 U/L	<50 U/L
Bilirubin Total	0.4 mg/dL	0.2–1.2 mg/dL
Bilirubin Direct	0.1 mg/dL	<0.3 mg/dL

Five weeks after the initial hospitalization, the patient presented to the emergency care with fever and dyspnea. At this time, he was still taking 300 mg CsA and 8 mg methylprednisolone. A PCR test (long nasal swab) confirmed the SARS-CoV-2 infection. Computer tomography demonstrated typical lung infiltration (Figure 2). It had to be decided whether to continue or modify the immunosuppressive therapy or to interrupt cyclosporine A since cyclosporine interferes with the antiviral immune pathway [3]. We decided to halve the cyclosporine A dosage to 75 mg twice a day (Figure 3). The patient's clinical condition significantly improved within three days from the beginning of COVID-19 symptoms. The ulcer healed 8.5 weeks after the initial diagnosis (Figure 1b).

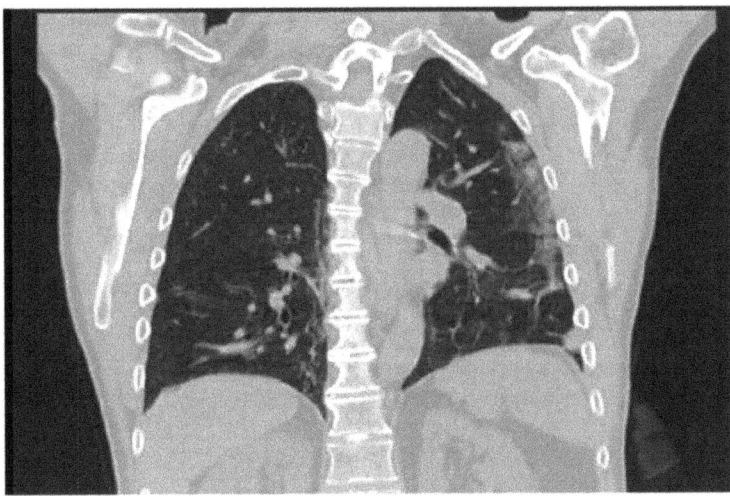

Figure 2. Typical COVID-19 lung infiltrates, five weeks after initial presentation.

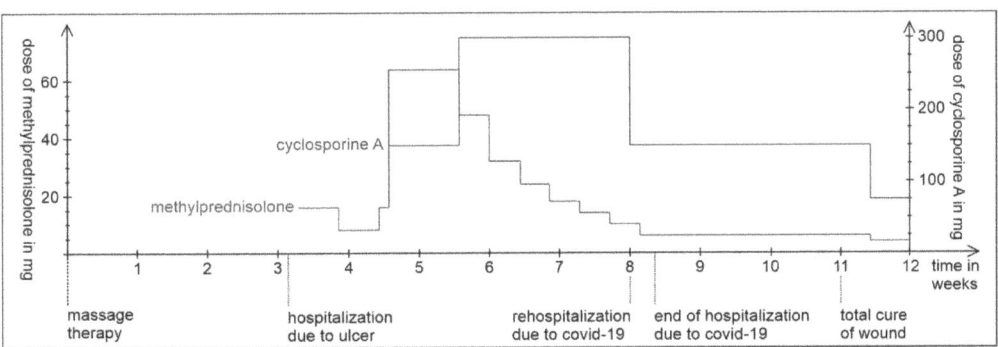

Figure 3. Timeline of patient's healing and the dose of methylprednisolone and cyclosporine A.

3. Discussion

Immunosuppressive therapy—mostly corticosteroids in combination with CsA—depending on the severity, the extent of the PG lesion, and previous conditions, is the cornerstone of the treatment in PG patients. In addition, proper local treatment, including adapted wound care to prevent secondary bacterial infection and slight compression, as well as administration of analgesics for pain relief, is important [16]. In the case of our patient, pain relief and reduction in wound size occurred after initiating the therapy with corticosteroids and CsA. At the time of treatment, the patient was not vaccinated yet, and as the patient contracted a COVID-19 infection, we needed to decide how to continue the immunosuppressive therapy.

Patients with severe COVID-19 infections may receive systemic corticosteroids in order to reduce the systemic inflammatory response that can lead to lung injury and multisystem organ dysfunction [4]. The uncontrolled proinflammatory response with the release of cytokines known as the cytokine storm is not well defined. It has been reported to occur after unsuccessful viral clearance and it might involve less specific defense mechanisms such as monocyte and macrophage activation [19]. The exact pathophysiologic mechanisms are unclear. One study reported elevated IL-6 levels in severely ill COVID-19 patients [20]. Conversely, another study on 46 critically ill COVID-19 patients showed no difference in levels of IL-6/8 and tumor necrosis factor (TNF), compared with other critically ill patients, and even lower levels than in critically ill patients with a septic shock [21].

How to deal with immune suppressive medication during COVID-19 infection is not standardized yet. One study on 374 clinician-reported psoriasis patients from 25 countries showed that the hospitalization rate due to COVID-19 was more frequent in patients using nonbiologic systemic therapy than in those using biologics (OR = 2.84; 95% CI = 1.31–6.18). Other risk factors in this study were older age, male sex, nonwhite ethnicity, and comorbid chronic lung disease [22]. Some studies advise withholding immune-modulating medication, with the exception of corticosteroids [5]. Contrarily, a recent position statement on immunotherapeutics in patients with inflammatory skin disease pointed out that limited data suggested there is no additional risk for patients using CsA. However, no dose-dependent advice was given in this paper [23]. CsA has already been used as a treatment for patients with COVID-19, as reported in the World Health Organization (WHO) guidelines [4,24,25]. CsA bind to cyclophilin, which theoretically inhibits SARS-CoV-2 replication [26]. In agreement, in another review, it was concluded as well that "there is no evidence that [the] use of cyclosporine possesses an additional risk for severe COVID-19" [27]. Other studies on immunosuppressives during COVID-19 infection suggest that cyclosporine A can potentially prevent acute respiratory failure and hyperinflammation-induced lung injury [28,29]. On the other hand, an increased risk of several viral infections is seen in organ transplant patients treated with CsA [30]. As a causative factor, CsA suppresses helping T cells and precursors of cytotoxic T lymphocytes and depresses the innate immune system by inhibition of natural killer cells, which are the most important immune cells in this regard, along with antibody-dependent cellular cytotoxicity and certain cytokines (IL-6, IL-2), prominently interferons. NF-κB suppression inhibits mainly the production of proinflammatory cytokines. An animal study demonstrated an inability to mount an effective immune response to viral infections with the administration of CsA [31]. Even though a potential beneficial effect of cyclosporine has been discussed in several studies, the experts are not yet unified regarding this topic. In addition, most studies do not give dose-dependent advice for CsA. When administrating CsA we have to keep in mind that it will inhibit establishing immune memory following COVID-19 infection or vaccination [32].

In the presented case, methylprednisolone and cyclosporine were the main therapy of the patient. Their specific immunosuppressive mechanisms are described in Figure 2. Methylprednisolone is a synthetic glucocorticoid and displays the same features (immunosuppressive, anti-inflammatory, and antiallergic) as cortisol. Corticosteroids inhibit both T and B cells. It rapidly reduces circulating T cells due to enhanced circulatory emigration, induction of apoptosis, inhibition of T-cell growth factors, and impaired release of cells from lymphoid tissues. Effects on B-cell function and immunoglobulin production are more delayed [33]. Potent suppressive effects on the effector functions of monocytes and neutrophils, as well as the suppression of NF-κB and activator protein- 1 (AP-1), are of great importance because they inhibit many inflammatory and immune modulators as a result of modulation of the expression of pro-inflammatory cytokines such as IL-1b, TNFα, and IL-2 (Figure 4) [34]. As a result, the cellular and humoral immune reactions regress. In addition, suppression of NF-κB can suppress the synthesis of cyclooxygenase-2 (COX-2).

In conclusion, the glucocorticoid responsive genes encode a large array of effectors in the host antiviral defense system [35]. Synergistically, cyclosporine A binds to cyclophilin, which leads to an inhibition of calcineurin, leading additionally to inhibition of intracellular NF-κB (Figure 4) [3]. As a consequence, the transcription factor NF-AT cannot be dephosphorylated, and the cytokine IL-2 is produced in lower quantities. Consequently, T lymphocytes are activated less. Interestingly, a mutation in the NF-κB signaling pathway (critically important for regulation of the innate and adaptive immune responses) has been identified in a PG case report [36]. It has been postulated that observed effects of corticosteroids are dose dependent probably due to the variable dose-dependent affinity of target genomic sites for the glucocorticoid receptor and that some additional genes are affected as the concentration of glucocorticoid increases [34]. It has been proven that corticosteroids improve survival of critically ill COVID-19 patients; nevertheless, a recent study showed that a dose over 40 mg methylprednisolone equivalent dosing (MED) had a higher mortality rate [37]. In the aforementioned recent position statement, it was advised to continue corticosteroids at a lower dose < 10 mg prednisolone since it may suppress viral clearance [30].

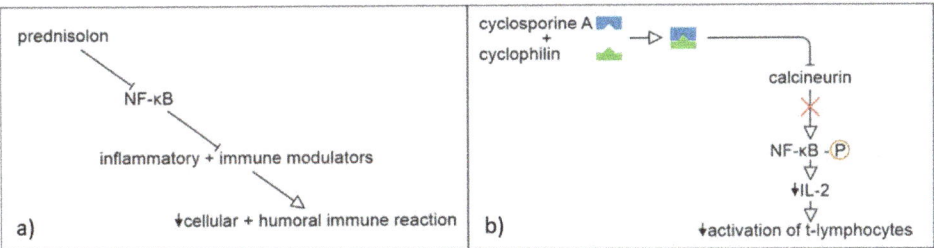

Figure 4. Effect of (**a**) prednisolone and (**b**) cyclosporine A.

Alternative treatment of pyoderma gangrenosum includes azathioprine, methotrexate, thalidomide, dapsone, mycophenolate mofetil, sulfasalazine, cyclophosphamides, colchicine, antitumor necrosis factor-alpha inhibitor (TNF-α), and intravenous immune globulin (IVIG). As our patient reacted well to the combinational therapy with cyclosporine and corticosteroids, alternative therapy was not taken into consideration. Additional therapeutic options include antibodies against IL-17, IL-12/IL-23, Il-6, IL-1β, IL-1 receptor I, as well as JAK1, 2, and 3 inhibitors [16,38–44]. For all the mentioned therapeutic options, and likewise for CsA, limited data demonstrated no risk for severe COVID-19 infection [30].

In conclusion, we cautiously advise the adaption of immune suppressive therapy in patients with pyoderma gangrenosum suffering from COVID-19. Adaptation should be performed according to the severity of the disease and the stage of treatment. In patients with symptomatic light to moderate infection, we suggest temporarily halving the CsA treatment in case of high dosage and lowering the corticosteroid dose.

Author Contributions: Conceptualization, M.L.; methodology, M.L., A.R., A.L., L.V. and M.R.M.; investigations, M.L., M.R.M. and A.L.; writing—original draft preparation, M.R.M. and M.L.; writing—review and editing, M.L., M.R.M., A.R., A.L. and L.V.; visualization, M.R.M. and M.L.; supervision, M.L., A.R. and A.L. All authors have read and agreed to the published version of the manuscript.

Funding: This research received no external funding.

Institutional Review Board Statement: The study was conducted according to the guidelines of the Declaration of Helsinki. Approval of the ethics committee was not needed considering the retrospective nature of the study and that the findings are a description of a single case report. This paper follows the rules of the Declaration of Helsinki. The patient involved in the research agreed to participate and agreed to provide case details and have the results of the research about them published.

Informed Consent Statement: Verbal and written informed consent was obtained from the subject involved in the study. Anyone involved in the research agreed to participate and agreed to provide case details and have the results of the research about them published.

Data Availability Statement: Most data are presented in the manuscript. Further details are available on request from the corresponding author. The data are not publicly available due to privacy restrictions.

Acknowledgments: We are grateful to Anne Piron for the histological analysis.

Conflicts of Interest: The authors declare no conflict of interest.

References

1. Yen, C.-C.; Lin, S.-Y.; Chen, S.-C.; Chiu, Y.-W.; Chang, J.-M.; Hwang, S.-J. COVID-19 vaccines in patients with maintenance hemodialysis. *J. Pers. Med.* **2021**, *11*, 789. [CrossRef] [PubMed]
2. Marzano, A.; Borghi, A.; Meroni, P.L.; Cugno, M. Pyoderma gangrenosum and its syndromic forms: Evidence for a link with autoinflammation. *Br. J. Dermatol.* **2016**, *175*, 882–891. [CrossRef] [PubMed]
3. Johnson, K.M.; Belfer, J.J.; Peterson, G.R.; Boelkins, M.R.; Dumkow, L.E. Managing COVID-19 in renal transplant recipients: A review of recent literature and case supporting corticosteroid-sparing immunosuppression. *Pharmacother. J. Hum. Pharmacol. Drug Ther.* **2020**, *40*, 517–524. [CrossRef] [PubMed]
4. Khurana, A.; Sethia, K. Using cyclosporine in the COVID era: An emergent need for caution. *J. Am. Acad. Dermatol.* **2020**, *83*, e315–e316. [CrossRef]
5. World Health Organization (WHO). Corticosteroids for COVID-19. In *Living Guid*; WHO: Geneva, Switzerland, 2020; pp. 1–25.
6. Sun, Y.; Zhou, J.; Ye, K. White blood cells and severe COVID-19: A mendelian randomization study WBC COVID-19 SNPs associated with WBC SNPs associated with COVID-19. *J. Pers. Med.* **2021**, *11*, 195. [CrossRef]
7. Zhou, F.; Yu, T.; Du, R.; Fan, G.; Liu, Y.; Liu, Z.; Xiang, J.; Wang, Y.; Song, B.; Gu, X.; et al. Clinical course and risk factors for mortality of adult inpatients with COVID-19 in Wuhan, China: A retrospective cohort study. *Lancet* **2020**, *395*, 1054–1062. [CrossRef]
8. Deutsche Dermatologische Gesellschaft, B. Deutsche Dermatologische Gesellschaft B. S1-Leitlinie Pyoderma Gangrenosum. 2020. AWMF. Available online: https://www.awmf.org/uploads/tx_szleitlinien/013-091l_S1_Pyoderma-gangrenosum_2020-10_1.pdf (accessed on 28 November 2021).
9. Monari, P.; Moro, R.; Motolese, A.; Misciali, C.; Baraldi, C.; Fanti, P.A.; Caccavale, S.; Puviani, M.; Olezzi, D.; Zampieri, P.; et al. Epidemiology of pyoderma gangrenosum: Results from an Italian prospective multicentre study. *Int. Wound J.* **2018**, *15*, 875–879. [CrossRef]
10. Powell, F.C.; Su, W.D.; Perry, H.O. Pyoderma gangrenosum: Classification and management. *J. Am. Acad. Dermatol.* **1996**, *34*, 392–395. [CrossRef]
11. Abenavoli, L.; Dastoli, S.; Bennardo, L.; Boccuto, L.; Passante, M.; Silvestri, M.; Proietti, I.; Potenza, C.; Luzza, F.; Nisticò, S.P. The skin in celiac disease patients: The other side of the coin. *Medicina* **2019**, *55*, 1–17. [CrossRef]
12. Maverakis, E.; Ma, C.; Shinkai, K.; Fiorentino, D.; Callen, J.P.; Wollina, U.; Marzano, A.V.; Wallach, D.; Kim, K.; Cheng, M.Y.; et al. Diagnostic criteria of ulcerative pyoderma gangrenosum: A Delphi consensus of international experts. *JAMA Dermatol.* **2018**, *154*, 461–466. [CrossRef]
13. Jockenhöfer, F.; Wollina, U.; Salva, K.; Benson, S.; Dissemond, J. The PARACELSUS score: A novel diagnostic tool for pyoderma gangrenosum. *Br. J. Dermatol.* **2018**, *180*, 615–620. [CrossRef] [PubMed]
14. Marzano, A.V.; Cugno, M.; Trevisan, V.; Fanoni, D.; Venegoni, L.; Berti, E.; Crosti, C. Role of inflammatory cells, cytokines and matrix metalloproteinases in neutrophil-mediated skin diseases. *Clin. Exp. Immunol.* **2010**, *162*, 100–107. [CrossRef] [PubMed]
15. Braswell, S.F.; Kostopoulos, T.C.; Ortega-Loayza, A.G. Pathophysiology of pyoderma gangrenosum (PG): An updated review. *J. Am. Acad. Dermatol.* **2015**, *73*, 691–698. [CrossRef] [PubMed]
16. Skopis, M.; Bag-Ozbek, A. Pyoderma gangrenosum: A review of updates in diagnosis, pathophysiology and management. *J* **2021**, *4*, 367–375. [CrossRef]
17. Wang, E.A.; Steel, A.; Luxardi, G.; Mitra, A.; Patel, F.; Cheng, M.Y.; Wilken, R.; Kao, J.; De Ga, K.; Sultani, H.; et al. Classic ulcerative pyoderma gangrenosum is a T Cell-Mediated disease targeting follicular adnexal structures: A hypothesis based on molecular and clinicopathologic studies. *Front. Immunol.* **2018**, *8*, 1980. [CrossRef]
18. Wise, C.A.; Gillum, J.D.; Seidman, C.E.; Lindor, N.M.; Veile, R.; Bashiardes, S.; Lovett, M. Mutations in CD2BP1 disrupt binding to PTP PEST and are responsible for PAPA syndrome, an autoinflammatory disorder. *Hum. Mol. Genet.* **2002**, *11*, 961–969. [CrossRef]
19. Merad, M.; Martin, J.C. Pathological inflammation in patients with COVID-19: A key role for monocytes and macrophages. *Nat. Rev. Immunol.* **2020**, *20*, 355–362. [CrossRef]
20. Sinha, P.; Matthay, M.A.; Calfee, C.S. Is a "Cytokine Storm" relevant to COVID-19? *JAMA Intern. Med.* **2020**, *180*, 1152–1154. [CrossRef]
21. Kox, M.; Waalders, N.J.B.; Kooistra, E.J.; Gerretsen, J.; Pickkers, P. Cytokine levels in critically Ill patients with COVID-19 and other conditions. *JAMA* **2020**, *324*, 1565–1567. [CrossRef]

22. Mahil, S.K.; Dand, N.; Mason, K.J.; Yiu, Z.Z.; Tsakok, T.; Meynell, F.; Coker, B.; McAteer, H.; Moorhead, L.; Mackenzie, T.; et al. Factors associated with adverse COVID-19 outcomes in patients with psoriasis—Insights from a global registry–based study. *J. Allergy Clin. Immunol.* **2021**, *147*, 60–71. [CrossRef]
23. Beecker, J.; Cooper, C.; Gisondi, P.; Gooderham, M.; Hong, C.H.; Kirchhof, M.G.; Lynde, C.W.; Maari, C.; Poulin, Y.; Puig, L. Position statement for a pragmatic approach to immunotherapeutics in patients with in flammatory skin diseases during the coronavirus disease 2019 pandemic and beyond. *J. Eur. Acad. Dermatol. Venereol.* **2021**, *35*, 797–806. [CrossRef] [PubMed]
24. Wang, C.; Rademaker, M.; Baker, C.; Foley, P. COVID-19 and the use of immunomodulatory and biologic agents for severe cutaneous disease: An Australian/New Zealand consensus statement. *Australas. J. Dermatol.* **2020**, *61*, 210–216. [CrossRef] [PubMed]
25. Guisado-Vasco, P.; Valderas-Ortega, S.; Carralón-González, M.M.; Roda-Santacruz, A.; González-Cortijo, L.; Sotres-Fernández, G.; Martí-Ballesteros, E.M.; Luque-Pinilla, J.M.; Almagro-Casado, E.; La Coma-Lanuza, F.J.; et al. Clinical characteristics and outcomes among hospitalized adults with severe COVID-19 admitted to a tertiary medical center and receiving antiviral, antimalarials, glucocorticoids, or immunomodulation with tocilizumab or cyclosporine: A retrospective observational study (COQUIMA cohort). *EClinicalMedicine* **2020**, *28*, 100591. [PubMed]
26. de Wilde, A.H.; Zevenhoven-dobbe, J.C.; van der Meer, Y.; Thiel, V.; Narayanan, K.; Makino, S.; Snijder, E.J.; van Hemert, M.J. Communication cyclosporin A inhibits the replication of diverse coronaviruses. *J. Gen. Virol.* **2011**, *92*, 2542–2548. [CrossRef]
27. Rochwerg, B.; Siemieniuk, R.A.; Agoritsas, T.; Lamontagne, F.; Askie, L.; Lytvyn, L.; Agarwal, A.; Leo, Y.-S.; Macdonald, H.; Zeng, L.; et al. A living WHO guideline on drugs for covid-19. *BMJ* **2020**, *370*, 1–14.
28. Poulsen, N.N.; von Brunn, A.; Hornum, M.; Blomberg Jensen, M. Cyclosporine and COVID-19: Risk or favorable? *Am. J. Transpl.* **2020**, *20*, 2975–2982. [CrossRef]
29. de Almeida, S.M.V.; Soares, J.C.S.; dos Santos, K.L.; Alves, J.E.F.; Ribeiro, A.G.; Jacob, Í.T.T.; da Silva Ferreira, C.J.; Santos, J.C.D.; de Oliveira, J.F.; de Lima, M.D.C.A. COVID-19 therapy: What weapons do we bring into battle? *Bioorg. Med. Chem.* **2020**, *28*, 115757. [CrossRef]
30. Khurana, A.; Saxena, S. Immunosuppressive agents for dermatological indications in the ongoing COVID-19 pandemic: Rationalizing use and clinical applicability. *Dermatol. Ther.* **2020**, *33*, e13639. [CrossRef]
31. Kim, J.H.; Perfect, J.R. Infection and cyclosporine. *Rev. Infect. Dis.* **1989**, *11*, 677–690. [CrossRef]
32. Rudnicka, L.; Glowacka, P.; Goldust, M.; Sikora, M.; Sar-Pomian, M.; Rakowska, A.; Samochocket, Z.; Olszewska, M. Cyclosporine therapy during the COVID-19 pandemic. *J. Am. Acad. Dermatol.* **2020**, *83*, e151–e152. [CrossRef]
33. Chatham, W.W.; Kimberly, R.P. Treatment of lupus with corticosteroids. *SAGE J.* **2001**, *10*, 140–147. [CrossRef] [PubMed]
34. Tsokos, G.C. *Principles of Molecular Rheumatology*; Humana Press: Totowa, NJ, USA, 2000; pp. 439–449.
35. Cour, M.; Ovize, M.; Argaud, L. Cyclosporine A: A valid candidate to treat COVID-19 patients with acute respiratory failure? *Crit. Care* **2020**, *24*, 1–3. [CrossRef] [PubMed]
36. Fang, R.; Wang, J.; Jiang, X.-Y.; Wang, S.-H.; Cheng, H.; Zhou, Q. Case report: A novel mutation in NFKB1 associated with pyoderma gangrenosum. *Front. Genet.* **2021**, *10*, 673453. [CrossRef] [PubMed]
37. Kumar, G.; Patel, D.; Hererra, M.; Jefferies, D.; Sakhuja, A.; Cpa, M.M.; Dalton, D.; Nanchal, R.; Guddati, A.K. Do high-dose corticosteroids improve outcomes in hospitalized COVID-19 patients? *J. Med. Virol.* **2022**, *1*, 372–379. [CrossRef]
38. McPHIE, M.L.; Kirchhof, M.G. Pyoderma gangrenosum treated with secukinumab: A case report. *SAGE Open Med. Case Rep.* **2020**, *1*, 2050313X20940430. [CrossRef]
39. Vallerand, I.A.; Hardin, J. Ustekinumab for the treatment of recalcitrant pyoderma gangrenosum: A case report. *SAGE Open Med. Case Rep.* **2019**, *1*, 2050313X19845206. [CrossRef]
40. McKenzie, F.; Arthur, M.; Ortega-Loayza, A.G. Pyoderma Gangrenosum: What Do We Know Now? *Curr. Dermatol. Rep.* **2018**, *7*, 147–157. [CrossRef]
41. Kolios, A.; Maul, J.-T.; Meier, B.; Kerl, K.; Traidl-Hoffmann, C.; Hertl, M.; Zillikens, D.; Röcken, M.; Ring, J.; Facchiano, A.; et al. Canakinumab in adults with steroid-refractory pyoderma gangrenosum. *Br. J. Dermatol.* **2015**, *173*, 1216–1223. [CrossRef]
42. Brenner, M.; Ruzicka, T.; Plewig, G.; Thomas, P.; Herzer, P. Targeted treatment of pyoderma gangrenosum in PAPA (pyogenic arthritis, pyoderma gangrenosum and acne) syndrome with the recombinant human interleukin-1 receptor antagonist anakinra. *Br. J. Dermatol.* **2009**, *161*, 1199–1201. [CrossRef]
43. Kochar, B.; Herfarth, N.; Mamie, C.; Navarini, A.A.; Scharl, M.; Herfarth, H.H. Tofacitinib for the treatment of pyoderma gangrenosum. *Clin. Gastroenterol. Hepatol.* **2019**, *17*, 991–993. [CrossRef]
44. Nasifoglu, S.; Heinrich, B.; Welzel, J. Successful therapy for pyoderma gangrenosum with a Janus kinase 2 inhibitor. *Br. J. Dermatol.* **2018**, *179*, 504–505. [CrossRef] [PubMed]

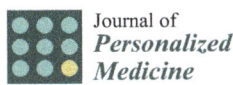
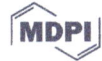

Review

Current Challenges in Deciphering Sutton Nevi—Literature Review and Personal Experience

Roxana Nedelcu [1,2], Alexandra Dobre [1,*], Alice Brinzea [1,2,3], Ionela Hulea [1], Razvan Andrei [4,5], Sabina Zurac [1,4], Mihaela Balaban [2], Mihaela Antohe [1,2], Lorena Manea [1,4,6], Andreea Calinescu [1,2], Anastasia Coman [1,2], Florentina Pantelimon [2], Adina Dobritoiu [2], Catalin Popescu [1,4], Raluca Popescu [1,4], Elena Balasescu [1], Daniela Ion [1] and Gabriela Turcu [1,2,4]

1. General Medicine, Carol Davila University of Medicine and Pharmacy, 050474 Bucharest, Romania; roxanaioana.nedelcu@yahoo.com (R.N.); brinzeaalice@gmail.com (A.B.); dr.ionelahulea@yahoo.com (I.H.); sabina_zurac@yahoo.com (S.Z.); dr.antohemihaela@gmail.com (M.A.); lor.manea@gmail.com (L.M.); andreea.calinescu0202@yahoo.com (A.C.); anastasia.hodorogea@gmail.com (A.C.); catalin.m.popescu@gmail.com (C.P.); rlc.popescu@gmail.com (R.P.); elena_balasescu@yahoo.com (E.B.); danielaion7@ymail.com (D.I.); dr.gabriela.turcu@gmail.com (G.T.)
2. Derma 360 Clinic, 11273 Bucharest, Romania; mihaela.cernat@gmail.com (M.B.); florentina.pantelimon@gmail.com (F.P.); adina_dobritoiu@yahoo.com (A.D.)
3. National Institute for Infectious Diseases, Outpatient Clinic, 021105 Bucharest, Romania
4. Department of Pathology and Dermatovenerology, Colentina Clinical Hospital, 020125 Bucharest, Romania; razvan.andrei.13@gmail.com
5. Synevo Medical Laboratory, 014192 Bucharest, Romania
6. Department of Dermatovenerology, Centre Hospitalier Régional D'orléans, 45100 Orléans, France
* Correspondence: alexandraa.dobre@yahoo.com; Tel.: +40-740-853-353

Citation: Nedelcu, R.; Dobre, A.; Brinzea, A.; Hulea, I.; Andrei, R.; Zurac, S.; Balaban, M.; Antohe, M.; Manea, L.; Calinescu, A.; et al. Current Challenges in Deciphering Sutton Nevi—Literature Review and Personal Experience. *J. Pers. Med.* **2021**, *11*, 904. https://doi.org/10.3390/jpm11090904

Academic Editors: Mircea Tampa, Monica Neagu, Constantin Caruntu, Simona Roxana Georgescu and Reginald M. Gorczynski

Received: 22 July 2021
Accepted: 6 September 2021
Published: 9 September 2021

Publisher's Note: MDPI stays neutral with regard to jurisdictional claims in published maps and institutional affiliations.

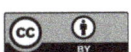

Copyright: © 2021 by the authors. Licensee MDPI, Basel, Switzerland. This article is an open access article distributed under the terms and conditions of the Creative Commons Attribution (CC BY) license (https://creativecommons.org/licenses/by/4.0/).

Abstract: Halo nevi, known as leukoderma acquisitum centrifugum, Sutton nevus, leukopigmentary nevus, perinevoid vitiligo, or perinevoid leukoderma, together with vitiligo and melanoma-associated hypopigmentation, belong to the group of dermatoses designated as immunological leukodermas. The etiology and pathogenesis of halo nevi has not been fully elucidated. There are several mechanisms through which a lymphocytic infiltrate can induce tumoral regression. In this review, we aimed to update the knowledge about Sutton nevi starting with the clinical appearance and dermoscopic features, continuing with information regarding conventional microscopy, immunohistochemistry, and the immunological mechanisms responsible for the occurrence of halo nevi. We also included in the article original unpublished results when discussing dermoscopic, pathologic and immunohistochemical results in halo nevi. Sutton nevi are valuable models for studying antitumor reactions that the human body can generate. The slow and effective mechanism against a melanocytic skin tumor can teach us important lessons about both autoimmune diseases and anticancer defenses.

Keywords: immune response; inflammation; Sutton nevi; halo nevi; skin tumor

1. Introduction

Leukoderma acquisitum centrifugum, later known as *Sutton nevus* or *halo nevus*, appeared in 1916 in the writings of Richard Lightburn Sutton [1,2]. The recognition of Dr. Richard Lightburn Sutton's work from whom the clinical entity takes its name has its root in describing and observing for the first time the disease in two of his patients [1,2]. Sutton described two cases of peculiar brown maculo-papules, but he considered the lesions to be clinical variants of vitiligo. He introduced his cases of abnormal pigmentation with a review of the cellular origins of pigmentation and vitiligo. It was only later that John H. Stokes made the correlation of *leukoderma acquisitum centrifugum* with melanocytic nevi [3].

With no gender or racial predilection, Sutton nevi are found in approximately 1% of young adults. The mean age at onset is thought to be 15 years. It is unusual and a sign of suspicion if a depigmentation around a nevus is found in an older patient [4,5].

The most common sites for Sutton nevi are the back, followed by head and neck [6,7]. The halo phenomenon can develop around preexisting junctional or compound nevi. [8].

Attempts have been made to better understand the natural evolution of halo nevi, by describing and didactically dividing the disease into four stages [8,9]: Stage I corresponds to the presence of the characteristic depigmented rim around the nevus; Stage II, with loss of pigment within the central nevus surrounded by a depigmented rim; Stage III is described by the presence of a circular area of depigmentation with the total disappearance of the nevus; Stage IV corresponds to the repigmentation phase, with normal appearing skin. The changes can develop for over 10 years.

2. Why Measure the Diameter?—The Average Size of Halo Nevi, the Relationship between the Halo and the Nevus

The stages mentioned above are variable with every patient and natural evolution of Sutton nevi has not yet been fully deciphered. The presence of halo depigmentation correlates with the onset of nevus regression, evolving towards total resorption of the melanocytic lesion with the possibility of repigmentation after many years. Complete regression of the central nevus has been reported in over 50% of cases [10]. Even if it is known that the halo phenomenon has four clinical stages of evolution, an unusual clinical evolution with repigmentation of the nevus component was also reported [11,12].

The size of the hypomelanotic halo varies and the most frequently reported values in the literature were between 0.5 and 5 cm [13]. At present, there are few data in the literature related to the factors that influence the diameter of the halo, the significance of this diameter and the possible correlations between the diameter of the nevus and the diameter of the halo. Rongioletti et al. were among the few authors who studied these possible correlations. They calculated a correlation coefficient and showed the existence of a linear and highly significant direct link between these two parameters. Thus, the larger the nevus, the larger its halo. They were also the ones who described the "melanocyte antigenic unit" (melanocyte antigenic unit—MAU). It consists of melanocytes with radial disposition from the central melanocytic lesion, having the same phenotype and being functionally dependent on the central nevus. This concept provides a valid explanation for the etiopathogenesis of the recurrent melanocytic nevus and also seems to provide useful information in understanding the link between melanoma margins and tumor thickness [14]. Further studies are still needed to explore in more detail the connection between the halo and the thickness of the central nevus.

3. Dermoscopic Pattern—Same Look as in Common Nevi?

For the last few years, dermoscopy has been shown to be one of the most helpful tools used to diagnose and monitor skin tumors. Despite the fact that the Sutton nevus is a benign lesion, the diagnostic process is often challenging, because it may present clinical, dermoscopical and histopathological structures that resemble melanoma. Furthermore, dermoscopic features that characterize this type of nevi have not yet been described in detail, so we will present you hereunder a comparison between the actual data from the literature and our own personal findings.

We retrospectively analyzed 32 digital dermoscopic images of Sutton nevi from 17 patients. The diagnosis was made by experienced dermatologists and was mostly based on clinical and dermoscopic examination. All nevi were checked with a hand-held DermLite DL4W dermoscope and stored afterwards as digital images in a computer database. Of the 17 patients, 11 (64.7%) were women and six (35.3%) were men. The mean age at presentation was 26.05 years (median 29; range 9–50), somewhat higher than previous studies (18.2%; 22.4%) [15,16]. The most frequent Fitzpatrick skin phototype we found was type III (15/17; 88.22%), followed by type II (2/17; 11.8%). Between 25% and 50% of people with Sutton nevi have been described with more than one nevus [8]. In our group, the ratio of solitary to multiple nevi was 11:6, even though most occurred as single lesions. Out of the 32 halo nevi, 20 (62.5%) were located on the chest, five (15.6%) were located in the lumbar region, three (9.4%) were located on the abdomen, two (6.62%) in the head region and two (6.62%) on upper extremities. Indeed, a predilection for the trunk has been reported in the literature [13].

The appearance of the nevi varied between flat (n = 25, 72.1%), elevated (n = 4, 12.5%) and central elevated (n = 3, 9.4%). The first dermoscopic aspects that we analyzed were size and color. Similarly to previously published studies, the mean diameter of the central nevus was 5.22 mm (range 3–10) [8]. Most were light brown (n = 11), but we also observed brown (n = 6), pink (n = 2), or multicolored (n = 3) nevi. Additionally, nine were fully regressed with a residual white halo and one was fully regressed with total repigmentation of the skin.

Next, we analyzed the halo of the nevi and we observed a particularity. According to Sutton and the existing literature, the surroundings of the central nevus should be a completely well-circumscribed depigmentation area [13]. In our case, this classical uniformly annular halo was not seen in all nevi. For 21 (65.6%) of them, we observed a symmetrical white rim (Figure 1a); for seven (21.9%) an asymmetrical white rim (Figure 1b); whereas two (6.25%) had just a local white patch (Figure 1c) and two (6.25%) nevi lacked any halo or depigmented area (Figure 1d). A recent study described two other particular types of halo: one with visible telangiectasis and a pinkish surrounding halo [15]. The mean diameter of Sutton nevi for our group was 12.06 mm (range 5–19 mm).

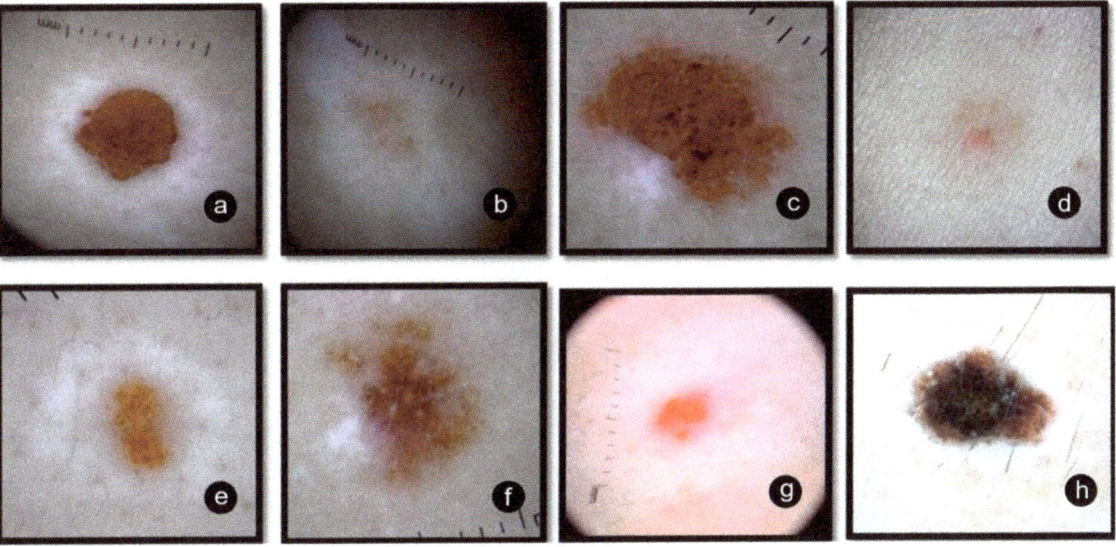

Figure 1. (**a**) Sutton nevus with symmetrical white rim; (**b**) Sutton nevus with asymmetrical white rim; (**c**) Sutton nevus with regional white patch; (**d**) Sutton nevus with no depigmentation area; (**e**) Complex pattern: reticulo-globular; (**f**) Complex pattern: globular-homogeneous with blue white veil and peppering; (**g**) Homogeneous pattern with coma-like vessels; (**h**) Multicomponent pattern: inverse network with peripheral globular-homogeneous.

In terms of global structure, out of the 32 nevi, 16 (50%) were symmetrical, six (18.75%) were asymmetrical and 10 (31.25%) were fully regressed. Of the regressed nevi, nine had a residual white halo and one was completely repigmented. We also found out that 14/32 (43.75%) nevi had developed poliosis. Generally, the diagnosis of these cases is clinical, but given the several worrisome dermoscopic findings, we had to excise three nevi for histopathological diagnosis (Figure 1d,f).

In Table 1, we present a synopsis of the dermoscopic pattern we found in our group of patients. Half of the nevi had a uniform distribution of pigmentation, 31.25% had no pigmentation, 9.4% were multifocal hyper/hypopigmented and fewer were the central hyperpigmented annular type (6.25%) and eccentric hyperpigmented type (3.1%). Homogeneous (62.5%) and globular (37.5%) patterns were most frequently encountered; findings that support the established literature [17]. Reticular pattern was seen in three nevi (9.4%), one of which had diffuse typical network, another had inverse network and the last one had patchy peripheral typical network. In regard to structureless pattern, 18 nevi had just one homogeneous color and two had two homogeneous colors. Of 12 nevi with globular pattern, seven had regular globules, four had irregular globules and one had cobblestone pattern.

Table 1. Dermoscopic features of our investigated patient group with Sutton nevi.

Global Structure	
Symmetric	16/32 (50%)
Asymmetric	6/32 (18.75%)
Regressed	10/32 (31.25%)
Size- mean, median, min, max (mm)	5.22, 5, 3, 10
Distribution of Pigmentation	
Uniform	16/32 (50%)
Centralhyperpigmentedannular type	2/32 (6.25%)
Eccentric hyperpigmented type	1/32 (3.1%)
Multifocalhyper/hypopigmentedtype	3/32 (9.4%)
No pigmentation	10/32 (31.25%)
Structural Patterns	
Globular	**12/32 (37.5%)**
Regular	7/32 (21.9%)
Irregular	4/32 (12.5%)
Cobblestone	1/32 (3.1%)
Network	**3/32 (9.4%)**
Typical	1/32 (3.1%)
Inverse	1/32 (3.1%)
Patchy Peripheral	1/32 (3.1%)
Homogeneous	**20/32 (62.5%)**
One Color	18/32 (56.25%)
Two Colors	2/32 (6.25%)
Regression	**25/32 (59.4%)**
Partial	15/32 (46.9%)
Total	10/32 (31.25%)
Local Features	
Vascular Pattern—Coma-Like Vessels	5/32 (15.6%)
Poliosis	14/32 (43.75%)
Regression Structures	
Blue White Veil	1/32 (3.1%)
Peppering	2/32 (6.25%)
Surrounding Halo	
Symmetric	21/32 (65.6%)
Asymmetric	7/32 (21.9%)
Regional	2/32 (6.25%)
Without	2/32 (6.25%)
Size- mean, median, min, max (mm)	12.06, 12, 5, 19

We could only establish the global pattern for 22 nevi, since 10 were fully regressed. Complex patterns were most common (11/32); two nevi were reticulo-globular and nine were globular-homogeneous (one of them had also two local regression structures; blue white veil and blue pepper-like granules). Of the 32 nevi, 10 were homogeneous (31.25%), five of which also presented local features (four with coma-like vessels and one with blue pepper-like granules). The least frequent pattern was the multicomponent one (1/32), which presents a combination of globular, reticular and homogeneous features.

After analyzing the dermoscopic pattern of all nevi, we were able to categorize them into four stages. The proportion of each nevus stage was represented in Figure 2.

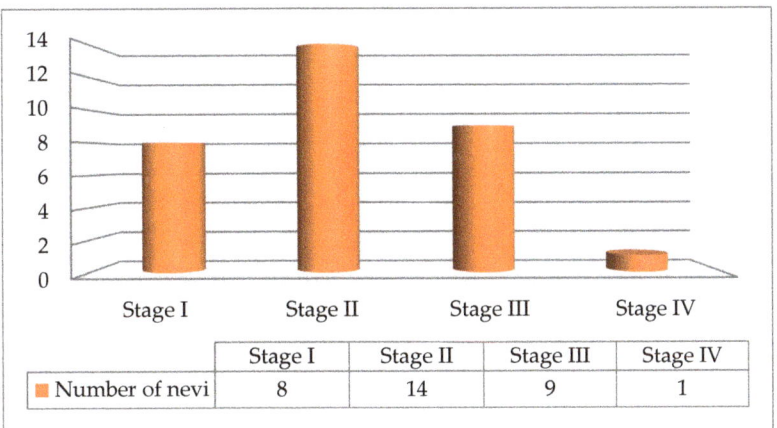

Figure 2. Stages proportion in our investigated group with Sutton nevi.

Finally, it must be underlined that depigmentation may occur around the lesion, within it as focal white patches, at distance from halo nevi [18], or it may not be visible at all. The different types of achromatic halo that depend on age are shown in Figure 3. It is worth noting that all patients below the age of 15 had nevi with a symmetrical halo (4/4), a proportion which decreased for patients aged between 15 and 30; they also presented nevi with focal white depigmentation ($n = 2$), with asymmetrical halo ($n = 1$) and without any depigmentation ($n = 2$). In the group of patients aged over 30 the ratio of symmetrical (4/10) and asymmetrical (6/20) halo was reversed.

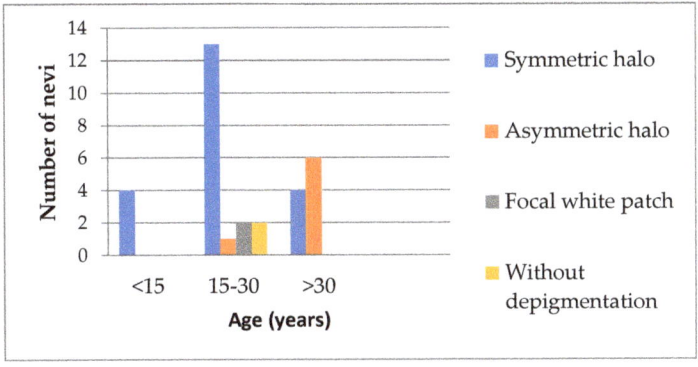

Figure 3. Types of depigmented rim depending on age.

Moreover, Figure 4 shows the occurrence of dermoscopic patterns depending on age. We noticed that the number of regressed nevi increases with age. Nevertheless, atypical

Sutton nevi were especially found in the group of patients aged 15 to 30 years. Two of them had a focal depigmentation area (Figure 1c,f) and one did not present with any patch of depigmentation (Figure 1d). Additionally, two nevi had local regression structures such as blue white veil and peppering (Figure 1d,f) and one had a multicomponent concentric pattern (Figure 1h). Even though dermoscopy allows a more accurate diagnosis of melanocytic skin lesions, when evaluation emphasizes atypia, a subsequent histopathologic diagnosis should be considered [19]. We want to highlight the fact that sometimes it is really hard to distinguish between halo nevus from an area of melanoma regression, and the patient age should not be the main criteria when deciding to perform a biopsy [16]. Our analysis is limited by the rarity of this dermatological entity and implicitly, the low number of patients included in this study.

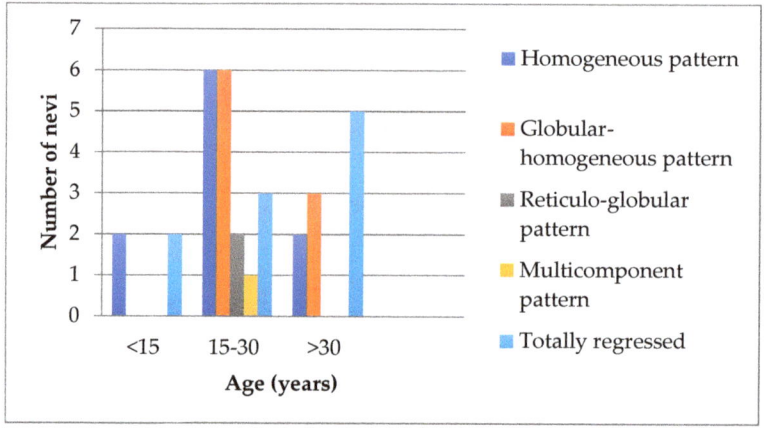

Figure 4. Dermoscopic patterns depending on age.

4. The Microscopic Features—What Matters in Atypical Tumors?

From a clinical point of view, halo nevi develop in several stages, depending on which the dermoscopic appearance is different, as we detailed above. Histologically, four forms are described without always having a dermoscopic correspondence: (a) inflammatory, (b) noninflammatory, (c) halo nevus without halo, (d) halo dermatitis around a melanocytic nevus, and a classification focused on inflammatory infiltrate is presented below [20,21]. The clinical correlation is very important because some nevi may demonstrate marked inflammation, but, clinically, no halo is visible, and other, noninflammatory halo nevi, may demonstrate a halo, but histologically no inflammatory infiltrate.

The diagnosis of halo nevus is usually considered an easy one, based only on the clinical aspect. However, atypical presentations, at the beginning of the depigmentation or repigmentation can be challenging even on dermoscopy and reflectance confocal microscopy and the lesion needs to be excised to rule out melanoma [22]. Bruges et al. estimated that atypical halo nevi represent about 1.4% of all atypical benign nevi excised [22]. Regression structures identified on dermoscopy may also generate histopathological controversy [23].

Halo phenomenon refers to the presence of a dense lymphohistiocytic infiltrate that can be associated with congenital melanocytic nevi, Spitz nevi, congenital giant nevocellular nevi, balloon cell nevi, or atypical nevi, and it can be prominent even before the clinical evidence of the depigmentation [24,25]. The inflammatory infiltrate has a different density, composition and distribution in different stages of the regression. In 1994, Akasu et al. characterized four stages of the process and more the one can be present at a time in a single lesion: In stage I (pre-regression) intact nests can be found and no atypia, and the inflammatory infiltrate (CD3 positive more than 50%, CD4 positive approximate 25%, few

Langerhans cells) surrounds nevus nests. Stage II (early regression) is defined by the presence of nests with ragged edges mild nuclear atypia and the inflammatory infiltrate (similar lymphocytes distribution and increased number of S-100 protein-positive Langerhans cells) surrounds and invades nevus nests. Stage III (late regression) is characterized by single or ill-defined clusters, with nuclear atypia and a dense infiltrate within nevus clusters (numerous enlarged FXIII$_a$—positive cells and numerous S-100 protein—positive epidermal Langerhans cells). In Stage IV (complete regression), there are no nevus cells, moderate dermal inflammatory infiltrate, along with flattening of the epidermis and neovascularization in the superficial dermis [26].

Studies have shown that halo nevi exhibited a broad spectrum of atypia (mild, moderate, severe), so halo nevi should not be regarded as a single clinicopathological entity [27].

The etiology and pathogenesis of halo nevi has not been fully elucidated. Two theories have been discussed as pathogenic mechanism: the antibody theory and the cytotoxic T cell response. The antibody theory has been downplayed, because it has been shown that activated and cell proliferating lymphocytes disappeared after excision of the halo nevus [28]. Mononuclear infiltrates in halo nevus consist of about 80% of T cell lymphocytes, mainly CD8 + T cell. Most T cells are positive for granzyme B, perforin, and Fas ligand, illustrating their cytotoxic activity [29].

Immunohistochemical studies suggest a stronger cytotoxic response (higher prevalence of granzyme) in halo nevi compared with melanoma, and a higher immune-regulatory mechanism (higher prevalence of PD1) in halo nevi [30]. Additionally, the number of CD8 + cells overcome the number of CD4 + T cells in halo nevi.

The most challenging differential diagnosis of halo nevi is malignant melanoma with regression. There are some architectural differences such as: the proliferating cell type, the distribution and type of the inflammatory infiltrate, and the effect of the tumor cells destruction. In halo nevi, the atypical cells are in the junctional nests and upper portion of the nevus with maturation toward the base of lesion. The inflammatory infiltrate in early regression stages of melanoma may look similar to the one in halo nevi. FOXP3 regulatory T cells are highly expressed in early stages of halo nevi [31], while in regression areas of melanoma, a small number of regulatory T cells was described [31,32]. The inflammatory cell infiltrate is distributed in a band-like pattern, symmetrically around the nevus, while in regressing primary melanoma it is asymmetric, surrounding only some segments of the tumor [33].

The autoimmune phenomena may induce reactive atypia and affect the architecture of the nevocytes, making the differential diagnosis even more challenging. Traditionally, regression in nevi is not accompanied by fibrosis, contrary to melanoma where there are thick collagen bundles. Some studies have demonstrated that in the late stages of regression, nevi can be thin and delicate collagen bundles suggesting a feedback mechanism or balance between apoptotic factors and tolerogenic factors [34]. Although this difference is not completely understood, antifibrotic cytokine tumor necrosis factor (TNF-α) was significantly highly expressed in halo nevus than in melanoma, while fibrogenic cytokines were more frequently expressed in melanoma [33].

HMB45 staining can be useful in distinguishing the two entities. Typically, in halo nevus, lesional melanocytes are HBM45-positive in the superficial dermis and HMB45-negative in the deep dermis. On the other hand, in melanoma, HMB45 staining can be either irregular or diffusely positive throughout the lesion or can be negative [25,35]. Atypical distribution of HMB45 positivity was described in halo nevi and more accurate tests are necessary to descriminate between halo nevus and melanoma [25].

In the recent years, complementary preferentially expressed antigen in melanoma (PRAME) was used to help differentiate benign from malignant melanocytes, as it is rarely expressed in nevi [36].

We present below the unpublished histopathological and immunohistochemical aspects (Figures 5–7) from the case of a 29-year-old patient, with atypical features, clinically and dermoscopically (Figure 1f).

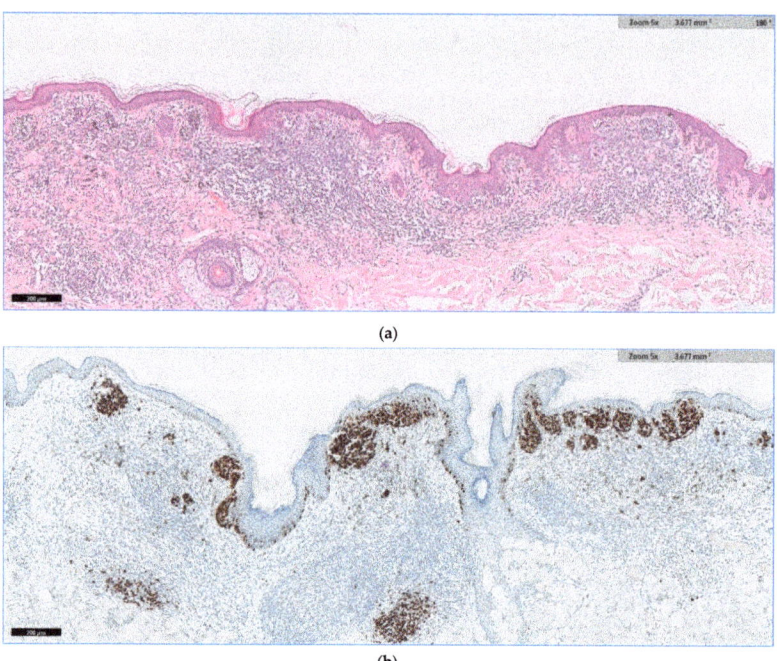

Figure 5. (a) HE and (b) SOX10. Melanocytic lesion with irregular distribution of nests at the dermal–epidermal junction and dense chronic inflammation (halo type) within the dermis, partially obscuring the dermal component.

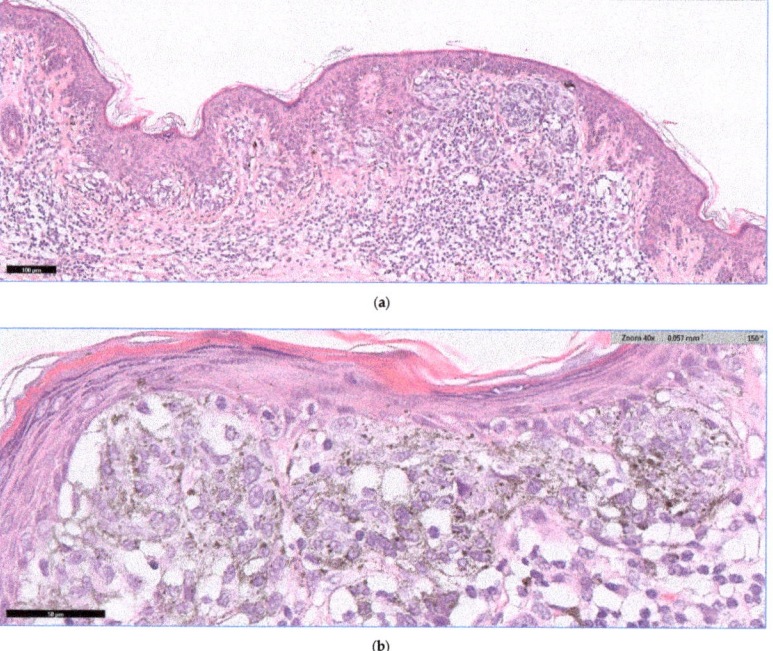

Figure 6. (a,b) HE. Fusion of junctional melanocytic nests with low-grade dysplasia.

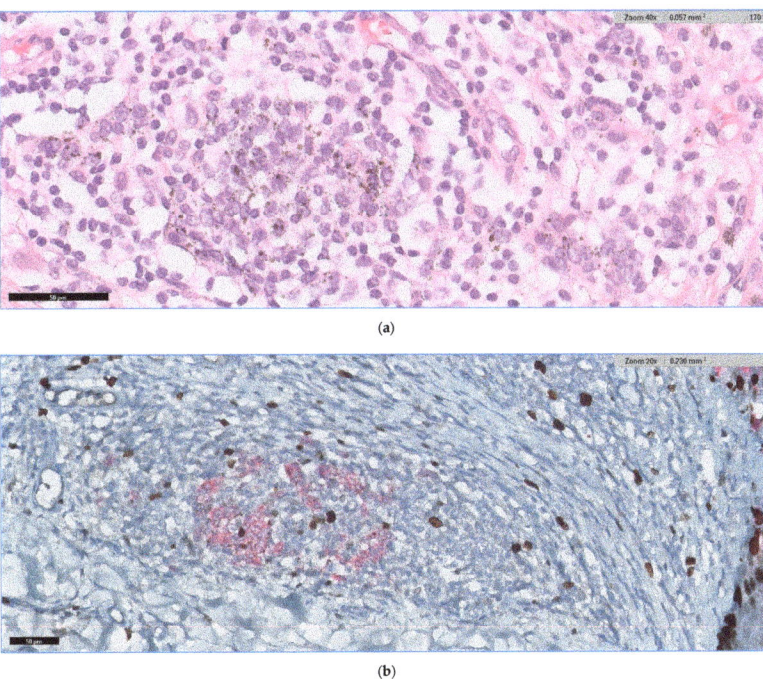

Figure 7. (**a**) HE and (**b**) Ki67-Mart1 dual stain. The halo phenomenon showing lymphocytic inflammation intermigled with benign nevus cells.

5. Association with Diseases—What to (Not) Investigate?

There are many diseases that have been described in individuals with Sutton nevi, such as vitiligo, thyroid diseases, and neoplasia [18,19,37,38]. Among them, vitiligo is the most frequently seen [19]. The association with malignant diseases needs further investigation.

Even though studies have focused on finding out whether patients with halo nevi are susceptible to developing vitiligo, a consensus is lacking. When associated with vitiligo, halo nevi tend to appear earlier in life [18,37]. In other words, the lower the age of the patient with halo nevi, the greater the risk of developing vitiligo. The idea that multiple halo nevi rather than a single lesion associate with vitiligo was suggested by many authors in studies involving children [39] and adults [37]. On the other hand, van Geel et al. considered that the risk of vitiligo decreased when the number of halo nevi was greater than three [18].

Zhou et al. demonstrated that patients with halo nevi and Koebner phenomenon had a greater risk of vitiligo [37]. Moreover, a patient with halo nevi has an increased risk of contracting vitiligo if a member of his family has vitiligo [37].

Great significance was given to studies that involve pediatric patients with vitiligo and halo nevi. A study showed that halo nevi were present in more than a quarter of children with vitiligo [40]. Many of them supported the idea that pediatric patients with vitiligo were more affected by halo nevi than adults with the same disease [39]. The scientific work conducted by Cohen et al. showed that male children with vitiligo were more affected by halo nevi [40]. Moreover, the pediatric patients that had only vitiligo were younger at the moment of the diagnosis than the patients who had both diseases at the same time [40]. A higher incidence of halo nevi was observed in children with generalized vitiligo than in those with more localized forms (segmental and focal) [40]. The idea that children with generalized vitiligo were more prone to develop halo nevi was highlighted in other articles [41].

Autoimmune diseases, especially Hashimoto's thyroiditis, were more frequently seen in patients with both halo nevi and vitiligo when compared to halo nevi without vitiligo [37]. Considering the fact that vitiligo can be associated with a thyroid pathology, the authors suggested that blood tests should be recommended for patients with Sutton nevi thyroid, in order to estimate the risk of vitiligo [37].

Halo nevi can also appear as an adverse effect of a treatment. Immunotherapy-induced halo nevi was described in patients treated with atezolizumab [42] and ipilimumab [43].

As far as it is known in the literature, the presence of Sutton nevi does not carry an additional risk for the appearance of primary melanoma. However, the link between neoplasia and eruptive Sutton nevi was discussed by Lorentzen in a case series study, where 16 patients with eruptive halo nevi were followed for six years [38]. All the patients were adults and most of their nevi (>80%) had become Sutton nevi [38]. No immunotherapy was administered prior to the appearance of the lesions. During this period, eight patients developed a malignant disease. There was an increased incidence of melanoma (955 times higher than expected) and cancer overall (papillary thyroid cancer, neuroendocrine lung tumor, lung metastases from melanoma) [38].

6. Key Antimelanocyte Immune Reaction Lesson

The etiology and pathogenesis of halo nevi has not been fully elucidated. There are several mechanisms through which a lymphocytic infiltrate can induce tumoral regression. The marked inflammatory infiltrate seen in the histopathological examination suggests an immune-based mechanism. Two theories have been discussed as pathogenic mechanism: the antibody theory and the cytotoxic T cell response. The antibody theory has been downplayed, because it has been shown that activated and cell proliferating lymphocytes disappeared after excision of the halo nevus [28]. Mononuclear infiltrates in halo nevus consist of about 80% of T cell lymphocytes, mainly CD8 + T cell. Most of the T cells are positive for granzyme B, perforin, and Fas ligand, illustrating their cytotoxic activity [29].

In this review, we aimed to update the knowledge about Sutton nevi starting with the clinical appearance, the dermoscopic features, continuing with information regarding conventional microscopy, immunohistochemistry, and the immunological mechanisms responsible for the occurrence of halo nevi. We also included in the article original unpublished results when discussing dermoscopic, pathologic and immunohistochemical results in halo nevi.

Sutton nevi are valuable models for studying the antitumor reactions that the human body can generate. The slow and effective mechanism against a melanocytic skin tumor can teach us important lessons about both autoimmune diseases and anticancer defenses.

Author Contributions: R.N., A.D. (Alexandra Dobre), A.B., I.H., R.A., S.Z., M.B., M.A., L.M., A.C. (Andreea Calinescu), A.C. (Anastasia Coman), F.P., A.D. (Adina Dobritoiu), C.P., R.P., E.B., D.I., G.T. have equal contribution to this paper. They contributed to conceptualization, design of the study, interpretation of the data and revising it critically for important intellectual content. All authors have read and agreed to the published version of the manuscript.

Funding: This research received no external funding.

Institutional Review Board Statement: The study was conducted according to the guidelines of the Declaration of Helsinki, and approved by the Ethics Committee of UMF (PO-35-F-03 December 2017).

Informed Consent Statement: Informed consent was obtained from all subjects involved in the study.

Conflicts of Interest: The authors declare no conflict of interest.

References

1. Nazzaro, G.; Rovaris, M. The men or women behind nevi: Richard Sutton. *JAMA Dermatol.* **2014**, *150*, 302. [CrossRef]
2. Steffen, C.; Thomas, D. The man behind the eponyms: Richard L Sutton: Periadenitis mucosa necroticarecurrens (Sutton's ulcer) and leukoderma acquisitumcentrifugum-Sutton's (halo) nevus. *Am. J. Dermatopathol.* **2003**, *25*, 349–354. [CrossRef] [PubMed]
3. Stokes, J.H. Clinical note on leukoderma acquisitumcontrifugum. *Arch. Derm. Syphilol.* **1923**, *8*, 178.
4. Kopf, A.W.; Morrill, S.D.; Silberberg, I. Broad spectrum of leukoderma acquisitumcentrifugum. *Arch. Dermatol.* **1965**, *92*, 14–33. [CrossRef]
5. Rivers, J.K.; MacLennan, R.; Kelly, J.W.; Lewis, A.E.; Tate, B.J.; Harrison, S.; McCarthy, W.H. The eastern Australian childhood nevus study: Prevalence of atypical nevi, congenital nevus-like nevi, and other pigmented lesions. *J. Am. Acad. Derm.* **1995**, *32*, 957–963. [CrossRef]
6. Larsson, P.; Liden, S. Prevalence of skin diseases among adolescents 12–16 years of age. *Acta Derm. Venereol.* **1980**, *60*, 415–423. [PubMed]
7. Mollet, I.; Ongenae, K.; Naeyaert, J.M. Origin, Clinical Presentation, and Diagnosis of Hypomelanotic Skin Disroders. *Derm. Clin.* **2007**, *25*, 363–371. [CrossRef]
8. Ortonne, J.P.; Passeron, T. Vitiligo and other disorders of hypopigmentation. In *Textbook of Dermatology*, 3rd ed.; Bologna, J.L., Jorizzo, J.L., Schaffer, J.V., Eds.; Elsevier Saunders: Philadelphia, PA, USA, 2012; pp. 1023–1048.
9. Aouthmany, M.; Weinstein, M.; Zirwas, M.J.; Brodell, R.T. The natural history of halo nevi: A retrospective case series. *J. Am. Acad. Derm.* **2012**, *67*, 582–586. [CrossRef]
10. Frank, S.B.; Cohen, H.J. The Halo Nevus. *Arch. Dermatol.* **1964**, *89*, 367–373. [CrossRef] [PubMed]
11. Soyer, H.P.; Argenziano, G.; Hofmann-Wellenhof, R.; Johr, R.H. *Color Atlas of Melanocytic Lesions of the Skin*; Springer: Berlin/Heidelberg, Germany, 2007; pp. 124–128.
12. Inamadar, A.C.; Palit, A.; Athanikar, S.B.; Sampagavi, V.V.; Deshmukh, N.S. Unusual course of a halo nevus. *Pediatr. Derm.* **2003**, *20*, 542–543. [CrossRef]
13. Speeckaert, R.; Van Geel, N.; Vermaelen, K.V.; Lambert, J.; Van Gele, M.; Speeckaert, M.M.; Brochez, L. Immune reactions in benign and malignant melanocytic lesions: Lessons for immunotherapy. *Pigment Cell Melanoma Res.* **2011**, *24*, 334–344. [CrossRef] [PubMed]
14. Rongioletti, F.; Cecchi, F.; Rebora, A. Halo phenomenon in melanocytic nevi (Sutton's nevi). Does the diameter matter? *J. Eur. Acad. Dermatol. Venereol.* **2011**, *25*, 1231–1232. [CrossRef]
15. Kaminska-Winciorek, G.; Szymszal, J. Dermoscopy of halo nevus in own observation. *Postepy Derm. Alergol.* **2014**, *31*, 152–158. [CrossRef] [PubMed]
16. Kolm, I.; Di Stefani, A.; Hofmann-Wellenhof, R.; Fink-Puches, R.; Wolf, I.H.; Richtig, E.; Smolle, J.; Kerl, H.; Soyer, H.P.; Zalaudek, I. Dermoscopy patterns of halo nevi. *Arch. Derm.* **2006**, *142*, 1627–1632. [CrossRef] [PubMed]
17. Larre Borges, A.; Zalaudek, I.; Longo, C.; Dufrechou, L.; Argenziano, G.; Lallas, A.; Piana, S.; Moscarella, E. Melanocytic nevi with special features: Clinical-dermoscopic and reflectance confocal microscopic findings. *J. Eur. Acad. Derm. Venereol.* **2014**, *28*, 833–845. [CrossRef] [PubMed]
18. Van Geel, N.; Speeckaert, R.; Lambert, J.; Mollet, I.; De Keyser, S.; De Schepper, S.; Brochez, L. Halo naevi with associated vitiligo-like depigmentations: Pathogenetic hypothesis. *J. Eur. Acad. Derm. Venereol.* **2011**, *26*, 755–761. [CrossRef]
19. Nedelcu, R.I.; Zurac, S.A.; Brinzea, A.; Cioplea, M.D.; Turcu, G.; Popescu, R.; Popescu, C.M.; Ion, D.A. Morphological features of melanocytic tumors with depigmented halo: Review of the literature and personal results. *Rom J. Morphol. Embryol.* **2015**, *56*, 659–663.
20. Naveh, H.P.; Rao, U.N.M.; Butterfield, L.H. Melanoma-associated leukoderma—Immunology in black and white? *Pigment Cell Melanoma Res.* **2013**, *26*, 796–804. [CrossRef]
21. Babu, A.; Bhat, M.R.; Dandeli, S.; Ali, N.M. Throwing Light onto the Core of a Halo Nevus: A New Finding. *Indian J. Derm.* **2016**, *61*, 238. [CrossRef] [PubMed]
22. Brugues, A.; Ribero, S.; Da Silva, V.M.; Aguilera, P.; Garcia, A.P.; Alos, L.; Malvehy, J.; Puig, S.; Carrera, C. Sutton Naevi as Melanoma Simulators: Can Confocal Microscopy Help in the Diagnosis? *Acta Derm. Venereol.* **2020**, *100*, adv00134. [CrossRef]
23. Ferrara, G.; Argenziano, G.; Soyer, H.P.; Corona, R.; Sera, F.; Brunetti, B.; Cerroni, L.; Chimenti, S.; El Shabrawi-Caelen, L.; Ferrari, A.; et al. Dermoscopic and histopathologic diagnosis of equivocal melanocytic skin lesions: An interdisciplinary study on 107 cases. *Cancer* **2002**, *95*, 1094–1100. [CrossRef]
24. Bayer-Garner, I.B.; Ivan, D.; Schwartz, M.R.; Tschen, J.A. The immunopathology of regression in benign lichenoid keratosis, keratoacanthoma and halo nevus. *Clin. Med. Res.* **2004**, *2*, 89–97. [CrossRef]
25. Ruby, K.N.; Li, Z.; Yan, S. Aberrant expression of HMB45 and negative PRAME expression in halo nevi. *J. Cutan. Pathol.* **2021**, *48*, 519–525. [CrossRef]
26. Akasu, R.; From, L.; Kahn, H.J. Characterization of the mononuclear infiltrate involved in regression of halo nevi. *J. Cutan. Pathol.* **1994**, *21*, 302–311. [CrossRef] [PubMed]
27. De Schriver, S.; Theate, I.; Vanhooteghem, O. Halo Nevi Are Not Trivial: About 2 Young Patients of Regressed Primary Melnaoma That Simulates Halo Nevi. *Case Rep. Derm.* **2021**, *2021*, 6672528.

28. Speeckaert, R.; Van Geel, N.; Luiten, R.M.; Van Gele, M.; Speeckaert, M.; Lambert, J.; Vermaelen, K.; Tjin, E.P.M.; Borchez, L. Melanocyte-specific Immune Response in a Patient with Multiple Regressing Nevi and a History of Melanoma. *Anticancer Res.* **2011**, *31*, 3697–3703. [PubMed]
29. Musette, P.; Bachelez, H.; Flageul, B.; Delarbre, C.; Kourilsky, P.; Dubertret, L.; Gachelin, G. Immune-Mediated Destruction of Melanocytes in Halo Nevi Is Associated with the Local Expansion of a Limited Number of T Cell Clones. *J. Immunol.* **1999**, *162*, 1789–1794. [PubMed]
30. Botella-Estrada, R.; Kutzner, H. Study of the immunophenotype of the inflammatory cells in melanomas with regression and halo nevi. *Am. J. Derm.* **2015**, *37*, 376–380. [CrossRef] [PubMed]
31. Park, H.S.; Jin, S.A.; Choi, Y.D.; Shin, M.H.; Lee, S.E.; Yun, S.J. Foxp3(+) regulatory T cells are increased in the early stages of halo nevi: Clinicopathological features of 30 halo nevi. *Dermatology* **2012**, *225*, 172–178. [CrossRef]
32. Cioplea, M.; Nichita, L.; Georgescu, D.; Sticlaru, L.; Cioroianu, A.; Nedelcu, R.; Turcu, G.; Rauta, A.; Mogodici, C.; Zurac, S.; et al. FOXP3 in Melanoma with Regression: Between Tumoral Expression and Regulatory T Cell Upregulation. *J. Immunol. Res.* **2020**, *2020*. [CrossRef]
33. Moretti, S.; Spallanzani, A.; Pinzi, C.; Prignano, F.; Fabbri, P. Fibrosis in regressing melanoma versus nonfibrosis in halo nevus upon melanocyte disappearance: Could it be related to a different cytokine microenvironment? *J. Cutan. Pathol.* **2007**, *34*, 301–308. [CrossRef]
34. Martín, J.M.; Rubio, M.; Bella, R.; Jordá, E.; Monteagudo, C. Regresióncompleta de nevosmelanocíticos: Correlaciónclínica, dermatoscópica e histológica de una serie de 13 casos. *Actas Dermo-Sifiliográficas* **2012**, *103*, 401–410. [CrossRef]
35. Uguen, A.; Talagas, M.; Costa, S.; Duigou, S.; Bouvier, S.; De Braekeleer, M.; Marcorelles, P. A p16-Ki-67-HMB45 immunohistochemistry scoring system as an ancillary diagnostic tool in the diagnosis of melanoma. *Diagn. Pathol.* **2015**, *10*, 195. [CrossRef] [PubMed]
36. Lezcano, C.; Jungbluth, A.A.; Nehal, K.S.; Hollmann, T.J.; Busam, K.J. PRAME expression in melanocytic tumors. *Am. J. Surg. Pathol.* **2018**, *42*, 1456–1465. [CrossRef]
37. Zhou, H.; Wu, L.C.; Chen, M.K.; Liao, Q.M.; Mao, R.X.; Han, J.D. Factors Associated with Development of Vitiligo in Patients withHalo Nevus. *Chin. Med. J.* **2017**, *130*, 2703–2708. [CrossRef]
38. Lorentzen, H.F. Eruptive Halo Naevi: A Possible Indicator of Malignant Disease in a Case Series of Post-adolescent Patients. *Acta Derm. Venereol.* **2020**, *100*, adv00228. [CrossRef]
39. Patrizi, A.; Bentivogli, M.; Raone, B.; Dondi, A.; Tabanelli, M.; Neri, I. Association of halo nevus/i and vitiligo in childhood: A retrospective observational study. *J. Eur. Acad. Dermatol. Venereol.* **2013**, *27*, e148–e152. [CrossRef] [PubMed]
40. Cohen, B.E.; Mu, E.W.; Orlow, S.J. Comparison of Childhood Vitiligo Presenting with or without Associated Halo Nevi. *Pediatr Derm.* **2016**, *33*, 44–48. [CrossRef] [PubMed]
41. Lin, X.; Tang, L.Y.; Fu, W.W.; Kang, K.F. Childhood vitiligo in China: Clinical profiles and immunological findings in620 cases. *Am. J. Clin. Derm.* **2011**, *12*, 277–281. [CrossRef]
42. Birnbaum, M.R.; Ma, M.W.; Casey, M.A.; Amin, B.D.; Jacobson, M.; Cheng, H.; McLellan, B.N. Development of Halo Nevi in a Lung Cancer Patient: A Novel Immune-Related Cutaneous Event from Atezolizumab. *J. Drugs Derm.* **2017**, *16*, 1047–1049.
43. Plaquevent, M.; Greliak, A.; Pinard, C.; Duval-Modeste, A.B.; Joly, P. Simultaneous long-lasting regression of multiple nevi and melanoma metastases after ipilimumab therapy. *Melanoma Res.* **2019**, *29*, 311–312. [CrossRef] [PubMed]

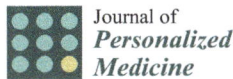

Review

Current Trends in Advanced Alginate-Based Wound Dressings for Chronic Wounds

Andreea Barbu [1,2,*], Bogdan Neamtu [1,3,4,*], Marius Zăhan [2], Gabriela Mariana Iancu [3,5], Ciprian Bacila [3] and Vioara Mireșan [2]

1. Pediatric Research Department, Pediatric Clinical Hospital Sibiu, 550166 Sibiu, Romania
2. Faculty of Animal Science and Biotechnologies, University of Agricultural Sciences and Veterinary Medicine Cluj-Napoca, 400372 Cluj-Napoca, Romania; mzahan@usamvcluj.ro (M.Z.); vioara.miresan@usamvcluj.ro (V.M.)
3. Faculty of Medicine, "Lucian Blaga" University of Sibiu, 550169 Sibiu, Romania; gabriela.iancu@ulbsibiu.ro (G.M.I.); ciprian.bacila@ulbsibiu.ro (C.B.)
4. Faculty of Engineering, "Lucian Blaga" University of Sibiu, 550025 Sibiu, Romania
5. Dermatology Clinic, County Clinical Emergency Hospital, 550245 Sibiu, Romania
* Correspondence: ing.andreea.barbu@gmail.com (A.B.); bogdan.neamtu@ulbsibiu.ro (B.N.); Tel.: +40-748063335 (A.B.); +40-773994375 (B.N.)

Citation: Barbu, A.; Neamtu, B.; Zăhan, M.; Iancu, G.M.; Bacila, C.; Mireșan, V. Current Trends in Advanced Alginate-Based Wound Dressings for Chronic Wounds. *J. Pers. Med.* **2021**, *11*, 890. https://doi.org/10.3390/jpm11090890

Academic Editors: Mircea Tampa, Monica Neagu, Constantin Caruntu and Simona Roxana Georgescu

Received: 15 August 2021
Accepted: 5 September 2021
Published: 7 September 2021

Publisher's Note: MDPI stays neutral with regard to jurisdictional claims in published maps and institutional affiliations.

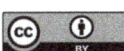

Copyright: © 2021 by the authors. Licensee MDPI, Basel, Switzerland. This article is an open access article distributed under the terms and conditions of the Creative Commons Attribution (CC BY) license (https://creativecommons.org/licenses/by/4.0/).

Abstract: Chronic wounds represent a major public health issue, with an extremely high cost worldwide. In healthy individuals, the wound healing process takes place in different stages: inflammation, cell proliferation (fibroblasts and keratinocytes of the dermis), and finally remodeling of the extracellular matrix (equilibrium between metalloproteinases and their inhibitors). In chronic wounds, the chronic inflammation favors exudate persistence and bacterial film has a special importance in the dynamics of chronic inflammation in wounds that do not heal. Recent advances in biopolymer-based materials for wound healing highlight the performance of specific alginate forms. An ideal wound dressing should be adherent to the wound surface and not to the wound bed, it should also be non-antigenic, biocompatible, semi-permeable, biodegradable, elastic but resistant, and cost-effective. It has to give protection against bacterial, infectious, mechanical, and thermal agents, to modulate the level of wound moisture, and to entrap and deliver drugs or other molecules This paper explores the roles of alginates in advanced wound-dressing forms with a particular emphasis on hydrogels, nanofibers networks, 3D-scaffolds or sponges entrapping fibroblasts, keratinocytes, or drugs to be released on the wound-bed. The latest research reports are presented and supported with in vitro and in vivo studies from the current literature.

Keywords: alginate; biomaterial; dressing; fibers; hydrogel; nanofibers; commercially available; wound care; wound healing

1. Introduction

Chronic wounds represent a major public health issue, with an extremely high cost worldwide. In the USA, chronic wounds affect 1% of the total population, in Europe the incidence is 4 million cases per year which implies a rate of about 0.8%, in Australia 0.86%, in China 0.8–1%, and in India 0.6–1% [1,2]. In healthy individuals, the wound healing process takes place in different stages: inflammation, cell proliferation (fibroblasts and keratinocytes of the dermis), and finally remodeling of the extracellular matrix (equilibrium between metalloproteinases and their inhibitors). In the case of chronic wounds, a chronic inflammatory status is noted, so it takes a longer time to reach the cell proliferation and remodeling (healing) phases. Chronic inflammation favors exudate persistence. The bacterial film has a special importance in the dynamics of chronic inflammation in wounds that do not heal. Clinical studies showed that over 60% of chronic wounds presented a biofilm. Current research envisages advanced wound-dressings to address these disadvantages. These wound-dressings should act by removing the biofilm pathogenic bacteria and modulating the inflammation. Many in vitro and in vivo studies centered upon creating new or better biopolymer-based materials for wound healing in recent years. An ideal wound dressing should adhere to the wound surface and not to the wound bed, it should also be non-antigenic, biocompatible, semi-permeable, biodegradable, elastic but resistant, and cost-effective. It has to give protection against bacterial, infectious, mechanical, and thermal agents, to modulate the level of wound moisture, and to entrap and deliver drugs or other molecules [3–5]. Alginate, chitosan, collagen, and cellulose are the most used biomaterials for wound-dressing products [3,6–10]. Of these, alginate is by far the most commonly biomaterial among other bioproducts with wound healing properties [3,6,7].

Because of its hydrophilic nature, alginate is capable to take multiple forms [11–14] (beads, blends, dressings, electrospun scaffolds, flexible fibers, films, foams, gels, hydrogels, injections, microparticles, microspheres, nanoparticles, polyelectrolyte complex, powders, ropes, sheets, sponges) that could be applied on post-traumatic wounds or exuding wounds (ulcers) while decreasing contamination [15–18], either as a stand-alone biomaterial, or in various combinations.

This review focuses on the roles of alginates in advanced wound-dressing forms with a particular emphasis on hydrogels, nanofibers networks, 3D-scaffolds or sponges entrapping fibroblasts, keratinocytes, or drugs to be released on the wound-bed. The latest research reports are presented and supported with in vitro and in vivo studies from the current literature.

2. Chronic Wounds Mechanisms and Alginates Roles

Wound healing mechanisms involve multiple cellular events, while also being related to the biodynamic of the bacterial film on the wound surface. Inflammation occurs as a result of the inflammatory response of keratinocytes (at the edge of the wound), cytokines, and growth factors during thermal and cellular processes. The cells involved are leukocytes and fibroblasts [19–21]. Leukocytes (polymorphonuclear leukocytes-PMN, macrophages, lymphocytes) secrete biomarkers such as IL-1, IL-6, TNF-α, with role for the maintenance of inflammation. Platelets, epithelial cells, endothelial cells, and macrophages secrete growth factors, PDGF (platelets derived growth factors), TGF-β (tumoral growth factor-β), β-FGF(fibroblast growth factor-beta), VEGF-(vascular endothelial growth factor, hypoxia-induced), KGF (keratinocytes growth factors), metalloproteinases-MMPs, and their inhibitors—TIMPs. More than 20 types of matrix metalloproteins have been described to be involved in extracellular matrix (ECM) proliferation [22–24].

A fibroblast's function is to remodel the extracellular matrix and to secrete growth factors. Proliferation is the most critical stage, since the ECM is formed, and the collagen synthesis, reepithelization, and angiogenesis processes begin [25]. Remodeling is represented by the moment when collagen reshapes, the vessels mature and regress from the injured area. Eventually, the reepithelization process takes place [26].

A mechanism implicated in unhealing of wounds seems to point out the fact that fibroblasts are unresponsive to growth factors and cytokines. In patients with chronic wounds, increased levels of IL-1 β, IL-6, TNF-α, and an abnormally high ratio MMPs/TIMPs have been found, as demonstrated by computational models, as well. The liquid in chronic wound with its cytokinic composition seems to inhibit the proliferation of dermal fibroblasts by their arrest in the G0/G1 cell cycle by activating an intracellular molecular pathway mediated by Ras protein [27]: (1) High Mobility Group Box Protein 1 (HMGB1) and the analogues involved in wound repair; (2) cell growth mechanisms regulating given by Ras protein. The study of cell matrix and of the ration between metalloproteinases/their inhibitors seems to have a crucial importance in understanding the chronic wounds physiopathology.

Alginates were proved to exhibit: (1) anti-microbial (Gram-positive—Staphylococcus, *Bacillus cereus*; Gram-negative—*E. coli*, *Pseudomonas aeruginosa*, and *Acinetobacter* spp. [9,28,29]); (2) antifungal—*Candida albicans* [9,30,31]; (3) antiviral—*Herpeviridae, Rhabdoviridae, Flaviviridae*, and *Togaviridae*, due to sulfated polymeric chain [9,32]; (4) antianaphylactic; (5) anti-inflammatory, immuno-modulatory by induction of nitric-oxide (NO), reactive oxygen species (ROS), TNF-α, NF-KB release from macrophages, the MAPK signaling pathway; (6) antioxidant; (7) hemostatic by platelets activation and thrombin clot generation; (8) regenerative/angiogenetic properties [28,29,32–36]. Infection is one of the leading causes for a wound to become chronic [34,37] thus making alginate a good candidate when discussing its possible use as a wound dressing especially in hydrogel forms or more advanced solutions such as electrospun nanofibers networks, 3D-scaffolds and sponges entrapping fibroblasts, keratinocytes, or drugs to be released on the wound-bed.

3. Alginate Physical Properties

Alginates (ALG), are linear water soluble high swelling natural anionic polysaccharides obtained from brown algae cell walls and from some bacteria strains such as *Pseudomonas* or *Azotobacter* [6,38–40]. They are biopolymers consisting of 1,4-linked β-D-mannuronic acid (M) and 1,4 α-L-guluronic acid (G) monomers [9,30,39,41]. These monomers are grouped in block-like patterns which can be heterogenous (MG) or homogenous (poly-M, poly-G) (Figure 1). When it comes to terminology, alginate usually refer to alginic acid, and its derivatives [6,9,32,42]. To become water soluble for viscous solutions alginic acid should be converted into ALG esters and monovalent salts like sodium alginate or calcium alginate. The viscosity of sodium alginate aqueous solution (1% w/v) for example, is highly dynamic ranging between 20 and 400 mPa·s at 20 °C. By tuning the ALG concentration viscosity and other physicochemical properties are influenced [9,43].

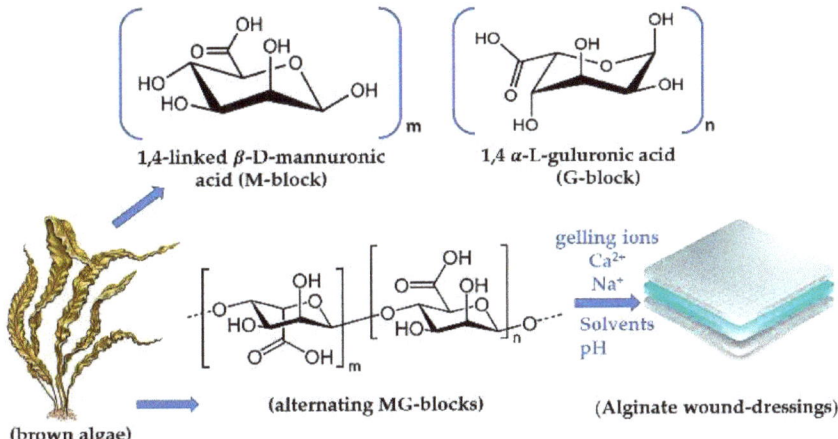

Figure 1. Alginates' blocks in the polymeric chain.

The parameters to modulate ALG's solubility are represented by structure, the carboxylic groups states (protonated/deprotonated), ionic strength, concentration, temperature, the amount of the 'gelling ions' such as Ca^{2+} and Na^+, the solvents, and pH. At a pKa under 3.28–3.65 the solubility is highly affected and the polymer precipitates [9,32]. ALG's solubility also changes when long alkyl or aromatic groups are attached to their backbone. Then, the presence of protonated carboxylic groups in ALG's structure comes with the loss of water or any other solvent solubility. Environmental pH also influences ALG mucoadhesive capacity where the polymers carboxyl groups bind with mucin, and if it is higher, the carboxylic groups become deprotonated [9,15,32,42,44].

The gelling ions trigger a cross-link process of the ALG chains and eventually the gelation process [9,32]. Modulating the G-blocks, M-Blocks, or MG-block concentration in the technological process, different gel patterns can be obtained: stiffer, elastic, or flexible [9,32]. When the alginate is fully crosslinked, the gel will be more rigid, with a higher Young's modulus and lower elongation which affects its tensile strength. The higher the Ca^{2+} concentration the better water resistance and swelling behavior is observed, while in thin films more translucent and clear behavior was noticed [9].

With an impressive swelling capacity (20 times their own weight) ALG weakly jellify in the wound environment, providing moisture and stimulating epidermis regeneration [6,9,40]. ALG are acknowledged to have an excellent biocompatibility and it seems that the adverse events were related to the alginate's (unobserved) impurities that were added unintentionally in the wound-dressings [9,15,42]. The most used alginate types in wound healing studies are the calcium and the sodium alginate, depending on the wound type or the desired dressing form. The physicochemical properties are correlated with the amount of ALG, more ALG will lead to the viscosity and the bead size to increase [43,45,46]. The used concentration of ALG varies from 0.001% w/v to 95% depending on the dressing type [47–49].

The ALG wound dressings have the ability of exchanging the 'gelling ions' with the wound fluids with a direct application in infected wounds. For example, calcium alginate makes a reliable non-woven wound dressing with the ability to exchange Na^+ in exuding or infected wounds. Consequently, this wound dressing type does not adhere to the wound-bed and the removal is painless. The new formed tissue will not be affected by washing away the alginate fibers. Moreover, there is a self-adherence process in the peri-wound area with a good cover of the affected area [9,15].

In the case of sodium alginate salts, only the water solubility is maintained. It dissolves completely in water but not in organic solvents. Nevertheless, sodium alginate has better gel-forming characteristics [9]. To date, at pH of 1.2 spray-dried particles of sodium alginate consisting of hydrophilic matrix controlled-release form, have a longer release time for the entrapped drugs, forming gels in aqueous media. The speed and the drugs' absorption rate depend of the wound pH and drug type, but also on the solubility of the alginate salt [9,50]. Some authors state that an alginate-based dressing should be changed every week or when the gel loses its viscos properties [51].

4. Alginate-Based Hydrogels for Wound Healing

One of the most promising alginate forms being used in helping wound healing is the hydrogel because it keeps the moisture and absorbs the excessive exudate, it reduces local pain because it has a cooling effect, it does not adhere to the wound bed and it can hold active compounds such as various drugs, signaling molecules, or stem cells. Their disadvantages are their price and their mechanical instability [52,53]. Their structure influences the obtained gel. Repeating M-blocks have a better water retaining ability that transforms into a softer and more elastic gel, whereas repeating G-blocks will give gels a good mechanical resistance, but they will be stiff, and more MG-blocks will lead to a more flexible gel (Figure 2). ALG rich in M-blocks makes soft flexible gels, while ALG in rich G-blocks make firm gels after they absorb wound secretions [11,23,32,42,49,54]. ALG with high G content reveals interesting in situ gel formation properties with superior results after using a gel instead of a solution for ocular drug delivery, being conditioned by pH and temperature [32,55,56]. An oxidized alginate and borax hydrogel dressing obtained directly in situ with a WVTR (water vapor transmission rate) of 2686 ± 124 $g/m^2/day$, was applied on rats, proving that the antiseptic properties of borax helped completely heal the wound within two weeks [57].

If the gelation rate is slow, the gel will be uniform and will have a good mechanical resistance [32,49,54]. To make that happen, one might add phosphate buffer or lower the temperature. Alginate's gelation rate might be slowed by adding cryoprotectants such as tetrasodium pyrophosphate and di- or trisodium phosphate. ALG also turns into hydrogels after rehydration [32,49,54].

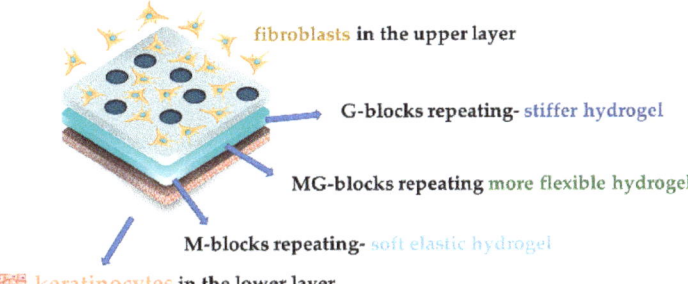

Figure 2. A 3D model of porous hydrogel with fibroblasts and keratinocytes.

Porous 3D hydrogel calcium alginate (Ca ALG) has great swelling capacity in wounds, providing slow drug release, and it is used to entrap cells for tissue regeneration and engineering, as a physical support for cells or tissue or as a hurdle between two media, because it protects the cells from the host's immune system until it reaches the targeted area. A great example is represented by the encapsulated fibroblasts into a dual-layered structure made from alginate hydrogel with apical keratinocytes [32,58,59]. Also, a hydrogel film based on poly (N-vinyl caprolactam)-calcium alginate (PVCL/PV-Ca ALG) loaded with thrombin receptor agonist peptide (TRAP) has shown a beneficial effect on wound healing and tissue regeneration [11].

A relatively recent study compared a sodium alginate-acacia gum-based hydrogel loaded with zinc oxide nanoparticles (ZnO-NPs) to only ZnO-NPs by their healing effects and activity against *B. cereus* and *P. aeruginosa*. The authors have started from the premise that zinc helps wound healing by having antipathogenic properties, helping reepithelization and reducing the inflammation and bacterial growth in leg ulcers. This study used sheep fibroblasts and concluded that the hydrogel had less cytotoxicity than the use of only zinc oxide nanoparticles, if the concentration is carefully monitored. The hydrogel also demonstrated better results against both aforementioned rod-shaped bacteria. A complete new monolayer was observed if the plate was treated with the hydrogel, whereas the same concentration of only the nanoparticles led to cell death [29]. Also, Neacsu et al. [60] mention a study by Mohandas et al. [61] that concluded that the use of ZnO-NPs in an alginate hydrogel did have antibacterial effects against *E. coli* and *S. aureus*, but their used concentration had potentially cytotoxic effects.

When a Na ALG, chitin/chitosan, and fucoidan (60:20:2:4 w/w) hydrogel sheet (ACF-HS) was applied on rats with full thickness wounds in an in vivo cytotoxicity assay study, it provided a moist wound environment, showing easy application and removal, and enhanced cell migration [42,62–66]. The study involved Sprague Dawley rats treated with mitomycin C (wound-healing inhibitor) or Kaltostat® (alginate-based fiber, for the positive control) and ACF hydrogel sheets were applied before being sealed with a plastic sheet [63]. Because the wounds exuded heavily the alginate-chitosan/chitin-fucoidan hydrogel sheets were replaced on day 3. The dressings were removed on day 7 and the established observation period was 18 days. The ACF-HS treated wounds displayed better healing, based on histological examinations. The wound closure and contraction, granulation, capillary formation and re-epithelization started with day 7, whether or not the wound was previously treated with mitomycin C, and the latter process was enhanced after the dressing was removed from the inhibited-healing wound, making ACF-HS a good candidate for wounds with impaired healing [63,64]. The recently developed alginate-based hydrogels are summarized in Table 1.

Table 1. Alginate-based hydrogels used for wound healing.

Composition	Study Type/Target	Ref.
1% w/v Na ALG—0.1% w/v acacia gum—1 mg/mL ZnO-NPs	Characterization, healing effects and cytotoxicity on sheep fibroblasts, antibacterial activity	[29]
0.5–2.5% w/v LF 200S ALG hydrogel emulsion + 0.9, 1.4, 2.8% Tween 80/Span 20/isopropyl myristate oil/Ketoprofen ratio 26:1.25:4:1 Ca^{2+}/D (+) gluconic acid δ-lactone molar ratio: 1:2 Ketoprofen microemulsion: 0.9, 1.4, 2.8%	Characterization, drug release, scattering patterns	[56]
alginate dialdehyde (ADA)—gelatin—0.1 M borax	Characterization and in vivo study on rat model	[57]
60:20:2:4 w/w Na ALG—chitin/chitosan—fucoidan hydrogel sheet	Sprague-Dawley rats with full thickness wounds, gives a moist wound environment, easy application and removal, migration, cytotoxicity assay	[62–66]
encapsulated TRAP—0.5% w/w chitosan—PV-Ca ALG hydrogel film	C57 black 6/CBA mice wound healing	[67]
10 g ALG—4 mg trypan blue, 10 g ALG—10 μg VEGF	Drug release: in vitro and in vivo on NOD and SCID mice, angiogenesis	[68]
1% heparin—1% Na ALG—bFGF	Characterization, angiogenesis and bFGF release profile in Wistar rats	[69]
10 & 15% Polyvinyl pyrrolidone—0.5 and 1% ALG—0, 30, 50, 70, and 100 ppm Ag-NPs.	Characterization, crosslinking degree, antimicrobial activity. Best results: 0.5% ALG, 15% PVP, 70 ppm Ag-NPs	[48]
Polyurethane foam—pH-sensitive Na ALG-bentonite hydrogels 1:0, 0.7:0.3, 0.5:0.5, 0.3:0.7	Characterization, drug release from foam, cytotoxicity	[70]
Micro-emulsion 20% Tea tree oil—1% w/v ALG hydrogel	Characterization, oil dispersion, antimicrobial effect	[71]
10% Na ALG sulfate—CM11 peptide	Mouse wound healing	[72]
ALG—k-CG ratio: 5:5, 7:3, 8:2 ALG—i-CG ratio: 5:5, 7:3, 8:2	Formation and characterization; cytotoxicity, cell encapsulation	[73]
VEGF—2 wt % Na ALG, VEGF—0.05% chitosan—2 wt % Na ALG VEGF—heparin-coated chitosan—2 wt % Na ALG	In vitro drug release	[74]
2 wt % ALG—trypan blue, 2 wt % ALG—methylene blue, 2 wt % ALG—VEGF	In vitro drug release	[75,76]
PEG diacrylate—thiolated ALG bilayered hydrogel with small extracellular vesicles (sEVs)	Characterization, rats and rabbit full thickness wound size reduction, sEVs release, angiogenesis, collagen arrangement	[77]
Sr^{2+} loaded Na ALG aldehyde—polyetherimide (PEI)	Characterization, hydrogel self-healing behavior, in vitro cell response, cytotoxicity, rat wound healing	[78]

5. Alginate-Based Beads and Microcapsules for Wound Healing

The microcapsules (around 200 μm) and beads are obtained either by using $CaCl_2$ as a cross-linking agent, or they can be obtained by dripping a liquid polysaccharide solution in an acidic (pH < 4) gelling solvent [15]. The bead size is also influenced by the gravity force and the resisting interfacial tension force when the droplet is falling in the liquid [45]. Furthermore, alginate beads [79], obtained through emulsion or extrusion, have the ability to entrap drugs, proteins, growth factors such as the platelet-derived growth factor (PDGF) and/or other wound healing promotors. One example is the alginate-chitosan polyelectrolyte membranes, with or without silver sulfadiazine (AgSD), and the chitosan–fibrin–sodium alginate hydrogel that displayed wound healing properties [11], as seen in Table 2.

Table 2. Alginate-based beads and microcapsules used for wound healing.

Composition	Study Type/Target	Ref.
3.5% Na ALG—3% KCl—3.5% k-CG—3% CaCl$_2$ Na ALG/k-CG weight ratio: 10:0, 9:1, 8:2, 7:3, 6:4, 5:5, 4:6, 3:7, 2:8, 1:9, 0:10	Characterization and thermostability	[80]
ALG—k-CG ratio: 5:5, 7:3, 8:2 ALG—i-CG ratio: 5:5, 7:3, 8:2	Formation and characterization; cytotoxicity, cell encapsulation	[73]
3% w/v diclofenac—1–3% w/v Na CMC—0.5% w/v AlCl$_3$ 6H$_2$O 3% w/v diclofenac—1–3% w/v Na ALG—5% w/v AlCl$_3$	Drug content and particle size, disintegration, friability and in vitro dissolution test, in vivo test on beagles	[50,81]
Na ALG/k-CG %: 100, 75:25, 50:50, 25:75 + 0.125 g Fe$_3$O$_4$	Hydrogel magnetic beads characterization, drug release, swelling	[82]
2% w/v high M Na ALG—VEGF	In vitro drug analysis	[83]
Beads of 1% Ca ALG—0.25% platelet lysate—0.03% vancomycin hydrochloride	Particle characterization, drug and PDGF AB release, PBS absorption, cell proliferation	[84]

6. Alginate-Based Nanofibers and Fibers for Wound Healing

When discussing the average diameter of alginate-based nanofibers obtained after electro-spinning authors mention a myriad of dimensions, ranging from 70 to almost 200 nm, as follows: 93 ± 22 nm after lavender oil was added to a Na ALG-Polyvinyl alcohol (PVA) blend; 100.35 ± 12.79 nm for a Na ALG-PVA; 105 nm for Na ALG—polyethylene oxide/glycol (PEO) blend, 175 ± 75 nm Na ALG-PVA-moxifloxacin hydrochloride [85]; 151 ± 19 nm for Na ALG-PEO [86]; 190–240 nm Na Alg-PVA [87]; 196.4 nm for a collagen-alginate [88]. The alginate-based fibers can be obtained either by spinning in an aqueous media or by extrusion. The average diameter of these fibers depends on the gauge of the used extrusion device, ranging from 70 μm up to 0.1 mm for the extruded ones, whereas fibers obtained in a coagulation bath had a diameter of 6 mm [89]. Liao et al. [90] mentions fibers with an average diameter of 10–20 μm.

A bio-polymeric system, effective in chronic wound therapy, remains a challenge. Bioactive functionalized bio-polymeric supports based on nanofibers, with integrated antibacterial components, is an area of extremely high interest, both in chemical and biopharmaceutical terms. This is because the changes in nanofibers diameters affect the rate of controlled release of the active agent within the nanofibers network [91].

When the alginate fiber dressings make contact with a wound, the space in-between its fibers will close and the bacteria will be trapped in this wound dressing because of the water intake and thus the fiber swelling [34].

Alginate-based nanofibers are obtained through electrospinning. This process takes place after high voltage electrical current passes through a liquid drop that becomes charged, and because of the antagonistic tension surface and electrostatic forces, the drop will elongate until it reaches the nanofiber state [92] (Figure 3).

The molecular weight and viscosity of the ingredients influence the resulting nanofibers [23]. Sodium alginate (Na ALG) cannot form electrospun nanofibers on its own [86,87] but the possibilities regarding the blends are numerous (Table 3). If Na ALG is blended with PEO or PVA, then the resulting nanofibers are smooth [86,93,94] and ZnO nanoparticles can be cross-linked to the mat for an antibacterial effect. When a 1:1 ratio of PVA and Na ALG was used, under a 17 kV treatment at a 0.1 mL/h rate with the collector being 5 cm away from the needle, the resulting average diameter of the nanofibers was 190–240 nm [87]. Alginate fibers can also be treated with silver nanoparticles (AgNPs) either from a silver nitrate solution or Ag^+/Ag^0 ions and have antimicrobial and antifungal properties [34].

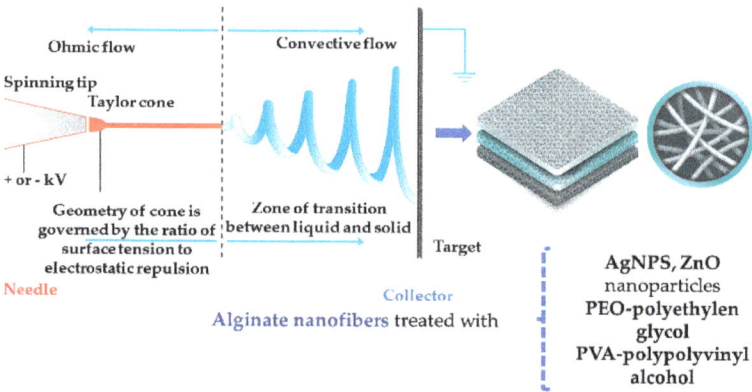

Figure 3. Electrospun ALG nanofibers.

PVA-Na ALG nanofibers were also generated through electrospinning at 15 kV, a flow rate of 0.5 mL/h and 15 cm away from the syringe tip and ciprofloxacin was incorporated in the created patch through active loading. The diameter of the resulting PVA-Na ALG nanofibers was 200–300 nm and it increased after the drug was loaded. These drug-loaded nanofibers showed encouraging results in an in vivo wound healing study when applied as a composite nanofiber patch following the Higuchi and Korsmeyer–Peppas drug-releasing models [95].

During an in vitro study PEO and Na ALG were used to create nanofibers at a 1:1 ratio. By adding DMSO and Triton X-100 the surface tension and the viscosity of the solution lowered. The conditions for obtaining nanofibers with an average diameter of 151 ± 19 nm were 20 kV through an 18G needle, the collector being 20 cm away from the source in a 30% humidity area. If cross-linkers like 1M calcium nitrate tetrahydrate ($Ca(NO_3)_2$) and glutaraldehyde ($C_5H_8O_2$) treat the fibers they become thinner ($Ca(NO_3)_2$ average diameter of 149 ± 69 nm versus $C_5H_8O_2$ average diameter 130 ± 51 nm), have better tensile strength and degradation rate, while losing their flexibility. The addition of 0.1 vol % poly-L-lysine increased the fibroblast cell attachment and their proliferation, showing the feasibility of using this type of nanofibers in other wound healing studies [86,94].

In another study, performed by Kataria et al. [95], 0.5 cm deep and 4 cm^2 incisions were inflicted on male rabbits in a study that compared the wound healing ability of ciprofloxacin loaded- and non-loaded PVA with or without Na ALG electrospun composite nanofiber transdermal patches. The changes of the wound site were observed every 5 days for a total of 20 days and the best results were recorded the used transdermal patch was the drug-loaded PVA-Na ALG dressing. This result was proven after both histological and biochemical assays, when the complete healing of the wounded area was seen after 17 days, and the maximum amounts of collagen and hydroxyproline in the wound bed were measured after 20 days. Another advantage of the alginate-based dressing was its ability to be removed by dissolution because of its gel-forming property.

Table 3. Alginate-based nanofibers and fibers used for wound healing.

Composition	Study Type/Target	Ref.
2% Na ALG solution—16% PVA solution—0.5, 1, 2, 5% ZnO-NPs; Na ALG/PVA ratio 1:1	Composite nanofiber characterization, antibacterial effect, cell adhesion potential, cytotoxicity	[11,87]
Na ALG from unmodified methacrylated ALG—1% w/v RGD-modified methacrylated ALG—methacrylated heparin—4% w/v PEO; Na ALG/PEO ratio 1:1	Nanofiber characterization, cell interaction, adhesion and proliferation, binding and releasing heparin tests	[28,96]
4 wt % Na ALG—5 wt % PEO—0.5 wt % Triton X-100—5 wt % DMSO; Na ALG/PEO ratios: 65:35, 50:50, 35:65	Nanofiber characterization, fibroblast proliferation	[86,94]
8 wt % PVA—2% w/w Na ALG—3.2% w/v ciprofloxacin; PVA/Na ALG ratio: 5.5:1	Nanofiber characterization, swelling, drug incorporation and release; in vivo tests on rabbits: drug release, wound healing	[94,95]
1, 2, 3% wt of Na ALG—PEO—0.3 wt % Lecithin—5% w/w CaCl$_2$; 1, 2, 3% wt of Na ALG/PEO weight % ratios: 1:1, 2:1, 3:1, 1:2, 2:2, 3:2	Solution characterization: viscosity, conductivity; Nanofiber characterization: structure, water absorption, fibroblast attachment	[93,94]
6% w/v Na ALG—0.1, 0.15, 2% chitin whisker Chitin whisker/ALG weight ratio: 0.05–2%	Whiskers and fibers characterization	[62,65,97]
ZnCl$_2$—Ca ALG fibers	Antimicrobial and immuno-modulatory effects for wound healing keratinocyte migration, ppm Zn release	[11,42,89,98,99]
AgNO$_3$—6% Ca ALG fibers	Antimicrobial effect	[11,89,98,100]
0.5–0.75% w/v Chitosan—0.5–1% w/v ALG—Dexamethasone/BSA/PDGF-bb/Avidin fibers	Drug incorporation and release, PDGF-bb bioactivity	[49,90]
0, 0.014, 0.041% w/v Chitosan—0.001% w/v Na ALG—Ninhydrin—CaCl$_2$ in fibers	Filament characterization	[49,101]
1.5 w % Na ALG—Ag-NPs in crosslinked fibers	Wound healing effect on SKH-1 mice	[102]

An uniform morphology of the nanofibers can also be obtained by adding lecithin as a natural surfactant [93], or arginine–glycine–aspartic acid (RGD) [103].

Nanofibers can also be obtained by mixing methacrylated alginate, RGD-modified methacrylated alginate and PEO at 10.4 kV, with a flow rate of 0.6 mL/h and the collector being placed at 15 cm away from the syringe tip. The interesting part about this blend was the UV treatment with 365 nm UV light at <1 mW/cm^2 that can or cannot be followed by the PEO extraction. The resulting photo-cross-linked nanofibers can also be coated with gold. Before the cross-linking the fiber diameters were between 185.5 ± 37 and 195.4 ± 23 nm, after cross-linking the fiber diameters were between 182.2 ± 36 and 190.4 ± 30 nm, but the PEO extraction lead to a diameter increase due to nanofiber swelling, ranging between 256.3 ± 43 and 297.9 ± 42 nm [96]. When this study used PEO/methacrylated heparin-, RGD-modified-, or unmodified methacrylated alginate-based nanofibers, it concluded that—by adding methacrylated heparin—the stress–strain curves are influenced, therefore making the elongation at break significantly lower and the tensile strength and Young's modulus significantly greater than those observed for the unmodified or RGD-modified methacrylated alginate-based nanofibers [96].

7. Other Alginate-Based Dressings

Among the alginate-based wound healing blends (Table 4) are gelatin-alginate sponges, alginate-scaffolds based on antisense oligo-deoxynucleotides (asODN) linking to Connexin 43 (Cx43) [11,104], viscose/Ag NPs/ALG/nicotinamide/CaCl$_2$ fabrics [105]. The 3D bi-layered scaffold made of polyethylene glycol (PEG)-chitosan hydrogel and chitosan-alginate can also help tissue regeneration after injury by holding fibroblasts on the upper surface and keratinocytes on the lower one [106,107].

The wound pH is a reliable factor when discussion the healing status, because it shifts from high when infected to low when healed either naturally or because it was modulated through applying different treatments [108–110]. Polyethylene oxide–alginate wafers loaded with diclofenac and streptomycin show controlled drug release at room temperature, in simulated wound fluid (BSA, $CaCl_2$, NaCl, $C_4H_{11}NO_3$) conditions at pH 7.5. The diffusion of both drugs from the annealed wafers takes place slowly, making them potentially useful in highly exuding wounds [23,111]. Because wound pH-variation has a strong effect on the healing process, researchers also developed, through microfluidic spinning using their electrostatic interactions, a mesoporous particle hydrogel alginate-based flexible microfiber linked to a pH-responsive dye linked onto a transparent medical tape place on top of a wound, in order to observe the pH modifications in real-time [112].

A 3D porous sponge was obtained after a pre-gelled (with bivalent cations) alginate was frozen and then lyophilized. The type and concentration of both alginate and cross-linkers, as well as the freezing protocol influenced the mechanical properties as well as the size (70–300 µm) and display pattern of the pores. This pore size was appropriate for fibroblast seeding [113]. On the other hand, when comparing the tensile strength for G-ALG and M-ALG sponge dressings with different ALG concentrations, the elongation at fracture was not influenced by the alginate concentration, whereas Young's modulus and the maximum stress at fracture increased with it [114].

Table 4. Other alginate-based dressings used for wound healing.

Composition	Study Type/Target	Ref.
Na ALG—0.1% w/v I-labeled SDF-1 plasmid Na ALG—0.0001% w/v (1 ng/µL) I-labeled SDF-1 protein	Acute surgical wounds on Yorkshire pigs: SDF-1 release kinetics, wound healing rate, scar formation	[42,115]
Viscose/silver/ALG Vis/Ag-NPs/ALG Viscose/silver/ALG/nicotinamide Viscose/silver/ALG/nicotinamide/$CaCl_2$ 0.5–1.5% w/w Na ALG in nonwoven fabric	Burn—diabetic rats	[105]
Chitosan 4% w/v—1% w/w CH_3COOH—4% ALG Chitosan 4% w/v—1% w/w CH_3COOH—4% CG w/v—5.7% NaCl	Comparative drug release system study: swelling, Diltiazem HCl-loaded tablet formulation, dissolution in 1:1 complex systems	[116]
Ca ALG versus silicone-coated polyamide net	Comparative randomized trial: healing and slippage rate, removal discomfort degree on skin graft donor sites	[117,118]
2% w/v Na ALG—pH-responsive dye—glycerol 0–60% w/v	Flexible microfibers description, real-time pH modifications on the pig wound site	[112]
collagen—0.5, 1.0, 1.5, 2.0, 3.0, 4.0, 5.0% alginic acid, at 3:1 ratio in cross-linked sheet	Sheet characterization	[98,119]
75% Alginic acid solution 2% w/v— 45S5 bioactive glass—25% cell suspension	VEGF secretion, cell viability, cytotoxicity	[120]
Polyox®—CG—Streptomycin—Diclofenac (0.75:0.25:0.3:0.25 g) Polyox®—0.5 g Na ALG—Streptomycin—Diclofenac (0.5:0.5:0.25:0.1 g)	Wafer characterization, adhesion, drug release, swelling	[23,111]
2% w/v Alginic acid—murine antisense nucleotides (Cx43asODN) based scaffolds	Wounded ICR mice: inflammatory response, re-epithelization	[11,104]
20 µg Smad3 ASOs in Na ALG and chitosan 1:1, 1:2, 1:4, 1:8, 1:16 ALG/chitosan ratio in PEC	Scaffold characterization, wound healing in C57BL/6 mice	[40,62,65]
gelatin—1 wt % Na ALG (with or without 0.4 mg/cm^2 AgSD) sponge	Wistar rat wound healing	[11,98,121]

Table 4. Cont.

Composition	Study Type/Target	Ref.
1% solution silk fibroin—1% solution alginic acid in 10:0, 5:5 and 0:10 ratios sponge	Sprague Dawley rats full thickness wound	[98,122]
2 or 4% w/v high G and high M ALG—0.1–10% w/w PEG—9.5% w/v poly(D,L-lactide-co-glycolide) (PLGA)—0.5% w/v insulin microparticles in sponge	Sponge characterization: density, tensile strength, water vapor transmission rate and absorption capacity. In vitro study: interaction with HaCaT cells, insulin release	[23,114]
Chitosan—1% w/w Na ALG—hematoxylin-eosin—DHEA—AgSD in PEC sponge	Microscope assay, in vitro drug release, cytotoxicity, antibacterial effect, in vivo burn healing on BALB/C mice	[49,123]
ALG—0.2, 0.4% chitosan—0.1, 0.5% all-trans retinoic acid (ATRA). 1:10 ATRA/ALG ratio in microparticles	Microparticles characterization, encapsulation efficiency, dermal localization, ATRA skin release	[42,124]
2% Na ALG (61% M and 39% G)—2–4 µg VEGF in microspheres	In vitro drug release, in vivo angiogenesis	[125]

PEG addition to the aforementioned sponge increases the flexibility while having a plasticizing effect. Furthermore, its concentration and molecular weight significantly modifies the tensile strength of the sponge. For low molecular weight PEG of 1.45 kDa a concentration increases from 0.1% to 1% leads to a lower Young's modulus, maximum stress at fracture and elongation at fracture. For high molecular weight PEG (10 kDa) the concentration increases from 0.1% to 1% leads to an increase for Young's modulus and maximum stress at fracture, while the elongation at fracture is significantly lower. While comparing the results between the uses of different molecular weight PEG in the sponge, the one with a molecular weight of 1.45 kDa displayed higher tensile strength values than the 10 kDa PEG. PEG addition to the M-ALG sponges also increases the WVTR and decreases the water absorption capacity, regardless of its molecular weight, but the observed values for WVTR (16.7 ± 0.4 before PEG addition and (22.9 ± 0.8)–(28.8 ± 2.1) after PEG addition) were almost double the recommended values (8–10 mg/cm^2/h) [114].

8. Commercially Available Pharmaceutical Alginate-Based Products

The list of commercially available alginate-based wound dressing is growing fast (Table 5), while the most recent FDA approval available on-line at this time was given to Luofucon® Extra Silver Alginate Dressing (Prescribed only—PO) and Luofucon® Antibacterial Alginate Wound Dressing (Over-The-Counter—OTC) [126,127]. The researchers state the dressings proved their activity against *E. coli*, *E. faecalis*, *K. pneumoniae*, Methicillin-resistant *S. aureus* (MRSA), *P. aeruginosa*, *S. aureus*, *S. pyogenes*, and Vancomycin-resistant *Enterococcus* (VRE). Silver creates a barrier against a broad spectrum of bacteria [128] for as long as seven days [126].

Enzymes were added into a PEG-alginate hydrogel called Flaminal® Forte that underwent human clinical trials for treating partial thickness burns [129] and had better results than the Ag sulfadiazine-based one (Flamazine®), regarding the times it needed to be changed [130]. When a patient is unable to move, pressure ulcers may appear. Such a case was also healed after several dressings were applied, including a honey-loaded alginate-based product, named Algivon® [131,132]. An improved version of this dressing, Algivon® Plus, showed good clinical results when applied on chronic wounds [133]. Algivon® Ribbon or Plus is also used for diabetic, pressure, and leg ulcers, fungating lesions, infected, cavity, and chronic or complicated surgical wounds and abrasions [32,131,133–136]. On the other hand, another Manuka honey loaded calcium alginate-based wound dressing is Activon® Tube or Tulle for diabetic and leg ulcers, pressure sores, and malodorous, infected, dry, sloughy, or necrotic wounds [135,137–139].

Recently, researchers have studied the effect of treating human skin lesions, produced by an atypical form of Henoch–Shönlein purpura, with three hyaluronic acid-based commercially available products Hyalomatrix PA® (a 3D matrix of a hyaluronic acid ester

(Hyaff) and a transparent film), Hyalogran®, and Jaloskin®, which were maintained on the wound site for various time periods in a consecutive order. One of the treatments, Hyalogran®, was an alginate-hyaluronan dressing made of sodium alginate and Hyaff [140]. After the eschar resection, wound debridement, and 21 days of the first dressing, the next step was applying the second one for two weeks, and the third for an unmentioned period. After two months from the first treatment the wound was completely healed [140], with minimal scaring and thus confirming the benefits of wound treatments involving hyaluronic acid in combination with sodium alginate. Silvercel®, another commercially available alginate-based non-adherent dressing, was used in a wound healing study, when it was applied twice a week on a diabetic patient with a repetitive non-infected venous leg ulcer and the wound healed in 14 day [141].

Table 5. Alginate-based commercially available pharmaceutical products used in wound healing.

Name	Composition/Target	Study Type/Effects	Ref.
ALGS6 Ag (Prescribed/Over-The-Counter)	Ca ALG fiber—Lyocell fiber—1.7% Ag$^+$ Surgical, traumatic, acute and chronic wounds, ulcers, first and second degree burns; Minor cuts, burns	Exudate absorption, gel forming, wound healing promoter if changed weekly	[142]
Aquacel™ Ag EXTRA™ Hydrofiber™ (Prescribed/OTC)	Bi-layer Na ALG CMC—Ag$^+$—strengthening fibers; Surgical, traumatic, exuding, infected, and painful wounds, second degree burns, ulcers or for minor cuts or burns	Bacterial inhibition, absorbs the wound exudate while forming a gel, it must be changed every 1–2 weeks	[142]
Calgitrol™ foam or SilverSite™	Ag+ in Ag ALG—Ca ALG—polyurethane foam	Antimicrobial effect, cytotoxicity	[23,143–145]
Fibracol 10% Ca ALG in Fibracol Plus® dressing	90% Collagen—10% Ca ALG; Exuding full- and partial-thickness wounds, second degree burns; diabetic, pressure, and venous ulcers	Clinical Trial: healing time of diabetic foot ulcers	[16,32,146]
Flaminal® gel	ALG—PEG matrix—notatin—lactoperoxidase—guaiacol; burns, post-surgery wounds, diabetic, leg and pressure ulcers. If used with H_2O_2 and SCN- it has a bacteriostatic effect against both gram-positive and gram-negative bacteria.	Antimicrobial and bacteriostatic effect, wound surface moisturizer, exudate absorber, debrides necrotic tissue	[32,129,147,148]
Guardix-SG®	Na ALG—poloxamer—$CaCl_2$; post-surgery (silicone implantation, blepharoplasty)	In vivo post-surgery studies on rabbits: thermosensitive gel, mechanical barrier formation, suppression of capsular contracture, reduced inflammation and fibrosis	[32,149,150]
Hyalogran® dressing	Hyaluronic acid ester—Na ALG; Leg and pressure sores, diabetic and ischemic wounds (with slough or necrosis)	Exudate absorption, gel transformation, necrotic tissue removal	[32,140]
Kaltostat®	80% High G Ca ALG—20% NaALG; Acute and chronic wounds with moderate to heavy exudate	Wound healing	[6,28,49,62–65,151]
Luofucon® Antibacterial Alginate Wound Dressing (OTC)	Ca ALG—Ag; minor cuts, abrasions, and burns	Changed daily it has antibacterial effect and promotes wound healing	[126]

Table 5. *Cont.*

Name	Composition/Target	Study Type/Effects	Ref.
Luofucon® Extra Silver Alginate Dressing (PO)	Ca ALG—Ag; moderate to heavily exuding wounds, ulcers, trauma-inflicted or post-operative wounds, infected wounds, grafts	Antibacterial effect for seven days and it promotes wound healing	[126]
Medihoney® (gel, hydrogel or paste)	Ca ALG—Manuka honey; ulcers: hemorrhagic, heavily exuding, diabetic foot, leg (arterial or venous), pressure (partial or full-thickness) ulcers. First and second partial thickness burns. Surgical and traumatic wounds	Antibacterial effect	[3,23]
Purilon Gel®	Na CMC—Ca ALG; Used with another dressing for first and second degree burns or sloughy and necrotic wounds	Wound surface moisturizer	[32,147,152,153]
Saf-gel®	Carbomer propylene glycol sodium—Ca ALG; Abrasions, cuts, sloughy and necrotic wounds, second degree burns, non-infected diabetic foot ulcers, and pressure and venous ulcers	Wound healing and surface moisturizer.	[32,147,154]
SeaSorb® fine foam sheet	Na ALG/Ca ALG—polyethylene net; Heavily exuding wounds: cavity wounds, second degree burns, diabetic, leg and pressure ulcers, spina bifida	Human clinical trials: fiber to gel transformation, tolerance, healing rate with reduced exudate, maceration and pain intensity	[32,155,156]
Silvercel™	36% Ca ALG with high G—6% CMC—28% Ag (111 mg Ag/100 cm^2)—30% EasyLift Precision Film (Acelity/Systagenix)	Pig and human trials, wound healing	[141,157–162]
Tromboguard® bi-layer dressing	Polyurethane sponge—chitosan + Na ALG + Ca ALG + Ag$^+$; Traumatic and post-surgery wounds	Antibacterial effect and strong hemostatic	[32]

Other commercially available dressings contain both ALG and silver, like Aquacel™ Ag EXTRA™ Hydrofiber™ or ALGS6 Ag Alginate Wound Dressing have similar wound healing characteristics [142]. Various other commercially available alginate-based dressings that were included in a multiple comparative studies were Suprasorb® A (100% ALG), Suprasorb® A—Ag (ALG—ionic Ag), and LG—nano Ag® Acticoat Absorbent with SILCRYST™, for their anti-microbial effect, binding to elastase capacity, MMP-2, TNF-α and IL-8, antioxidant ability, cytotoxicity, and effect on HaCaT keratinocytes, showing promising results [42,163,164].

9. Conclusions

The development of alginate-based biomaterials for wound healing has an accelerated pace. The last years gave patients hopes for receiving better treatment for their wounds because the development of a wound dressing that might actually become a true 'ideal dressing' seems to be in hands reach. The versatility of alginate-based wound dressings, the promising results after both in vivo and in vitro trials and the cost-effectiveness of obtaining them makes alginate one of the favorites when choosing the material that could act both as a support and as a carrier for the bio-active compounds that have to reach a wound.

Author Contributions: Conceptualization, A.B. and B.N.; Methodology, A.B. and B.N.; Formal analysis A.B. and B.N.; Investigation, A.B. and B.N.; Resources, A.B.; Data curation, A.B. and B.N.; Writing—original draft preparation, A.B., B.N., M.Z., G.M.I., C.B. and V.M.; Writing—review and editing A.B., B.N., M.Z., G.M.I., C.B. and V.M.; Visualization, A.B. and B.N.; Supervision, V.M.; Project administration, A.B. All authors have read and agreed to the published version of the manuscript.

Funding: This research received no external funding.

Institutional Review Board Statement: Not applicable.

Informed Consent Statement: Not applicable.

Acknowledgments: This work has been conducted in the Pediatric Clinical Hospital Sibiu, within the Research and Telemedicine Center in Neurological Diseases in Children—CEFORATEN. This study is part of the doctoral thesis of the Andreea Barbu, under the supervision of Vioara Mireșan.

Conflicts of Interest: The authors declare no conflict of interest.

References

1. Sen, C.K.; Gordillo, G.M.; Roy, S.; Kirsner, R.; Lambert, L.; Hunt, T.K.; Gottrup, F.; Gurtner, G.C.; Longaker, M.T. Human Skin Wounds: A Major Snoballing Threat to Public Health and Economy. *Wound Repair Regen.* **2009**, *17*, 763–771. [CrossRef]
2. Chandran, S.; Seetharaman, A.; Rajalekshmi, G.; Pandimadevi, M. Potential wound healing materials from the natural polymers—A review. *Int. J. Pharma. Bio Sci.* **2015**, *6*, 1365–1389.
3. Das, S.; Baker, A.B. Biomaterials and Nanotherapeutics for Enhancing Skin Wound Healing. *Front. Bioeng. Biotechnol.* **2016**, *4*, 82. [CrossRef] [PubMed]
4. Erdogan, I.; Bayraktar, O.; Uslu, M.E.; Tuncel, O. Wound Healing Effects of Various Fractions of Olive Leaf Extract (OLE) on Mouse Fibroblasts. *Rom. Biotechnol. Lett.* **2018**, *23*, 14217–14228. [CrossRef]
5. Miricioiu, M.G.; Niculescu, V.C.; Filote, C.; Raboaca, M.S.; Nechifor, G. Coal fly ash derived silica nanomaterial for mmms-application in CO_2/CH_4 separation. *Membranes* **2021**, *11*, 78. [CrossRef]
6. Aramwit, P. Introduction to biomaterials for wound healing. In *Wound Healing Biomaterials*; Elsevier Ltd.: London, UK, 2016; Volume 2, pp. 3–38. ISBN 9780081006061.
7. Liu, J.; Zheng, H.; Dai, X.; Sun, S.; Machens, H.G.; Schilling, A.F. Biomaterials for Promoting Wound Healing in Diabetes. *J. Tissue Sci. Eng.* **2017**, *8*, 193–196. [CrossRef]
8. Mihai, M. Novel biocompatible chitosan based multilayer films. *Rom. Biotechnol. Lett.* **2011**, *16*, 6313–6321.
9. Barbu, A.; Neamțu, M.B.; Zăhan, M.; Mireșan, V. Trends in alginate-based films and membranes for wound healing. *Rom. Biotechnol. Lett.* **2020**, *25*, 1683–1689. [CrossRef]
10. Alizadehgiashi, M.; Nemr, C.R.; Chekini, M.; Ramos, D.P.; Mittal, N.; Ahmed, S.U.; Khuu, N.; Kelley, S.O.; Kumacheva, E. Multifunctional 3D-Printed Wound Dressings. *ACS Nano* **2021**, *15*, 12375–12387. [CrossRef]
11. Chaudhari, A.A.; Vig, K.; Baganizi, D.R.; Sahu, R.; Dixit, S.; Dennis, V.; Singh, S.R.; Pillai, S.R. Future prospects for scaffolding methods and biomaterials in skin tissue engineering: A review. *Int. J. Mol. Sci.* **2016**, *17*, 1974. [CrossRef] [PubMed]
12. Chin, C.Y.; Gan, J.E. Formulation and characterisation of alginate hydrocolloid film dressing loaded with gallic acid for potential chronic wound healing. *F1000Research* **2021**, *10*, 451. [CrossRef]
13. Snyder, D.; Sullivan, N.; Margolis, B.D.; Schoelles, K. Skin substitutes for treating chronic wounds—Technical brief. In *Technology Assessment Program—Technical Brief*; Project ID No. WNDT0818. (Prepared by the ECRI Institute-Penn Medicine Evidence-Based Practice Center under Contract No. HHSA 290-2015-00005-I); Agency for Healthcare Research and Quality: Rockville, MD, USA, February 2020. Available online: http://www.ahrq.gov/research/findings/ta/index.html (accessed on 31 May 2021).
14. Koga, A.Y.; Felix, J.C.; Silvestre, R.G.M.; Lipinski, L.C.; Carletto, B.; Kawahara, F.A.; Pereira, A.V. Evaluation of wound healing effect of alginate film containing aloe vera gel and cross-linked with zinc chloride. *Acta Cir. Bras.* **2020**, *35*, 1–11. [CrossRef] [PubMed]
15. Clark, M. Technology update: Rediscovering alginate dressings. *Wounds Int.* **2012**, *3*, 3–6. [CrossRef]
16. Dumville, J.; O'Meara, S.; Deshpande, S.; Speak, K. Alginate dressings for healing diabetic foot ulcers. *Cochrane Database Syst. Rev.* **2013**, *6*, CD009110. [CrossRef] [PubMed]
17. Radu, C.-D.; Parteni, O.; Sandu, I.G.; Lisa, G.; Munteanu, C.; Lupu, V.V. Specific characterization of a multilayer biomaterial controlled release of tacrolimus. *Rev. Chim.* **2016**, *67*, 199–204.
18. Samimi, M.; Validov, S. Characteristics of pDNA-loaded chitosan/alginate-dextran sulfate nanoparticles with high transfection efficiency. *Rom. Biotechnol. Lett.* **2018**, *23*, 13996–14006. [CrossRef]
19. Yussof, S.J.M.; Omar, E.; Pai, D.R.; Sood, S. Cellular events and biomarkers of wound healing. *Indian J. Plast. Surg.* **2012**, *45*, 220–228. [CrossRef]
20. Nagaraja, S.; Wallqvist, A.; Reifman, J.; Mitrophanov, A.Y. Computational Approach To Characterize Causative Factors and Molecular Indicators of Chronic Wound Inflammation. *J. Immunol.* **2014**, *192*, 1824–1834. [CrossRef]
21. Mathew-Steiner, S.S.; Roy, S.; Sen, C.K. Collagen in wound healing. *Bioengineering* **2021**, *8*, 63. [CrossRef]
22. Chen, F.M.; Liu, X. Advancing biomaterials of human origin for tissue engineering. *Prog. Polym. Sci.* **2016**, *53*, 86–168. [CrossRef]
23. Boateng, J.; Catanzano, O. Advanced Therapeutic Dressings for Effective Wound Healing—A Review. *J. Pharm. Sci.* **2015**, *104*, 3653–3680. [CrossRef]

24. Matei, A.M.; Caruntu, C.; Tampa, M.; Georgescu, S.R.; Matei, C.; Constantin, M.M.; Constantin, T.V.; Calina, D.; Ciubotaru, D.A.; Badarau, I.A.; et al. Applications of nanosized-lipid-based drug delivery systems in wound care. *Appl. Sci.* **2021**, *11*, 4915. [CrossRef]
25. Pastar, I.; Stojadinovic, O.; Yin, N.C.; Ramirez, H.; Nusbaum, A.G.; Sawaya, A.; Patel, S.B.; Khalid, L.; Isseroff, R.R.; Tomic-Canic, M. Epithelialization in Wound Healing: A Comprehensive Review. *Adv. Wound Care* **2014**, *3*, 445–464. [CrossRef]
26. Orsted, H.L.; Keast, D.; Forest-lalande, L. Basic Principles of Wound Healing An understanding of the basic physiology of wound healing provides. *Wound Care Can.* **2011**, *9*, 4–12.
27. Ching, C.S.; Phillips, T.J.; Howard, C.E.; Panova, I.P.; Hayes, C.M.; Asandra, A.S.; Park, H.Y. Chronic wound fluid suppresses proliferation of dermal fibroblasts through a Ras-mediated signaling pathway. *J. Investig. Dermatol.* **2005**, *124*, 466–474. [CrossRef]
28. De Jesus Raposo, M.F.; De Morais, A.M.B.; De Morais, R.M.S.C. Marine polysaccharides from algae with potential biomedical applications. *Mar. Drugs* **2015**, *13*, 2967. [CrossRef]
29. Raguvaran, R.; Manuja, B.K.; Chopra, M.; Thakur, R.; Anand, T.; Kalia, A.; Manuja, A. Sodium alginate and gum acacia hydrogels of ZnO nanoparticles show wound healing effect on fibroblast cells. *Int. J. Biol. Macromol.* **2017**, *96*, 185–191. [CrossRef]
30. Badea, V.; Paula Balaban, D.P.; Rapeanu, G.; Amariei, C.; Badea, C.F. The antibacterial activity evaluation of Cystoseira barbata biomass and some alginates upon bacteria from oropharyngeal cavity. *Rom. Biotechnol. Lett.* **2009**, *14*, 4851–4857.
31. Spadari, C.d.C.; Lopes, L.B.; Ishida, K. Potential use of alginate-based carriers as antifungal delivery system. *Front. Microbiol.* **2017**, *8*, 97. [CrossRef]
32. Szekalska, M.; Pucilowska, A.; Szymanska, E.; Ciosek, P.; Winnicka, K. Alginate: Current Use and Future Perspectives in Pharmaceutical and Biomedical Applications. *Int. J. Polym. Sci.* **2016**, *2016*, 7697031. [CrossRef]
33. Ueno, M.; Oda, T. Effects of Alginate Oligosaccharides on the Growth of Marine Microalgae. In *Marine Algae Extracts: Processes, Products, and Applications*; Kim, S.-K., Chojnacka, K., Eds.; Wiley-VCH: Weinheim, Germany, 2015; Volumes 1–2, pp. 213–226. ISBN 9783527679577.
34. Wiegand, C.; Hipler, U.C. Polymer-based biomaterials as dressings for chronic stagnating wounds. *Macromol. Symp.* **2010**, *294*, 1–13. [CrossRef]
35. Pawar, H.V.; Tetteh, J.; Boateng, J.S. Preparation, optimisation and characterisation of novel wound healing film dressings loaded with streptomycin and diclofenac. *Colloids Surf. B Biointerfaces* **2012**, *102*, 102–110. [CrossRef]
36. Liakos, I.; Rizzello, L.; Scurr, D.J.; Pompa, P.P.; Bayer, I.S.; Athanassiou, A. All-natural composite wound dressing films of essential oils encapsulated in sodium alginate with antimicrobial properties. *Int. J. Pharm.* **2014**, *463*. [CrossRef]
37. Raducu, L.; Cozma, C.N.; Balcangiu-Stroescu, A.E.; Avino, A.; Tanasescu, A.D.; Balan, D.G.; Jecan, C.R. Our Experience in Chronic Wounds Care with Polyurethane Foam. *Rev. Chim.* **2018**, *69*, 585–586. [CrossRef]
38. Mushollaeni, W. The physicochemical characteristics of sodium alginate from Indonesian brown seaweeds. *Arab. J. Chem.* **2011**, *5*, 349–352.
39. Ivancic, A. Recent Trends in Alginate, Chitosan and Alginate-Chitosan Antimicrobial Systems. *Chem. J. Mold.* **2017**, *11*, 17–25. [CrossRef]
40. Hong, H.J.; Jin, S.E.; Park, J.S.; Ahn, W.S.; Kim, C.K. Accelerated wound healing by smad3 antisense oligonucleotides-impregnated chitosan/alginate polyelectrolyte complex. *Biomaterials* **2008**, *29*, 4831–4837. [CrossRef] [PubMed]
41. Rhein-Knudsen, N.; Ale, M.T.; Ajalloueian, F.; Meyer, A.S. Characterization of alginates from Ghanaian brown seaweeds: Sargassum spp. and Padina spp. *Food Hydrocoll.* **2017**, *71*, 236–244. [CrossRef]
42. Lee, K.Y.; Mooney, D.J. Alginate: Properties and biomedical applications. *Prog. Polym. Sci.* **2012**, *37*, 106–126. [CrossRef]
43. Lotfipour, F.; Mirzaeei, S.; Maghsoodi, M. Evaluation of the effect of $CaCl_2$ and alginate concentrations and hardening time on the characteristics of Lactobacillus acidophilus loaded alginate beads using response surface analysis. *Adv. Pharm. Bull.* **2012**, *2*, 71–78. [CrossRef]
44. Pawar, S.N. Chemical Modification of Alginates in Organic Media. Ph.D. Thesis, Virginia Polytechnic Institute and State University, Blacksburg, VA, USA, 2013.
45. Maritz, J.; Krieg, H.M.; Yeates, C.A.; Botes, A.L.; Breytenbach, J.C. Calcium alginate entrapment of the yeast Rhodosporidium toruloides for the kinetic resolution of 1,2-epoxyoctane. *Biotechnol. Lett.* **2003**, *25*, 1775–1781. [CrossRef]
46. Nicolae, V.; Neamtu, B.; Picu, O.; Stefanache, M.A.M.; Cioranu, V.S.I. The comparative evaluation of salivary biomarkers (Calcium, Phosphate, Salivary pH) in Cario-resistance versus Cario-activity. *Rev. Chim.* **2016**, *67*, 821–824.
47. Pereira, R.; Carvalho, A.; Vaz, D.C.; Gil, M.H.; Mendes, A.; Bártolo, P. Development of novel alginate based hydrogel films for wound healing applications. *Int. J. Biol. Macromol.* **2013**, *52*, 221–230. [CrossRef] [PubMed]
48. Singh, R.; Singh, D. Radiation synthesis of PVP/alginate hydrogel containing nanosilver as wound dressing. *J. Mater. Sci. Mater. Med.* **2012**, *23*, 2649–2658. [CrossRef] [PubMed]
49. Smith, A.M.; Moxon, S.; Morris, G.A. Biopolymers as wound healing materials. In *Wound Healing Biomaterials*; Ågren, M., Ed.; Woodhead Publishing: Cambridge, UK, 2016; Volume 2, pp. 261–287. ISBN 9780081006061.
50. Bhardwaj, T.R.; Kanwar, M.; Lal, R.; Gupta, A. Natural gums and modified natural gums as sustained release carriers. *Drug Dev. Ind. Pharm.* **2000**, *26*, 1025–1038. [CrossRef]
51. Stoica, A.E.; Chircov, C.; Grumezescu, A.M. Nanomaterials for Wound Dressings: An Up-to-Date Overview. *Molecules* **2020**, *25*, 2699. [CrossRef]

52. Koehler, J.; Brandl, F.P.; Goepferich, A.M. Hydrogel wound dressings for bioactive treatment of acute and chronic wounds. *Eur. Polym. J.* **2018**, *100*, 1–11. [CrossRef]
53. Rezvani Ghomi, E.; Khalili, S.; Nouri Khorasani, S.; Esmaeely Neisiany, R.; Ramakrishna, S. Wound dressings: Current advances and future directions. *J. Appl. Polym. Sci.* **2019**, *136*, 47738. [CrossRef]
54. Augst, A.D.; Kong, H.J.; Mooney, D.J. Alginate Hydrogels as Biomaterials. *Macromol. Biosci.* **2006**, *6*, 623–633. [CrossRef]
55. Coviello, T.; Matricardi, P.; Marianecci, C.; Alhaique, F. Polysaccharide hydrogels for modified release formulations. *J. Control. Release* **2007**, *119*, 5–24. [CrossRef]
56. Josef, E.; Zilberman, M.; Bianco-Peled, H. Composite alginate hydrogels: An innovative approach for the controlled release of hydrophobic drugs. *Acta Biomater.* **2010**, *6*, 4642–4649. [CrossRef] [PubMed]
57. Balakrishnan, B.; Mohanty, M.; Umashankar, P.R.; Jayakrishnan, A. Evaluation of an in situ forming hydrogel wound dressing based on oxidized alginate and gelatin. *Biomaterials* **2005**, *26*, 6335–6342. [CrossRef] [PubMed]
58. Da Silva, L.P.; Cerqueira, M.T.; Correlo, V.M.; Reis, R.L.; Marques, A.P. Engineered hydrogel-based matrices for skin wound healing. In *Wound Healing Biomaterials*; Agren, M., Ed.; Elsevier Ltd.: London, UK, 2016; Volume 2, pp. 227–250. ISBN 9780081006061.
59. Chicea, D.; Neamtu, B.; Chicea, R.; Chicea, L.M. The application of AFM for biological samples imaging. *Dig. J. Nanomater. Biostruct.* **2010**, *5*, 1015–1022.
60. Neacsu, I.-A.; Melente, A.E.; Holban, A.-M.; Ficai, A.; Ditu, L.-M.; Kamerzan, C.-M.; Tihăuan, B.M.; Nicoara, A.I.; Bezirtzoglou, E.; Chifiriuc, M.-C. Novel hydrogels based on collagen and ZnO nanoparticles with antibacterial activity for improved wound dressings. *Rom. Biotechnol. Lett.* **2019**, *24*, 317–323. [CrossRef]
61. Mohandas, A.; Kumar, S.; Raja, B.; Lakshmanan, V.-K.; Jayakumar, R. Exploration of alginate hydrogel/nano zinc oxide composite bandages for infected wounds. *Int. J. Nanomed.* **2015**, *10*, 53–66. [CrossRef]
62. Jayakumar, R.; Prabaharan, M.; Kumar, P.T.S.; Nair, S.V.; Furuike, T.; Tamura, H. Novel Chitin and Chitosan Materials in Wound Dressing. In *Biomedical Engineering, Trends in Materials Science*; Laskovski, A., Ed.; InTech: Rijeka, Croatia, 2011; ISBN 9789537619824.
63. Murakami, K.; Aoki, H.; Nakamura, S.; Nakamura, S.-i.; Takikawa, M.; Hanzawa, M.; Kishimoto, S.; Hattori, H.; Tanaka, Y.; Kiyosawa, T.; et al. Hydrogel blends of chitin/chitosan, fucoidan and alginate as healing-impaired wound dressings. *Biomaterials* **2010**, *31*, 83–90. [CrossRef]
64. Murakami, K.; Ishihara, M.; Aoki, H.; Nakamura, S.; Nakamura, S.I.; Yanagibayashi, S.; Takikawa, M.; Kishimoto, S.; Yokoe, H.; Kiyosawa, T.; et al. Enhanced healing of mitomycin C-treated healing-impaired wounds in rats with hydrosheets composed of chitin/chitosan, fucoidan, and alginate as wound dressings. *Wound Repair Regen.* **2010**, *18*, 478–485. [CrossRef]
65. Jayakumar, R.; Prabaharan, M.; Kumar, S.P.T.; Nair, S.V.; Tamura, H. Biomaterials based on chitin and chitosan in wound dressing applications. *Biotechnol. Adv.* **2011**, *29*, 322–337. [CrossRef]
66. Rayyif, S.M.I.; Mohammed, H.B.; Curuțiu, C.; Bîrcă, A.C.; Grumezescu, A.M.; Vasile, B.Ș.; Dițu, L.M.; Lazăr, V.; Chifiriuc, M.C.; Mihăescu, G.; et al. ZnO Nanoparticles-Modified Dressings to Inhibit Wound Pathogens. *Materials* **2021**, *14*, 3084. [CrossRef]
67. Strukova, S.M.; Dugina, T.N.; Chistov, I.V.; Lange, M.; Markvicheva, E.A.; Kuptsova, S.; Zubov, V.P.; Glusa, E. Immobilized thrombin receptor agonist peptide accelerates wound healing in mice. *Clin. Appl. Thromb.* **2001**, *7*, 325–329. [CrossRef]
68. Lee, K.Y.; Peters, M.C.; Anderson, K.W.; Mooney, D.J. Controlled growth factor release from synthetic extracellular matrices. *Nature* **2000**, *408*, 998–1000. [CrossRef] [PubMed]
69. Tanihara, M.; Suzuki, Y.; Yamamoto, E.; Noguchi, A.; Mizushima, Y. Sustained release of basic fibroblast growth factor and angiogenesis in a novel covalently crosslinked gel of heparin and alginate. *J. Biomed. Mater. Res.* **2001**, *56*, 216–221. [CrossRef]
70. Oh, S.T.; Kim, W.R.; Kim, S.H.; Chung, Y.C.; Park, J.S. The preparation of polyurethane foam combined with pH-sensitive alginate/bentonite hydrogel for wound dressings. *Fibers Polym.* **2011**, *12*, 159–165. [CrossRef]
71. Catanzano, O.; Straccia, M.C.; Miro, A.; Ungaro, F.; Romano, I.; Mazzarella, G.; Santagata, G.; Quaglia, F.; Laurienzo, P.; Malinconico, M. Spray-by-spray in situ cross-linking alginate hydrogels delivering a tea tree oil microemulsion. *Eur. J. Pharm. Sci.* **2015**, *66*, 20–28. [CrossRef] [PubMed]
72. Babavalian, H.; Latifi, A.M.; Shokrgozar, M.A.; Bonakdar, S.; Mohammadi, S.; Moghaddam, M.M. Analysis of healing effect of alginate sulfate hydrogel dressing containing antimicrobial peptide on wound infection caused by methicillin-resistant Staphylococcus aureus. *Jundishapur J. Microbiol.* **2015**, *8*, e28320. [CrossRef]
73. Popa, E.G.; Gomes, M.E.; Reis, R.L. Cell delivery systems using alginate-carrageenan hydrogel beads and fibers for regenerative medicine applications. *Biomacromolecules* **2011**, *12*, 3952–3961. [CrossRef]
74. Lee, K.W.; Yoon, J.J.; Lee, J.H.; Kim, S.Y.; Jung, H.J.; Kim, S.J.; Joh, J.W.; Lee, H.H.; Lee, D.S.; Lee, S.K. Sustained release of vascular endothelial growth factor from calcium-induced alginate hydrogels reinforced by heparin and chitosan. *Transplant. Proc.* **2004**, *36*, 2464–2465. [CrossRef]
75. Lee, K.Y.; Peters, M.C.; Mooney, D.J. Controlled drug delivery from polymers by mechanical signals. *Adv. Mater.* **2001**, *13*, 837–839. [CrossRef]
76. Drury, J.L.; Mooney, D.J. Hydrogels for tissue engineering: Scaffold design variables and applications. *Biomaterials* **2003**, *24*, 4337–4351. [CrossRef]

77. Shen, Y.; Xu, G.; Huang, H.; Wang, K.; Wang, H.; Lang, M.; Gao, H.; Zhao, S. Sequential Release of Small Extracellular Vesicles from Bilayered Thiolated Alginate/Polyethylene Glycol Diacrylate Hydrogels for Scarless Wound Healing. *ACS Nano* **2021**, *15*, 6352–6368. [CrossRef]
78. Lu, W.; Bao, D.; Ta, F.; Liu, D.; Zhang, D.; Zhang, Z.; Fan, Z. Multifunctional Alginate Hydrogel Protects and Heals Skin Defects in Complex Clinical Situations. *ACS Omega* **2020**, *5*, 17152–17159. [CrossRef]
79. Peretz, S.; Cinteza, O. Removal of some nitrophenol contaminants using alginate gel beads. *Colloids Surf. A Physicochem. Eng. Asp.* **2008**, *319*, 165–172. [CrossRef]
80. Mohamadnia, Z.; Zohuriaan-Mehr, M.J.; Kabiri, K.; Jamshidi, A.; Mobedi, H. Ionically cross-linked carrageenan-alginate hydrogel beads. *J. Biomater. Sci. Polym. Ed.* **2008**, *19*, 47–59. [CrossRef] [PubMed]
81. Al-Hosny, E.A.; Al-Helw, A.R.M.; Al-Dardiri, M.A. Comparative study of in-vitro release and bioavailability of sustained release diclofenac sodium from certain hydrophilic polymers and commercial tablets in beagle dogs. *Pharm. Acta Helv.* **1997**, *72*, 159–164. [CrossRef]
82. Mahdavinia, G.R.; Rahmani, Z.; Karami, S.; Pourjavadi, A. Magnetic/pH-sensitive κ-carrageenan/sodium alginate hydrogel nanocomposite beads: Preparation, swelling behavior, and drug delivery. *J. Biomater. Sci. Polym. Ed.* **2014**, *25*, 1891–1906. [CrossRef]
83. Peters, M.C.; Isenberg, B.C.; Rowley, J.A.; Mooney, D.J. Release from alginate enhances the biological activity of vascular endothelial growth factor. *J. Biomater. Sci. Polym. Ed.* **1998**, *9*, 1267–1278. [CrossRef]
84. Mori, M.; Rossi, S.; Bonferoni, M.C.; Ferrari, F.; Sandri, G.; Riva, F.; Del Fante, C.; Perotti, C.; Caramella, C. Calcium alginate particles for the combined delivery of platelet lysate and vancomycin hydrochloride in chronic skin ulcers. *Int. J. Pharm.* **2014**, *461*, 505–513. [CrossRef]
85. Aderibigbe, B.A.; Buyana, B. Alginate in wound dressings. *Pharmaceutics* **2018**, *10*, 42. [CrossRef]
86. Leung, V.; Hartwell, R.; Elizei, S.S.; Yang, H.; Ghahary, A.; Ko, F. Postelectrospinning modifications for alginate nanofiber-based wound dressings. *J. Biomed. Mater. Res. Part B Appl. Biomater.* **2014**, *102*, 508–515. [CrossRef]
87. Shalumon, K.T.; Anulekha, K.H.; Nair, S.V.; Nair, S.V.; Chennazhi, K.P.; Jayakumar, R. Sodium alginate/poly(vinyl alcohol)/nano ZnO composite nanofibers for antibacterial wound dressings. *Int. J. Biol. Macromol.* **2011**, *49*, 247–254. [CrossRef] [PubMed]
88. Alven, S.; Nqoro, X.; Aderibigbe, B.A. Polymer-based materials loaded with curcumin for wound healing applications. *Polymers* **2020**, *12*, 2286. [CrossRef] [PubMed]
89. Qin, Y. Alginate fibers: An overwiew of the production processes and applications in wound management. *Polym. Int.* **2008**, *57*, 171–180. [CrossRef]
90. Liao, I.C.; Wan, A.C.A.; Yim, E.K.F.; Leong, K.W. Controlled release from fibers of polyelectrolyte complexes. *J. Control. Release* **2005**, *104*, 347–358. [CrossRef] [PubMed]
91. Konwarh, R.; Misra, M.; Mohanty, A.K.; Karak, N. Diameter-tuning of electrospun cellulose acetate fibers: A Box-Behnken design (BBD) study. *Carbohydr. Polym.* **2013**, *92*, 1100–1106. [CrossRef]
92. Ågren, M.S. *Wound Healing Biomaterials Volume 2: Functional Biomaterials*; Elsevier: London, UK, 2016; Volume 2, ISBN 9780081006061.
93. Park, S.A.; Park, K.E.; Kim, W.D. Preparation of Sodium Alginate/Poly(ethylene oxide) Blend Nanofibers with Lecithin. *Macromol. Res.* **2010**, *18*, 891–896. [CrossRef]
94. Norouzi, M.; Boroujeni, S.M.; Omidvarkordshouli, N.; Soleimani, M. Advances in Skin Regeneration: Application of Electrospun Scaffolds. *Adv. Healthc. Mater.* **2015**, *4*, 1114–1133. [CrossRef]
95. Kataria, K.; Gupta, A.; Rath, G.; Mathur, R.B.; Dhakate, S.R. In vivo wound healing performance of drug loaded electrospun composite nanofibers transdermal patch. *Int. J. Pharm.* **2014**, *469*, 102–110. [CrossRef]
96. Jeong, S.I.; Jeon, O.; Krebs, M.D.; Hill, M.C.; Alsberg, E. Biodegradable photo-crosslinked alginate nanofibre scaffolds with tuneable physical properties, cell adhesivity and growth factor release. *Eur. Cells Mater.* **2013**, *24*, 331–343. [CrossRef]
97. Watthanaphanit, A.; Supaphol, P.; Tamura, H.; Tokura, S.; Rujiravanit, R. Fabrication, Structure, and Properties of Chitin Whisker-Reinforced Alginate Nanocomposite Fibers. *J. Appl. Polym. Sci.* **2008**, *110*, 890–899. [CrossRef]
98. Mogoşanu, G.D.; Grumezescu, A.M. Natural and synthetic polymers for wounds and burns dressing. *Int. J. Pharm.* **2014**, *463*, 127–136. [CrossRef] [PubMed]
99. Agren, M. Zinc in Wound repair. *Arch. Derm.* **1999**, *135*, 1273–1274. [CrossRef] [PubMed]
100. Pielesz, A.; Machnicka, A.; Sarna, E. Antibacterial activity and scanning electron microscopy (SEM) examination of alginate-based films and wound dressings. *Ecol. Chem. Eng. S* **2011**, *18*, 197–210.
101. Tamura, H.; Tsuruta, Y.; Tokura, S. Preparation of chitosan-coated alginate filament. *Mater. Sci. Eng. C* **2002**, *20*, 143–147. [CrossRef]
102. Neibert, K.; Gopishetty, V.; Grigoryev, A.; Tokarev, I.; Al-Hajaj, N.; Vorstenbosch, J.; Philip, A.; Minko, S.; Maysinger, D. Wound-healing with mechanically robust and biodegradable hydrogel fibers loaded with silver nanoparticles. *Adv. Healthc. Mater.* **2012**, *1*, 621–630. [CrossRef] [PubMed]
103. Kibungu, C.; Kondiah, P.P.D.; Kumar, P.; Choonara, Y.E. This Review Recent Advances in Chitosan and Alginate-Based Hydrogels for Wound Healing Application. *Front. Mater.* **2021**, *8*, 1960. [CrossRef]
104. Gilmartin, D.J.; Alexaline, M.M.; Thrasivoulou, C.; Phillips, A.R.J.; Jayasinghe, S.N.; Becker, D.L. Integration of scaffolds into full-thickness skin wounds: The connexin response. *Adv. Healthc. Mater.* **2013**, *2*, 1151–1160. [CrossRef]

105. Montaser, A.S.; Abdel-Mohsen, A.M.; Ramadan, M.A.; Sleem, A.A.; Sahffie, N.M.; Jancar, J.; Hebeish, A. Preparation and characterization of alginate/silver/nicotinamide nanocomposites for treating diabetic wounds. *Int. J. Biol. Macromol.* **2016**, *92*, 739–747. [CrossRef]
106. Tsao, C.T.; Leung, M.; Chang, J.Y.-F.; Zhang, M. A simple material model to generate epidermal and dermal layers in vitro for skin regeneration. *J. Mater. Chem. B* **2014**, *2*, 5256–5264. [CrossRef]
107. Zhang, H.; Cheng, J.; Ao, Q. Preparation of alginate-based biomaterials and their applications in biomedicine. *Mar. Drugs* **2021**, *19*, 264. [CrossRef]
108. Kelso, M. *The Importance of Acidic pH on Wound Healing the Importance of Acidic pH on Wound Healing—Why All the (pH)uss about Microenvironments?* Wound Care Advisor: Doylestown, PA, USA, 2018; Available online: http://woundcareadvisor.com/wp-content/uploads/2018/09/Why-All-the-pHuss-About-Microenvironments.pdf (accessed on 31 May 2019).
109. Martinotti, S.; Calabrese, G.; Ranzato, E. Honey and Wound Healing: New Solutions from an Old Remedy. In *Wound Healing: Cellular Mechanisms, Alternative Therapies and Clinical Outcomes*; Nova Science Publishers, Inc.: London, UK, 2015; pp. 43–48. ISBN 9781634634755.
110. Ono, S.; Imai, R.; Ida, Y.; Shibata, D.; Komiya, T.; Matsumura, H. Increased wound pH as an indicator of local wound infection in second degree burns. *Burns* **2015**, *41*, 820–824. [CrossRef]
111. Pawar, H.V.; Boateng, J.S.; Ayensu, I.; Tetteh, J. Multifunctional medicated lyophilised wafer dressing for effective chronic wound healing. *J. Pharm. Sci.* **2014**, *103*, 1720–1733. [CrossRef]
112. Tamayol, A.; Akbari, M.; Zilberman, Y.; Comotto, M.; Lesha, E.; Serex, L.; Bagherifard, S.; Chen, Y.; Fu, G.; Ameri, S.K.; et al. Flexible pH-Sensing Hydrogel Fibers for Epidermal Applications. *Adv. Healthc. Mater.* **2016**, *5*, 711–719. [CrossRef] [PubMed]
113. Venugopal, V. *Marine Products for Healthcare: Functional and Bioactive Nutraceutical Compounds from the Ocean*; CRC Press Taylor & Francis Group: Boca Raton, FL, USA, 2009; ISBN 978-1-4200-5263-3.
114. Hrynyk, M.; Martins-Green, M.; Barron, A.E.; Neufeld, R.J. Alginate-PEG sponge architecture and role in the design of insulin release dressings. *Biomacromolecules* **2012**, *13*, 1478–1485. [CrossRef] [PubMed]
115. Rabbany, S.Y.; Pastore, J.; Yamamoto, M.; Miller, T.; Rafii, S.; Aras, R.; Penn, M. Continuous delivery of stromal cell-derived factor-1 from alginate scaffolds accelerates wound healing. *Cell Transplant.* **2010**, *19*, 399–408. [CrossRef] [PubMed]
116. Tapia, C.; Escobar, Z.; Costa, E.; Sapag-Hagar, J.; Valenzuela, F.; Basualto, C.; Gai, M.N.; Yazdani-Pedram, M. Comparative studies on polyelectrolyte complexes and mixtures of chitosan-alginate and chitosan-carrageenan as prolonged diltiazem clorhydrate release systems. *Eur. J. Pharm. Biopharm.* **2004**, *57*, 65–75. [CrossRef]
117. White, R.; Cowan, T.; Glover, D. Supporting evidence-based practice: A clinical review of TLC technology. *J. Wound Care* **2011**, *1*, 1–36.
118. O'Donoghue, J.M.; O'Sullivan, S.T.; O'Shaughnessy, M.; O'Connor, T.P.F. Effects of a silicone-coated polyamide net dressing and calcium alginate on the healing of split skin graft donor sites: A prospective randomised trial. *Acta Chir. Plast.* **2000**, *42*, 3–6.
119. Mitra, T.; Sailakshmi, G.; Gnanamani, A.; Raja, S.T.K.; Thiruselvi, T.; Gowri, V.M.; Selvaraj, N.V.; Ramesh, G.; Mandal, A.B. Preparation and characterization of a thermostable and biodegradable biopolymers using natural cross-linker. *Int. J. Biol. Macromol.* **2011**, *48*, 276–285. [CrossRef] [PubMed]
120. Keshaw, H.; Forbes, A.; Day, R.M. Release of angiogenic growth factors from cells encapsulated in alginate beads with bioactive glass. *Biomaterials* **2005**, *26*, 4171–4179. [CrossRef] [PubMed]
121. Choi, Y.S.; Lee, S.B.; Hong, S.R.; Lee, Y.M.; Song, K.W.; Park, M.H. Studies on gelatin-based sponges. Part III: A comparative study of cross-linked gelatin/alginate, gelatin/hyaluronate and chitosan/hyaluronate sponges and their application as a wound dressing in full-thickness skin defect of rat. *J. Mater. Sci. Mater. Med.* **2001**, *12*, 67–73. [CrossRef]
122. Roh, D.H.; Kang, S.Y.; Kim, J.Y.; Kwon, Y.B.; Hae, Y.K.; Lee, K.G.; Park, Y.H.; Baek, R.M.; Heo, C.Y.; Choe, J.; et al. Wound healing effect of silk fibroin/alginate-blended sponge in full thickness skin defect of rat. *J. Mater. Sci. Mater. Med.* **2006**, *17*, 547–552. [CrossRef] [PubMed]
123. Kim, H.J.; Lee, H.C.; Oh, J.S.; Shin, B.A.; Oh, C.S.; Park, R.D.; Yang, K.S.; Cho, C.S. Polyelectrolyte complex composed of chitosan and sodium alginate for wound dressing application. *J. Biomater. Sci. Polym. Ed.* **1999**, *10*, 543–556. [CrossRef]
124. Lira, A.A.M.; Rossetti, F.C.; Nanclares, D.M.A.; Neto, A.F.; Bentley, M.V.L.B.; Marchetti, J.M. Preparation and characterization of chitosan-treated alginate microparticles incorporating all-trans retinoic acid. *J. Microencapsul.* **2009**, *26*, 243–250. [CrossRef]
125. Elçin, Y.M.; Dixit, V.; Gitnick, G. Extensive in vivo angiogenesis following controlled release of human vascular endothelial cell growth factor: Implications for tissue engineering and wound healing. *Artif. Organs* **2001**, *25*, 558–565. [CrossRef]
126. Huizhou Foryou Medical Devices Co., Ltd. Luofucon Extra Silver Alginate Dressing (Rx Only)/Luofucon Antibacterial Alginate Wound Dressing (OTC) 2018. Available online: https://www.accessdata.fda.gov/cdrh_docs/pdf17/K172554.pdf (accessed on 31 May 2021).
127. Luofucon PHMB Alginate Dressing (Rx Use) Premarket Notification. Available online: https://www.accessdata.fda.gov/scripts/cdrh/cfdocs/cfpmn/pmn.cfm?ID=K201016 (accessed on 31 May 2021).
128. Avino, A.; Cozma, C.-N.; Balcangiu-Stroescu, A.-E.; Tanasescu, M.-D.; Balan, D.G.; Timofte, D.; Stoicescu, S.M.; Hariga, C.-S.; Ionescu, D. Our Experience in Skin Grafting and Silver Dressing for Venous Leg Ulcers. *Rev. Chim.* **2019**, *70*, 742–744. [CrossRef]

129. Rashaan, Z.M.; Krijnen, P.; van den Akker- van Marle, M.E.; van Baar, M.E.; Vloemans, A.F.P.; Dokter, J.; Tempelman, F.R.H.; van der Vlies, C.H.; Breederveld, R.S. Clinical effectiveness, quality of life and cost-effectiveness of Flaminal® versus Flamazine® in the treatment of partial thickness burns: Study protocol for a randomized controlled trial. *Trials* **2016**, *17*, 122. [CrossRef] [PubMed]
130. Rashaan, Z.M.; Krijnen, P.; Kwa, K.A.A.; van der Vlies, C.H.; Schipper, I.B.; Breederveld, R.S. Flaminal® versus Flamazine® in the treatment of partial thickness burns: A randomized controlled trial on clinical effectiveness and scar quality (FLAM study). *Wound Repair Regen.* **2019**, *27*, 257–267. [CrossRef] [PubMed]
131. Porter, M.; Kelly, J. Pressure Ulcer Treatment in a Patient with Spina Bifida. *Nurs. Stand.* **2014**, *28*, 60–69. [CrossRef]
132. Vivcharenko, V.; Przekora, A. Modifications of wound dressings with bioactive agents to achieve improved pro-healing properties. *Appl. Sci.* **2021**, *11*, 4114. [CrossRef]
133. Rafter, L.; Reynolds, T.; Collier, M.; Rafter, M.; West, M. A clinical evaluation of Algivon® Plus manuka honey dressings for chronic wounds. *Wounds UK* **2017**, *13*, 132–140.
134. Parker, J. Debridement of Chronic Leg Ulcers with Algivon. 2012. Available online: https://nl.advancismedical.com/uploads/files/documents/resources/UK/Debridement%20of%20chronic%20leg%20ulcers%20Algivon-%20Jane%20Parker.pdf (accessed on 28 August 2018).
135. Activon® Manuka Honey. Available online: http://www.advancis.co.uk/uploads/files/files/ActivonWoundDressingGuide2015-A5V3.pdf (accessed on 27 August 2018).
136. Algivon®—Alginate Dressing Impregnated with 100% Manuka Honey. Available online: http://www.advancis.co.uk/uploads/files/documents/resources/UK/AlgivonFactsheet.pdf (accessed on 27 August 2018).
137. Preston, G. The Use of Activon® Tulle on a Venous Ulcer. Available online: https://uk.advancismedical.com/uploads/files/documents/resources/UK/Use%20of%20Activon%20Tulle%20on%20a%20venous%20ulcer(1).pdf (accessed on 28 August 2018).
138. Activon® Tulle. Available online: http://www.advancis.co.uk/uploads/files/documents/resources/UK/ActivonTulle.pdf (accessed on 27 August 2018).
139. Activon Tulle—Activon—Manuka Honey Dressings. Available online: http://www.advancis.co.uk/products/activon-manuka-honey/activon-tulle (accessed on 27 August 2018).
140. Carella, S.; Maruccia, M.; Fino, P.; Onesti, M.G. An atypical case of Henoch-Shönlein purpura in a young patient: Treatment of the skin lesions with hyaluronic acid-based dressings. *In Vivo* **2013**, *27*, 147–152. [PubMed]
141. Clark, R.; Bradbury, S. SILVERCEL® Non-Adherent made easy. *Wounds Int.* **2010**, *1*, 1–6.
142. Rego, A. ALGS6 Ag Alginate Wound Dressing & AQUACEL Ag EXTRA Hydrofiber Dressing with Silver and Strengthening Fiber 2017. Available online: https://www.accessdata.fda.gov/cdrh_docs/pdf17/K172570.pdf (accessed on 29 August 2018).
143. Scherr, G.H. Silver Alginate Foam Dressing: Silversite or Calgitrol 2006. pp. 202–211. Available online: https://www.accessdata.fda.gov/cdrh_docs/pdf4/K041268.pdf (accessed on 29 August 2018).
144. Bhende, S.; Rothenburger, S. In Vitro Antimicrobial Effectiveness of 5 Catheter Insertion-Site Dressings. *J. Assoc. Vasc. Access* **2007**, *12*, 227–231. [CrossRef]
145. Ullman, A.; Cooke, M.; Rickard, C. Examining the role of securement and dressing products to prevent central venous access device failure: A narrative review. *J. Assoc. Vasc. Access* **2015**, *20*, 99–110. [CrossRef]
146. Donaghue, V.; Chrzan, J.; Rosenblum, B.; Giurini, J.; Habershaw, M.; Veves, A. Evaluation of a collagen-alginate wound dressing in the management of diabetic foot ulcers. *Adv. Wound Care* **1998**, *11*, 114–119. [PubMed]
147. Sussman, C.; Bates-Jensen, B. *Wound Care—A Collaborative Practice Manual for Health Professionals*, 4th ed.; Sussman, C., Bates-Jensen, B.M., Eds.; Wolters Kluwer Health/Lippincott Williams & Wilkins: Baltimore, MD, USA; Philadelphia, PA, USA, 2012; Volume 3, ISBN 9788578110796.
148. White, R. Flaminal: A novel approach to wound bioburden control. *Wounds UK* **2006**, *2*, 64–69.
149. Park, S.O.; Han, J.; Minn, K.W.; Jin, U.S. Prevention of capsular contracture with Guardix-SG® after silicone implant insertion. *Aesthetic Plast. Surg.* **2013**, *37*, 543–548. [CrossRef]
150. Sohn, E.J.; Ahn, H.B.; Roh, M.S.; Ryu, W.Y.; Kwon, Y.H. Efficacy of temperature-sensitive guardix-sg for adhesiolysis in experimentally induced eyelid adhesion in rabbits. *Ophthal. Plast. Reconstr. Surg.* **2013**, *29*, 458–463. [CrossRef]
151. Kaltostat—Product Sheet 2011. Available online: https://marketingworld.convatec.com/MarketPortCore/MediaFile/DownloadByApplication?applicationToken=dc038e44b0b0ee4d8616f7b6880b24551bfecf237645a04fb5b76ab792a36858&itemId=82f0feec-e798-41e6-8f81-e16dfd5f8757&mediaFileId=c4dca46b-d305-489c-b2cc-1b74979e08 (accessed on 30 August 2018).
152. Boateng, J.S.; Matthews, K.H.; Stevens, H.N.E.; Eccleston, G.M. Wound healing dressings and drug delivery systems: A review. *J. Pharm. Sci.* **2008**, *97*, 2892–2923. [CrossRef]
153. Caló, E.; Khutoryanskiy, V.V. Biomedical applications of hydrogels: A review of patents and commercial products. *Eur. Polym. J.* **2015**, *65*, 252–267. [CrossRef]
154. Fonder, M.A.; Lazarus, G.S.; Cowan, D.A.; Aronson-Cook, B.; Kohli, A.R.; Mamelak, A.J. Treating the chronic wound: A practical approach to the care of nonhealing wounds and wound care dressings. *J. Am. Acad. Dermatol.* **2008**, *58*, 185–206. [CrossRef] [PubMed]
155. Bale, S.; Baker, N.; Crook, H.; Rayman, A.; Rayman, G.; Harding, K.G. Exploring the use of an alginate dressing for diabetic foot ulcers. *J. Wound Care* **2001**, *10*, 81–84. [CrossRef] [PubMed]

156. Ausili, E.; Paolucci, V.; Triarico, S.; Maestrini, C.; Murolo, D.; Focarelli, B.; Rendeli, C. Treatment of pressure sores in spina bifida patients with calcium alginate and foam dressings. *Eur. Rev. Med. Pharmacol. Sci.* **2013**, *17*, 1642–1647.
157. Kammerlander, G.; Afarideh, R.; Baumgartner, A.; Berger, M.; Fischelmayer, K.; Hirschberger, G.; Hangler, W.; Huber, A.; Kramml, M.; Locherer, E.; et al. Silvercel: Level two—Case studies. Clinical experiences of using a silver hydroalginate dressing in Austria, Switzerland & Germany. *J. Wound Care* **2008**, *17*, 384–388. [PubMed]
158. Meaume, S.; Vallet, D.; Nguyen Morere, M.; Téot, L. Silvercel: Level one—RCT Study Evaluation of a silver-releasing hydroalginate dressing in chronic wounds with signs of local infection. *J. Wound Care* **2005**, *14*, 411–419. [CrossRef]
159. Bell, A.; Hart, J. Silvercel: Level three—In vivo studies. Evaluation of two absorbent silver dressings in a porcine partial-thickness excisional wound model. *J. Wound Care* **2007**, *16*, 445–453. [CrossRef]
160. Edwards, J. Use of SILVERCEL® NON-ADHERENT on burn wounds: A case series. *Wounds UK* **2013**, *9*, 81–84.
161. Silvercel Guidelines. Available online: www.woundsinternational.com/uploads/resources/d426e9e2f7575b30a7a42c5f5bbdb82a.pdf (accessed on 27 August 2018).
162. Gray, D. Silvercel™ non-adherent dressing: Taking the pain out of antimicrobial use. *Wounds UK* **2009**, *5*, 118–120.
163. Wiegand, C.; Heinze, T.; Hipler, U.C. Comparative in vitro study on cytotoxicity, antimicrobial activity, and binding capacity for pathophysiological factors in chronic wounds of alginate and silver-containing alginate. *Wound Repair Regen.* **2009**, *17*, 511–521. [CrossRef]
164. Boonkaew, B.; Barber, P.M.; Rengpipat, S.; Supaphol, P.; Kempf, M.; He, J.; John, V.T.; Cuttle, L. Development and characterization of a novel, antimicrobial, sterile hydrogel dressing for burn wounds: Single-step production with gamma irradiation creates silver nanoparticles and radical polymerization. *J. Pharm. Sci.* **2014**, *103*, 3244–3253. [CrossRef]

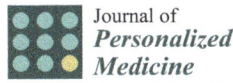 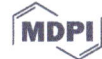

Article

Unconventional Therapy with IgY in a Psoriatic Mouse Model Targeting Gut Microbiome

Mihaela Surcel [1], Adriana Munteanu [1,2], Gheorghita Isvoranu [3], Alef Ibram [4], Constantin Caruntu [5], Carolina Constantin [1,6] and Monica Neagu [1,2,6,*]

1. Immunology Department, "Victor Babes" National Institute of Pathology, 99-101 Spl. Independentei, 050096 Bucharest, Romania; msurcel2002@yahoo.com (M.S.); iadinuta@yahoo.com (A.M.); caroconstantin@gmail.com (C.C.)
2. Faculty of Biology, Doctoral School of Biology, University of Bucharest, 91-95 Spl. Independentei, 030018 Bucharest, Romania
3. Animal Husbandry, "Victor Babes" National Institute of Pathology, 99-101 Spl. Independentei, 050096 Bucharest, Romania; gina_isvoranu@yahoo.com
4. Research Laboratory, Romvac Company SA, 077190 Voluntari, Romania; mustafa_alef@yahoo.com
5. Department of Physiology, "Carol Davila" University of Pharmacy and Medicine, 37 Dionisie Lupu Street, 020021 Bucharest, Romania; costin.caruntu@gmail.com
6. Department of Pathology, Colentina University Hospital, 020125 Bucharest, Romania
* Correspondence: neagu.monica@gmail.com

Abstract: Psoriasis has a multifactorial pathogenesis and recently it was shown that alterations in the skin and intestinal microbiome are involved in the pathogenesis of psoriasis. Therefore, microbiome restoration becomes a promising preventive/therapy strategy in psoriasis. In our pre-clinical study design using a mice model of induced psoriatic dermatitis (Ps) we have tested the proof-of-concept that IgY raised against pathological human bacteria resistant to antibiotics can alleviate psoriatic lesions and restore deregulated immune cell parameters. Besides clinical evaluation of the mice and histology of the developed psoriatic lesions, cellular immune parameters were monitored. Immune cells populations/subpopulations from peripheral blood and spleen cell suspensions that follow the clinical improvement were assessed using flow cytometry. We have quantified T lymphocytes (CD3ε^+) with T-helper (CD4$^+$CD8$^-$) and T-suppressor/cytotoxic (CD8a$^+$CD4$^-$) subsets, B lymphocytes (CD3ε^-CD19$^+$) and NK cells (CD3ε^-NK1.1$^+$). Improved clinical evolution of the induced Ps along with the restoration of immune cells parameters were obtained when orally IgY was administered. We pin-point that IgY specific compound can be used as a possible pre-biotic-like alternative adjuvant in psoriasis.

Keywords: IgY; psoriatic dermatitis; imiquimod; inflammation; C57 BL/6 mice

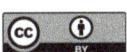

1. Introduction

Psoriasis (Ps) is a complex and heterogeneous disease that affects not only the skin of the patients but echoes also on several other organs [1]. Recognized as a chronic autoimmune inflammatory disease, mediated mainly by T cells, Ps has important systemic manifestation [2], being frequently associated with psychological, metabolic, arthritic and cardiovascular comorbidities. Ps associated pathologies can lead to increased mortality and alters the clinical management of the patients. Ps affects 0.5–1% of children and in the world's population the prevalence raises around 2–3%. Prevalence of Ps varies depending on age, sex, geography, ethnicity, genetic and environmental factors [3]. Although it can occur at any age, the most common cases are reported before the age of 35, an age range that affects highly active individuals [4].

The causes of Ps have not yet been fully elucidated. Besides genetic predisposition and environmental factors, an inefficient immune system is highly involved in Ps onset. Among the triggers or aggravating factors of Ps we can mention air pollutants and exposure to sunlight, prolonged exposure to UV radiation [5], administration of certain drugs (β-blockers, lithium) [6], smoking [7], obesity [8] and alcohol consumption [9]. Streptococcal infections, involved in both acute and chronic forms of the disease [10] and mental stress are also factors that have with critical roles in the initiation, development and exacerbation of Ps [11].

The assessment of Ps severity is mainly based on clinical indicators [12], but the golden standard remains the PASI score (Psoriasis Area Severity Index) [13], which combines the severity (erythema, scaling, induration) and the percentage of affected area.

19In Ps pathogenesis are involved both innate (NK cells, macrophages, dendritic cells) and adaptive immune cells (T lymphocytes), as well as non-immune cells (keratinocytes), their interactions being mediated by pro-inflammatory cytokines/chemokines that maintain the chronic inflammatory state [14,15]. Among the biological therapies currently available, TNF-α inhibitors [16–18], IL-23 inhibitors [19–22], IL-17 inhibitors [23–25] are the ones that entered the standard care of Ps. New treatments that address immune pathways and are currently undergoing clinical trials include RORγt inhibitors [26], IL-36 Receptor antagonist [27], Janus Kinase (JAK) inhibitors [28], TYK2/JAK1 inhibitor [29], Rho-Associated Kinase (ROCK2) inhibitor [30], Sphingosine-1-Phosphate (S1P) agonist [31] and aryl hydrocarbon receptor (AhR) agonists [32]. All current therapies display adverse effects, such as nasopharyngitis, upper respiratory tract infections, fatigue, headache and even tuberculosis, therefore adjuvant therapies that can aid the standard ones are searched.

Immunoglobulin Y (IgY) has important characteristics like high tolerability, being essentially a component of the human diet. Hence, it can be used even in subjects that are allergic to egg components because the purified IgY does not contain allergenic ovalbumin [33]. Since IgY cannot link to the Fc receptors or to the complement system expressed by the mammalian cells, administering IgY does not trigger adverse effects [34,35]. A report published more than 20 years ago has shown in animal models that purified IgY does not trigger an IgE response, therefore no allergic reaction [36]. Moreover, the systemic administration of IgY has shown that this Ig can have anti-viral and/or anti-bacterial potency [37]. IgY can neutralize bacteria and viruses, hindering their replication [38,39] therefore passive immunization can be used in humans because it will rapidly give a positive clinical response. In the last decade, IgY has gained an increased scientific attention due to its specific characteristic and biological potency [40].

In Ps, association of bacterial strains residing in the digestive tract of patients was reported, staring from the incidence of *H. pylori* [41], of *Candida albicans* [42] and ending with the major gut dysbiosis registered in these patients, dysbiosis that can influence the skin microbiota favoring thus flare-up of the psoriatic events [43].

Our previously published work has shown that in psoriatic dermatitis murine models, although involving just a psoriatic-like skin lesion, significant alterations of lymphocytes percentages and important changes in NK cell phenotype, in both peripheral blood and spleen were found [43,44]. Considering all the accumulated data, we have initiated in the current study a Ps experimental model in which an adjuvant therapy using oral IgY developed against several pathogenic bacteria to evaluate the potency to alleviate the psoriatic lesions and to restore the immune-related mechanisms. Imiquimod murine model (IMQ-1-isobutyl-1H-imidazo[4,5-c]quinolin-4-amine) was used to develop the experimental psoriatic dermatitis and further evaluate if the orally given IgY treatment would clinically improve the experimental Ps and would restore the cellular immune parameters.

2. Materials and Methods

2.1. Immunoglobulin Y

IgY was isolated from the yolk of hyperimmune eggs laid by chickens immunized with human pathogenic bacteria that are antibiotic-resistant, namely groups of pathogens with a high rate of antibiotic resistance responsible for the majority of nosocomial infections. IgY was obtained according to the methodology described in the patent [45]. The obtained IgY is an original product of the ROMVAC Company and is part of the IMUNOINSTANT brand having a European trademark (EUIPO). IgY that was used is a mix of antibodies raised against the following antibiotic-resistant strains Salmonella spp (enteritidis, typhimurium), Streptococcus pneumoniae, Clostridium difficile, Staphylococcus aureus, Pseudomonas aeruginosa, Enterococcus faecalis, Klebsiella pneumoniae, Acinetobacter baumannii, Escherichia coli [46].

2.2. Animal Model

C57 BL/6 mice (Jackson Laboratory, Bar Harbor, ME), males and females, aged 10–11 weeks, were provided by the Animal Husbandry from Victor Babeș National Institute of Pathology. The animals were kept in an open cage system, in optimal conditions (temperature $22 \pm 2\ °C$, humidity $55 \pm 10\%$, artificial ventilation, 12/12-light/dark cycle) and fed (standard granulated fodder) and watered (filtered and sterilized water) *ad libitum*. The mice were monitored daily. The experiments were conducted in accordance with recognized principles of laboratory animal care in the framework of EU Directive 2010/63/EU [45] and the study was comprised in a research project that was approved by the Ethics Committee from Victor Babeș Institute (Approval no 88/20 January 2021) and National Sanitary Veterinary and Food Safety Authority (Approval no 598/8 February 2021).

The experimental murine model of psoriatic dermatitis was performed according to the protocols previously described [43,44,47].

Four groups of C57 BL/6 mice, were constituted as follows:
- Ps group (8 mice-1:1 sex ratio, with a mean weight 20.4 ± 2.9 g) received a daily topical dose of 62.5 mg IMQ-based cream (5% Aldara Cream, Meda AB Sweden) on the shaved back region, for 6 consecutive days. The daily dose contains 3.125 mg of active compound. The mice that were designed for clinical and immunological evaluation were sacrificed on day 7 of the experiment;
- IgY-treated Ps group (12 mice-1:1 sex ratio, with a mean weight 21.33 ± 2.14 g) with induced psoriatic dermatitis as described above, received (starting with day 7) a gavage dose of 37.5 µg IgY, for 5 consecutive days; the dose matches the dose of IgY given to a human adult (g/kg) according to a study case [48]. Mice were sacrificed on day 20, the day on which it was macroscopically assessed that experimental psoriatic dermatitis was remitted;
- Naturally remitted Ps group (8 mice—1:1 sex ratio, with a mean weight 17.87 ± 0.81 g) with induced psoriatic dermatitis were allowed to heal naturally and were sacrificed on day 22—the day on which the natural remission was assessed macroscopically;
- Control group (8 mice—1:1 sex ratio, with a mean weight 20.26 ± 1.36 g). Healthy mice with no treatment housed and fed in the same room with all the presented experimental groups and subjected to the same manipulation as the IgY-treated group but with sham gavage.

2.3. Scoring Severity of IMQ-Induced Skin Inflammation and Healing Assesment

The severity of IMQ-induced skin inflammation and the progress of the disease, were daily evaluated using three in vivo parameters-erythema, thickening and skin scaling. These parameters were scored daily on a 0–4 scale such as 0—no change, 1—mild change, 2—marked change; 3—significant change, 4—severe change. By summing erythema, thickening and skin scaling daily scores, a modified PASI score was calculated (0–12 scale).

The body weight of the animals was monitored during the experiments (Scientech SL 3100D, Boulder, CO, USA). For the mice from IgY-treated Ps group the body weight was recorded at the beginning of the experiment (day 1), day 7 (beginning of IgY treatment), at the end of IgY treatment (day 12) and before being humanely euthanized—day 20—when it was macroscopically appreciated that the induced psoriasis disappeared. The mice from naturally remitted Ps group were allowed to heal naturally and weighed at the beginning of the experiment (day 1), after IMQ-based cream application (day 7) and before euthanization—day 22—when it was macroscopically appreciated that the effects produced by IMQ-based cream disappeared. The mice from Ps group were weighed at the beginning of the experiment (day 1) and before sacrifice (day 7).

2.4. Sampling of Biological Material and Processing of Samples

At the end of experiments, the animals were anesthetized with ketamine/acepromazine/xylazine cocktail (ketamine 80 mg/kg, Richterpharma ag, Wells, Austria; acepromazine 6 mg/kg, Vetoquinol SA, Lure, France; xylazine 1 mg/kg, Bioveta SA, Czech Republic) for blood, spleen and skin sample collection. Peripheral blood was collected by intra-cardiac puncture in K2-EDTA coated tubes (SARSTEDT AG & CO. KG, Nümbrecht, Germany). Spleens were weighed (Balance AEP-1500A, Adam Equipment Co., Ltd., Kingston, UK) for splenomegaly evaluation and processed in order to isolate the spleen cells. The spleens were collected in 5% FBS RPMI 1640 media (Biochrom AG GmbH, Berlin, Germany), passed through a 70 µm cell strainer (BD Falcon -BD Biosciences, San Jose, CA, USA), cells centrifuged for 5 min at $350 \times g$ (20 °C) and resuspended in RBC Lysis Buffer (BioLegend, San Diego, CA, USA). After 5 min on ice, 10 mL Cell Staining Buffer (BioLegend, San Diego, CA, USA) was added in order to stop the lysis and centrifuged for 5 min at $350 \times g$ (20 °C). The pellet was resuspended twice in Cell Staining Buffer, for a final concentration of 1×10^6 cells/mL. Skin samples were collected and processed (fixed in 10% buffered formalin, embedded in paraffin, sectioned in 5 µm sections) for hematoxylin and eosin (H&E) staining, prior to histopathological evaluation (Olympus BX43 with CellSens Dimension Program, Tokyo, Japan).

2.5. Flow Cytometry Analysis

Lymphocyte immunophenotyping performed from peripheral blood and spleen cell suspension were done for all experimental groups by flow cytometry, using a BD FACSCanto II cytometer (BD Biosciences, San Jose, CA, USA). We have quantified T lymphocytes ($CD3\varepsilon^+$), with T helper ($CD4^+CD8^-$) and T suppressor/cytotoxic ($CD8a^+CD4^-$) subsets, B lymphocytes ($CD3\varepsilon^- CD19^+$), NK cells ($CD3\varepsilon^- NK1.1^+$), and the expression levels of several maturation markers (CD49b, CD27, CD11b, CD43, KLRG1) and activation (CD69, CD28, CD11c, NKp46) markers on NK cells were assessed.

Both types of samples (peripheral blood and spleen cell suspension) were incubated with TruStain fcX (anti-mouse CD16/32, isotype Rat IgG2a, λ) Antibody (BioLegend, San Diego, CA, USA) for 7 min on ice and stained in the dark for 20 min at room temperature with the following monoclonal antibodies conjugated with fluorochromes: 0.5 µL Alexa Fluor 647 anti-mouse CD3ε (clone 145-2C11, isotype Armenian Hamster IgG); 0.5 µL Alexa Fluor 488 anti-mouse CD8a (clone 53–6.7, isotype Rat IgG2a, κ); 1.25 µL PE-Cy7 anti-mouse CD4 (clone GK1.5, isotype Rat IgG2b, κ); 1,25 µL PerCP-Cy5.5 anti-mouse CD19 (clone 6D5, isotype Rat IgG2a, κ); 1,25 µL PE anti-mouse NK1.1 (clone PK136, isotype Mouse IgG2a, κ); 0.5 µL FITC anti-mouse CD3ε (clone 145-2C11, isotype Armenian Hamster IgG); 2.5 µL Brilliant Violet 510 anti-mouse NK1.1 (clone PK136, isotype Mouse IgG2a, κ); 0.6 µL PerCP/Cy5.5 anti-mouse/rat/human CD27 (clone LG.3A10, isotype Armenian Hamster IgG); 0.6 µL APC/Cy7 anti-mouse CD43 (clone RA3-6B2, isotype Rat IgG2a, κ); 1.25 µL PE anti-mouse CD28 (clone 37.51, isotype Syrian Hamster IgG); 2.5 µL PE/Cy7 anti-mouse CD69 (clone H1.2F3, isotype Armenian Hamster IgG); 2.5 µL PE/Cy7 anti-mouse CD335 (NKp46) (clone 29A1.4, isotype Rat IgG2a, κ); 2.5 µL PerCP/Cy5.5 anti-mouse CD11c (clone N418, isotype Armenian Hamster IgG) (all from BioLegend, San Diego, CA, USA); 2.5 µL eFluor 450 anti-mouse CD49b (clone DX5, isotype Rat IgM, κ); 0.3 µL APC anti-mouse CD11b (clone M1/70, isotype Rat IgG2b, κ); 0.6 µL PE anti-mouse KLRG1 (clone 2F1, isotype Syrian Hamster IgG) (all from eBioscience Inc, San Diego, CA, USA). Red blood cells lysis was performed with BD FACS Lysing Solution (BD Biosciences, San Jose, CA, USA) for 10 min in the dark at room temperature, followed by centrifugation for 5 min at $350 \times g$ and two washing steps with Cell Staining Buffer. Flow cytometry analysis was preceded by daily check-up of cytometer performances (BD Cytometer Setup and Tracking Beads Kit, BD Biosciences, San Jose, CA, USA) and compensation of spectral overlaps (UltraComp eBeads, Invitrogen by Thermo Fischer Scientific, San Diego, CA, USA). Unlabeled cells were used as negative control. Data were acquired and analyzed using BD FACSDiva v 6.1 software (BD Biosciences, San Jose, CA, USA).

2.6. Statistical Analysis

The results were expressed as mean values ± SD, and Microsoft Excel (Microsoft, Redmond, CA, USA) was used for data analysis. Student's *t*-test (two-tailed, assuming equal variance) was used to compare the experimental groups, and a *p*-value less than 0.05 was considered statistically significant. T-CD4$^+$ and T-CD8a$^+$ were expressed as percentages of CD3ε^+ lymphocytes (mean values ± SD), B and NK cells as percentages of CD3ε^- lymphocytes (mean values ± SD), and the expressions of maturation and activation markers on NK cells, as percentages of NK1.1$^+$ cells gated from CD3ε^- lymphocytes (mean values ± SD).

3. Results

3.1. IMQ-Based Experimental Murine Model of Psoriatic Dermatitis

The experimental model of psoriatic dermatitis was performed to evaluate the effect of the IgY treatment on Ps-specific skin and systemic lesions. The murine model of psoriatic dermatitis previously described [43,44,47], used IMQ-based cream applied on the back skin area for 6 consecutive days in order to induce an extensive psoriatic-like reaction. Animals were monitored daily, and the severity of skin inflammation induced by applying IMQ-based cream was assessed based on daily scores of erythema, thickening and skin scaling, PASI score, splenomegaly evaluation and histopathological assessment. Erythema, thickening and scaling of the back skin were daily scored on a 0–4 scale (0—no change, 1—mild change, 2—marked change; 3—significant change, 4—severe change) and the evolution of these scores is shown in Figure 1a. Table S1 presents the individual PASI scores for all the animals within the groups.

Starting with day 2, signs of inflammation were visible and increased in intensity until the end of the application. The skin on the back region of the mice began to show signs of erythema, thickening, and scaling that became visible from day 3 of the experiment. As a measure of the disease severity, a modified PASI score (0–12 scale) was calculated daily, by summing erythema, thickening and skin scaling daily scores. The PASI cumulative score had a progressive evolution, reaching high values at the end of the applications (Figure 1b).

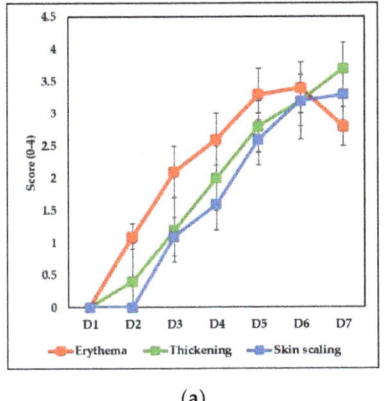

(a)

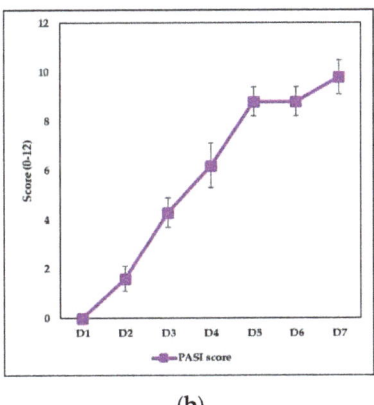

(b)

Figure 1. *Cont.*

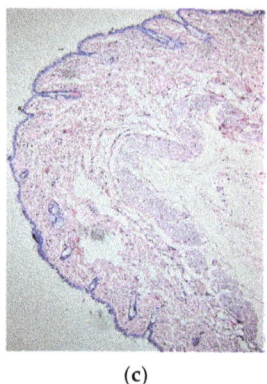 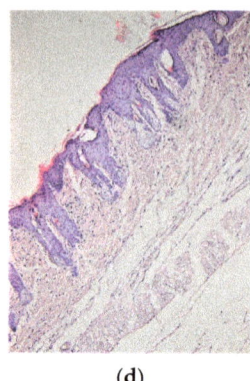

(c) (d)

Figure 1. Evolution of in vivo parameters and histopathological assessment of dorsal skin samples. (**a**) In vivo measurements scores for erythema (0 ± 0; 1.1 ± 0.2; 2.1 ± 0.4; 2.6 ± 0.4; 3.3 ± 0.4; 3.4 ± 0.4; 2.8 ± 0.4), thickening (0 ± 0; 0.4 ± 0.6; 1.2 ± 0.4; 2 ± 0.4; 2.8 ± 0.4; 3.3 ± 0.4; 3.7 ± 0.4) and skin scaling (0 ± 0; 0 ± 0; 1.1 ± 0.3; 1.6 ± 0.4; 2.6 ± 0.4; 3.2 ± 0.5; 3.5 ± 0.3) scores; (**b**) PASI scores (0 ± 0; 1.5 ± 0.6; 4.4 ± 0.6; 6.2 ± 0.8; 8.7 ± 0.6; 8.7 ± 0.6; 9.9 ± 0.7). The results are presented as mean score ± SD; n = 28 (n = number of mice; D = day); (**c**) H&E staining of the back skin samples provided from normal mouse (control group); (**d**) H&E staining of the back skin samples provided from IMQ-induced mouse (Ps group). IMQ-based cream induces hyperkeratosis, parakeratosis, acanthosis and elongation of rete ridges.

Skin inflammation induced by IMQ-based cream was histopathologically assessed. Skin samples harvested from all groups were collected at the end of experiment, fixed in 10% buffered formaldehyde and incorporated into paraffin; the paraffin blocks were sectioned (5 µm thick sections), stained with hematoxylin-eosin and examined by pathologist. Histopathological evaluation revealed hyperkeratosis, parakeratosis, acanthosis and elongation of the red ridges, histopathological features typical for human psoriatic lesions (Figure 1d). None of these features were observed in healthy mice (control group) (Figure 1c). Individual data for the assessment of all histological parameters and individual mice are presented in Table S2 (Supplementary Material).

3.2. IgY Treatment-Induced Changes in Experimental Murine Model of Psoriatic Dermatitis

For naturally remitted Ps group, the mice were allowed to heal naturally and erythema, thickening and skin scaling were daily observed in order to appreciate the day when the effects produced by applying of IMQ-based cream disappeared. The mice were weighed at the beginning of the experiment (day 1), after IMQ-based cream treatment (day 7) and before sacrifice—day 22—when the natural remission of the IMQ-skin effects was noticed.

For IgY-treated Ps group, mice received a dose of IgY by gavage for 5 consecutive days, The evolution of the three in vivo parameters (erythema, thickening and skin scaling) was monitored and we established that the skin healing took place in day 20, 2 days earlier than naturally remitted Ps group. The body weight was recorded at the beginning of the experiment (day 1), day 7 (beginning of IgY treatment), at the end of IgY treatment (day 12) and before sacrifice—day 20—when it was macroscopically appreciated that the IMQ-skin effects disappeared.

Body weight (Figure 2a,b) revealed a decrease after the IMQ topical application (day 7) for both IgY-treated Ps group and naturally remitted Ps group. For the IgY-treated Ps group (Figure 2a) the values decrease until the end of the IgY treatment and at the end of the experiment, for both experimental groups, weight increases were recorded.

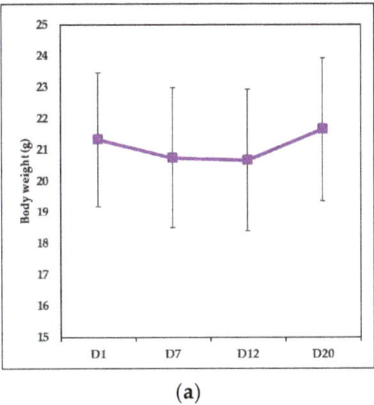
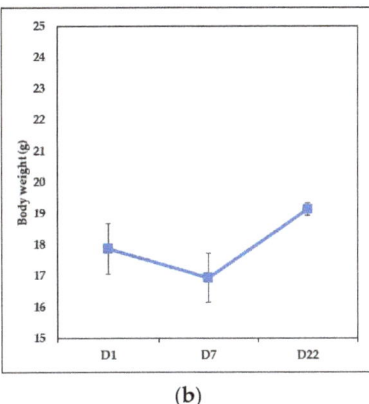

Figure 2. Evolution of the body weight (**a**) Evolution of the body weight for IgY-treated Ps group ($n = 12$)-day 1 (21.33 ± 2.14), day 7 (20.74 ± 2.24), day 12 (20.66 ± 2.27), day 20 (21.65 ± 2.28) (**b**) Evolution of the body weight for naturally remitted Ps group ($n = 8$)-day 1 (17.87 ± 0.81), day 7 (16.93 ± 0.78), day 22 (19.13 ± 0.21). The results are presented as mean ± SD; n = number of mice; D = day.

In order to assess the involvement of the triggered Ps on the secondary immune organs, splenomegaly evaluation was performed. Spleens were weighed separately and the ratio between spleen weight (SW) and body weight (BW) was calculated. Spleen weight was significantly higher in Ps group (0.22 ± 0.02, $p = 2.19 \times 10^{-9}$) as compared to controls (0.08 ± 0.01) (Figure 3e). The measurements also showed that in IMQ-mice, SW/BW ratio is almost 3 times higher than in healthy mice (0.011 ± 0.001 versus 0.0039 ± 0.0002, $p = 2.21 \times 10^{-8}$) (Figure 3f).

The SW/BW parameter was evaluated also for IgY-treated group. As mentioned above, a marked splenomegaly was noticed in IMQ-based experimental model of psoriatic dermatitis, namely spleen weights and SW/BW were about three times higher for Ps group as compared to control group. In the IgY-treated group there is a clear reduction of the splenomegaly. Figure 3a–d presents the macroscopic images of spleens and Figure 3e shows the mean values of spleen weights for all experimental groups.

As a measure of splenomegaly, SW/BW ratio was calculated for all groups and IgY-treated Ps group and naturally remitted Ps group were compared to control and Ps groups (Figure 3f).

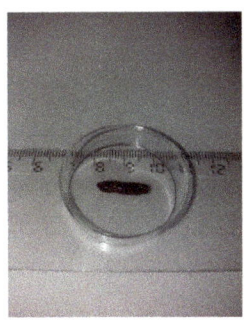
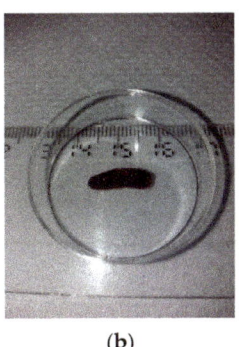
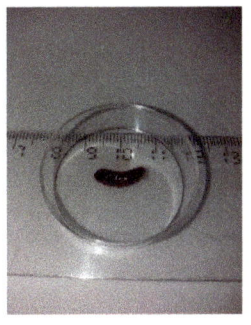
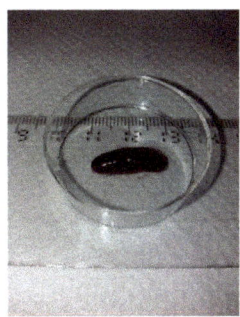

Figure 3. *Cont.*

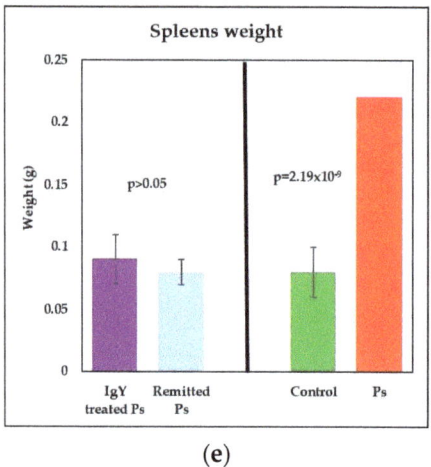
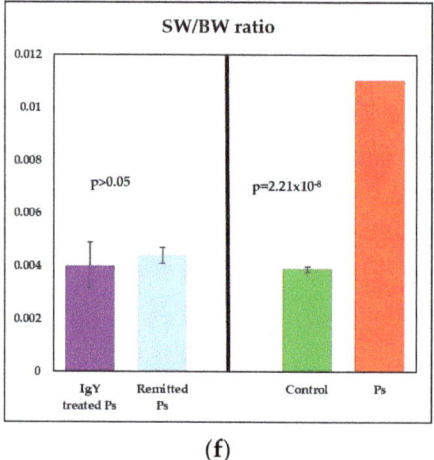

Figure 3. Representative images for the assessment of splenomegaly reduction. Spleens harvested from (**a**) mouse from IgY – treated Ps group; (**b**) mouse naturally remitted Ps group; (**c**) mouse from control group; (**d**) mouse from Ps group; (**e**) The weight of the spleens for IgY – treated Ps group (n = 12) (0.09 ± 0.02) as compared to naturally remitted Ps group (n = 8) (0.08 ± 0.01), control group (n = 8) (0,08 ± 0.01) and Ps group (n = 8) (0.22 ± 0.02); (**f**) SW/BW ratio for IgY-treated Ps group (n = 12) (0.0040 ± 0.0009) as compared to naturally remitted Ps group (n = 8) (0.0044 ± 0.0003), control group (n = 8) (0.0040 ± 0.0009) and Ps group (n = 8) (0.011 ± 0.001). The results are presented as mean ± SD; n = number of mice.

At the end of the experiment, values for both spleen weight and SW/BW ratio after IgY treatment were identical or statistically equivalent to the values recorded for the control group Additionally, there are no statistically significant differences between IgY-treated Ps group and naturally remitted Ps group, for both spleen weight and SW/BW ratio. Thus, the splenomegaly observed after the induction of Ps (respectively, after applying the IMQ-based cream for 6 consecutive days) was completely remitted.

3.3. IgY Treatment-Induced Changes in Lymphocyte Distribution in Peripheral Blood and Spleen Cell Suspensions in Experimental Murine Model of Psoriatic Dermatitis

To evaluate the immune cells populations/subpopulations that follow the clinical improvement of the induced psoriasis lymphocyte immunophenotyping was performed by flow cytometry from both peripheral blood and spleen cell suspensions. For all experimental groups we quantified T lymphocytes (CD3ε^+), with T-helper (CD4$^+$CD8$^-$) and T-suppressor/cytotoxic (CD8a$^+$CD4$^-$) subsets, B lymphocytes (CD3ε^-CD19$^+$) and NK cells (CD3ε^-NK1.1$^+$).

Therefore, a statistically significant lower percentages of T-CD4+ (p = 0.007) and signifi-cantly increased of T-CD8a+ lymphocytes (p = 0.007 vs) were obtained (Figure 4a). As a consequence of the changes observed in T subsets distribution, the T-CD4+/T-CD8+ ratio was decreased in Ps group as compared to control group (p = 0.003) (Figure 5a). Also, a decreased percentage of B lymphocytes (p = 1.1 × 10^{-6}) and a significantly increased of NK1.1+ cells percentages (p = 0.0001) were registered (Figure 6a).

The main changes observed in spleen cell suspensions were statistically significant in Ps group, namely lower percentages of T-CD4$^+$ (p = 0.02) and B lymphocytes (p = 4 × 10^{-7}), (Figures 4b and 6b). T-CD4$^+$/T-CD8$^+$ ratio is decreased in Ps mice as compared to control group but not statistically significant (Figure 5b).

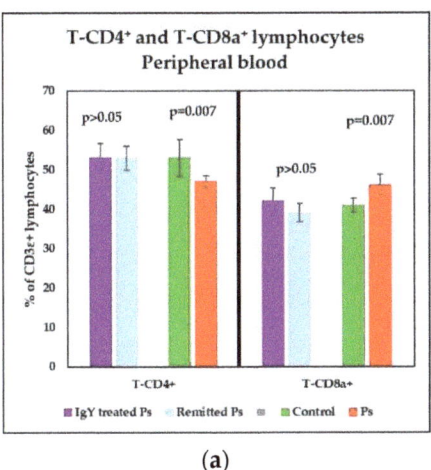
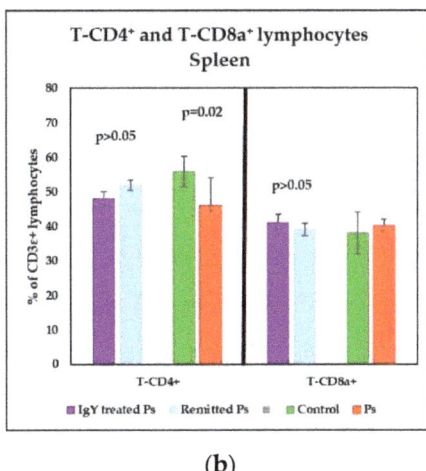

Figure 4. Distribution of T-CD4⁺ and T-CD8a⁺ lymphocytes in peripheral blood and spleen cell suspension. (**a**) Peripheral blood-distribution of T-CD4⁺ and T-CD8a⁺ lymphocytes for IgY-treated Ps group (n = 12) (53 ± 3.6 and 42 ± 3.3) as compared to naturally remitted Ps group (n = 8) (53 ± 3 and 39 ± 2.4), control group (n = 8) (53 ± 4.7 and 41 ± 1.8) and Ps group (n = 8) (47 ± 1.5 and 46 ± 2.8); (**b**) Spleen cell suspension-distribution of T-CD4⁺ and T-CD8a⁺ lymphocytes for IgY-treated Ps group (n = 12) (48 ± 2.2 and 41 ± 2.3) as compared to naturally remitted Ps group (n = 8) (52 ± 1.5 and 39 ± 1.8), control group (n = 8) (56 ± 4.3 and 38 ± 6.1) and Ps group (n = 8) (46 ± 8.1 and 40 ± 1.9). The results (% of CD3ε⁺ lymphocytes) are presented as mean ± SD; n = number of mice).

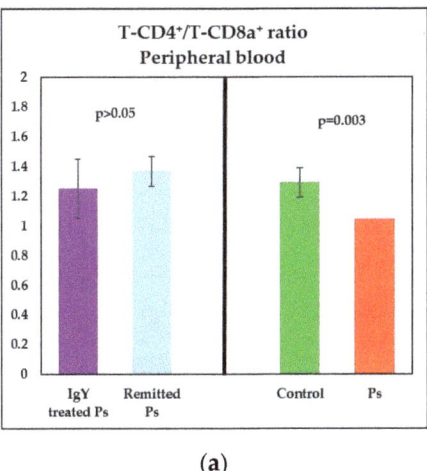
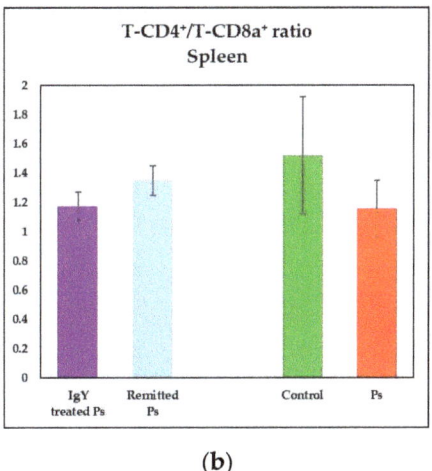

Figure 5. Distribution of T-CD4⁺/T-CD8a⁺ ratio in peripheral blood and spleen cell suspension. (**a**) Peripheral blood-distribution of T-CD4⁺/T-CD8a⁺ ratio for IgY-treated Ps group (n = 12) (1.25 ± 0.2) as compared to naturally remitted Ps group (n = 8) (1.37 ± 0.1), control group (n = 8) (1.29 ± 0.2) and Ps group (n = 8) (1.04 ± 0.1); (**b**) Spleen cell suspension–distribution of T-CD4⁺/T-CD8a⁺ ratio for IgY-treated Ps group (n = 12) (1.17 ± 0.1) as compared to naturally remitted Ps group (n = 8) (1.35 ± 0.1), control group (n = 8) (1.52 ± 0.4) and Ps group (n = 8) (1.15 ± 0.2). The results are presented as mean ± SD; n = number of mice).

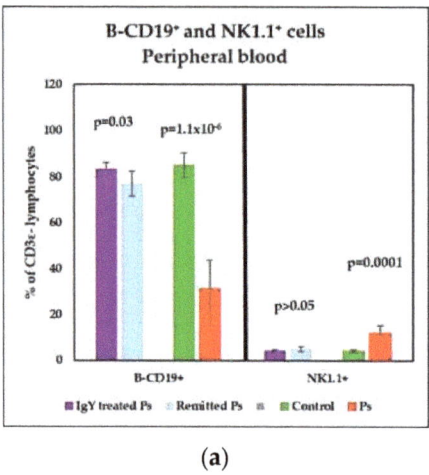
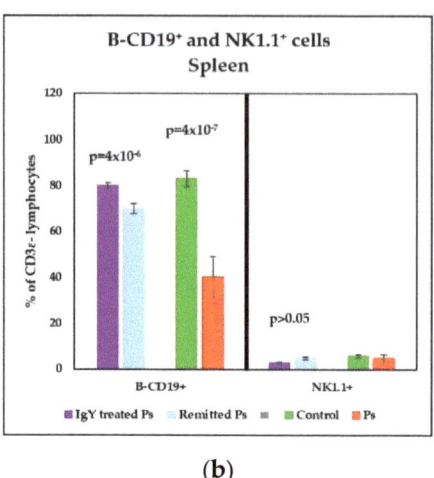

Figure 6. Distribution of B-CD19$^+$ and NK1.1$^+$ cells in peripheral blood and spleen cell suspension. (**a**) Peripheral blood–distribution of B-CD19$^+$ and NK1.1$^+$ cells for IgY-treated Ps group (n = 12) (83 ± 3.2 and 4 ± 0.7) as compared to naturally remitted Ps group (n = 8) (77 ± 5.5 and 5 ± 1.1), control group (n = 8) (85 ± 5.3 and 4 ± 0.7) and Ps group (n = 8) (31 ± 12.8 and 12 ± 3.3); (**b**) Spleen cell suspension–distribution of B-CD19$^+$ and NK1.1$^+$ cells for IgY-treated Ps group (80 ± 1 and 3 ± 0.4) as compared to naturally remitted Ps group (70 ± 2.1 and 5 ± 0.5), control group (83 ± 3.6 and 6 ± 0.8) and Ps group (40 ± 9 and 5 ± 1.8). The results (% of CD3ε^- lymphocytes) are presented as mean ± SD; n = number of mice.

Analysis of T-CD4$^+$ and T-CD8a$^+$ lymphocyte subsets in peripheral blood revealed normalization of mean percentage values of these parameters for both IgY-treated Ps group and naturally remitted Ps group (Figure 4a). There were statistically significant differences between the values of T-CD4$^+$ and T-CD8a$^+$ subsets for Ps group and IgY-treated Ps group (p = 0.002 for T-CD4$^+$ and p = 0.04 for T-CD8a$^+$), and naturally remitted Ps group (p = 0.002 for T-CD4$^+$ and p = 0.006 for T-CD8a$^+$), respectively, comparable to the differences observed between Ps group and controls for the investigated parameters. No statistically significant differences were observed between IgY-treated Ps group and naturally remitted Ps group for these T-subsets. Furthermore, no statistically significant differences were observed between IgY-treated Ps group and control group for T-CD4$^+$ and T-CD8a$^+$ subsets (p > 0.05), thus statistically underlining the normalization of these values after IgY treatment.

Data obtained for T-CD4$^+$ and T-CD8a$^+$ subpopulations in spleen cell suspensions revealed a tendency to normalization for both IgY-treated Ps group and naturally remitted Ps group (Figure 4b). For T-CD8a$^+$ lymphocytes, no statistically significant differences were observed between the IgY-treated Ps group and control group. Although the values of T-CD4$^+$ subset obtained for IgY-treated Ps group were significantly lower than control (p = 0.006), no statistically significant differences were observed between the IgY-treated Ps group and naturally remitted Ps group for T-CD4$^+$ and T-CD8a$^+$ subsets.

Analysis of the T-CD4$^+$/T-CD8a$^+$ ratio in the peripheral blood revealed the normalization of the mean values for both IgY-treated Ps group and naturally remitted Ps group (Figure 5a). There were statistically significant differences between Ps group and naturally remitted Ps groups (p = 0.0003), respectively IgY-treated Ps group (p = 0.01), and no statistically significant differences between control group and IgY-treated Ps group, respectively naturally remitted Ps group. The value of the T-CD4$^+$/T-CD8a$^+$ ratio for IgY-treated group was almost identical to control group (1.25 vs. 1.29).

A tendency of normalization of T-CD4$^+$/T-CD8a$^+$ ratio values was also noticed in spleen cell suspensions for both experimental groups. Although the values obtained for IgY-treated Ps group were significantly lower than control (p = 0.04), no statistically significant differences were observed between the IgY-treated Ps group and naturally remitted Ps group for T-CD4$^+$/T-CD8a$^+$ ratio.

Analysis of B-CD19$^+$ and NK1.1$^+$ cells in peripheral blood revealed normalization of these parameters for both IgY-treated Ps group and naturally remitted Ps group (Figure 6a). Statistically significant differences were observed between the Ps group and the naturally remitted Ps group ($p = 0.0003$ for B-CD19$^+$ and $p = 0.01$ for NK1.1$^+$), respectively, and the IgY-treated Ps group ($p = 1 \times 10^{-8}$ for B-CD19$^+$ and $p = 9.8 \times 10^{-6}$ for NK1.1$^+$). Although for both experimental groups B-CD19$^+$ and NK1.1$^+$ normalization in peripheral blood was noticed, it is important that the values normalization obtained for IgY-treated Ps group is more pronounced, and the days necessary for skin healing is reduced compared to the naturally remitted Ps group. The normalization of values for the IgY-treated group is also supported by the fact that no statistically significant differences were obtained between the IgY-treated group and controls.

The main change observed in the cellular population of the spleen was the normalizing of B-CD19$^+$ cells revealed by a significant increase of B lymphocyte percentages in both IgY-treated Ps group and naturally remitted Ps group (Figure 6b). Statistically significant differences were observed between Ps group and the naturally remitted Ps group ($p = 0.0006$), respectively IgY-treated Ps ($p = 2.1 \times 10^{-9}$) group, differences were also noticed between the Ps group and controls ($p = 4 \times 10^{-7}$). Although for both experimental groups, the normalization of B-CD19$^+$ values from spleen cell suspension were observed, once more the normalization is enhanced for IgY-treated Ps group, and less healing days necessary compared to naturally remitted Ps group. No statistically significant differences were obtained for B-CD19$^+$ lymphocytes between IgY-treated Ps group and controls ($p > 0.05$), the values obtained being comparable. For NK1.1$^+$ cells, there is a tendency to normalize their values, and it was more pronounced in this case for the naturally remitted Ps group, but no statistically significant differences were observed between the IgY-treated Ps group and naturally remitted Ps group.

3.4. IgY Treatment-Induced Changes in NK Phenotype in Peripheral Blood and Spleen Cell Suspensions in Experimental Murine Model of Psoriatic Dermatitis

The expressions on NK cells of CD49b, CD11b, CD43, CD27, KLRG1-maturation markers, on CD69, CD28, CD11c, NKp46-activation markers, respectively, were quantified for all experimental groups.

The analysis of maturation markers in peripheral blood (Figure 7) showed a significant tendency to increase their expression on NK cells as compared to control group and the differences between the experimental groups were statistically significant ($p = 0.01$; $p = 0.0009$; $p = 0.01$). The level of CD49b on NK cells is significant reduced in Ps group. The percentages of NK1.1$^+$CD11b$^+$ cells in Ps group are higher than controls, but without statistical significance. In spleen cell suspension (Figure 8), analysis of maturation markers revealed the same tendency of variation: increased values for CD11b, CD27, KLRG1 levels on NK cells and lower values for CD49b and CD43 in Ps mice as compared to controls. Only for CD49b and KLRG1 the differences were statistically significant ($p = 0.01$; $p = 0.008$).

Analysis of CD69, CD11c and CD28 (activation markers) on NK1.1$^+$ cells in peripheral blood revealed significantly increased values in Ps group $p = 8.5 \times 10^{-11}$; $p = 9.5 \times 10^{-9}$; $p = 0.003$) compared to controls; the expression of NKp46 on NK1.1$^+$ cells is lower in Ps mice as compared to controls and the differences between the experimental groups were statistically significant ($p = 0.001$) (Figure 9). We found the same tendency of variation for activation markers in spleen cell suspensions (Figure 10): significantly increased values for CD69, CD11c and CD28 in Ps group ($p = 4.1 \times 10^{-12}$; $p = 2.1 \times 10^{-7}$; $p = 0.0001$) compared to controls; the expression of NKp46 on NK1.1$^+$ cells is lower in Ps mice as compared to controls, and the differences between the experimental groups were statistically significant ($p = 0.0003$).

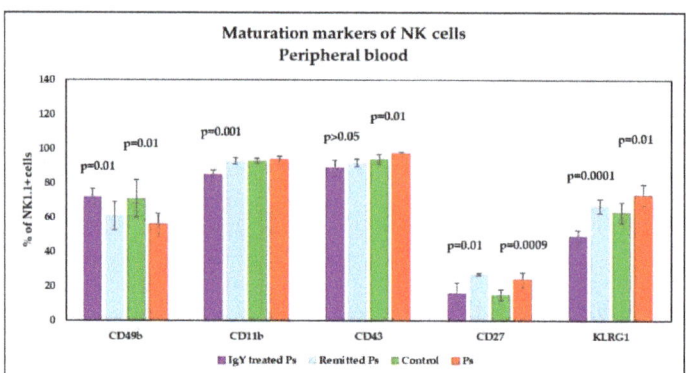

Figure 7. Expression of maturation markers on NK cells in peripheral blood. Expression of CD49b, CD11b, CD43, CD27 and KLRG1 levels on NK1.1$^+$ cells for IgY-treated Ps group (n = 12) (72 ± 4.7; 85 ± 2.7; 89 ± 4.6; 16 ± 6.1; 49 ± 3.7) as compared to naturally remitted Ps group (n = 8) (61 ± 8.3; 93 ± 1.8; 92 ± 2.1; 27 ± 0.8; 67 ± 4.1), control group (n = 8) (71 ± 11; 93 ± 1.5; 94 ± 2.7; 15 ± 3; 63 ± 6) and Ps group (n = 8) (56 ± 6.5; 94 ± 1.8; 97 ± 1.3; 24 ± 4.1; 73 ± 6.6). The results (% of NK1.1$^+$ cells) are presented as mean ± SD; n = number of mice).

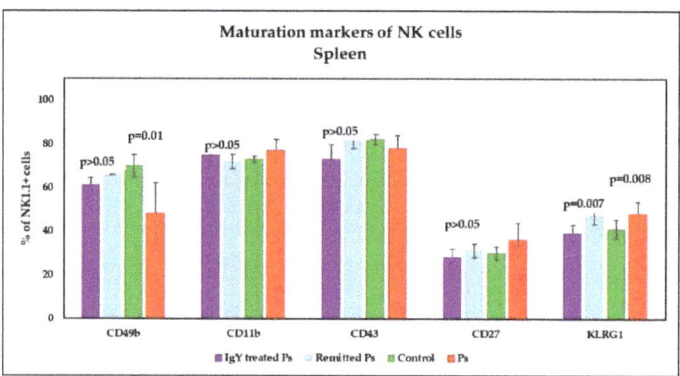

Figure 8. Expression of maturation markers on NK cells in spleen cell suspensions. Expression of CD49b, CD11b, CD43, CD27 and KLRG1 levels on NK1.1$^+$ cells for IgY-treated Ps group (n = 12) (61 ± 3.7; 75 ± 3.1; 73 ± 6.8; 28 ± 3.9; 39 ± 3.9) as compared to naturally remitted Ps group (n = 8) (66 ± 0.2; 72 ± 3.2; 82 ± 4.1; 31 ± 3.1; 47 ± 3.7), control group (n = 8) (70 ± 5.1; 73 ± 1.4; 82 ± 2.3; 30 ± 2.9; 41 ± 4.3) and Ps group (n = 8) (48 ± 13.9; 77 ± 5.2; 78 ± 6; 36 ± 7.8; 48 ± 5.4). The results (% of NK1.1$^+$ cells) are presented as mean ± SD; n = number of mice).

Analysis of NK cell maturation markers in peripheral blood (Figure 7) revealed a normalization of values for NK1.1$^+$CD49$^+$ and NK1.1$^+$CD27$^+$ cells in the IgY-treated Ps group. As there are statistically significant differences (p = 0.01 and p = 0.0009) obtained for these parameters between the Ps and control groups, after application of the IgY treatment we did not find statistical differences when comparing the values obtained for IgY-treated Ps group and controls. The expression of CD11b, CD43 and KLRG1 markers on NK1.1$^+$ cells is significantly lower for IgY-treated Ps group as compared to control group. For the naturally remitted Ps group, the values for CD49b, CD11b, CD43 and KLRG1 are normalized when comparing the values obtained for naturally remitted Ps group and controls. The expression of CD27 on NK1.1$^+$ cells was still significantly increased (p = 0.0003) for the naturally remitted Ps group, being almost equal to that obtained for the Ps group.

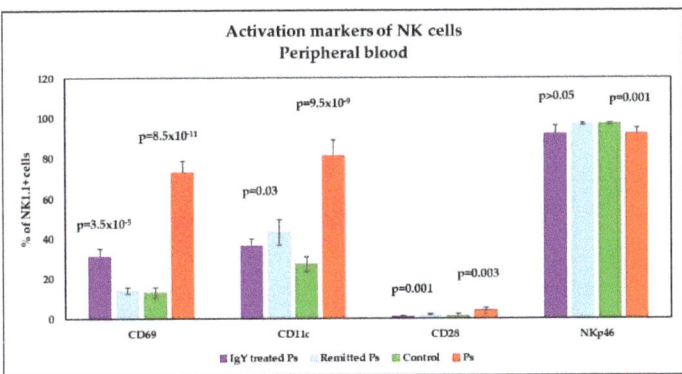

Figure 9. Expression of activation markers on NK cells in peripheral blood. Expression of CD69, CD11c, CD28 and NKp46 levels on NK1.1$^+$ cells for IgY-treated Ps group (n = 12) (31 ± 4; 36 ± 3.8; 1 ± 0.5; 92 ± 4.2) as compared to naturally remitted Ps group (n = 8) (14 ± 1.6; 43 ± 6.4; 2 ± 0.3; 97 ± 0.6), control group (n = 8) (13 ± 2.6; 27 ± 3.7; 1.2 ± 1.2; 97 ± 0.5) and Ps group (n = 8) (73 ± 5.7; 81 ± 8.1; 4 ± 1.5; 92 ± 3.2). The results (% of NK1.1$^+$ cells) are presented as mean ± SD; n = number of mice.

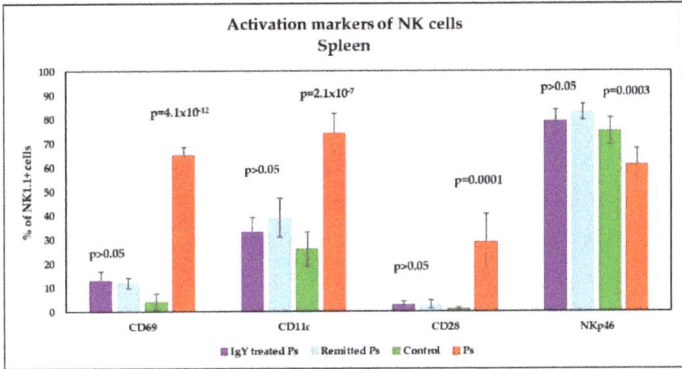

Figure 10. Expression of activation markers on NK cells in spleen cell suspensions. Expression of CD69, CD11c, CD28 and NKp46 levels on NK1.1$^+$ cells for IgY-treated Ps group (n = 12) (13 ± 3.8; 33 ± 6.2; 3 ± 1.2; 79 ± 5) as compared to naturally remitted Ps group (n = 8) (12 ± 2.2; 39 ± 8.1; 3 ± 1.8; 83 ± 3.2), control group (n = 8) (4 ± 3.5; 26 ± 7.1; 1 ± 0.7; 75 ± 5.7) and Ps group (n = 8) (65 ± 3.5; 74 ± 8.2; 29 ± 11.5; 61 ± 6.8). The results (% of NK1.1$^+$ cells) are presented as mean ± SD; n = number of mice.

In the spleen (Figure 8), the analysis of CD11b, CD27 and KLRG1 maturation markers revealed the normalization of their expression on NK cells following IgY treatment when comparing to control group. CD43 expression on NK cells decreased after IgY treatment. There were no statistically significant differences between IgY-treated Ps group and naturally remitted Ps group for CD49b, CD11b, CD43 and CD27 on NK cells.

Analysis of the expression of activation markers on NK1.1$^+$ cells in peripheral blood after IgY treatment revealed the normalization of CD28 values when compared to controls. For CD69 and CD11c levels in IgY-treated Ps group we observed a significant decreasing trend compared to Ps group but the expressions of these NK markers are significantly increased compared to control group (Figure 9). Although there is no statistically significant difference between the IgY-treated Ps group and naturally remitted Ps group for NKP46 expression, its expression on NK cells after IgY treatment is comparable to Ps group, namely below normal limits. For naturally remitted Ps group, the values of all activation markers have normalized when comparing to controls, except for CD11c, whose expression is significantly increased compared to control group and IgY-treated Ps group ($p = 0.001$ and $p = 0.03$, respectively).

Analysis of the expression of CD69, CD11c and CD28 activation markers on NK1.1$^+$ cells in spleen showed a pronounced decreasing trend for both IgY-treated mice and naturally remitted Ps group, toward normalization of their values (Figure 10). For CD11c expression, there is no statistically significant difference between IgY-treated Ps group and control group, while for naturally remitted Ps group, there are still significant differences ($p = 0.03$), when compared to controls. For all activation markers there are no statistically significant difference between IgY-treated Ps group and naturally remitted Ps group. NKp46 expression on NK cells have normalized in both IgY-treated group and naturally remitted Ps group as compared to the control group. Normalization of NKp46 values is more evident after IgY treatment.

4. Discussion

Psoriasis affecting the health of numerous individuals world-wide has a multifactorial pathogenesis and the exact triggering factor remains still unclear, As the skin is the major human organ with multiple functions, Ps instalment would trigger complex systemic disturbances. Alterations in the skin and intestinal microbiome are involved in the pathogenesis of psoriasis, therefore microbiome restoration becomes a promising preventive/therapy strategy in psoriasis [49].

Several years ago, it was shown that the overall microbial diversity is increased in the psoriatic plaque [50]. More recent studies proclaim an abnormal gut/skin microbiome as a potential driving force of systemic inflammation underlying Ps. It is hypothesized a gut-skin axis to be involved in Ps etiology as gut microbiota dysbiosis may alter systemic immunity and diminishes skin's physiological functions [42,51]. Regarding therapy strategies, Ps treatment resembles bowel disease and could implicate appropriate antibiotics to restore a normal flora, and also the use of prebiotics might be an alternative avenue to explore [52]. Therefore, aiding current therapies with adjuvant compounds becomes a necessity. As IgY is gaining new therapeutical potential in the anti-viral and anti-bacterial fight and acknowledging all the accumulated data, we have initiated in a psoriasis experimental model an adjuvant therapy using oral IgY developed against several pathogenic bacteria to evaluate the potency to alleviate the psoriatic lesions and to restore the cellular immune-related mechanisms.

The IMQ-induced psoriasiform dermatitis model [47] represents one of the most used inducible systems in studying Ps due to its reduced cost, rapid induction of skin inflammation and high reproducibility. Topical application of IMQ in animal models induce the formation of cutaneous lesions similar with human Ps plaque, [53–55]. group [53,54], Splenomegaly, as an indicator of intense lymphocyte activation, was observed in all experimental groups in which psoriatic dermatitis was induced. As recently published, splenomegaly is a characteristic of this animal model [56] and it is an indicator that although the induction of lesions was topical there is a systemic immune response. Following oral therapy with IgY or naturally healing, the values of spleen weight and SW / BW ratio were identical to the control group values. Practically, the splenomegaly installed after 6 consecutive days of IMQ-based cream topical application was completely remitted, for both experimental groups.

As reported in Ps patients [57], peripheral and spleen immune cell deregulations were found. As previously reported also by other groups [58] lower percentages of T-CD4$^+$ and B lymphocytes, while the percentages of T-CD8a$^+$ lymphocytes and NK1.1$^+$ cells were significantly increased. As a consequence, the T-CD4$^+$/T-CD8$^+$ ratio was significant decreased in Ps mice. The main changes observed in spleen cell suspensions were statistically significant, namely lower percentages of T-CD4$^+$ and B lymphocytes for Ps group as compared to controls. T-CD4$^+$/T-CD8$^+$ ratio is decreased in Ps mice, but the differences between the experimental groups were not statistically significant. The values obtained for these immunological parameters are comparable to the results published by our research team for psoriatic dermatitis mice model in which the IMQ-based cream was applied for 5 consecutive days [44] and with other group's results [59].

Analysis of T-CD4$^+$ and T-CD8a$^+$ lymphocyte subsets in peripheral blood revealed normalization of these parameters for IgY-treated Ps, naturally remitted Ps and control groups. T-CD8a$^+$ lymphocytes, identified in spleen cell suspensions in the IgY-treated Ps group are identical to the control group. Although the values of T-CD4$^+$ subset obtained for IgY-treated Ps group were significantly lower than control ($p = 0.006$), no statistically significant differences were observed between the IgY-treated Ps group and naturally remitted Ps group for T-CD4$^+$ subset. Recent findings have shown that T-CD8$^+$ cells are involved in psoriasiform skin inflammation and that memory T cells are involved in the pathogenesis of psoriasis, especially its recurrence. Therefore, normalization of these values brings clear clinical benefit [60].

As expected, the T-CD4$^+$/T-CD8a$^+$ ratio in peripheral blood also revealed the normalization pattern of IgY-treated Ps group compared to naturally remitted Ps or control group. A tendency of normalization was also noticed in spleen cell suspensions for both experimental groups. Although T-CD4$^+$/T-CD8a$^+$ ratio for IgY-treated Ps group were significantly lower than control ($p = 0.04$), no statistically significant differences were observed between the IgY-treated Ps group and naturally remitted Ps group.

Even though B-CD19$^+$ and NK1.1$^+$ normalization in peripheral blood was noticed the normalization for IgY-treated Ps group is more pronounced.

The main change observed in the spleen cell suspension was the normalizing of B–CD19$^+$ cells by significant increase of B lymphocyte percentages in both IgY-treated Ps group and naturally remitted Ps group. B cells have an important role in the protection against different infectious and inflammatory diseases, but there are very few reports on B lymphocytes involvement in Ps. The regulatory sub-population of B cells, B$_{regs}$ were found decreased in Ps patients [61] and moreover, it was shown that B$_{regs}$ may positively influence the course of Ps by producing IL-10 [62,63]. Therefore, the B cells increase that we have noticed in the treated group could account for the clinical improvement of the induced Ps.

For NK1.1$^+$ cells, there is a tendency to normalize the values, in the naturally remitted Ps group, with no statistically significant differences when compared to IgY-treated Ps group. The role of NK cells in Ps development is not fully elucidated. Although NK cells are recruited in human psoriatic lesions and in the induced Ps in mice, the studies regarding NK cells involvement in Ps do not abound [64]. The level of maturation marker CD49b on NK cells is significantly reduced in the Ps group. In spleen cell suspension, analysis of maturation markers revealed the same tendency of variation: increased values for CD11b, CD27, KLRG1 levels on NK cells and lower values for CD49b and CD43 in Ps mice as compared to controls. Only for CD49b and KLRG1 the differences were statistically significant.

Analysis of activation markers CD69, CD11c and CD28 on NK1.1$^+$ cells in peripheral blood revealed significantly increased values in Ps group compared to controls; the expression of NKp46 on NK1.1$^+$ cells is lower in Ps mice as compared to controls, and the differences between the experimental groups were statistically significant. Published studies report controversial results regarding NK cells in Ps and the matter is still subject of debate [65–67].

We found the same tendency of variation for activation markers in spleen cell suspensions, namely significantly increased values for CD69, CD11c and CD28 in Ps group compared to controls along with decreased expression of NKp46 on NK1.1+, with statistically significant differences. As a major activating receptor, NKp46, is an NK cell specific surface marker involved in all NK physiological immune processes [68] therefore an indicator that NK cells are mis-functioning due to the induced Ps.

In IgY-treated Ps group, NK cell maturation markers assessed in the peripheral blood revealed a normalization of values for NK1.1$^+$CD49$^+$ and NK1.1$^+$CD27$^+$ cells. Thus, the statistically significant differences obtained for these parameters between the Ps and control groups subside after IgY treatment. For naturally remitted Ps group, the values for CD49b, CD11b, CD43 and KLRG1 are as well normalized when compared to controls. As already mentioned, it should be noted that the healing period was longer for naturally remitted Ps group compared to the IgY-treated group. The expression of CD27 on NK1.1$^+$ cells was still significantly increased for the naturally remitted Ps group, being almost equal to that obtained for Ps group. NK maturation in periphery is characterized by an upregulation of CD11b, CD43, KLRG1, and Ly49 receptors, and a downregulation of CD27 [69,70], therefore we can speculate that even in clinically remitted psoriatic lesions the NK population remains alert to any psoriatic-dependent antigen.

In spleen cell suspension, analysis of CD11b, CD27 and KLRG1 maturation markers revealed the normalization of their expression on NK cells following IgY treatment compared to the control group. CD43 expression on NK cells decreased after IgY treatment. In contrast to the periphery, in the spleen, no statistically significant differences between IgY-treated Ps group and naturally remitted Ps group for CD49b, CD11b, CD43 and CD27 on NK cells was found. Yet again we can speculate that while NK residing in the secondary immune organs, such as the spleen, have normalized their parameters while in the periphery there are still populations that patrol in search of a psoriatic-like antigen.

Analysis of the expression of activation markers on NK1.1$^+$ cells in peripheral blood after IgY treatment revealed the normalization of CD28 values when compared to controls. For CD69 and CD11c levels in IgY-treated Ps group we observed a significant decreasing trend compared to Ps group, but the expressions of these markers on NK cells are significantly increased compared to control group. Although there is no statistically significant difference between IgY-treated Ps group and naturally remitted Ps group for NKP46, its expression on NK cells after IgY treatment is comparable to the Ps group, namely below normal limits. For naturally remitted Ps group, the values of all activation markers have normalized, except for CD11c, whose expression is significantly increased compared to control group and IgY-treated Ps group. Several years ago, it was reported that the CD56$^+$CD16$^+$CD11c$^+$ NK population are endowed with important characteristics such as IFN-γ production, tumor cell cytotoxicity and promotion of $\gamma\delta$ T lymphocyte proliferation [71]. Therefore, in our experimental model NK cells retain their activation capacity as proven by CD11c expression.

In spleen cell suspensions analysis of the expression of CD69, CD11c and CD28 activation markers on NK1.1$^+$ cells showed a pronounced decreasing trend for IgY-treated mice normalizing their values. For CD11c expression, there is no statistically significant difference between IgY-treated Ps group and control group ($p > 0.05$), while for naturally remitted Ps group, there are still significant differences. For all activation markers there are no statistically significant difference between IgY-treated Ps group and naturally remitted Ps group. NKp46 expression on NK cells have normalized in both IgY-treated group and naturally remitted Ps group as compared to the control group. Normalization of NKp46 values is more obvious after IgY treatment.

Study limitations. We acknowledge some limitations of our study. Thus, as human Ps is a complex auto-immune disease comprising, as presented, various triggering factors, the mice model is an induced one, therefore it misses probably more complex relations gut-skin interrelation. Another limitation of the study is that the IgY compound is designed for human ingestion as it is comprised out of IgY developed against antibiotic-resistant bacteria, therefore there could be bacterial strains that were missed in our mice model. Yet, in our model the Ps lesions subside earlier than the naturally remitted group probably as the utilized IgY is most probably restoring the digestive track microbiota. This limitation is overridden by the findings that mouse and human gut microbiota have similarity at the genus level [72]. Moreover, the mouse gut microbiota has similar functionality with the human one [73,74], therefore we can speculate in our experimental model that at least for some of the gut bacteria the IgY compound restored the microbiota inducing hence the solving of the induced psoriasis.

Perspectives. Far from being exhaustive, our work can open new perspective in Ps therapy. Therefore, we can foresee application in human psoriasis by first establishing the patients gut microbiota, then inoculating hens with the bacteria and isolating the raised IgY. Then, in conjunction with the standard psoriasis therapy, purified IgY can be ingested in doses matching the ones tested within our work. As shown, IgY preparations are non-allergenic and have high biocompatibility. Hence, one can imagine in the future adjuvant setting in which personalized IgY could aid the established therapy, alleviate the psoriatic lesions and improve the overall health status of the patient.

5. Conclusions

Ps affecting the health of numerous individuals worldwide has a multifactorial pathogenesis and recently it was shown that alterations in the skin and intestinal microbiome are involved in the pathogenesis of Ps, therefore microbiome restoration becomes a promising preventive/therapy strategy in this pathology. In our pre-clinical design study, using a mice model of induced psoriatic dermatitis, we have tested the proof-of-concept that IgY raised against pathological human bacteria resistant to antibiotics can alleviate psoriatic lesions and restore immune parameters. We pin-pointed that the IgY specific compound can be a possible pre-biotic alternative adjuvant in Ps. As IgY preparation can be raised against individualized microbiome using this compound can open also the personalized medicine domain in Ps.

Supplementary Materials: The following are available online at https://www.mdpi.com/article/10.3390/jpm11090841/s1, Table S1: Individual experimental data for erythema (E), skin scaling (S), thickening (T) and PASI score. Table S2: Individual histological parameters for each mouse from groups control, naturally remitted, psoriasis and IgY treated (- represents the absence of the investigated parameter, + low presence; ++ medium presence; +++ intense presence; ++++ extremely high presence).

Author Contributions: Conceptualization, M.S., C.C. (Carolina Constantin) and M.N.; methodology, M.S., A.M., G.I., C.C. (Carolina Constantin) and A.I.; writing—original draft preparation, M.S., A.M.; writing—review and editing, C.C. (Constantin Caruntu), M.S. and M.N.; supervision, M.N. All authors have read and agreed to the published version of the manuscript.

Funding: This research was funded by Competitiveness Operational Program (COP), IntelBiomed project, SMIS code 105631, ID: P_40_197, Grant No. 52/2016, and by Romanian Ministry of Research, Innovation and Digitization, grant PN 19.29.01.01 and PN 19.29.02.03.

Institutional Review Board Statement: The study was approved by the Ethics Committee from Victor Babeș Institute (no 88/20 January 2021) and National Sanitary Veterinary and Food Safety Authority (no 598/8 February 2021).

Informed Consent Statement: Not applicable.

Data Availability Statement: The datasets used and/or analyzed during current study are available from corresponding author on reasonable request.

Acknowledgments: Authors would like to thank Emilia Manole (Victor Babes National Institute of Pathology) for the histology of the skin sections. Authors would also like to thank all the technicians from the Animal Husbandry (Victor Babes National Institute of Pathology) for their resilience and patience to follow all the technicalities of this animal model design.

Conflicts of Interest: The authors declare no conflict of interest.

Abbreviations

APC, Allophycocyanin; BD, Becton Dickinson; B_{regs}, regulatory B cells; CD, Cluster of Differentiation; DC, Dendritic Cell; FACS, Fluorescence-Activated Cell Sorting; FBS, Fetal Bovine Serum; H&E, Haematoxylin-Eosin; FITC, Fluorescein Isothiocyanate; IFN, Interferon; Ig, Immunoglobulin; IL,

Interleukin; IMQ, Imiquimod; JAK, Janus Kinase; K2-EDTA, Kalium 2 EthyleneDiamine TetraAcetate; KLRG1, Killer Cell Lectin-Like Receptor G1; NK, Natural Killer cells; PASI, Psoriasis Area Severity Index; PE, Phycoerythrin; PE/Cy, Phycoerythrin Complex with Cyanine; PerCP/Cy, Peridinin Chlorophyll Protein Complex with Cyanine; R, Receptor; RORγt, Retinoic acid receptor-related orphan nuclear receptor gamma t; RPMI, Roswell Park Memorial Institute; SD, Standard Deviation; SW/BW, Spleen Weight/Body Weight; Th, Helper T Cells; TLR, Toll-Like Receptor; TNF, Tumor Necrosis Factor; UV, Ultraviolet.

References

1. Guo, R.; Zhang, T.; Meng, X.; Lin, Z.; Lin, J.; Gong, Y.; Liu, X.; Yu, Y.; Zhao, G.; Ding, X.; et al. Lymphocyte Mass Cytometry Identifies a CD3⁻CD4⁺ Cell Subset with a Potential Role in Psoriasis. *JCI Insight* **2019**, *4*. [CrossRef] [PubMed]
2. Nestle, F.O.; Kaplan, D.H.; Barker, J. Psoriasis. *N. Engl. J. Med.* **2009**, *361*, 496–509. [CrossRef] [PubMed]
3. Parisi, R.; Symmons, D.P.M.; Griffiths, C.E.M.; Ashcroft, D.M.; Identification and Management of Psoriasis and Associated ComorbidiTy (IMPACT) Project Team. Global Epidemiology of Psoriasis: A Systematic Review of Incidence and Prevalence. *J. Investig. Dermatol.* **2013**, *133*, 377–385. [CrossRef] [PubMed]
4. Parisi, R.; Iskandar, I.Y.K.; Kontopantelis, E.; Augustin, M.; Griffiths, C.E.M.; Ashcroft, D.M. National, Regional, and Worldwide Epidemiology of Psoriasis: Systematic Analysis and Modelling Study. *BMJ* **2020**, *369*, m1590. [CrossRef]
5. Wolf, P.; Weger, W.; Patra, V.; Gruber-Wackernagel, A.; Byrne, S.N. Desired Response to Phototherapy vs Photoaggravation in Psoriasis: What Makes the Difference? *Exp. Dermatol.* **2016**, *25*, 937–944. [CrossRef]
6. Fry, L.; Baker, B.S. Triggering Psoriasis: The Role of Infections and Medications. *Clin. Dermatol.* **2007**, *25*, 606–615. [CrossRef]
7. Naldi, L. Psoriasis and Smoking: Links and Risks. *Psoriasis* **2016**, *6*, 65–71. [CrossRef]
8. Wheatley, R.; Brooks, J.; Stumpf, B.; Boh, E. Obesity, Diet, and Inflammation in Psoriasis. *J. Psoriasis Psoriatic Arthritis* **2017**, *2*, 97–101. [CrossRef]
9. Farkas, A.; Kemény, L. Alcohol, Liver, Systemic Inflammation and Skin: A Focus on Patients with Psoriasis. *Skin Pharmacol. Physiol.* **2013**, *26*, 119–126. [CrossRef]
10. Wolk, K.; Mallbris, L.; Larsson, P.; Rosenblad, A.; Vingård, E.; Ståhle, M. Excessive Body Weight and Smoking Associates with a High Risk of Onset of Plaque Psoriasis. *Acta Derm.-Venereol.* **2009**, *89*, 492–497. [CrossRef]
11. Snast, I.; Reiter, O.; Atzmony, L.; Leshem, Y.A.; Hodak, E.; Mimouni, D.; Pavlovsky, L. Psychological Stress and Psoriasis: A Systematic Review and Meta-Analysis. *Br. J. Dermatol.* **2018**, *178*, 1044–1055. [CrossRef]
12. Finlay, A.Y.; Khan, G.K. Dermatology Life Quality Index (DLQI)—A Simple Practical Measure for Routine Clinical Use. *Clin. Exp. Dermatol.* **1994**, *19*, 210–216. [CrossRef] [PubMed]
13. Langley, R.G.; Ellis, C.N. Evaluating Psoriasis with Psoriasis Area and Severity Index, Psoriasis Global Assessment, and Lattice System Physician's Global Assessment. *J. Am. Acad. Dermatol.* **2004**, *51*, 563–569. [CrossRef] [PubMed]
14. Georgescu, S.-R.; Tampa, M.; Caruntu, C.; Sarbu, M.-I.; Mitran, C.-I.; Mitran, M.-I.; Matei, C.; Constantin, C.; Neagu, M. Advances in Understanding the Immunological Pathways in Psoriasis. *Int. J. Mol. Sci.* **2019**, *20*, 739. [CrossRef] [PubMed]
15. Surcel, M.; Huica, R.; Constantin, C.; Ursaciuc, C.; Neagu, M. Biomarkers Insights in Psoriasis-Regulatory Cytokines. *Curr. Biomark.* **2017**, *7*, 3–11. [CrossRef]
16. Gall, J.S.; Kalb, R.E. Infliximab for the Treatment of Plaque Psoriasis. *Biologics* **2008**, *2*, 115–124. [CrossRef]
17. Alwawi, E.A.; Mehlis, S.L.; Gordon, K.B. Treating Psoriasis with Adalimumab. *Ther. Clin. Risk Manag.* **2008**, *4*, 345–351. [CrossRef]
18. Blauvelt, A.; Reich, K.; Lebwohl, M.; Burge, D.; Arendt, C.; Peterson, L.; Drew, J.; Rolleri, R.; Gottlieb, A.B. Certolizumab Pegol for the Treatment of Patients with Moderate-to-Severe Chronic Plaque Psoriasis: Pooled Analysis of Week 16 Data from Three Randomized Controlled Trials. *J. Eur. Acad. Dermatol. Venereol.* **2019**, *33*, 546–552. [CrossRef]
19. Farhi, D. Ustekinumab for the Treatment of Psoriasis: Review of Three Multicenter Clinical Trials. *Drugs Today* **2010**, *46*, 259–264. [CrossRef]
20. Nogueira, M.; Torres, T. Guselkumab for the Treatment of Psoriasis—Evidence to Date. *Drugs Context* **2019**, *8*, 212594. [CrossRef]
21. Witjes, H.; Khatri, A.; Diderichsen, P.M.; Mandema, J.; Othman, A.A. Meta-Analyses of Clinical Efficacy of Risankizumab and Adalimumab in Chronic Plaque Psoriasis: Supporting Evidence of Risankizumab Superiority. *Clin. Pharmacol. Ther.* **2020**, *107*, 435–442. [CrossRef]
22. Blauvelt, A.; Sofen, H.; Papp, K.; Gooderham, M.; Tyring, S.; Zhao, Y.; Lowry, S.; Mendelsohn, A.; Parno, J.; Reich, K. Tildrakizumab Efficacy and Impact on Quality of Life up to 52 Weeks in Patients with Moderate-to-Severe Psoriasis: A Pooled Analysis of Two Randomized Controlled Trials. *J. Eur. Acad. Dermatol. Venereol.* **2019**, *33*, 2305–2312. [CrossRef]
23. López-Ferrer, A.; Vilarrasa, E.; Puig, L. Secukinumab (AIN457) for the Treatment of Psoriasis. *Expert Rev. Clin. Immunol.* **2015**, *11*, 1177–1188. [CrossRef]
24. Papp, K.A.; Leonardi, C.L.; Blauvelt, A.; Reich, K.; Korman, N.J.; Ohtsuki, M.; Paul, C.; Ball, S.; Cameron, G.S.; Erickson, J.; et al. Ixekizumab Treatment for Psoriasis: Integrated Efficacy Analysis of Three Double-Blinded, Controlled Studies. *Br. J. Dermatol.* **2018**, *178*, 674–681. [CrossRef]

25. Foulkes, A.C.; Warren, R.B. Brodalumab in Psoriasis: Evidence to Date and Clinical Potential. *Drugs Context* **2019**, *8*, 212570. [CrossRef] [PubMed]
26. Pandya, V.B.; Kumar, S.; Sachchidanand; Sharma, R.; Desai, R.C. Combating Autoimmune Diseases With Retinoic Acid Receptor-Related Orphan Receptor-γ (RORγ or RORc) Inhibitors: Hits and Misses. *J. Med. Chem.* **2018**, *61*, 10976–10995. [CrossRef] [PubMed]
27. Bachelez, H.; Choon, S.-E.; Marrakchi, S.; Burden, A.D.; Tsai, T.-F.; Morita, A.; Turki, H.; Hall, D.B.; Shear, M.; Baum, P.; et al. Inhibition of the Interleukin-36 Pathway for the Treatment of Generalized Pustular Psoriasis. *N. Engl. J. Med.* **2019**, *380*, 981–983. [CrossRef] [PubMed]
28. Schwartz, D.M.; Kanno, Y.; Villarino, A.; Ward, M.; Gadina, M.; O'Shea, J.J. JAK Inhibition as a Therapeutic Strategy for Immune and Inflammatory Diseases. *Nat. Rev. Drug Discov.* **2017**, *16*, 843–862. [CrossRef] [PubMed]
29. Page, K.M.; Suarez-Farinas, M.; Suprun, M.; Zhang, W.; Garcet, S.; Fuentes-Duculan, J.; Li, X.; Scaramozza, M.; Kieras, E.; Banfield, C.; et al. Molecular and Cellular Responses to the TYK2/JAK1 Inhibitor PF-06700841 Reveal Reduction of Skin Inflammation in Plaque Psoriasis. *J. Investig. Dermatol.* **2020**, *140*, 1546–1555.e4. [CrossRef]
30. Zanin-Zhorov, A.; Weiss, J.M.; Trzeciak, A.; Chen, W.; Zhang, J.; Nyuydzefe, M.S.; Arencibia, C.; Polimera, S.; Schueller, O.; Fuentes-Duculan, J.; et al. Cutting Edge: Selective Oral ROCK2 Inhibitor Reduces Clinical Scores in Patients with Psoriasis Vulgaris and Normalizes Skin Pathology via Concurrent Regulation of IL-17 and IL-10. *J. Immunol.* **2017**, *198*, 3809–3814. [CrossRef] [PubMed]
31. Vaclavkova, A.; Chimenti, S.; Arenberger, P.; Holló, P.; Sator, P.-G.; Burcklen, M.; Stefani, M.; D'Ambrosio, D. Oral Ponesimod in Patients with Chronic Plaque Psoriasis: A Randomised, Double-Blind, Placebo-Controlled Phase 2 Trial. *Lancet* **2014**, *384*, 2036–2045. [CrossRef]
32. Robbins, K.; Bissonnette, R.; Maeda-Chubachi, T.; Ye, L.; Peppers, J.; Gallagher, K.; Kraus, J.E. Phase 2, Randomized Dose-Finding Study of Tapinarof (GSK2894512 Cream) for the Treatment of Plaque Psoriasis. *J. Am. Acad. Dermatol.* **2019**, *80*, 714–721. [CrossRef]
33. Rahman, S.; Van Nguyen, L.; Icatlo, F.C., Jr.; Umeda, K.; Kodama, Y. Oral Passive IgY-Based Immunotherapeutics. *Hum. Vaccines Immunother.* **2013**, *9*, 1039–1048. [CrossRef] [PubMed]
34. Torché, A.-M.; Le Dimna, M.; Le Corre, P.; Mesplède, A.; Le Gal, S.; Cariolet, R.; Le Potier, M.-F. Immune Responses after Local Administration of IgY Loaded-PLGA Microspheres in Gut-Associated Lymphoid Tissue in Pigs. *Vet. Immunol. Immunopathol.* **2006**, *109*, 209–217. [CrossRef]
35. Kovacs-Nolan, J.; Mine, Y. Egg Yolk Antibodies for Passive Immunity. *Annu. Rev. Food Sci. Technol.* **2012**, *3*, 163–182. [CrossRef] [PubMed]
36. Akita, E.M.; Jang, C.B.; Kitts, D.D.; Nakai, S. Evaluation of Allergenicity of Egg Yolk Immunoglobulin Y and Other Egg Proteins by Passive Cutaneous Anaphylaxis. *Food Agric. Immunol.* **1999**, *11*, 191–201. [CrossRef]
37. Vega, C.G.; Bok, M.; Vlasova, A.N.; Chattha, K.S.; Fernández, F.M.; Wigdorovitz, A.; Parreño, V.G.; Saif, L.J. IgY Antibodies Protect against Human Rotavirus Induced Diarrhea in the Neonatal Gnotobiotic Piglet Disease Model. *PLoS ONE* **2012**, *7*, e42788. [CrossRef] [PubMed]
38. Xu, Y.; Li, X.; Jin, L.; Zhen, Y.; Lu, Y.; Li, S.; You, J.; Wang, L. Application of Chicken Egg Yolk Immunoglobulins in the Control of Terrestrial and Aquatic Animal Diseases: A Review. *Biotechnol. Adv.* **2011**, *29*, 860–868. [CrossRef] [PubMed]
39. Constantin, C.; Neagu, M.; Diana Supeanu, T.; Chiurciu, V.; Spandidos, D.A. IgY—Turning the Page toward Passive Immunization in COVID-19 Infection (Review). *Exp. Ther. Med.* **2020**, *20*, 151–158. [CrossRef] [PubMed]
40. Michael, A.; Meenatchisundaram, S.; Parameswari, G.; Subbraj, T.; Selvakumaran, R.; Ramalingam, S. Chicken Egg Yolk Antibodies (IgY) as an Alternative to Mammalian Antibodies. *Indian J. Sci. Technol.* **2010**, *3*, 468–474. [CrossRef]
41. Yu, M.; Zhang, R.; Ni, P.; Chen, S.; Duan, G. Helicobacter Pylori Infection and Psoriasis: A Systematic Review and Meta-Analysis. *Medicina* **2019**, *55*, 645. [CrossRef] [PubMed]
42. de Jesús-Gil, C.; Sans-de San Nicolàs, L.; Ruiz-Romeu, E.; Ferran, M.; Soria-Martínez, L.; García-Jiménez, I.; Chiriac, A.; Casanova-Seuma, J.M.; Fernández-Armenteros, J.M.; Owens, S.; et al. Interplay between Humoral and CLA+T Cell Response against Candida albicans in Psoriasis. *Int. J. Mol. Sci.* **2021**, *22*, 1519. [CrossRef] [PubMed]
43. Visser, M.J.E.; Kell, D.B.; Pretorius, E. Bacterial Dysbiosis and Translocation in Psoriasis Vulgaris. *Front. Cell Infect. Microbiol.* **2019**, *9*, 7. [CrossRef] [PubMed]
44. Surcel, M.; Huică, R.-I.; Munteanu, A.N.; Isvoranu, G.; Pîrvu, I.R.; Ciotaru, D.; Constantin, C.; Bratu, O.; Căruntu, C.; Neagu, M.; et al. Phenotypic Changes of Lymphocyte Populations in Psoriasiform Dermatitis Animal Model. *Exp. Ther. Med.* **2019**, *17*, 1030–1038. [CrossRef] [PubMed]
45. Surcel, M.; Munteanu, A.N.; Huică, R.-I.; Isvoranu, G.; Pîrvu, I.R.; Constantin, C.; Bratu, O.; Căruntu, C.; Zahareasu, I.; Sima, L.; et al. Reinforcing Involvement of NK Cells in Psoriasiform Dermatitis Animal Model. *Exp. Ther. Med.* **2019**, *18*, 4956–4966. [CrossRef] [PubMed]
46. Pătrașcu, I.V.; Chiurciu, V.; Chiurciu, C.; Topilescu, G. Procedure to Obtain and Use Hen Egg Immunoglobulins (IgY). RO129645 A0, 2014 00156, 30 July 2014.
47. Pătrașcu, I.V.; Chiurciu, V.; Chiurciu, C.; Topilescu, G. Method for Immunobiological Assay of Chicken Immunoglobulins Specific Activity. RO129677 A0, 2014 00179, 30 July 2014.

48. van der Fits, L.; Mourits, S.; Voerman, J.S.A.; Kant, M.; Boon, L.; Laman, J.D.; Cornelissen, F.; Mus, A.-M.; Florencia, E.; Prens, E.P.; et al. Imiquimod-Induced Psoriasis-like Skin Inflammation in Mice Is Mediated via the IL-23/IL-17 Axis. *J. Immunol.* **2009**, *182*, 5836–5845. [CrossRef]
49. Chiurciu, C.; Chiurciu, V.; Sima, L.; Mihai, I.; Patrascu, I.V. Production and Use of Personalized (Ovopatch) Hyperimmune Egg in the Treatment of Psoriasis. RO 130965 A0, 2015 00735, 30 March 2016.
50. Chen, L.; Li, J.; Zhu, W.; Kuang, Y.; Liu, T.; Zhang, W.; Chen, X.; Peng, C. Skin and Gut Microbiome in Psoriasis: Gaining Insight Into the Pathophysiology of It and Finding Novel Therapeutic Strategies. *Front. Microbiol.* **2020**, *11*, 589726. [CrossRef]
51. Takemoto, A.; Cho, O.; Morohoshi, Y.; Sugita, T.; Muto, M. Molecular Characterization of the Skin Fungal Microbiome in Patients with Psoriasis. *J. Dermatol.* **2015**, *42*, 166–170. [CrossRef]
52. Salem, I.; Ramser, A.; Isham, N.; Ghannoum, M.A. The Gut Microbiome as a Major Regulator of the Gut-Skin Axis. *Front. Microbiol.* **2018**, *9*, 1459. [CrossRef]
53. Haines Ely, P. Is psoriasis a bowel disease? Successful treatment with bile acids and bioflavonoids suggests it is. *Clin. Dermatol.* **2018**, *36*, 376–389. [CrossRef]
54. Bocheńska, K.; Smolińska, E.; Moskot, M.; Jakóbkiewicz-Banecka, J.; Gabig-Cimińska, M. Models in the Research Process of Psoriasis. *Int. J. Mol. Sci.* **2017**, *18*, 2514. [CrossRef] [PubMed]
55. Hawkes, J.E.; Adalsteinsson, J.A.; Gudjonsson, J.E.; Ward, N.L. Research Techniques Made Simple: Murine Models of Human Psoriasis. *J. Investig. Dermatol.* **2018**, *138*, e1–e8. [CrossRef] [PubMed]
56. Yuan, J.; Ni, G.; Wang, T.; Mounsey, K.; Cavezza, S.; Pan, X.; Liu, X. Genital Warts Treatment: Beyond Imiquimod. *Hum. Vaccines Immunother.* **2018**, *14*, 1815–1819. [CrossRef] [PubMed]
57. Jabeen, M.; Boisgard, A.-S.; Danoy, A.; El Kholti, N.; Salvi, J.-P.; Boulieu, R.; Fromy, B.; Verrier, B.; Lamrayah, M. Advanced Characterization of Imiquimod-Induced Psoriasis-Like Mouse Model. *Pharmaceutics* **2020**, *12*, 789. [CrossRef]
58. Alecu, M.; Ursaciuc, C.; Surcel, M.; Coman, G.; Ciotaru, D.; Dobre, M. CD28 T-cell costimulatory molecule expression in pemphigus vulgaris. *J. Eur. Acad. Dermatol. Venereol.* **2009**, *23*, 288–291. [CrossRef]
59. Prietl, B.; Treiber, G.; Mader, J.K.; Hoeller, E.; Wolf, M.; Pilz, S.; Graninger, W.B.; Obermayer-Pietsch, B.M.; Pieber, T.R. High-Dose Cholecalciferol Supplementation Significantly Increases Peripheral CD4+ Tregs in Healthy Adults without Negatively Affecting the Frequency of Other Immune Cells. *Eur. J. Nutr.* **2014**, *53*, 751–759. [CrossRef]
60. Shin, S.-H.; Kim, H.-Y.; Yoon, H.-S.; Park, W.-J.; Adams, D.R.; Pyne, N.J.; Pyne, S.; Park, J.-W. A Novel Selective Sphingosine Kinase 2 Inhibitor, HWG-35D, Ameliorates the Severity of Imiquimod-Induced Psoriasis Model by Blocking Th17 Differentiation of Naïve CD4 T Lymphocytes. *Int. J. Mol. Sci.* **2020**, *21*, 8371. [CrossRef] [PubMed]
61. Chen, Y.; Yan, Y.; Liu, H.; Qiu, F.; Liang, C.-L.; Zhang, Q.; Huang, R.-Y.; Han, L.; Lu, C.; Dai, Z. Dihydroartemisinin Ameliorates Psoriatic Skin Inflammation and Its Relapse by Diminishing CD8+ T-Cell Memory in Wild-Type and Humanized Mice. *Theranostics* **2020**, *10*, 10466–10482. [CrossRef]
62. Kahlert, K.; Grän, F.; Muhammad, K.; Benoit, S.; Serfling, E.; Goebeler, M.; Kerstan, A. Aberrant B-Cell Subsets and Immunoglobulin Levels in Patients with Moderate-to-Severe Psoriasis. *Acta Derm.-Venereol.* **2019**, *99*, 226–227. [CrossRef]
63. Alrefai, H.; Muhammad, K.; Rudolf, R.; Pham, D.A.T.; Klein-Hessling, S.; Patra, A.K.; Avots, A.; Bukur, V.; Sahin, U.; Tenzer, S.; et al. NFATc1 Supports Imiquimod-Induced Skin Inflammation by Suppressing IL-10 Synthesis in B Cells. *Nat. Commun.* **2016**, *7*, 11724. [CrossRef]
64. Grän, F.; Kerstan, A.; Serfling, E.; Goebeler, M.; Muhammad, K. Current Developments in the Immunology of Psoriasis. *Yale J. Biol. Med.* **2020**, *93*, 97–110.
65. Polese, B.; Zhang, H.; Thurairajah, B.; King, I.L. Innate Lymphocytes in Psoriasis. *Front. Immunol.* **2020**, *11*, 242. [CrossRef] [PubMed]
66. Kucuksezer, U.C.; Aktas Cetin, E.; Esen, F.; Tahrali, I.; Akdeniz, N.; Gelmez, M.Y.; Deniz, G. The Role of Natural Killer Cells in Autoimmune Diseases. *Front. Immunol.* **2021**, *12*, 79. [CrossRef] [PubMed]
67. Luci, C.; Gaudy-Marqueste, C.; Rouzaire, P.; Audonnet, S.; Cognet, C.; Hennino, A.; Nicolas, J.-F.; Grob, J.-J.; Tomasello, E. Peripheral Natural Killer Cells Exhibit Qualitative and Quantitative Changes in Patients with Psoriasis and Atopic Dermatitis. *Br. J. Dermatol.* **2012**, *166*, 789–796. [CrossRef] [PubMed]
68. Dunphy, S.E.; Sweeney, C.M.; Kelly, G.; Tobin, A.M.; Kirby, B.; Gardiner, C.M. Natural Killer Cells from Psoriasis Vulgaris Patients Have Reduced Levels of Cytotoxicity Associated Degranulation and Cytokine Production. *Clin. Immunol.* **2017**, *177*, 43–49. [CrossRef]
69. Hadad, U.; Thauland, T.; Butte, M.; Porgador, A.; Martinez, O.; Krams, S. NKp46 Clusters at the NK Cell Immune Synapse Regulate Specific Effector Functions. In Proceedings of the 2015 American Transplant Congress, Philadelphia, PA, USA, 2–6 May 2015.
70. Abel, A.M.; Yang, C.; Thakar, M.S.; Malarkannan, S. Natural Killer Cells: Development, Maturation, and Clinical Utilization. *Front. Immunol.* **2018**, *9*, 1869. [CrossRef]
71. Ramírez-Ramírez, D.; Vadillo, E.; Arriaga-Pizano, L.A.; Mayani, H.; Estrada-Parra, S.; Velasco-Velázquez, M.A.; Pérez-Tapia, S.M.; Pelayo, R. Early Differentiation of Human CD11c+NK Cells with Γδ T Cell Activation Properties Is Promoted by Dialyzable Leukocyte Extracts. *J. Immunol. Res.* **2016**, *2016*, 4097642. [CrossRef]
72. Hugenholtz, F.; de Vos, W.M. Mouse models for human intestinal microbiota research: A critical evaluation. *Cell. Mol. Life Sci.* **2018**, *75*, 149–160. [CrossRef]

73. Xiao, L.; Feng, Q.; Liang, S.; Sonne, S.B.; Xia, Z.; Qiu, X.; Li, X.; Long, H.; Zhang, J.; Zhang, D.; et al. A catalog of the mouse gut metagenome. *Nat. Biotechnol.* **2015**, *33*, 1103–1108. [CrossRef]
74. Wang, J.; Lang, T.; Shen, J.; Dai, J.; Tian, L.; Wang, X. Core Gut Bacteria Analysis of Healthy Mice. *Front. Microbiol.* **2019**, *10*, 887. [CrossRef] [PubMed]

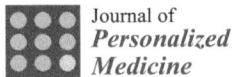

Article

Cellular Response against Oxidative Stress, a Novel Insight into Lupus Nephritis Pathogenesis

Corina Daniela Ene [1,*], Simona Roxana Georgescu [2,*], Mircea Tampa [3,*], Clara Matei [4], Cristina Iulia Mitran [5], Madalina Irina Mitran [5], Mircea Nicolae Penescu [1,6] and Ilinca Nicolae [2]

1. Department of Nephrology, Davila Clinical Hospital of Nephrology, 010731 Bucharest, Romania; mirceapenescu4@gmail.com
2. Department of Dermatology, Victor Babes Clinical Hospital of Tropical and Infectious Diseases, 030303 Bucharest, Romania; drnicolaei@yahoo.ro
3. Department of Dermatology, Carol Davila University of Medicine and Pharmacy, 020021 Bucharest, Romania
4. Department of Dermatology, Colentina Clinical Hospital, 020125 Bucharest, Romania; matei_clara@yahoo.com
5. Department of Microbiology, Carol Davila University of Medicine and Pharmacy, 020021 Bucharest, Romania; cristina.iulia.mitran@gmail.com (C.I.M.); madalina.irina.mitran@gmail.com (M.I.M.)
6. Department of Nephrology, Carol Davila University of Medicine and Pharmacy, 020021 Bucharest, Romania
* Correspondence: koranik85@yahoo.com (C.D.E.); srg.dermatology@gmail.com (S.R.G.); dermatology.mt@gmail.com (M.T.)

Abstract: The interaction of reactive oxygen species (ROS) with lipids, proteins, nucleic acids and hydrocarbonates promotes acute and chronic tissue damage, mediates immunomodulation and triggers autoimmunity in systemic lupus erythematous (SLE) patients. The aim of the study was to determine the pathophysiological mechanisms of the oxidative stress-related damage and molecular mechanisms to counteract oxidative stimuli in lupus nephritis. Our study included 38 SLE patients with lupus nephritis (LN group), 44 SLE patients without renal impairment (non-LN group) and 40 healthy volunteers as control group. In the present paper, we evaluated serum lipid peroxidation, DNA oxidation, oxidized proteins, carbohydrate oxidation, and endogenous protective systems. We detected defective DNA repair mechanisms via 8-oxoguanine-DNA-glycosylase (OGG1), the reduced regulatory effect of soluble receptor for advanced glycation end products (sRAGE) in the activation of AGE-RAGE axis, low levels of thiols, disulphide bonds formation and high nitrotyrosination in lupus nephritis. All these data help us to identify more molecular mechanisms to counteract oxidative stress in LN that could permit a more precise assessment of disease prognosis, as well as developing new therapeutic targets.

Keywords: systemic lupus erythematous; lupus nephritis; lipid peroxidation; DNA oxidation; oxidized proteins; carbohydrate oxidation; antioxidative stress strategies; biomarkers

1. Introduction

Systemic lupus erythematosus (SLE) is a chronic autoimmune disease with complex pathogenesis, characterized by formation of autoantibodies against normal structures of the body such as skin, joints, blood elements, kidney, and central nervous system, with a heterogeneity of clinical manifestations. Skin lesions are frequent, such as symmetric malar erythema, photo sensibility, hyperkeratosis, ecchymosis, oral or mucosal ulcerations, alopecia. Proteinuria or nephrotic syndrome, changes in urinary sediment, increase in serum creatinine and arterial hypertension are clinical manifestations of lupus nephritis [1,2]. SLE—Autoimmune prototype disease—is characterized by abnormal responses of T and B immune cells with excessive synthesis of autoantibodies and immune circulant complexes [3] associated with nonimmune factors [4,5].

SLE clinical evolution is variable, being influenced by genetic factors, external factors, and human body resources. The pathogenic mechanism is promoted by the UV exposure of keratinocytes. Keratinocyte activation induces chemokines synthesis (CXCL5, CXCL8, CXCL20), production of adhesion molecules, apoptosis, keratinocyte photodistruction, release of nuclear and cytoplasmic antigens, and immune response initiation. These pathogenic events are processed by dermic and epidermic macrophages and presented to dermal naïve T lymphocytes. In SLE-related skin lesions, vacuolar and hydropic degeneration of keratinocytes and lymphocytic infiltration in papillary dermis could be found. Direct immunofluorescence reveals deposition in band of antibodies and complement to the dermo–epidermic junction. The cascade of autoantibodies induces the formation of circulant immune complexes, with preferential deposition in the synovial joint and glomeruli. The forms of LE limited to skin can evolve to SLE [6,7].

Oxidative stress in SLE was intensively studied during years. Reactive oxygen species (ROS) interaction with lipids, proteins, nucleic acids and hydro carbonates promotes acute and chronic tissue damage, mediates immunomodulation and trigger autoimmunity in SLE subjects [8–11]. Moreover, for their viability and correct functions, the cells develop endogenous strategies for suppression or modulating oxidative stress [3,12–14]. High levels of oxidative and nitrosative stress markers were determined in SLE patients with high disease activity. Still, oxidative stress influence immune and nonimmune cells on determining the disease phenotype in each subject [12]. An imbalance in oxidant/antioxidant equilibrium in autoimmune disease by endogenous or exogenous toxic factors exposure, by alteration of tissue damage response/repair mechanisms induces an aberrant activity of innate and adaptative immune response, high production of autoantibodies, multiple lesions of tissues and organs [4]. The bidirectional relation between oxidative stress and immune response, considered as part of autoimmune physiopathology, could change the paradigm of a disease characterized by perturbation of immune system and high production of autoantibodies [5,15–17].

A large diversity of lipoperoxides were detected in SLE in extracellular fluids and in blood. They influence disease expression by their effect on immune and non-immune cells [16,18]. Lipid peroxidation generates a variety of metabolites, the best known being saturated monoaldehydes; unsaturated aldehydes; dicarbonyls; malondialdehyde; 4-oxo-2-nonenal; hydroxydialdehydes (4-hydroxy-2-nonenal, 4-hydroxy-2-hexenal); oxidized phospholipids [8,19–21]. High levels of oxidative and nitrosative stress were detected in patients with active SLE, suggesting a link between lipoperoxidation and disease activity. Increased activity of malondialdehyde (MDA), 4-hydroxy-2-nonenal (HNE), MDA-protein adduct, HNE-protein adduct, superoxide dismutase (SOD), nitric oxide synthase (INOS), anti-MDA and anti-HNE antibodies were correlated in SLE patients with SLEDAI over 6 [9,16,21]. These lipoperoxides' destructive effect could be limited by defense mechanisms of the human organism, such as lipoperoxides metabolization by oxide reductase (aldoceto-reductase, aldehyde-dehydrogenase, alcohol-dehydrogenase, glutathione-S-transferase) and cellular antioxidant defense mechanisms that include enzymes (SOD, chloramphenicol acetyltransferase—CAT, glutathione peroxidase—GPx, reductase—GR, S-transferases—GST, tioredoxin-reductase, hemoxigenase), non-enzymes (A, C, E vitamins), and carotenoids, flavonoids, glutathione and other antioxidant minerals [13,18]. Defense mechanism disruption was associated with clinical complications of SLE [10,11,16]. Isoprostan F2 (8-iso-PGF2) levels, a results of lipid peroxidation, was correlated with disease activity in SLE subjects. Moreover, high levels of MDA, F2-Isoprostan, nitric oxide and low levels of reduced glutathione were determined in patients with lupus nephritis [16].

In SLE, oxidative stress is involved in the formation of advanced glycation end products (AGEs) and advanced lipoperoxidation end products (ALEs), compounds with proinflammatory characteristics. AGEs and ALEs synthesis is realized through condensation reactions between electrophile and nucleophile reactants [17,21–25]. AGEs and ALEs are immunogen and they determine antibodies synthesis. AGEs initiate signaling cascades by specific receptors named RAGE. No data could be found in the literature about a receptor-mediated mechanism regarding the destructive effect of ALEs [21]. RAGE polymorphisms were associated with SLE susceptibility and lupus nephritis [26]. sRAGE could exert benefic effects by preventing proinflammatory signaling, they act as bait receiver [25,27–31].

In systemic autoimmune diseases, ROS and RNS overproduction induce DNA integrity alteration, damage of DNA response and repair (DDR/R) mechanisms, accumulation of mono- and double catenary cytosolic DNA, activation of stimulator of interferon genes (STING), synthesis of type 1 interferon [32]. DDR/R recognize defects during cell cycle and assures their correct reparation. In case of unrepaired lesions, the cell transmits the mutant genome to its descendants, otherwise it is neutralized by apoptosis or senescence [3,32,33].

The most frequent oxidative lesion in aerobe organisms is the formation of 7,8-dihydro-8-oxo-2′-deoxyguanosin (8-oxo-dG or 8-OH dG) [17,34,35]. In normal cells, during DNA replication, 2-deoxyguaninae (dG) is associated with 2′-deoxycitosine (dC). In tissues with high levels of oxidative stress, dG could wrongly link 2′-deoxyadenine (dA) and could induce $G \rightarrow C$ at $T \rightarrow A$ transversion. If 8-OHdG is not efficiently eliminated, it accumulates in tissue and induces genomic instability and cells dysfunctions [17,32,33,35]. Usually, 8-oxoguanine-DNA-glycosylase (OGG1) is responsible for 8-OH-dG clean-up. OGG1 deficit induces high levels of 8-OH-dG in DNA. OGG1 overexpression in mitochondria improves its function, cell survival and reduces the number of DNA lesions by 8-OH-dG reparation in oxidative stress conditions, in vitro. These data suggest that OGG1 could play a protective role in inflammatory diseases. OGG1 polymorphism could offer susceptibility to lupus nephritis and modulate 8-OH-d G serum level in SLE patients [36–38].

Carbonylated proteins, nitrotyrosine and oxidated glutathione are stable chemical products and they are used as biomarkers in SLE [16]. Increased levels of nitrates, nitrites, homocysteine and oxidated serum proteins are associated with tissue lesions and SLE activity. High SLEDAI was correlated with low serum albumin in lupus nephritis [15]. Some studies in the last few years showed that thiol-disulfides interconversion plays a crucial role in antioxidant defense, apoptosis, detoxification, transcription, enzymatic activity regulation [20,37,38].

All these data suggest that SLE patients have high risk of developing oxidative stress-associated inflammatory response. The effects of pharmacological therapies on oxidative stress depend on chemical characteristics of reactive metabolites and action mechanisms consequences. Based on these data, the present study tries to determine a pattern of oxidative stress markers and endogenous strategies for suppression/modulating oxidative stress in SLE patients. The aim of the study was to detect deficiencies in protective system of cells in order to minimize the consequences of oxidative stress and to identify individualized pharmacological targets in SLE patients.

2. Results

2.1. Clinical Characteristics of the Studied Groups

The paraclinical characteristics of the studied groups are presented in Table 1. Classic biomarkers of lupus activity such as anti-ds DNA, UACR, C1q, C3 and C4 complement proteins were assessed. dsDNA was statistically significantly higher in LN and non-LN groups when compared with control group ($p < 0.05$), but it did not vary between SLE groups ($p > 0.05$). Urinary albumin: creatinine ratio was statistically significantly higher in LN group than in non-LN group ($p < 0.05$) or in control group ($p < 0.05$). C1q, C3 and C4 complement proteins were statistically significantly higher in LN group than in non-LN group ($p < 0.05$) or in control group ($p < 0.05$). Leucocytes and Hemoglobin were statistically significantly lower in SLE groups compared with the control group ($p < 0.05$), but without statistical variation between LN and non-LN subjects ($p > 0.05$). Albumin was statistically significantly lower in SLE groups, when compared with control ($p < 0.05$) and also in LN compared with non-LN group ($p < 0.05$). The estimated glomerular filtration rate was found to be lower in LN group than in non-LN group ($p < 0.05$) or in control group ($p < 0.05$). Renal tubular injury was evaluated by measuring the urinary levels of b2-microglobulin, that was found to be higher in LN group than in non-LN group

($p < 0.05$) or in control group ($p < 0.05$). Inflammation was assessed by determination of erythrocyte sedimentation rate and C reactive protein, and we found high inflammation in SLE groups compared with control ($p < 0.05$), but no significant variation between SLE groups ($p > 0.05$).

Table 1. Patients' characteristics.

Characteristics	SLE–Non-LN	LN	Control	p Significance
Number of patients	44	38	40	0.47
Women:Men ratio	2/1	2/1	2/1	0.89
Age (years)	42.6 ± 6.3	44.8 ± 5.5	43.7 ± 6.2	0.56
Disease duration (years)	6.4 ± 1.3	6.7 ± 1.1	–	0.28
SLEDAI	6.2 ± 4.7	7.4 ± 5.3	–	0.35
dsDNA (IU/mL)	320.1 ± 122.4	342.7 ± 98.2	80.2 ± 16.2	**0.02**
BMI (Kg/mp)	22.9 ± 1.7	23.0 ± 2.1	22.0 ± 3.3	0.64
Leucocytes (cells/mmc)	3800 ± 2008	4050 ± 1040	5860 ± 1070	**0.03**
Haemoglobin (g/L)	10.3 ± 1.1	10.8 ± 0.8	12.8 ± 1.2	**0.02**
Phosphorus (mg/dL)	3.6 ± 0.7	3.6 ± 0.9	3.7 ± 0.6	0.41
Calcium (mg/dL)	9.11 ± 0.4	9.18 ± 0.6	9.22 ± 0.57	0.28
LDH (U/L)	297 ± 65	307 ± 63	316 ± 57	0.08
Glycemia (mg/dL)	84.1 ± 11.3	78.7 ± 13.7	82.7 ± 11.4	0.11
ASAT (U/L)	19.4 ± 11.2	17.2 ± 8.4	19.2 ± 8.7	0.24
ALAT (U/L)	17.1 ± 13.2	16.2 ± 6.2	20.2 ± 10.3	0.08
Cholesterol (mg/dL)	152.5 ± 21.2	146.2 ± 24.1	142.5 ± 19.9	0.07
Triglycerides (mg/dL)	89.5 ± 12.7	81.4 ± 10.5	86.7 ± 15.5	0.23
Albumin (g/dL)	3.26 ± 0.25	3.68 ± 0.34	4.01 ± 0.44	**<0.04**
Urea (mg/dL)	35.4 ± 11.4	34.6 ± 0.7	30.2 ± 0.9	0.08
Creatinine (mg/dL)	1.0 ± 0.22	1.28 ± 0.11	0.77 ± 0.12	**0.02**
eGFR (mL/min/1.73 mp)	91.45 ± 12.23	82.17 ± 17.12	97.82 ± 7.22	**0.02**
Uric acid (mg/dL)	4.2 ± 1.3	3.8 ± 1.0	4.2 ± 1.2	0.13
UACR (mg/g creatinine)	10.81 ± 3.88	19.84 ± 2.97	7.34 ± 0.22	**0.03**
Haematuria (sw-RBC/camp)	5 ± 4	16 ± 7	3 ± 1	**0.02**
Leucocyturia (sw-leuc/camp)	5.3 ± 1.1	6.8 ± 0.9	3.8 ± 2.7	0.07
Urinary b2-microglobulin (mg/L)	0.22 ± 0.07	0.38 ± 0.14	0.12 ± 0.04	**0.04**
ESR (mm/h)	21.7 ± 17.1	24.5 ± 11.0	5.7 ± 5.0	**0.02**
CRP (mg/dL)	1.04 ± 0.72	1.29 ± 0.35	0.14 ± 0.12	**0.02**
C3 (mg/dL)	82.4 ± 21.2	70.5 ± 15.8	98.5 ± 25.1	**0.03**
C4 (mg/dL)	10.2 ± 1.7	7.4 ± 1.3	19.4 ± 9.3	**0.01**
C1q (mg/dL)	4.22 ± 0.95	3.02 ± 1.1	15.4 ± 6.3	**0.04**

SLEDAI—Systemic Lupus Erythematosus Disease Activity Index, BMI—body mass index; LDH—lactatdehydrogenase; ASAT—aspartate aminotransferase; ALAT—alanyl aminotransferase; eGFR—estimated glomerular filtration rate; UACR—urinary albumin: creatinine ratio; ESR—erythrocyte sedimentation rate; CRP—C reactive protein; p—statistical significance.

The clinical manifestations of SLE in non-LN and LN groups and the associated comorbidities are presented in Table 2.

Table 2. Clinical characteristics of the SLE groups.

Clinical Characteristics	SLE—Non-LN	LN	p Significance
Number of patients	44	38	0.47
Constitutional symptoms (fatigue, fever, weight loss)	40	33	0.07
Mucocutaneous (malar rash, alopecia, mucosal ulcers, discoid lesions)	41	3	**0.02**
Musculoskeletal (arthritis/arthralgia, myositis, avascular necrosis)	21	10	0.05
Neuropsychiatric involvement (depression, seizures, demyelinating syndromes, peripheral neuropathy)	3	1	0.26
Pulmonary manifestations (pleural effusion)	1	—	0.68
Cardiac manifestation (pericarditis)	1	—	0.68
Co-morbidities			
Arterial Hypertension	14	29	**0.04**
Heart failure	4	1	0.08
History of myocardial infarction	2	—	0.16
Chronic pulmonary disease	3	1	0.21
Diabetes mellitus without organ damage	2	1	0.37
Hepatic steatosis	3	1	0.22
Osteoporosis	1	3	0.18

2.2. Lipid Peroxidation Pattern in the Studied Groups

We evaluated lipid peroxidation pattern by determining serum levels of 4-HNE (μg/mL), TBARs (μmol/L), MDA (ng/mL), F2-Isoprostan (pg/mL) and ImAnOx (μmol/L). 4-HNE levels had an increase with 28.9% in non-LN group ($p > 0.05$) and with 43.22% in LN group ($p < 0.05$), when compared with control group. TBARs levels were statistically significantly higher with 52.76% in non-LN group ($p < 0.05$) and with 71.35% in LN group ($p < 0.01$), when compared with control group. MDA increased with 93.3% in non-LN group ($p < 0.05$) and with 73.9% in LN group ($p < 0.05$) compared with control group. F2-Isoprostan also increased with 240% in LN group ($p < 0.01$) and with 334% in non-LN group ($p < 0.01$) compared with control group ($p < 0.01$). ImAnOx decreased with statistical significance with 33.6% in LN group ($p < 0.01$), and 14.3% in non-LN group ($p < 0.01$) compared with control group. When comparing LN and non-LN groups, we detected a statistically significant increase in F2-Isoprostan and TBARS and decrease in ImAnOx in LN group ($p < 0.05$). 4-HNE, TBARs and F2-Isoprostan had statistically significantly higher levels, while ImAnOx had statistically significantly lower levels in type IV lupus nephritis patients, when compared with SLE non-LN control group. When comparing SLE–LN patients with type IV lupus nephritis patients, we did not detect any statistically significant variations. All results are presented in Table 3.

2.3. DNA Oxidation in Studied Groups

Oxidative DNA damage was evaluated by serum levels of 8-OHdG (ng/mL) and OGG1 status. 8-OHdG increased 1.16-fold in non-LN group ($p < 0.01$), 1.17-fold in LN group ($p < 0.01$), respectively 1.16 in type IV lupus nephritis ($p < 0.05$) compared with control group. There were no statistically significant variations between LN, type IV nephritis subjects and non-LN group. OGG1 did not vary significantly between non-LN and the control group, but in LN group it decreased 1.23-fold when compared with the control group ($p < 0.001$) and 1.28-fold when compared with non-LN group ($p < 0.001$). OGG1 did not vary significantly between SLE–LN and type IV LN subjects. All results are presented in Table 4.

Table 3. Lipid peroxidation pattern in the studied group.

Metabolites	SLE–Non LN	SLE–LN	Type IV Lupus Nephritis	Control	$p1$	$p2$
4-HNE (µg/mL)	18.17 ± 4.02	20.18 ± 6.08	19.92 ± 5.88	14.09 ± 1.42	0.04	AB = 0.04 AC = 0.04 AD = 0.04 BC = 0.07 BD = 0.02 CD = 0.02
TBARs (µmol/L)	3.04 ± 0.51	3.41 ± 0.66	3.39 ± 0.62	1.99 ± 0.14	0.03	AB = 0.04 AC = 0.03 AD = 0.006 BC = 0.05 BD = 0.003 CD = 0.004
MDA (ng/mL)	38.02 ± 5.37	35.11 ± 5.94	36.12 ± 6.01	20.18 ± 1.22	0.04	AB = 0.08 AC = 0.07 AD = 0.02 BC = 0.06 BD = 0.04 CD = 0.04
8-Isoprostan (pg/mL)	21.80 ± 6.14	27.87 ± 6.15	28.19 ± 5.88	6.41 ± 0.72	0.007	AB = 0.02 AC = 0.03 AD = 0.007 BC = 0.05 BD = 0.002 CD = 0.003
ImAnOx (µmol/L)	259.3 ± 61.2	201.0 ± 77.4	197.12 ± 72.3	302.6 ± 13.1	0.0004	AB = 0.03 AC = 0.04 AD = 0.001 BC = 0.04 BD = 0.0005 CD = 0.0004

4-HNE—4-hydroxy-2-nonenal, TBARs—Thiobarbituric acid reactive substances, MDA—Malondialdehyde, ImAnOX—Total antioxidative capacity, SLE—Systemic lupus erythematosus, LN—Lupus nephritis, p—Statistical significance, $p1$—Triple comparison of the groups, $p2$—Pairwise comparison of the groups, A—SLE non-LN, B—LN, C—type IV lupus nephritis, D—Control.

Table 4. DNA oxidation in studied groups.

Metabolite	SLE–Non LN	SLE–LN	Type IV Lupus Nephritis	Controls	$p1$	$p2$
8-OHdG (ng/mL)	3.58 ± 0.68	3.61 ± 0.81	3.59. ± 0.88	3.06 ± 0.43	0.007	AB = 0.08 AC = 0.08 AD = 0.005 BC = 0.07 BD = 0.005 CD = 0.005
OGG1 (pg/mL)	20.80 ± 2.26	16.21 ± 3.31	16.32 ± 3.61	20.04 ± 1.07	0.0006	AB = 0.0007 AC = 0.004 AD = 0.0004 BC = 0.09 BD = 0.0006 CD = 0.0005

8-OHdG—7,8-dihydro-8-oxo-2′-deoxyguanosine, OGG1—8-oxoguanine-DNA-glycosylase, SLE—Systemic lupus erythematosus, LN—Lupus nephritis, p—Statistical significance, $p1$—Triple comparison of the groups, $p2$—Pairwise comparison of the groups, A—SLE non-LN, B—LN, C—type IV lupus nephritis, D—Control.

2.4. Carbohydrate Oxidation in Studied Groups

Carbohydrate oxidation status was evaluated by assessment of serum pentosidine (ng/mL) and AGE (ng/mL)- sRAGE (pg/mL) axis. Pentosidine levels were 249% higher in non-LN group ($p < 0.01$), 276% higher in LN group ($p < 0.01$), and 278% higher in the type IV nephritis cohort ($p < 0.01$) when compared with the control group. Pentosidine did not vary significantly between LN, non-LN group and type IV nephritis groups. AGE levels were 216% higher in non-LN group ($p < 0.01$), 243% in LN group ($p < 0.01$), and 267% in type IV nephritis ($p < 0.01$), when compared with control group. sRAGE decreased with 7.6% in non-LN group ($p < 0.001$), with 5.8% in LN group ($p < 0.001$), with 5.5% in type IV nephritis ($p < 0.001$), when compared with the control group. Pentosidine, AGE and sRAGE vary insignificantly both between LN–Non-LN group, and LN–Type IV nephritis group. All results are presented in Table 5.

Table 5. Carbohydrate oxidation in studied groups.

Metabolite	SLE–Non LN	SLE–LN	Type IV Lupus Nephritis	Controls	p1	p2
Pentosidine (ng/mL)	3.91 ± 0.79	4.22 ± 0.85	4.26 ± 0.88	1.12 ± 0.13	0.002	AB = 0.05 AC = 0.06 AD = 0.009 BC = 0.18 BD = 0.006 CD = 0.005
AGE (ng/mL)	38.11 ± 4.61	41.38 ± 4.02	42.29 ± 4.62	12.04 ± 1.82	0.004	AB = 0.08 AC = 0.06 AD = 0.005 BC = 0.05 BD = 0.008 CD = 0.007
sRAGE (pg/mL)	963.1 ± 164.3	982.4 ± 201.7	986.12 ± 206.01	1043 ± 123.1	0.0009	AB = 0.06 AC = 0.05 AD = 0.001 BC = 0.07 BD = 0.0008 CD = 0.0004

AGE—Advanced glycation end products, sRAGE—Soluble receptor for advanced glycation end products—Systemic lupus erythematosus, LN—Lupus nephritis, p—Statistical significance, $p1$—Triple comparison of the groups, $p2$—Pairwise comparison of the groups, A—SLE non-LN, B—LN, C—type IV lupus nephritis, D—control.

2.5. Oxidized Protein Pattern in the Studied Groups

Protein oxidation was evaluated by serum levels of 3-nitrotyrosine (μmol/L), carbonylated proteins (PCO-μmol/L), native thiols (NT-μmol/L), total thiols (TT-μmol/L), disulphides (DS-μmol/L) and DS/NT, DS/TT and NT/TT ratios. Nitrotyrosine increased 2.23-fold in non-LN group ($p < 0.001$), and 3-fold in LN group ($p < 0.001$) when compared with control group. Nitrotyrosine varied statistically significantly between LN and non-LN group ($p < 0.001$). PCO increased 1.54-fold in non-LN group ($p < 0.01$), and 1.67-fold in LN group ($p < 0.01$) when compared with control group. PCO also varied statistically significantly between LN and non-LN group ($p < 0.01$). NT decreased by 1.12-fold in non-LN group ($p < 0.001$), and 1.23-fold in LN group ($p < 0.001$) when compared with the control group. NT varied statistically significantly between LN and non-LN group ($p < 0.001$). TT decreased 1-fold in non-LN group ($p < 0.001$), and 1.13-fold in LN group ($p < 0.001$) when compared with the control group. TT varied statistically significantly between LN and non-LN group ($p < 0.001$). DS increased 1.31-fold in non-LN group ($p < 0.001$), and 1.63-fold in LN group ($p < 0.001$) when compared with control group. DS varied statistically significantly between LN and non-LN group ($p < 0.001$). DS/NT increased 1.48-fold in non-LN group ($p < 0.001$), and 2.02-fold in LN group ($p < 0.001$) when compared with control group. DS/NT varied statistically significantly between LN and non-LN group ($p < 0.001$). DS/TT increased 1.58-fold in non-LN group ($p < 0.001$), and 2.06-fold in LN group ($p < 0.001$) when compared with the control group. DS/TT varied statistically significantly between LN and non-LN group ($p < 0.001$). NT/TT decreased 1.04-fold in non-LN group ($p < 0.001$), and 1.09-fold in LN group ($p < 0.001$) when compared with the control group. NT/TT varied statistically significantly between LN and non-LN group ($p < 0.001$). 3-NT, PCO, NT, TT, DS and DS/NT, DS/TT and NT/TT ratios had similar statistical variations when compared type IV lupus nephritis with SLE and controls and no statistical variations when compared with SLE–LN. All results are presented in Table 6.

Table 6. Oxidized protein pattern in the studied groups.

Metabolite	SLE–Non LN	SLE–LN	Type IV Lupus Nephritis	Controls	p1	p2
Nitrotyrosine (μmol/L)	0.29 ± 0.04	0.40 ± 0.11	0.39 ± 0.09	0.13 ± 0.02	0.0003	AB = 0.0003 AC = 0.0004 AD = 0.0004 BC = 0.31 BD = 0.0002 CD = 0.0004
PCO (μmol/L)	34.82 ± 5.84	37.72 ± 6.01	38.79 ± 6.11	22.51 ± 2.21	0.007	AB = 0.009 AC = 0.008 AD = 0.005 BC = 0.05 BD = 0.004 CD = 0.003
NT (μmol/L)	355.92 ± 8.53	324.21 ± 19.32	324.40 ± 18.81	401.83 ± 4.89	0.0008	AB = 0.005 AC = 0.004 AD = 0.0004 BC = 0.09 BD = 0.0007 CD = 0.008
TT (μmol/L)	407.23 ± 7.40	388.12 ± 6.89	387.99 ± 6.42	440.89 ± 4.78	0.0004	AB = 0.0008 AC = 0.0005 AD = 0.0004 BC = 0.09 BD = 0.0002 CD = 0.0002
DS (μmol/L)	25.65 ± 1.62	31.95 ± 2.97	31.40 ± 3.01	19.50 ± 0.53	0.0003	AB = 0.0006 AC = 0.0004 AD = 0.0004 BC = 0.12 BD = 0.0004 CD = 0.0005
DS/NT	7.21 ± 0.55	9.84 ± 0.72	9.47 ± 0.56	4.85 ± 0.15	0.0008	AB = 0.0005 AC = 0.0007 AD = 0.0002 BC = 0.22 BD = 0.0003 CD = 0.0003
DS/TT	6.30 ± 0.42	8.23 ± 0.76	8.34 ± 0.61	3.98 ± 1.27	0.0006	AB = 0.0007 AC = 0.0005 AD = 0.0004 BC = 0.08 BD = 0.0005 CD = 0.0004
NT/TT	87.39 ± 0.85	83.35 ± 0.94	83.69 ± 0.72	91.15 ± 0.25	0.0003	AB = 0.0007 AC = 0.0006 AD = 0.0003 BC = 0.07 BD = 0.0002 CD = 0.0004

PCO—Carbonylated proteins, NT—Native thiol, TT—Total thiol, DS—Disulphide, SLE—Systemic lupus erythematosus, LN—Lupus nephritis, p—Statistical significance, $p1$—Triple comparison of the groups, $p2$—Pairwise comparison of the groups, A—SLE non-LN, B—LN, C—type IV lupus nephritis, D—Control.

2.6. Correlation Analysis between the Different Parameters Studied in SLE Patients

The correlation between some parameters were studied both in SLE patients, and LN-SLE patients by Pearson coefficient. Correlations of different parameters in SLE patients are presented in Tables 7 and 8. We detected a negative, statistically significant correlation between ImAnOx and 4-HNE, TBARs, MDA, 8-oxo-dG and PCO. OGG-1 correlated negatively with statistical significance with 8-oxo-dG. NT and TT correlated negatively with statistical significance with 4-HNE, nitrotyrosine and PCO. DS correlated positively with statistical significance with TBARs, AGE, nitrotyrosine and PCO. DS/NT correlated positively, while DS/TT corelated negatively with nitrotyrosine and PCO. NT/TT negatively correlated with pentosidine, nitrotyrosine and PCO. sRAGE correlated negatively with pentosidine and AGE. Correlations of different parameters in LN patients are presented in Table 6. ImAnOx and 4-HNE, TBARs, MDA, F2Isoprostan, 8-oxo-dG and PCO. OGG-1 correlated negatively with statistical significance with 8-oxo-dG. NT and TT correlated negatively with statistical significance with 4-HNE, nitrotyrosine and PCO. DS correlated positively with statistical significance with TBARs, F2Isoprostan, 8-oxo-dG, pentosidine, AGE, nitrotyrosine and PCO. DS/NT correlated negatively with nitrotyrosine and PCOm while DS/TT corelated negatively only with PCO. NT/TT negatively correlated with pentosidine and PCO. sRAGE correlated negatively with pentosidine and AGE.

Table 7. Correlation analysis between studied parameters in SLE patients.

Metabolite	ImAnOx	OGG-1	NT	TT	DS	DS/NT	DS/TT	NT/TT	sRAGE
4-HNE	r = −0.42 p = 0.02	NS	r = −0.43 p = 0.02	r = −0.31 p = 0.04	NS	NS	NS	NS	NS
TBARs	r = −0.37 p = 0.02	NS	NS	NS	r = 0.26 p = 0.05	NS	NS	NS	NS
MDA	r = −0.23 p = 0.03	NS	NS	NS	NS	NS	NS	NS	NS
F2Isoprostan	NS	NS	NS	NS	NS	NS	NS	NS	NS
8-oxo-dG	r = −0.14 p = 0.04	r = −0.26 p = 0.04	NS	NS	NS	NS	NS	NS	NS
Pentosidine	NS	NS	NS	NS	NS	NS	NS	r = −0.34 p = 0.007	r = −0.29 p = 0.03
AGE	NS	NS	NS	NS	r = 0.45 p = 0.01	NS	NS	NS	r = −0.57 p = 0.007
Nitrotyrosine	NS	NS	r = −0.44 p = 0.006	r = −0.26 p = 0.008	r = 0.52 p = 0.002	r = 0.53 p = 0.01	r = −0.28 p = 0.04	NS	NS
PCO	r = −0.71 p = 0.0006	NS	r = −0.49 p = 0.02	r = −0.63 p = 0.006	r = 0.58 p = 0.03	r = 0.32 p = 0.04	r = −0.23 p = 0.04	r = −0.21 p = 0.04	NS

4-HNE—4-hydroxy-2-nonenal, TBARs—Thiobarbituric acid reactive substances, MDA—Malondialdehyde, ImAnOX—Total antioxidative capacity, 8-Oxo-dG—7,8-dihydro-8-oxo-2′-deoxyguanosin, OGG1—8-oxoguanine-DNA-glycosylase, AGE—Advanced glycation end products, sRAGE—Soluble receptor for advanced glycation end products, PCO—Carbonylated proteins, NT—Native thiol, TT—Total thiol, DS—Disulphide, SLE—Systemic lupus erythematosus, LN—Lupus nephritis, p—Statistical significance.

Table 8. Correlation analysis between studied parameters in LN patients.

Metabolite	ImAnOx	OGG-1	NT	TT	DS	DS/NT	DS/TT	NT/TT	sRAGE
4-HNE	r = −0.73 p = 0.007	NS	r = −0.51 p = 0.02	r = −0.38 p = 0.03	NS	NS	NS	NS	NS
TBARs	r = −0.62 p = 0.004	NS		NS	r = 0.26 p = 0.05	NS	NS	NS	NS
MDA	r = −0.45 p = 0.004	NS	NS	NS	NS	NS	NS	NS	NS
F2Isoprostan	r = −0.79 p = 0.008	NS	NS	NS	r = 0.62 p = 0.01	NS	NS	NS	NS
8-oxo-dG	r = −0.38 p = 0.01	r = −0.88 p = 0.0005	NS	NS	r = 0.44 p = 0.01	NS	NS	NS	NS
Pentosidine	NS	NS	NS	NS	r = 0.37 p = 0.03	NS	NS	r = −0.28 p = 0.04	r = 0.91 p = 0.0007
AGE	NS	NS	NS	NS	r = 0.29 p = 0.03	NS	NS	NS	r = 0.86 p = 0.0004
Nitrotyrosine	NS	NS	r = −0.39 p = 0.004	r = −0.42 p = 0.0006	r = 0.73 p = 0.0003	r = −0.28 p = 0.03	NS	NS	NS
PCO	r = −0.84 p = 0.0005	NS	r = −0.67 p = 0.02	r = −0.73 p = 0.004	r = 0.86 p = 0.03	r = −0.12 p = 0.04	r = −0.31 p = 0.01	r = −0.29 p = 0.04	NS

4-HNE—4-hydroxy-2-nonenal, TBARs—Thiobarbituric acid reactive substances, MDA—Malondialdehyde, ImAnOX—Total antioxidative capacity, 8-Oxo-dG—7,8-dihydro-8-oxo-2′-deoxyguanosin, OGG1—8-oxoguanine-DNA-glycosylase, AGE—Advanced glycation end products, sRAGE—Soluble receptor for advanced glycation end products, PCO—Carbonylated proteins, NT—Native thiol, TT—Total thiol, DS—Disulphide, SLE—Systemic lupus erythematosus, LN—Lupus nephritis, p—statistical significance.

3. Discussion

The results of the present study showed that SLE patients have a high risk of inflammatory responses associated with oxidative stress. The assessment of oxidized metabolites pattern and endogenous strategies for suppression or modulating oxidative stress in SLE patients with or without renal impairment could be relevant in differential regulation of cellular response for preventing the progression of the renal manifestations. We determined a large panel of oxidative damage serum metabolites and endogenous protective mechanisms in SLE patients and a control group. The comparative analysis of oxidized metabolites pattern and antioxidative capacity in SLE with all type lupus nephritis, in type IV lupus nephritis, and in SLE without renal impairment aimed to determine possible deficiencies in protective system of the cells and some humoral biomarkers for detection of renal impairment in SLE patients.

The comparative analysis of lipoperoxidation process by simultaneous determination of 4-HNE, TBARs, MDA and F2-isoprostan in SLE patients and controls demonstrated higher levels of lipoperoxidation-derived reactive carbonyl species in SLE and LN compared with the control group. LN patients have statistically significantly higher levels of TBARs and F2-isoprostan, comparative with SLE non-LN patients. These major oxidative degradations were accompanied by low levels of ImAnOx in SLE patients versus controls. Serum antioxidants inactivation was more accentuated in LN patients compared with non-LN patients. ImAnOx capacity of blocking lipoperoxides formation or blocking lipids peroxidation propagation was demonstrated in this paper by negative association between lipid metabolites levels and antioxidant capacity of serum. Based on these results, we could appreciate that ImAnOx diminishing and F2-isoprostan increase are associated with LN development. As a parameter of oxidative deterioration, F2-isoprostan is considered by some publications as a useful oxidative stress biomarker [39,40]. F2 isoprostan varies according to pathologies; it has very low levels in cancer or cardiovascular diseases, very high in respiratory diseases and uro-genital disorders, or its value varies with clinical features [40] or inflammation, such as in SLE [39]. F2-isoprostan does not present specificity for oxidative stress due to the synthesis mechanisms. In our study, serum variability of F2-isoprostan in SLE and LN was caused by the level of oxidative stress, both SLE groups being characterized by a low inflammatory state. F2-isoprostan is useful in identifying patients at risk of developing LN.

Some studies show that lipid peroxidation plays a major role in SLE pathogenesis. SLE patients had higher levels of MDA and 8-OHdG and lower levels of TAS compared with controls. Circulant levels of MDA, 8-OhdG and TAS in patients with SLEDAI over six were statistically significant modified comparative with patients with SLEDAI below six. MDA presented a positive correlation and TAS a negative correlation with SLEDAI. Remarkable also is the high MDA/TAS ratio, in patients with neuro-psychiatric manifestations and vasculitis in SLE, high levels of oxidized low density lipoprotein cholesterol in SLE patients with thrombocytopenia and vasculitis [41]. Increases of MDA and 8-OhdG, and decreases of TAS were associated with disease activity. ROS role in SLE was evaluated by aldehydes specific immune complexes derived from lipids. These data sustain a possible relation between oxidative stress, anti-species carbonyl reactive, pathogenic mechanisms and prognosis in SLE [42]. A recent study evaluated oxidative stress markers, inflammation and biomarkers of activity in SLE and detected significant differences between active and inactive lupus nephritis for MDA, total and oxidated GSH, TAS, CRP, MCP 1, beta 2-microglobulin, urinary protein/creatinine ratio, dsDNA antibodies, anti-C1q antibodies and C3, C4. These data show a redox disequilibrium in patients with lupus nephritis determined by lipid peroxidation, process that affects glomerular basal membrane integrity and renal tubular function in these patients [43].

An interesting finding of our study, relevant for oxidative stress in SLE was represented by elevated oxidative DNA damage levels and defective DNA repair mechanisms via OGG1. Oxidative DNA lesions were overexpressed both in non-LN and LN groups comparative to controls. OGG1 has the ability to catalyze lesions excision of 8-oxo-dG type and assure genomic integrity in SLE patients. OGG1 capacity of DNA repair and of 8-oxo-dG serum levels modulating in LN patients is highly altered. Based on these results, we consider that 8-oxo-dG/OGG1 ratio could offer information about LN development risk. DNA alteration by oxidative stimuli, DNA repair mechanisms dysfunctions and immune response alteration in cellular defense were intensively studied in the last years [3]. DNA alteration could induce aberrant activation of innate immunity, and, associated with chronic inflammation, could stimulate DDR/R network. ROS and RNS generated by inflammatory cells promote 8-oxo-dG and 8-nitro-dG overexpression resulting in the alteration of the repair mechanisms of DNA lesions. Still, in SLE, there is proved a bidirectional interaction between DDR/R and immune response induced by oxidative stress. DDR/R network and immune innate response act synergistically for the survival of all living organisms. Epigenetically regulated functional abnormalities of DNA repair mechanisms could lead to increased accumulation of DNA lesions. This accumulation facilitates the production of autoantibodies, the generation of damaged cytosolic DNA and micronuclei that can act as powerful stimulators of the immune system by over-expression of the cGAS-STING-IRF3 path and the production of type I IFN, leading to the systemic expression of autoimmune diseases [3,14,32].

Rigorous research of carbohydrate oxidation in this study showed profound alteration of the AGE–RAGE axis in patients with SLE and LN. The harmful effect of AGE on human tissues was proved by excessive production of RAGE ligands in the studied patients. Thus, serum levels of AGE and pentosidine were significantly increased in patients with SLE and LN compared to control. The toxic action of AGE was limited by sRAGE. The protective effect of sRAGE was well expressed in patients with SLE. On the other hand, the ability of sRAGE to block activation of RAGE in patients with LN was affected. The different behavior of sRAGE in SLE with or without LN could be sustained by negative correlation between AGE, and pentosidine and sRAGE in non-LN patients and their positive association in LN patients. It can be interpreted that an increased amount of AGE in patients' blood leads to increased consumption of sRAGE. These findings support the quality of sRAGE as a biomarker to differentiate patients with SLE at risk of kidney injury. Recent findings suggest that the occurrence of SLE depends on the interactions between genetic background and risk factors, such as exposure to oxidative stimuli. Chronic inflammation associated with SLE disturbs the oxidant/antioxidant balance. These processes are related to the excess accumulation of AGE. Lately, the accumulation of AGE in the skin in patients with autoimmune diseases and the expression of corresponding receptors gain the attention of researchers. These AGE compounds could be found in inflamed tissues. The reference data present in the literature show a link between oxidative stress, AGE formation and autoimmune diseases such as SLE [44,45]. The most representative AGEs are pentosidine, carboxymethyllysine (CML) and carboxiethyllysine (CEL). The high levels of AGEs in patients' blood are still being discussed. Some authors indicated that there were no significant differences between SLE patients and controls regarding plasma levels of CML and CEL. AGE levels did not correlate with CRP. The authors suggested that AGE accumulated mainly in tissues and plasma proteins [45,46]. Additionally, the level of pentosidine did not increase in the blood of patients with SLE. Some patients with increased fructosamine showed remarkably high levels of pentosidine. Other authors demonstrated an increase in plasma AGE in patients with SLE. In addition, the levels of CML and pentosidine showed a positive correlation with the SLEDAI score.

Other RAGE ligands, such as S100A12 levels are similar in SLE and healthy subjects, while levels of S100A8/A9 and S100A12 correlate with cardiovascular risk in SLE patients [47–49]. RAGE ligands appear to be mostly related to inflammation, hyperglycation and cellular stress processes; expression of the receptor itself being directly related to inflammation [50,51].

sRAGE can bind to RAGE, blocking its functions and leading to an improved expression of the molecules involved in inflammation, adhesion and RAGE itself [47].

RAGE expression is also enhanced by TNF-α. It remains unknown whether patients with SLE have autoantibodies against RAGE/sRAGE, but sRAGE functions are insufficient studied in this pathology [9]. A low amount of sRAGE has been detected in Sjogren's syndrome, though a possible link between SLE and visual disturbances could be established [47]. Contradictory data on the level of sRAGE have been reported in SLE patients. Some authors have reported increased concentrations of sRAGE in the serum of lupus patients [45]. Additionally, sRAGE positively correlates with SLEDAI [52]. Other studies showed the decreased levels of sRAGE in the plasma of SLE patients compared to control. Notably, SLE patients treated or untreated have similar levels of sRAGE, while subjects who received long-term treatment have a higher concentration of soluble receptor than subjects receiving short-term one. Short-term treatment induces a rapid decrease in sRAGE levels compared to long-term one. It is suggested that the receptor has a different role in the initial and progressive stage of the disease [47,48]. In addition, patients with SLE who have antiphospholipid antibodies (APA) or antiphospholipid syndrome (APS) have shown a decrease in sRAGE plasma levels compared to control [53]. sRAGE level is associated with leukocytes lymphocytes, neutrophils and monocytes number and with C4 levels, but it does not correlate with the presence of autoantibodies. sRAGE therefore participates in the development of inflammation and the recruitment of leukocytes. RAGE and sRAGE have the ability to interact with each other and with multiple ligands, and they are directly related to the immune. These processes increase the oxidative stress in the body. AGE and RAGE with sRAGE deficiency can cause the formation of neoepitopes, and of autoantibodies [47].

Finally, we found that changes in oxidative proteins and TDH regulators play a central role in the cellular response to oxidative stress. In this paper, it was found that 3-nitrotyrosine, carbonylated proteins and disulfides were overexpressed in patients with SLE and LN compared to the healthy population. The circulating level of 3-nitrothyrosine was significantly increased in patients with LN versus patients with SLE non-LN. The ability of TDH to maintain redox homeostasis of cells has also been demonstrated by the inverse association between the concentrations of sulfhydryl groups and oxidized proteins in both SLE and LN. Through their dynamics, the DS/TN, DS/TT, TN/TT ratios can be potential serum biomarkers that have managed to differentiate between SLE patients, those that will develop LN. Our findings suggest that protein oxidation may play a substantial role in the pathogenesis of chronic kidney damage in patients with SLE. These results reconfirm data from previously published studies regarding levels of multiple markers of protein oxidation. SOD and myeloperoxidase activities were increased, while thiol protein levels, glutathione peroxidase and catalase activities were reduced in serum of SLE patients compared to controls. Disease activity markers were positively correlated with erythrocyte sedimentation rate and carbonylated protein levels, 3-nitrosyrosine and CRP, and negatively correlated with protein thiol levels and SOD, glutathione peroxidase and catalase activities in patients with SLE. There were significant differences in serum levels of carbonylated proteins between patients with and without kidney disease [54].

Lipid peroxides (LOOH), advanced oxidation protein products (AOPP), nitrogen oxides (NOx), sulfhydryl groups (−SH), oxidative degradation products of deoxyribonucleic acid (DNA)/ribonucleic acid (RNA) and antioxidant parameter of radicals' uptake (TRAP) participates in SLE immune pathophysiology and modulates disease severity and adhesion molecule expression [55–57]. Another study showed that increased protein oxidation correlated with SLEDAI score and dsDNA levels [58]. Other publications have shown that oxidative stress is involved in the pathogenesis of LN. Higher levels of serum AOPP have been associated with an increased risk of LN. In contrast, neither high levels of dsDNA nor low levels of C3 were independent risk factors for LN [59]. Evaluation of the prooxidant–antioxidant balance (PAB) showed increased values in patients with SLE with alopecia, discoid rash, oral ulcers, arthritis and nephritis. These findings suggest that PAB measurement may be useful to show the state of oxidative stress in patients with SLE [60].

To resume, the present study is the first one in the literature that presents a pattern of oxidative stress markers and endogenous strategies for suppression/modulating oxidative stress in SLE patients. However, some limitations should be noted. Our study followed patients with SLE non-LN and LN, for a period of three years, only with chronic immunosuppressant treatment. Further studies with a larger number of patients with different therapeutic regimens should be developed. Most of the patients included in the study had type IV nephritis. For a better evaluation of oxidant/antioxidant axis in SLE a larger number of patients with all types of nephritis are needed, although it would be very hard to identify these patients because they have minimal symptoms. In LN patients, it is very important to identify as early as possible the patients at risk for LN development, in order to avoid invasive interventions and to establish an effective medical intervention.

4. Materials and Methods

4.1. Study Participants

The present study is prospective–observational and included 82 SLE patients and 40 healthy subjects. All the patients signed the informed consent, the Declaration of Helsinki from 1975 was respected. The study was developed between 2018 and 2021, and patients over 18 years old were selected from those who attended the Clinical Hospital of Nephrology "Carol Davila" and Clinical Hospital "Victor Babes". The study protocol was approved by the Ethics Committee of Clinical Hospital of Nephrology "Carol Davila" (11/23.07.2018). Of these 82 SLE patients, 44 had SLE with cutaneous and hematological determinations, but no lupus nephritis (non-LN group), while 38 had lupus nephritis (LN group) diagnosed by biopsy puncture and histological exam according to KDIGO guidelines. The activity and chronicity index of lupus nephritis was evaluated and it is presented in Table 9. In LN patients, 7% had type II LN, 18% had type III LN, 70% had type IV and 5% type V. SLE diagnosis was established according to Systemic Lupus International Collaborating Clinics/American College of Rheumatology criteria. The activity disease was based on clinical Systemic Lupus Erythematosus Disease Activity Index (SLEDAI). The time lapse of disease and ongoing treatment (non-steroidal anti-inflammatory drugs, corticosteroids, hydroxychlorochine, immunosuppressant drugs such as azathioprine, mycophenolate mophetil, antihypertensive therapy) were recorded for each patient. The exclusion criteria were the presence of any cardiovascular, hepatic, thyroid, gastrointestinal, or oncological disease, any viral or bacterial infections in the last three months, tobacco use, drug abuse, alcoholism, use of vitamin or other antioxidant supplements, and pregnancy.

Table 9. Activity and chronicity index in lupus nephritis.

NIH Activity Indices		Number of Patients
Endocapillary proliferation	0	—
	1	4
	2	15
	3	19
Glomerular leucocyte infiltration	0	1
	1	4
	2	12
	3	15
Hialin deposits/wire loops	0	9
	1	14
	2	10
	3	5

Table 9. Cont.

NIH Activity Indices		Number of Patients
Fibrinoid necrosys (x2)	0	7
	1	11
	2	8
	3	9
Cellular of fibrocellular crescents (x2)	0	16
	1	10
	2	7
	3	5
Interstitial inflammation	0	-
	1	10
	2	16
	3	12
Chronicity indices		
Global glomerulosclerosys	0	21
	1	8
	2	5
	3	4
Fibrous crescents	0	27
	1	6
	2	3
	3	2
Tubular atrophy	0	24
	1	8
	2	4
	3	2
Interstitial fibrosis	0	15
	1	12
	2	6
	3	2
	4	3

4.2. Laboratory Data

The blood samples were collected from all the study participants, after signing the informed consent, who fasted 12 h, using a holder-vacutainer system and ×3000 g, for ten minutes, after one hour of keeping at room temperature. The sera were separated and frozen at −80 degrees before analyzing.

4-HNE and MDA were assessed by competitive ELISA method (semi-automatic Tecan analyzer). The wells were pre-coated with substrate and the final product colorimetric evaluation was made at 450 nm. The results were expressed as microgram/mL serum for 4-HNE and as nanogram/mL serum for MDA. MDA forms a complex with thiobarbituric acid reactive substances (TBARS) that is measured using the spectrophotometric method (BS-3000M Semi-Automatic Chemistry Analyzer) and read at a wave-length of 532 nm. The results were expressed as µmol/L serum. 8-Isoprostan was determined by competitive ELISA method (semi-automatic Tecan analyzer). The wells were pre-coated with substrate to acetylcholinesterase and the final product colorimetric evaluation was made at 412 nm. Results were expressed in pg/mL. ImAnOx was assessed by spectrophotometry (semi-automatic Tecan analyzer). by the reaction of antioxidants in the sample with a defined amount of exogenously provided hydrogen peroxide. The antioxidants in the sample eliminate a certain amount of the provided hydrogen peroxide. The residual H_2O_2 is determined photometrically at 450 nm. Results were expressed in μmol/L.

8-OHdG was determined by competitive ELISA method (semi-automatic Tecan analyzer). The wells were pre-coated with a target specific capture antibody and the final product colorimetric evaluation was made at 450 nm. Results were expressed in ng/mL. OGG1 was determined by ELISA method, quantitative sandwich (semi-automatic Tecan analyzer). The wells were pre-coated with a target specific capture antibody and the final product colorimetric evaluation was made at 450 nm. Results were expressed in pg/mL.

Pentosidine and AGEs were assessed by ELISA method (semi-automatic Tecan analyzer). The wells were pre-coated with a target specific capture antibody and the final product colorimetric evaluation was made at 450 nm. Results were expressed in ng/mL. sRAGE was determined using the sandwich ELISA method (immunoenzymatic kits-R&D SYSTEMS (DR600 and SRG00 kits), USA), the results were read at 450 nm, using a TECAN analyzer (Tecan, Switzerland). The sensitivity of the method was 16.14 pg/mL and assay range was between 78 and 5000 pg/mL.

Circulant 3-NT was determined by ELISA method using the R&D systems reactive (MAB3248 kit) and a TECAN analyzer (Tecan, Switzerland).

Carbonyl groups were assessed by spectrophotometric methods, in reaction with 2,4-dinythrophenylhydrasine that generated hydrazone, employing the HumanStar300 analyzer (HUMAN Gesellschaft für Biochemica und Diagnostica mbH, Weisbaden, Germany) and Merck reactives (MAK094 kit).

Thiol disulphide homeostasis parameters (TDHPs) were determined using a spectrophotometric method The dynamic and reducible disulfide bonds were transformed into free functional thiol groups by using sodium borohydride ($NaBH_4$, 10 mM) as follows:

$R-S_2-R' + NaBH_4 \rightarrow 2\ R-SH + BH_3 + Na$.

Subsequently, the amount of $NaBH_4$, which have not participated in the reaction, was removed with formaldehyde (10 mM, pH 8.2). The levels of native thiol (TN) and total thiol (TT) were assessed using 5,5'-dithiobis-2-nitrobenzoic acid (DTNB, 10 mM) as follows:

$R-SH + DTNB \rightarrow R-TNB + TNB$.

The final product, 2-nitro-5-thiobenzoate (TNB), ionized at alkaline pH and turned yellow. An automatic biochemistry analyzer (HumaSTAR 300, (HUMAN Gesellschaft für Biochemica und Diagnostica mbH, Weisbaden, Germany) and Merck reactives were used. This technique allows for the assessment of functional disulfide bonds in the sample. Disulfide (DS) level was calculated as half of the difference between TT and NT. The levels of TT, NT and DS were expressed as μmol/L serum. The disulfide/native thiol ratio (DS/NT), disulfide/total thiol ratio (DS/TT), and native thiol/total thiol ratio (NT/TT) were calculated and expressed as %. TDHPs were represented by:

- NT (-SH), determined by a spectrophotometric method;
- TT (-SH + -S-S-), determined by a spectrophotometric method;
- DS (-S-S), determined by calculation;
- DS/NT (-S-S- * 100/-SH) was calculated;
- DS/TT (-S-S- * 100/-SH + -S-S-) was calculated;
- NT/TT (-SH * 100/-SH + -S-S-) was calculated.

4.3. Statistical Analysis

We used mean and standard deviation for data presentation. We compared the data using either the analysis of variance (ANOVA) with Tukey post hoc test or Kruskal–Wallis test with Dunn's post hoc test for normally and non-normally distributed data. The relation between the studied parameters was assessed by Pearson's correlation coefficient, but before the assessment, data normality by the Kolmogorov–Smirnov test was evaluated. The level of significance (p) chosen was 0.05 (5%) and the confidence interval was 95% for hypothesis testing and the corresponding ethical approval code.

5. Conclusions

SLE is a chronic autoimmune disease with complex pathogenesis, characterized by oxidative stress and high inflammatory state. The cellular response to oxidative stimuli in this pathology is concreted in the amplification of oxidative degradation of lipids, proteins, nucleic acid, and hydro carbonates, and in alteration of endogenous strategies for suppressing/modulating oxidative stress. The defective DNA repair mechanism via OGG1, the reduced regulatory effect of sRAGE in the activation of AGE-RAGE axis, low levels of thiols, disulphide bonds formation and high nitrotyrosination are important characteristics of lupus nephritis in our study and they could explain alteration of renal architecture and development of renal injury in SLE. All these data help us to establish a panel of biomarkers in order to identify as early as possible the patients at risk for LN development, thus avoiding invasive interventions such as renal biopsy, and establishing an effective treatment as soon as possible from diagnosis. The identification of more molecular mechanisms to counteract oxidative stress in LN could permit a more precise assessment of disease prognosis, as well as the development of new therapeutic targets.

Author Contributions: All authors have equally contributed to the writing and editing of the manuscript. Conceptualization, C.D.E., and I.N.; methodology, I.N.; software, C.D.E.; validation, C.D.E., I.N., S.R.G., and M.N.P.; formal analysis, I.N.; investigation, C.D.E.; resources, M.T., S.R.G., C.M.; data curation, C.D.E., S.R.G.; writing—original draft preparation, C.D.E., C.I.M., M.I.M.; writing—review and editing, C.D.E., M.N.P., C.M., M.T.; visualization, S.R.G., C.I.M., M.I.M., C.M.; supervision, S.R.G., I.N., M.T. All authors have read and agreed to the published version of the manuscript.

Funding: This research received no external funding.

Institutional Review Board Statement: The study was conducted according to the guidelines of the Declaration of Helsinki, and approved by the Ethics Committee of Clinical Hospital of Nephrology "Carol Davila" (11/23.07.2018).

Informed Consent Statement: Informed consent was obtained from all subjects involved in the study.

Data Availability Statement: The data presented in this study are available on request from the corresponding author.

Conflicts of Interest: The authors declare no conflict of interest.

References

1. Piga, M.; Arnaud, L. The Main Challenges in Systemic Lupus Erythematosus: Where Do We Stand? *J. Clin. Med.* **2021**, *10*, 243. [CrossRef] [PubMed]
2. Crincoli, V.; Piancino, M.G.; Iannone, F.; Errede, M.; Di Comite, M. Temporomandibular Disorders and Oral Features in Systemic Lupus Erythematosus Patients: An Observational Study of Symp-toms and Signs. *Int. J. Med. Sci.* **2020**, *17*, 153–160. [CrossRef] [PubMed]
3. Souliotis, V.L.; Vlachogiannis, N.I.; Pappa, M.; Argyriou, A.; Ntouros, P.A.; Sfikakis, P.P. DNA Damage Response and Oxidative Stress in Systemic Autoimmunity. *Int. J. Mol. Sci.* **2020**, *21*, 55. [CrossRef]
4. Wang, L.; Law, H.K.W. Immune Complexes Impaired Glomerular Endothelial Cell Functions in Lupus Nephritis. *Int. J. Mol. Sci.* **2019**, *20*, 5281. [CrossRef] [PubMed]
5. Mendoza, F.G.; Sansón, S.P.; Rodríguez-Castro, S.; Crispín, J.C.; Rosetti, F. Mechanisms of Tissue Injury in Lupus Nephritis. *Trends Mol. Med.* **2018**, *24*, 364–378. [CrossRef]
6. Wolff, K.; Goldsmith, L.; Katz, S.; Gilchrest, B.; Paller, A.S.; Leffell, D. *Fitzpatrick's Dermatology in General Medicine*, 7th ed.; McGraw-Hill: New York, NY, USA, 2008.
7. Elder, D.E. *Lever's Histopathology of the Skin*, 7th ed.; Lippincott Williams & Wilkins: Philadelphia, PA, USA, 1999.
8. Marnett, L.J. Oxy radicals, lipid peroxidation and DNA damage. *Toxicology* **2002**, *181*, 219–222. [CrossRef]
9. Wang, G.; Pierangeli, S.S.; Papalardo, E.; Ansari, G.A.; Khan, M.F. Markers of oxidative and nitrosative stress in systemic lupus erythematosus: Correlation with disease activity. *Arthritis Rheum.* **2010**, *62*, 2064–2072. [CrossRef]
10. Avalos, I.; Chung, C.P.; Oeser, A.; Milne, G.L.; Morrow, J.D.; Gebretsadik, T.; Shintani, A.; Yu, C.; Stein, C.M. Oxidative stress in systemic lupus erythematosus: Relationship to disease activity and symptoms. *Lupus* **2007**, *16*, 195–200. [CrossRef]
11. Perl, A. Oxidative stress in the pathology and treatment of systemic lupus erythematosus. *Nat. Rev. Rheumatol.* **2013**, *9*, 674–686. [CrossRef] [PubMed]

12. Wang, Y.; Andrukhov, O.; Fan, X.R. Oxidative stress and antioxidant system in periodontitis. *Front. Physiol.* **2017**, *8*, 910. [CrossRef]
13. Ene, C.D.; Ceausu, E.; Nicolae, I.; Tampa, M.; Matei, C.; Georgescu, S.R. Ultraviolet radiation, Vitamin D and Autoimmune Disorders. *Rev. Chim. Buc.* **2015**, *66*, 1068–1073.
14. Lee, T.H.; Kang, T.H. DNA Oxidation and Excision Repair Pathways. *Int. J. Mol. Sci.* **2020**, *20*, 6092. [CrossRef] [PubMed]
15. Lalwani, P.; de Souza, G.K.; de Lima, D.S.; Passos, L.F.; Boechat, A.L.; Lima, E.S. Serum thiols as a biomarker of disease activity in lupus nephritis. *PLoS ONE* **2015**, *10*, e0119947. [CrossRef]
16. Shah, D.; Mahajan, N.; Sah, S.; Nath, S.K.; Paudial, B. Oxidative stress and its biomarkers in systemic lupus erythematosus. *J. Biomed. Sci.* **2014**, *21*, 23. [CrossRef] [PubMed]
17. Popp, H.D.; Kohl, V.; Naumann, N.; Flach, J.; Brendel, S.; Kleiner, H.; Weiss, C.; Seifarth, W.; Saussele, S.; Hofmann, W.K.; et al. DNA Damage and DNA Damage Response in Chronic Myeloid Leukemia. *Int. J. Mol. Sci.* **2020**, *21*, 1177. [CrossRef] [PubMed]
18. Tampa, M.; Nicolae, I.; Ene, C.D.; Sarbu, I.; Matei, C.; Georgescu, S.R. Vitamin C and thiobarbituric acid reactive substances (TBARS) in psoriasis vulgaris related to psoriasis area severity index (PASI). *Rev. Chim.* **2017**, *68*, 43–47. [CrossRef]
19. Mitran, M.I.; Nicolae, I.; Tampa, M.; Mitran, C.I.; Caruntu, C.; Sarbu, M.I.; Ene, C.D.; Matei, C.; Georgescu, S.R.; Popa, M.I. Reactive Carbonyl Species as Potential Pro-Oxidant Factors Involved in Lichen Planus Pathogenesis. *Metabolites* **2019**, *9*, 213. [CrossRef]
20. Van't Erve, T.J.; Kadiiska, M.B.; London, S.J.; Mason, R.P. Classifying oxidative stress by F2-isoprostane levels across human diseases: A meta-analysis. *Redox Biol.* **2017**, *12*, 582–599. [CrossRef]
21. Vistoli, G.; de Maddis, D.; Cipak, A.; Zarkovic, N.; Carini, M.; Aldini, G. Advanced glycoxidation and lipoxidation end products (AGEs and ALEs): An overview of their mechanisms of formation. *Free Radic. Res.* **2013**, *1*, 23–27. [CrossRef] [PubMed]
22. Eichhorst, A.; Daniel, C.; Rzepka, R.; Sehnert, B.; Nimmerjahn, F.; Voll, R.E.; Chevalier, N. Relevance of Receptor for Advanced Glycation end Products (RAGE) in Murine Antibody-Mediated Autoimmune Diseases. *Int. J. Mol. Sci.* **2019**, *20*, 3234. [CrossRef]
23. Viedma-Poyatos, Á.; González-Jiménez, P.; Langlois, O.; Company-Marín, I.; Spickett, C.M.; Pérez-Sala, D. Protein Lipoxidation: Basic Concepts and Emerging Roles. *Antioxidants* **2021**, *10*, 295. [CrossRef]
24. Manganelli, V.; Truglia, S.; Capozzi, A.; Alessandri, C.; Riitano, G.; Spinelli, F.R.; Ceccarelli, F.; Mancuso, S.; Garofalo, T.; Longo, A.; et al. Alarmin HMGB1 and Soluble RAGE as New Tools to Evaluate the Risk Stratification in Patients With the Antiphospholipid Syndrome. *Front. Immunol.* **2019**, *14*, 460. [CrossRef] [PubMed]
25. Mitran, C.; Nicolae, I.; Tampa, M.; Mitran, M.; Caruntu, C.; Sarbu, M.; Ene, C.D.; Matei, C.; Ionescu, C.; Georgescu, S.R.; et al. The Relationship between the Soluble Receptor for Advanced Glycation End Products and Oxidative Stress in Patients with Palmoplantar Warts. *Medicina* **2019**, *55*, 706. [CrossRef] [PubMed]
26. Martens, H.A.; Nienhuis, H.L.; Gross, S.; van der Steege, G.; Brouwer, E.; Berden, J.H.; de Sévaux, R.G.; Derksen, R.H.; Voskuyl, A.E.; Berger, S.P.; et al. Receptor for advanced glycation end products (RAGE) polymorphisms are associated with systemic lupus erythematosus and disease severity in lupus nephritis. *Lupus* **2012**, *21*, 959–968. [CrossRef] [PubMed]
27. Gowry, B.; Shahriman, A.B.; Paulraj, M. Electrical bio-impedance as a promising prognostic alternative in detecting breast cancer: A review. In Proceedings of the 2015 2nd International Conference on Biomedical Engineering (ICoBE), Penang, Malaysia, 30–31 March 2015; pp. 1–6.
28. Lee, S.W.; Park, K.H.; Park, S.; Kim, J.H.; Hong, S.Y.; Lee, S.K.; Choi, D.; Park, Y.B. Soluble receptor for advanced glycation end products alleviates nephritis in (NZB/NZW) F1 mice. *Arthritis Rheum.* **2013**, *65*, 1902–1912. [CrossRef]
29. Myles, A.; Viswanath, V.; Singh, Y.P.; Aggarwal, A. Soluble receptor for advanced glycation endproducts is decreased in patients with juvenile idiopathic arthritis (ERA category) and inversely correlates with disease activity and S100A12 levels. *J. Rheumatol.* **2011**, *38*, 1994–1999. [CrossRef]
30. Ma, C.Y.; Ma, J.L.; Jiao, Y.L.; Li, J.F.; Wang, L.C.; Yang, Q.R.; You, L.; Cui, B.; Chen, Z.J.; Zhao, Y.R. The plasma level of soluble receptor for advanced glycation end products is decreased in patients with systemic lupus erythematosus. *Scand. J. Immunol.* **2012**, *75*, 614–622. [CrossRef]
31. Pullerits, R.; Bokarewa, M.; Dahlberg, L.; Tarkowski, A. Decreased levels of soluble receptor for advanced glycation end products in patients with rheumatoid arthritis indicating deficient inflammatory control. *Arthritis Res. Ther.* **2005**, *7*, R817–R824. [CrossRef]
32. Peluso, M.; Russo, V.; Mello, T.; Galli, A. Oxidative Stress and DNA Damage in Chronic Disease and Environmental Studies. *Int. J. Mol. Sci.* **2020**, *21*, 6936. [CrossRef]
33. Tumurkhuu, G.; Chen, S.; Montano, E.N.; Ercan Laguna, D.; de Los Santos, G.; Yu, J.M.; Lane, M.; Yamashita, M.; Markman, J.L.; Blanco, L.P.; et al. Oxidative DNA Damage Accelerates Skin Inflammation in Pristane-Induced Lupus Model. *Front. Immunol.* **2020**, *11*, 554725. [CrossRef]
34. Nicolae, I.; Ene, C.D.; Matei, C.; Tampa, M.; Georgescu, S.R.; Ceausu, E. Effects of UV radiations and oxidative DNA adduct 8-hydroxy-2'-deoxyguanosine on the skin diseases. *Rev. Chim.* **2014**, *65*, 1036–1041.
35. Dinu, L.; Ene, C.D.; Nicolae, I.; Tampa, M.; Matei, C.; Georgescu, S.R. The serum levels of 8-hydroxy-deoxyguanosine under the chemicals influence. *Rev. Chim.* **2014**, *65*, 1319–1326.
36. Lee, Y.M.; Song, B.C.; Yeum, K.J. Impact of Volatile Anesthetics on Oxidative Stress and Inflammation. *Biomed Res. Int.* **2015**, 242709–242720. [CrossRef] [PubMed]
37. Wang, K.; Maayah, M.; Sweasy, J.B.; Alnajjar, K.S. The role of cysteines in the structure and function of OGG1. *J. Biol. Chem.* **2020**, *296*, 100093. [CrossRef]

38. Ene, C.D.; Penescu, M.N.; Georgescu, S.R.; Tampa, M.; Nicolae, I. Posttranslational Modifications Pattern in Clear Cell Renal Cell Carcinoma. *Metabolites* **2021**, *11*, 10. [CrossRef]
39. Clayton, D.B.; Stephany, H.A.; Ching, C.B.; Rahman, S.A.; Tanaka, S.T.; Thomas, J.C.; Pope, J.C., 4th; Adams, M.C.; Brock, J.W., 3rd; Clark, P.E.; et al. F2-isoprostanes as a biomarker of oxidative stress in the mouse bladder. *J Urol.* **2014**, *191* (Suppl. S5), 1597–1601. [CrossRef]
40. Milne, G.L.; Musiek, E.S.; Morrow, J.D. F2-isoprostanes as markers of oxidative stress in vivo: An overview. *Biomarkers* **2005**, *10*, 10–23. [CrossRef] [PubMed]
41. Shruthi, S.; Thabah, M.M.; Zachariah, B.; Negi, V.S. Association of Oxidative Stress with Disease Activity and Damage in Systemic Lupus Erythematosus: A Cross Sectional Study from a Tertiary Care Centre in Southern India. *Ind. J. Clin. Biochem.* **2020**. [CrossRef]
42. Wang, G.; Pierangeli, S.S.; Willis, R.; Gonzalez, E.B.; Petri, M.; Khan, M.F. Significance of Lipid-Derived Reactive Aldehyde-Specific Immune Complexes in Systemic Lupus Erythematosus. *PLoS ONE* **2016**, *11*, e0164739. [CrossRef]
43. Bona, N.; Pezzarini, E.; Balbi, B.; Daniele, S.M.; Rossi, M.F.; Monje, A.L.; Basiglio, C.L.; Pelusa, H.F.; Arriaga, S.M.M. Oxidative stress, inflammation and disease activity biomarkers in lupus nephropathy. *Lupus* **2020**, *29*, 311–323. [CrossRef]
44. Nowak, A.; Przywara-Chowaniec, B.; Tyrpień-Golder, K.; Nowalany-Kozielska, E. Systemic lupus erythematosus and glycation process. *Cent. Eur. J. Immunol.* **2020**, *45*, 93–98. [CrossRef] [PubMed]
45. Nienhuis, H.L.; de Leeuw, K.; Bijzet, J.; Smit, A.; Schalkwijk, C.G.; Graaff, R.; Kallenberg, C.G.; Bijl, M. Skin autofluorescence is increased in systemic lupus erythematosus but is not reflected by elevated plasma levels of advanced glycation endproducts. *Rheumatology* **2008**, *47*, 1554–1558. [CrossRef] [PubMed]
46. De Leeuw, K.; Graaff, R.; de Vries, R.; Dullaart, R.P.; Smit, A.J.; Kallenberg, C.G.; Bijl, M. Accumulation of advanced glycation endproducts in patients with systemic lupus erythematosus. *Rheumatology* **2007**, *46*, 1551–1556. [CrossRef] [PubMed]
47. Bayoumy, N.; El-Shabrawi, M.; Nada, H. A soluble receptor for advanced glycation end product levels in patients with systemic lupus erythematosus. *Arch. Rheumatol.* **2013**, *208*, 101–108. [CrossRef]
48. Tydén, H.; Lood, C.; Gullstrand, B.; Jönsen, A.; Nived, O.; Sturfelt, G.; Truedsson, L.; Ivars, F.; Leanderson, T.; Bengtsson, A.A. Increased serum levels of S100A8/A9 and S100A12 are associated with cardiovascular disease in patients with inactive systemic lupus erythematosus. *Rheumatology* **2013**, *52*, 2048–2055. [CrossRef] [PubMed]
49. Wang, H.; Zeng, Y.; Zheng, H.; Liu, B. Association Between sRAGE and Arterial Stiffness in Women with Systemic Lupus Erythematosus. *Endocr. Metab. Immun. Disord. Drug Targets* **2021**, *21*, 504–510. [CrossRef]
50. Sirois, C.M.; Jin, T.; Miller, A.L.; Bertheloot, D.; Nakamura, H.; Horvath, G.L.; Mian, A.; Jiang, J.; Schrum, J.; Bossaller, L.; et al. RAGE is a nucleic acid receptor that promotes inflammatory responses to DNA. *J. Exp. Med.* **2013**, *210*, 2447–2463. [CrossRef]
51. Schmidt, A.M.; Yan, S.D.; Yan, S.F.; Stern, D.M. The multiligand receptor RAGE as a progression factor amplifying immune and inflammatory responses. *J. Clin. Investig.* **2001**, *108*, 949–955. [CrossRef]
52. Abou-Raya, A.N.; Nabi Kamel, M.A.; Ghani Sayed, E.A.; Hamid El-Sharkawy, A.A. The plasma level of soluble receptor for advanced glycation end products in systemic lupus erythematosus patients and its relation to disease activity. *Alexandria J. Med.* **2016**, *52*, 151–157. [CrossRef]
53. Tang, K.T.; Hsieh, T.Y.; Chao, Y.H.; Lin, M.X.; Chen, Y.H.; Chen, D.Y.; Lin, C.C. Plasma levels of high-mobility group box 1 and soluble receptor for advanced glycation end products in primary antiphospholipid antibody syndrome patients. *PLoS ONE* **2017**, *12*, e0178404. [CrossRef]
54. Zhang, Q.; Ye, D.Q.; Chen, G.P.; Zheng, Y. Oxidative protein damage and antioxidant status in systemic lupus erythematosus. *Clin. Exp. Dermatol.* **2010**, *35*, 287–294. [CrossRef]
55. Scavuzzi, B.M.; Simão, A.N.C.; Iriyoda, T.M.V.; Lozovoy, M.A.B.; Stadtlober, N.P.; Franchi Santos, L.F.D.R.; Flauzino, T.; de Medeiros, F.A.; de Sá, M.C.; Consentin, L.; et al. Increased lipid and protein oxidation and lowered anti-oxidant defenses in systemic lupus erythematosus are associated with severity of illness, autoimmunity, increased adhesion molecules, and Th1 and Th17 immune shift. *Immunol. Res.* **2018**, *66*, 158–171. [CrossRef] [PubMed]
56. Georgescu, S.R.; Ene, C.D.; Tampa, M.; Matei, C.; Benea, V.; Nicolae, I. Oxidative stress-related markers and alopecia areata through latex turbidimetric immunoassay method. *Mater. Plast.* **2016**, *53*, 522–526.
57. Iriyoda, T.M.V.; Stadtlober, M.A.B.; Lozovoy, F.; Delongui, N.T.; Costa, E.M.V.; Reiche, I.; Dichi, A.N.C. Reduction of Nitric Oxide and DNA/RNA Oxidation Products Are Associated with Active Disease in Systemic Lupus Erythematosus Patients. *Lupus* **2017**, *26*, 1106–1111. [CrossRef] [PubMed]
58. Morgan, P.E.; Sturgess, A.D.; Davies, M.J. Increased levels of serum protein oxidation and correlation with disease activity in systemic lupus erythematosus. *Arthritis Rheum.* **2005**, *52*, 2069–2079. [CrossRef] [PubMed]
59. Xie, Z.; Zhang, M.; Zhao, B.; Wang, Q.; Li, J.; Liu, Y.Y.; Chen, Y.H. Advanced oxidation protein products as a biomarker of cutaneous lupus erythematosus complicated by nephritis: A case-control study. *Genet. Mol. Res.* **2014**, *13*, 9213–9219. [CrossRef]
60. Jafari, S.M.; Salimi, S.; Nakhaee, A.; Kalani, H.; Tavallaie, S.; Farajian-Mashhadi, F.; Zakeri, Z.; Sandoughi, M. Prooxidant-Antioxidant Balance in Patients with Systemic Lupus Erythematosus and Its Relationship with Clinical and Laboratory Findings. *Autoimmune Dis.* **2016**, *2016*, 4343514. [CrossRef]

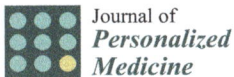

Article

Prevalence and Characteristics of Psoriasis in Romania—First Study in Overall Population

Alin Codruț Nicolescu [1], Ștefana Bucur [2,3,*], Călin Giurcăneanu [2,4], Laura Gheucă-Solovăstru [5], Traian Constantin [2,6], Florentina Furtunescu [2,7], Ioan Ancuța [2,8] and Maria Magdalena Constantin [2,3]

1. Roma Medical Center for Diagnosis and Treatment, 011773 Bucharest, Romania; nicolescualin66@yahoo.com
2. IIIrd Department, "Carol Davila" University of Medicine and Pharmacy, 050474 Bucharest, Romania; calin.giurcaneanu@gmail.com (C.G.); traianc29@yahoo.com (T.C.); florentina.furtunescu@umfcd.ro (F.F.); iancuta@hotmail.com (I.A.); drmagdadinu@yahoo.com (M.M.C.)
3. IInd Department of Dermatology, Colentina Clinical Hospital, 020125 Bucharest, Romania
4. Department of Dermatology, Elias University Emergency Hospital, 011461 Bucharest, Romania
5. Department of Dermatology, "Sf. Spiridon" Clinical Hospital, "Grigore T. Popa" University of Medicine and Pharmacy, 700115 Iași, Romania; lsolovastru13@yahoo.com
6. Department of Urology, "Th. Burghele" Hospital, 050652 Bucharest, Romania
7. Department of Public Health and Management, 050463 Bucharest, Romania
8. Department of Rheumatology, "Dr. I. Cantacuzino" Clinical Hospital, 020475 Bucharest, Romania
* Correspondence: stefanabucur11@gmail.com

Abstract: *Background:* Psoriasis is a chronic inflammatory disease characterized by an excessive hyperproliferation of keratinocytes and a combination of genetic, epigenetic, and environmental influences. The pathogenesis of psoriasis is complex and the exact mechanism remains elusive. *Objectives:* The study of the prevalence of psoriasis will allow the estimation of the number of people suffering from this condition at the national level, as well as the development and validation of a questionnaire to estimate the prevalence and the risk factors associated with the disease. *Methods:* A quantitative research was conducted at a national level among the target population in order to validate the questionnaire and estimate the national prevalence. *Results:* Declaratively, the prevalence of psoriasis in the studied group (N = 1500) is 4%, the first symptoms appearing around the age of 50, with a certified diagnosis being made on average at 55 years. The prevalence of psoriasis vulgaris was 4.99%. *Conclusions:* The results obtained will be useful in guiding future initiatives and communication campaigns related to this condition, and the methodological approach used will provide the opportunity to make recommendations for improving similar initiatives in the future.

Keywords: psoriasis vulgaris; prevalence; comorbidities; risk factors

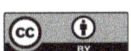

1. Introduction

Psoriasis is a chronic, inflammatory, genetically determined skin condition, with a frequency of 1–3% in the general population [1]. The onset of the disease frequently occurs around the age of 20 or around the age of 40, and the negative consequences of psoriasis should be emphasized: in young people at the beginning of their careers it often leads to their underestimation, and in working adults it often leads to premature retirement. Among the dermatological conditions, psoriasis takes the first place in terms of deterioration of life quality index, ahead of malignant skin diseases. Psoriasis impairment to psychological quality of life is comparable to cancer, myocardial infarction, and depression [2]. Psoriasis therefore has a debilitating influence both physically and mentally on the patient's daily life. Standard diagnostic criteria for epidemiological studies of psoriasis are currently lacking. In their absence, clinical examination and diagnosis of psoriasis by dermatologists provides the gold standard to underpin epidemiological research in psoriasis [3].

Psoriasis has been declared by the World Health Organization the fifth most important chronic non-contagious disease, along with diseases such as diabetes, cancer, cardiovascular or respiratory diseases. Statistics show that there are over 125 million patients in the world and Romania ranks first in Europe, having approximately 400,000 people with this condition [4]. A total of 20–30% of patients with psoriasis also develop psoriatic arthritis, which over time leads to severe, deforming joint injuries, which often cause disability [5]. In the absence of a set of specific criteria for the diagnosis of psoriatic arthritis, the most commonly used method for recognizing and monitoring this condition remains the clinical aspect [6].

In Romania, psoriasis remains a common, immune-mediated disease, with increasing prevalence. This publication quantifies the prevalence of psoriasis in Romania, its potentially genetic background, and the importance of environmental factors in triggering it [7], including the role of the diet [8,9] and other factors, such as vitamin D deficiency [10].

Psoriatic subjects represent an important target for health care issues and further epidemiological studies. The estimates provided can help guide countries and the international community when making public health decisions on the appropriate management of psoriasis.

2. Objectives

It is thought that there are more undiagnosed or untreated patients beyond those who have been diagnosed. This study aims to develop and validate a screening questionnaire for the early, presumptive identification of psoriasis in the general population and to estimate the prevalence of people suffering from this condition at a national level.

In order to achieve the objectives, quantitative research was conducted at a national level among the general adult population (people over 18 years old in urban and rural areas in Romania).

3. Materials and Methods

The study was performed in two stages. Stage 1 involved the development of the questionnaire and construction of the predictive model. Within this stage, the questionnaire was developed by a mixed team of experts (dermatologists, epidemiologists, sociologists), the methodology was finalized, and standardized working procedures were developed.

Stage 2 involved the validation of the questionnaire and the estimation of the national prevalence. At this stage, a national study was conducted on a representative sample of 1500 adult individuals. From this total of 1500 people to whom the questionnaire was applied, a subgroup of 500 people was randomly selected and received in addition a clinical examination aiming to diagnose the eventual presence of psoriasis.

Detailed description of the study.

The first stage of the study was conducted between November 2018–February 2019, on two groups of subjects: the group with psoriasis (288 patients with psoriasis selected from the offices of dermatologists from all over the country) and the control group (222 healthy people randomly selected from the general population). The inclusion criteria were: adults over 18 years old, from rural and urban areas in Romania, without a diagnosis of psoriasis (healthy group); or those with a previous diagnosis of psoriasis (affected group). The only exclusion criterion was represented by institutionalized persons. Both groups received a questionnaire applied through face-to-face interviews and underwent parallel dermatologic examination.

The questionnaire included three sections: (i) a general part referring to demographic characteristics; (ii) a screening part with specific questions regarding the existence of symptoms and the history of dermatological diseases; (iii) a section of a detailed characterization of the person from a social and clinical point of view. During this first stage, both the research tool (questionnaire) and the logistical organization and field activity management tools were tested. This activity was carried out by field operators with experience in conducting household surveys.

A predictive model has been elaborated by performing a logistic regression applied to the pilot data. The discriminative variables were: (1) the symptoms of psoriasis (presence and nature of skin and nail lesions, including the occurrence of stress for all forms of psoriasis) and the symptoms and signs of arthritis for the arthropathic form; (2) the presence of hereditary collateral antecedents; (3) smoking at the time of the study; (4) history of pharyngitis in childhood for the presence of arthropathy; (5) history of obesity, but not obesity at the time of the study; (6) depression due to the arthropathic nature of psoriasis; (7) treatment; (8) some psycho-emotional and contextual characteristics. The proposed questionnaire was reviewed and updated according to the relevant variables.

The second stage of the study was conducted in 2019 on a group of 1500 respondents over the age of 18 on a nationally representative group. The national study used a three-stage stratified probabilistic grouping model. The questionnaire was applied in a "face-to-face" interview by specialized interview operators. A total of 500 randomly selected individuals from this group underwent clinical examination performed by a dermatologist at the nearest medical unit to the home of the person included in the group. The application of the questionnaire at the same time with the performance of clinical examinations allowed the validation of the questionnaire and the establishment of its specific parameters (sensitivity, specificity, accuracy, predictive value).

In a further step, the prevalence of psoriasis was estimated at the national level.

The national sample selection used a stratified three-step probabilistic grouping pattern in which places were selected with PPS (probability proportional to size) in the first step. Households were systematically selected in the second step and only one individual from each household was selected by SRS (simple random sample) using mobile data collection devices. The first step consisted in the selection of localities (stratification was performed according to the environment of residence (urban or rural) and type of urban/rural locality: in urban areas, stratification was performed by size of locality: small town (less than 50,000 inhabitants), medium town (50,000–199,999 inhabitants) and large city (over 200,000 inhabitants). In rural areas, the stratification was carried out taking into account two types of rural localities: localities with up to 5000 inhabitants and localities with over 5000 inhabitants, depending on the number of questionnaires required, the sampling points were calculated for each locality. In the following step, starting from the selected group points, the systematic selection of households that were included in the research was performed. Prior to this stage, the households were identified and included in a list from which the selection of those that were part of the group was made (mapping and listing). In the last step, 1500 individuals were randomly selected.

The interviews were conducted with people over the age of 18 who actually lived at the address selected from the group. In each identified household, the questionnaire was applied to one person. If there were several eligible persons in the household (more than two over the age of 18) the questionnaire was applied to one person who was randomly selected. If the selected person was not at home at the time of the first visit and was absent for less than 30 days (the person was at work, on a delegation, on holiday etc.), a new visit to the household was scheduled. In this regard, at least three attempts (visits) were made to interview the selected person. The validation of the group was performed according to the official statistical data provided by the National Institute of Statistics [11].

Within the project, a software application was developed that allowed both data collection and management of the activity of conducting clinical examinations at a national level. The application was a client server type. The samples and the collected data were stored in the server component both after applying the questionnaire and as a result of clinical examinations. The clients of the application were represented by the face-to-face interview operators and by the doctors involved in performing the clinical examinations.

The coordination, monitoring, and supervision of the field activity were carried out by a field coordinator with experience. The activity which involved data collection at a local level was coordinated and supervised by the county coordinators, the data collection being ensured by a specialized network of interview operators. Dermatologists and nurses were recruited to perform clinical examinations from the dermatology medical offices who expressed their acceptance to participate in the study. After performing the clinical examinations, the specialists sent the results to the headquarters according to the established working procedures.

The statistical analysis was performed with the R system. Mean ± standard deviation and/or median have been calculated for the scale variables and proportions for the qualitative ones. Comparisons were performed using the t-test and ANOVA for quantitative research, normally distributed variables and the chi-square or Fisher test for qualitative. The logistic regression has been used to construct the predictive model. Sensitivity and specificity have been calculated for the questionnaire in relation to the gold standard dermatological diagnosis for psoriasis. A 95% confidence interval was calculated for the psoriasis prevalence in general population.

The demographic profile included: gender, age group, level of education, occupation, residence environment (urban, rural), region of economic development (Northeast, Southeast, South, Southwest, West, Northwest, Center, Bucharest). The clinical profile and personal medical history of the respondents included details on symptoms, frequency of symptoms, determining factors, associated conditions, previous diagnosis of dermatological disease, the age of onset of symptoms, personal medical history. The use of medical services for dermatological diseases was analyzed in terms of the following characteristics: previous treatments for dermatological conditions and their type, specific clinical examinations performed, accessed services.

The diagnosis in psoriasis for the subjects performing the dermatological examination was a clinical one (observation of erythematous and squamous patches, generalized or localized in specific areas, itching, burning or soreness, thickened, pitted or ridged nails, swollen and stiff joints). During the medical consultation, personal and family history and risk factors were also evaluated. A subgroup of 500 people randomly selected were invited to participate in a specialized clinical examination performed by a dermatologist in a medical office in order to analyze the association between the questionnaire and the real status of the subjects and to explore the validity and prediction of the questionnaire. The subgroup had similar geographic and demographic characteristics and similar history of the disease (Table 1).

Table 1. Comparative analysis of the groups according to the main demographic variables in stage 2 of the study.

Criteria	No.	%	No.	%	p-Value *
Region					
Bucharest-Ilfov	173	11.5%	58	11.6%	
Center	176	11.7%	59	11.8%	
Northeast	261	17.4%	87	17.4%	
Northwest	191	12.7%	63	12.6%	
South	220	14.7%	73	14.6%	
Southeast	193	12.9%	64	12.8%	
Southwest	146	9.7%	50	10.0%	
West	140	9.3%	46	9.2%	
Total	1500	100.0%	500	100.0%	>0.99
Environment					
Rural	638	42.5%	210	42.0%	
Urban	862	57.5%	290	58.0%	
Total	1500	100.0%	500	100.0%	0.834

Table 1. Cont.

Criteria	No.	%	No.	%	p-Value *
Gender					
Men	726	48.4%	241	48.2%	
Women	774	51.6%	259	51.8%	
Total	1500	100.0%	500	100.0%	0.938
Age groups					
18–29	264	17.6%	92	18.4%	
30–49	611	40.7%	202	40.4%	
50+	625	41.7%	206	41.2%	
Total	1500	100.0%	500	100.0%	0.921
Education					
No studies	2	0.1%	1	0.2%	
Primary	102	6.8%	35	7.0%	
Secondary	650	43.3%	222	44.4%	
Tertiary	746	49.7%	242	48.4%	
Total	1500	100.0%	500	100.0%	0.947
Declared diagnostic history					
Yes	63	4.2%	21	4.2%	
No	1437	95.8%	479	95.8%	
Total	1500	100.0%	500	100.0%	>0.99

* Test Chi^2.

Selected subjects were asked to give their consent for the examination. From the 500 selected subjects, 18 did not agree to participate to the clinical examination and another 21 agreed, but did not show up at the dermatologist. The study algorithm is shown in Figure 1.

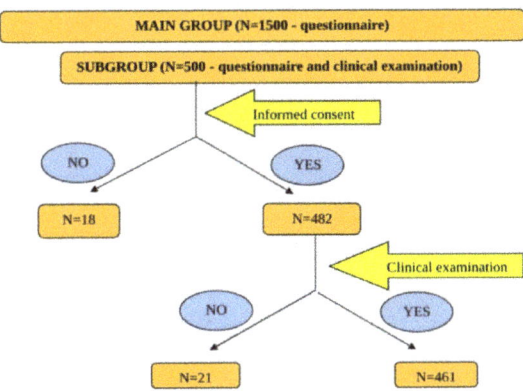

Figure 1. The study algorithm.

The diagnosis in psoriasis was a clinical one (observation of erythematous and squamous patches, generalized or localized in specific areas, itching, burning or soreness, thickened, pitted or ridged nails, swollen and stiff joints). During the medical consultation personal and family history and risk factors were also evaluated.

4. Results

Declaratively, the prevalence of psoriasis in the studied group (N = 1500) reached 4.2%, the first symptoms appearing around the age of 50 and a competent diagnosis being required by the patients around the age of 55. A series of studies carried out all over the world suggests that Caucasians are more affected than other races, with higher prevalence percentages, unlike Australian Aborigines, the pre-Colombian population of the New World, Andean Indians, Amerindians, Alaskan, Canadian, or Native Americans of the United States, where psoriasis has been reported to be extremely rare or absent [12]. Interestingly, late-onset psoriasis is slightly more common than the early-onset type, contrary to the often quoted convention that 75% of new psoriasis cases are present before the age of 40 [13].

Neither the environment, urban/rural, nor the type of locality presents statistical data or is associated with the presence of psoriasis for the 1500 individuals or for the 461 remaining subjects from the subgroup of 500 randomly selected individuals in the second stage of the study (Table 2). In contrast with an Italian study [14], psoriasis did not seem to be homogeneously distributed across the northern, central, and southern geographical areas of the country, findings which are similar to a study in Spain [15]. These variations in prevalence rates between regions are not unusual and are explained by different genetic and/or financial and stress conditions.

Table 2. Demographic characteristics depending on the presence of psoriasis vulgaris.

Variable	No.	%	p-Value–Nonhealthy-Healthy
Region			
Bucharest-Ilfov	56	12%	
Center	40	9%	
Northeast	87	19%	
Northwest	55	12%	
South	69	15%	0.089
Southeast	59	13%	
Southwest	49	11%	
West	46	10%	
Total	461	100%	
Environment			
Rural	194	42%	
Urban	267	58%	0.251
Total	461	100%	
Gender			
Men	221	48%	
Women	240	52%	0.104
Total	461	100%	
Age groups			
18–29	81	18%	
30–49	189	41%	0.188
50+	191	41%	
Total	461	100%	

Table 2. Cont.

Variable	No.	%	p-Value–Nonhealthy-Healthy
Education			
No studies	1	0%	
Primary	34	7%	
Secondary	201	44%	0.76
Tertiary	225	49%	
Total	461	100%	

The psoriatic patients, but not the healthy group, were usually supervised by the doctor, with a few exceptions (although they were selected by a doctor, perhaps the exceptions indicate a lack of understanding of the question). With rare exceptions, psoriatic patients report that they follow a treatment; no subject who is considered healthy is considered to be under treatment. Patients with psoriasis had significantly more frequent relatives with psoriasis than the healthy group.

Skin lesions appeared significantly more frequently in psoriatic patients than healthy people, but also in 3/4 of healthy people. Lesions of the elbows or knees have been reported very frequently by psoriatic patients and very rarely by healthy people. To a lesser extent, the lesions on the scalp, hands, feet, back, and to a very small extent other skin lesions had a differentiating value. An association with psoriasis in general is also observed for scales, pruritus, red areas, bleeding areas, frequent in psoriasis, but quite common in healthy people. The same association shows the disappearance with local treatment. Persistence of lesions does not appear to be associated with psoriasis, but the occurrence of lesions under stress, including pruritus, was reported more frequently by psoriatic patients. Increasing evidence over the past decade has shown that pruritus can be one of the most prevalent and burdensome symptoms associated with psoriasis, affecting almost every patient to some degree [16]. Spontaneous disappearance is relatively rare, but more common in healthy people. Small nail stains are reported significantly more frequently by psoriatic patients than healthy ones and nail loss is rare in both psoriatic and healthy individuals (Table 3).

Table 3. Results and data analysis of the national study (N = 1500 respondents).

Monitored by a Doctor	Local Treatment	Family Member with Psoriasis	Skin Lesions 25%		Types of Lesions 26%	Characteristics of the Lesions	Nail Changes
47.9%	44%	A form of psoriasis 9%	Hands 48%	Elbows 19%	Erythema 82%	Disappear spontaneously 52%	Nail yellowing 19%
75.8%—by a dermatologist	Only on lesions 88%	Psoriatic arthritis 2%	Feet 46%	Knees 17%	Pruritus 69%	Disappear and reappear depending on the local treatment 52%	Nail stains 19%
15.2%—by a family doctor	Phototherapy 17%		Face 30%	Nails 15%	Scales 33%	In correlation with stress 39%	Onychomadesis/nail loss 6%
6.1%—other doctors	NSAIDs 13%		Back 25%	Genitals 13%	Pigmentation disorders 29%	Persistent without improvement 36%	
	Other 4%		Abdomen 24%	Ears 9%	Papules/Pustules 18%		

Table 3. Cont.

Monitored by a Doctor	Local Treatment	Family Member with Psoriasis	Skin Lesions 25%		Types of Lesions 26%	Characteristics of the Lesions	Nail Changes
			Thorax 20%	All over the body 6%	Hemorrhagic areas 17%		
			Scalp 19%	Other areas 6%	Other 8%		

Comorbidities and strong related conditions are detailed in Table 4. Smoking is significantly more common in psoriatic patients than healthy people and also, the age of the onset of smoking does not make a difference. There is no difference between a former smoker or a passive smoker and the gross variables regarding the intensity of smoking exposure do not show, individually, differences between the studied groups. The link between alcohol consumption seems vague, the only more convincing association being with the concern of loved ones in the last year, which is significantly more common in those with psoriasis. The report of pharyngitis in childhood was insignificantly more frequent in psoriasis, but the reports of hospitalizations for pharyngitis in childhood were significantly more common in psoriasis. There were no significant differences in height, body weight, or maximum body mass in the groups. The diagnosis of depression as well as the treatment were significantly more frequently associated with psoriasis. Patients with mild psoriasis can experience psychiatric comorbidities; however, depression is more common in patients with severe psoriasis or psoriatic arthritis [17].

Table 4. Comorbidities and related conditions resulting from the national study (N = 1500 respondents).

Comorbidities and Related Conditions					
Arterial hypertension	31%	Following a treatment 82%			
Dyslipidemia	22%	Following a treatment 42%			
Diabetes mellitus	10%	Following a treatment 85%			
Depression/ Anxiety	10%	Following a treatment 45%			
Infections	30% pharyngitis and tonsillitis during childhood	12% hospitalized for these diseases			
Obesity	17% yes, 3% from childhood	1 out of 5 was diagnosed with obesity at some point in life			
Stress, life style	1 out of 3 cannot cope with the important things in life	2 out of 5 sometimes feel that the difficulties have accumulated to such an extent that they can no longer control them			
Alcohol	Never 23%	1 time/month 36%	2–4 times/month 29%	>4 times/month 12%	
Smoking	Average age of onset—20 years 45%	Currently smokers 51%	Average smoking period— 15 years	Passive smoking 25%	Exposure to smoke during childhood 74%

Of the 500 subjects selected for clinical examination, 461 attended the visit.

In this study group, the prevalence for psoriasis vulgaris was 4.99% (2.95: 7.03). The concordance between the initial diagnosis, established on the basis of the questionnaire and the final clinical diagnosis was 99.13% for psoriasis vulgaris. An acceptable sensitivity of the questionnaire more than 85% and a specificity of almost 100% were identified.

Regarding the treatment for psoriasis, only 2 of the clinically confirmed cases of the disease reported following treatment, while 7 did not receive treatment and 15 did not answer the question. Only one subject who considered himself healthy declared to be under treatment. Some psoriasis patients, even some dermatologists, are quite reluctant to undertake biologic therapy [18], even though it has demonstrated real efficacy in treatment of psoriasis and psoriatic arthritis [19], but novel biologics act by novel targets, technology, and mechanisms of action compared to previously approved biologics and the explosive development of biological therapy and the emergence of biosimilars, revolutionary tools against the most serious and provocative diseases which represent a significant success in the effort to provide advanced healthcare to patients all over the world [20–22]. To complete these results, an interesting study provides useful data on widely used biologic drugs and their tolerability, discontinuation rate, and the incurrence of severe adverse events [23].

We have detailed the data obtained from the national study regarding healthy and non-healthy groups in Table 5. Regarding the hereditary factors, patients with psoriasis significantly more frequently had relatives with psoriasis compared to those without disease. This result was also confirmed in the initial group. The frequency of reported skin and nail lesions differ significantly between the psoriatic patients and the disease-free, unlike the initial group in which the yellowing of the nails was significantly associated with the certified diagnosis of psoriasis. Regarding smoking, the only significant difference was identified for smoking exposure in the last 12 months, present in 21.1% of psoriatic patients and in none of the healthy patients. Moreover, alcohol consumption in the last year has never been significantly associated with an increased likelihood of the disease. Regarding infections, the data correspond to the results of stage 1. Many systemic therapies available for the management of psoriasis patients who cannot be treated with more conservative options, such as topical agents and/or phototherapy, can worsen or reactivate a chronic infection. Therefore, before administering immunosuppressive therapies it is mandatory to screen patients for some infections, including hepatitis B or C [24,25]. Metabolic syndrome is a highly prevalent, multifaceted condition characterized by a constellation of abnormalities that include abdominal obesity, hypertension, dyslipidemia, and elevated blood glucose [26]. The frequency of obesity was not significantly different between the psoriatic and the non-psoriatic patients (Table 5). Psychological stress has long been shown to play an important role in the natural history of psoriasis, but the details of this relationship remain to be clearly defined [27]. In the initial group, 5% of the interviewees stated that they often felt that they could not cope with the important things in life. In the diagnostic group, the proportion of those who chose the "very often" option on this question was 4.2% in non-patients and 8.7% in those with psoriasis, respectively. The difference did not reach statistical significance ($p = 0.342$).

Table 5. Results and data analysis of the national study (N = 1500 respondents).

	Nonhealthy		Healthy		*p*-Value
	Number	%	Number	%	
Hereditary factors					
Relative with psoriasis	17	70.8%	32	7.3%	<0.001
Skin and nail lesions					
Skin lesions	8	33.3%	118	27.0%	0.54
Nail lesions	4	16.7%	79	18.1%	0.58
Nail yellowing	4	16.7%	88	20.1%	0.46

Table 5. Cont.

	Nonhealthy		Healthy		p-Value
	Number	%	Number	%	
Onychomadesis	2	8.3%	23	5.3%	0.38
Smoking					
Ever smoked for at least 2 years	11	45.8%	165	37.8%	0.279
Currently smoker	3	12.5%	82	18.8%	0.248
Former smoker	8	33.3%	80	18.3%	0.179
Exposure in the last 12 months	0	0.0%	92	21.1%	0.004
Exposure in childhood	18	75.0%	325	74.4%	0.581
Alcohol					
Alcohol consumption ever in the last year	16	66.7%	332	76.0%	0.303
Infections					
Pharyngitis/tonsillitis during childhood	11	45.8%	102	23.3%	0.028
Hospitalization	6	25.0%	57	13.0%	0.009
Obesity					
BMI > 25	18	75.0%	224	51.3%	0.216
Ever been obese	8	33.3%	74	16.9%	0.053
Obesity during childhood	0	0.0%	18	4.1%	0.375
Arterial hypertension	9	37.5%	146	33.4%	0.663
Diabetes mellitus	4	16.7%	45	10.3%	0.307
Depression/Anxiety	5	20.8%	40	9.2%	0.073
Dyslipidemia	10	41.7%	115	26.3%	0.104

5. Discussion

In our study we elaborated a screening questionnaire for the early presumptive diagnosis of psoriasis and we applied this tool on a randomly selected sample of 1500 subjects from the general population.

In a second stage of the study, a group of 500 subjects (comparable to the initial sample by gender, age, area of residence, region, level of education) was selected to be examined clinically at the same time, for a certain diagnosis. Among the analyzed risk factors, a significantly higher presence of family history in patients was also confirmed, in accordance with the predictive model, while for the rest of the analyzed factors there were no significant differences between psoriatic and non-psoriatic patients.

Our study has some limitations related to the fact that only one third of the initial sample has received a medical examination due to feasibility reasons. We tried to minimize those limits by randomly selecting the subjects and therefore revealing the similarities of the two groups from demographic and geographical perspectives. Another limitation is related to the fact that only 23 patients with psoriasis have been identified in the subgroup of people with a medical examination. We used for comparisons in this case the Fisher test and the demographic and geographical characteristics did not differ significantly for psoriatic and non-psoriatic patients. Last but not least, we did not measure the concordance between different dermatologists who have been involved in the clinical diagnosis.

6. Conclusions

The pilot study demonstrated the ability of the questionnaire and the procedure for completing it to highlight the most expected associations based on the literature on the epidemiology of psoriasis.

Our study is the first attempt, upon our knowledge, to estimate the prevalence of psoriasis in Romania. The prevalence of psoriasis vulgaris measured within the second stage of the study was 4.99% and the proposed questionnaire was found to have a convenient sensitivity for psoriasis vulgaris (86.96%). The correlation between the declared diagnosis established on the basis of a questionnaire and the final clinical diagnosis was 99.13% for psoriasis vulgaris.

Further research is required to determine the reasons driving the increase in psoriasis prevalence over time. The results obtained in this study are intended to be a source of recommendations and suggestions for new initiatives, campaigns, and public policy proposals to address the various issues of these diseases.

Author Contributions: All authors had equal contribution. Conceptualization A.C.N., M.M.C., C.G., Ș.B.; data curation L.G.-S., T.C.; formal analysis A.C.N., M.M.C., F.F., I.A.; supervision A.C.N., M.M.C., T.C., C.G.; writing—original draft Ș.B., L.G.-S., T.C.; writing—review and editing M.M.C., T.C., Ș.B., F.F., I.A. All authors have read and agreed to the published version of the manuscript.

Funding: Romanian Society of Dermatology; Eli Lilly; Novartis; Abbvie; Johnson & Johnson.

Institutional Review Board Statement: The study was conducted according to the guidelines of the Declaration of Helsinki, and approved by the Ethics Committee of Scientific Research (no. 26/05.11.2018).

Informed Consent Statement: Informed consent was obtained from all subjects involved in the study.

Acknowledgments: The authors express their thanks for the support received from the Romanian Society of Dermatology, Totem Communication, Abbvie, Eli Lilly, Novartis, Johnson & Johnson.

Conflicts of Interest: No conflict of interest to declare.

Ethics Committee: The study has the approval of the Scientific Research Ethics Committee no. 26/05.11.2018.

References

1. Fernández-Armenteros, J.M.; Gómez-Arbonés, X.; Buti-Solé, M.; Betriu-Bars, A.; Sanmartin-Novell, V.; Ortega-Bravo, M.; Martínez-Alonso, M.; Casanova-Seuma, J.M. Epidemiology of Psoriasis. A Population-Based Study. *Actas Dermo-Sifiliogr.* **2019**, *110*, 385–392. [CrossRef] [PubMed]
2. Rapp, S.R.; Feldman, S.R.; Exum, M.; Fleischer, A.B.; Reboussin, D.M. Psoriasis causes as much disability as other major medical diseases. *J. Am. Acad. Dermatol.* **1999**, *41*, 401–407. [CrossRef]
3. Plunkett, A.; Marks, R. A review of the epidemiology of psoriasis vulgaris in the community. *Australas. J. Dermatol.* **1998**, *39*, 225–232. [CrossRef]
4. International Federation of Psoriasis Associations. World Psoriasis Day. Available online: https://ifpa-pso.com/our-actions/world-psoriasis-day (accessed on 6 May 2021).
5. Ocampo D, V.; Gladman, D. Psoriatic arthritis. *F1000Research* **2019**, *8*, 1665. [CrossRef]
6. Dinu, A.; Bucur, S.; Olteanu, R.; Constantin, T.; Raducan, A.; Baetu, M.; Constantin, M. Psoriatic arthritis: A permanent new challenge for dermatologists (Review). *Exp. Ther. Med.* **2019**, *20*, 47–51. [CrossRef] [PubMed]
7. Barrea, L.; Nappi, F.; Di Somma, C.; Savanelli, M.C.; Falco, A.; Balato, A.; Balato, N.; Savastano, S. Environmental Risk Factors in Psoriasis: The Point of View of the Nutritionist. *Int. J. Environ. Res. Public Health* **2016**, *13*, 743. [CrossRef] [PubMed]
8. Barrea, L.; Megna, M.; Cacciapuoti, S.; Frias-Toral, E.; Fabbrocini, G.; Savastano, S.; Colao, A.; Muscogiuri, G. Very low-calorie ketogenic diet (VLCKD) in patients with psoriasis and obesity: An update for dermatologists and nutritionists. *Crit. Rev. Food Sci. Nutr.* **2020**, 1–17. [CrossRef] [PubMed]
9. Barrea, L.; Muscogiuri, G.; Di Somma, C.; Annunziata, G.; Megna, M.; Falco, A.; Balato, A.; Colao, A.; Savastano, S. Coffee consumption, metabolic syndrome and clinical severity of psoriasis: Good or bad stuff? *Arch. Toxicol.* **2018**, *92*, 1831–1845. [CrossRef]
10. Barrea, L.; Savanelli, M.C.; Di Somma, C.; Napolitano, M.; Megna, M.; Colao, A.; Savastano, S. Vitamin D and its role in psoriasis: An overview of the dermatologist and nutritionist. *Rev. Endocr. Metab. Disord.* **2017**, *18*, 195–205. [CrossRef] [PubMed]
11. National Institute of Statistics. Tempo Online Statistics. Available online: http://statistici.insse.ro:8077/tempo-online/#/pages/tables/insse-table (accessed on 13 April 2020).
12. Raychaudhuri, S.P.; Farber, E.M. The prevalence of psoriasis in the world. *J. Eur. Acad. Dermatol. Venereol.* **2001**, *15*, 16–17. [CrossRef] [PubMed]
13. Schonmann, Y.; Ashcroft, D.M.; Iskandar, I.Y.K.; Parisi, R.; Sde-Or, S.; Comaneshter, D.; Batat, E.; Shani, M.; Vinker, S.; Griffiths, C.E.; et al. Incidence and prevalence of psoriasis in Israel between 2011 and 2017. *J. Eur. Acad. Dermatol. Venereol.* **2019**, *33*, 2075–2081. [CrossRef]

14. Finzi, A.F.; Benelli, C. A clinical survey of psoriasis in Italy: 1st AISP report. Interdisciplinary Association for the Study of Psoriasis. *J. Eur. Acad. Dermatol. Venereol.* **1998**, *10*, 125–129. [CrossRef] [PubMed]
15. Ferrandiz, C.; Bordas, X.; García-Patos, V.; Puig, S.; Pujol, R.M.; Smandia, A. Prevalence of psoriasis in Spain (Epiderma Project: Phase I). *J. Eur. Acad. Dermatol. Venereol.* **2001**, *15*, 20–23. [CrossRef]
16. Elewski, B.; Alexis, A.F.; Lebwohl, M.; Gold, L.S.; Pariser, D.; Del Rosso, J.; Yosipovitch, G. Itch: An under-recognized problem in psoriasis. *J. Eur. Acad. Dermatol. Venereol.* **2019**, *33*, 1465–1476. [CrossRef] [PubMed]
17. Koo, J.; Marangell, L.; Nakamura, M.; Armstrong, A.; Jeon, C.; Bhutani, T.; Wu, J. Depression and suicidality in psoriasis: Review of the literature including the cytokine theory of depression. *J. Eur. Acad. Dermatol. Venereol.* **2017**, *31*, 1999–2009. [CrossRef]
18. Abramovits, W.; Stevenson, L.C. A comparison of biologic therapies for psoriasis. *J. Am. Acad. Dermatol.* **2004**, *50*, P142. [CrossRef]
19. Olteanu, R.; Constantin, M.M.; Zota, A.; Dorobanțu, D.; Constantin, T.; Serban, E.D.; Bălănescu, P.; Mihele, D.; Solovastru, L. Original clinical experience and approach to treatment study with interleukine 12/23 inhibitor in moderate-to-severe psoriasis patients. *Farmacia* **2016**, *64*, 918–921.
20. Constantin, M.M.; Cristea, C.M.; Taranu, T. Biosimilars in dermatology: The wind of change. *Exp. Ther. Med.* **2019**, *18*, 911–915.
21. Olteanu, R.; Zota, A.; Constantin, M. Biosimilars: An Update on Clinical Trials (Review of Published and Ongoing Studies). *Acta Dermatovenerol. Croat. ADC* **2017**, *25*, 57–66.
22. Dattola, A.; Silvestri, M.; Tamburi, F.; Amoruso, G.F.; Bennardo, L.; Nisticò, S.P. Emerging role of anti-IL23 in the treatment of psoriasis: When humanized is very promising. *Dermatol. Ther.* **2020**, *33*, e14504. [CrossRef] [PubMed]
23. Iannone, L.F.; Bennardo, L.; Palleria, C.; Roberti, R.; De Sarro, C.; Naturale, M.D.; Dastoli, S.; Donato, L.; Manti, A.; Valenti, G.; et al. Safety profile of biologic drugs for psoriasis in clinical practice: An Italian prospective pharmacovigilance study. *PLoS ONE* **2020**, *15*, e0241575. [CrossRef] [PubMed]
24. Raducan, A.; Bucur, S.; Caruntu, C.; Constantin, T.; Nita, I.E.; Manolache, N.; Constantin, M.-M. Therapeutic management with biological anti-TNF-α agent in severe psoriasis associated with chronic hepatitis B: A case report. *Exp. Ther. Med.* **2019**, *18*, 895–899. [CrossRef] [PubMed]
25. Noe, M.H.; Grewal, S.K.; Shin, D.B.; Ogdie, A.; Takeshita, J.; Gelfand, J.M. Increased prevalence of HCV and hepatic decompensation in adults with psoriasis: A population-based study in the United Kingdom. *J. Eur. Acad. Dermatol. Venereol.* **2017**, *31*, 1674–1680. [CrossRef] [PubMed]
26. Sondermann, W.; Deudjui, D.D.; Körber, A.; Slomiany, U.; Brinker, T.; Erbel, R.; Moebus, S. Psoriasis, cardiovascular risk factors and metabolic disorders: Sex-specific findings of a population-based study. *J. Eur. Acad. Dermatol. Venereol.* **2019**, *34*, 779–786. [CrossRef] [PubMed]
27. Stewart, T.J.; Tong, W.; Whitfeld, M. The associations between psychological stress and psoriasis: A systematic review. *Int. J. Dermatol.* **2018**, *57*. [CrossRef] [PubMed]

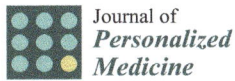

Article

Sea-Buckthorn Seed Oil Induces Proliferation of both Normal and Dysplastic Keratinocytes in Basal Conditions and under UVA Irradiation

Maria Dudau [1,2,†], Alexandra Catalina Vilceanu [2,†], Elena Codrici [1], Simona Mihai [1], Ionela Daniela Popescu [1], Lucian Albulescu [1], Isabela Tarcomnicu [3], Georgeta Moise [3], Laura Cristina Ceafalan [1,2], Mihail E. Hinescu [1,2], Ana-Maria Enciu [1,2,*] and Cristiana Tanase [1,4]

1. Victor Babes National Institute of Pathology, Biochemistry, 050096 Bucharest, Romania; maria.dudau@ivb.ro (M.D.); elena.codrici@ivb.ro (E.C.); simona.mihai@ivb.ro (S.M.); daniela.popescu@ivb.ro (I.D.P.); lucian.albulescu@ivb.ro (L.A.); laura.ceafalan@ivb.ro (L.C.C.); mhinescu@yahoo.com (M.E.H.); cristianatp@yahoo.com (C.T.)
2. Faculty of Medicine, Carol Davila University of Medicine and Pharmacy, 050474 Bucharest, Romania; alexandra.vilceanu@gmail.com
3. SC Cromatec Plus, 077167 Ilfov, Romania; isa.tarcomnicu@gmail.com (I.T.); georgeta.moise@scient.ro (G.M.)
4. Faculty of Medicine, Titu Maiorescu University, 031593 Bucharest, Romania
* Correspondence: ana.enciu@ivb.ro
† Equal contribution.

Abstract: Past decades demonstrate an increasing interest in herbal remedies in the public eye, with as many as 80% of people worldwide using these remedies as healthcare products, including those for skin health. Sea buckthorn and its derived products (oil; alcoholic extracts), rich in flavonoids and essential fatty acids, are among these healthcare products. Specifically, sea buckthorn and its derivatives are reported to have antioxidant and antitumor activity in dysplastic skin cells. On the other hand, evidence suggests that the alteration of lipid metabolism is related to increased malignant behavior. Given the paradoxical involvement of lipids in health and disease, we investigated how sea-buckthorn seed oil, rich in long-chain fatty acids, modifies the proliferation of normal and dysplastic skin cells in basal conditions, as well as under ultraviolet A (UVA) radiation. Using real-time analysis of normal and dysplastic human keratinocytes, we showed that sea-buckthorn seed oil stimulated the proliferation of dysplastic cells, while it also impaired the ability of both normal and dysplastic cells to migrate over a denuded area. Furthermore, UVA exposure increased the expression of CD36/SR-B2, a long-chain fatty acid translocator that is related to the metastatic behavior of tumor cells.

Keywords: sea-buckthorn seed oil; long-chain fatty acids; skin dysplastic keratinocytes; UVA; CD36; SR-B2

1. Introduction

Past decades show an increasing interest in herbal remedies in the public eye, and almost 80% of the population worldwide is now using them as healthcare products [1,2], particularly in developing countries. Sea buckthorn (*Elaeagnus rhamnoides* L.) is a unique medicinal and aromatic plant, frequently used as part of various pharmaceutical treatments, some of which are related to skin care. Sea-buckthorn-derived alcoholic extracts and seed oil were tested for antioxidant, antitumor and regenerative properties [3,4]. Most of these properties are related to its complex structure, rich in flavonoids and essential fatty acids (FA) [5]. Antioxidant activity was suggested as a protectant against different types of irradiation (gamma irradiation [6], UVA and UVB [3]), and, indeed, sea-buckthorn oil treatment showed increased antioxidant protection in irradiated keratinocytes [3]. Antitumor activity of sea-buckthorn-derived products was mostly related to their phenolic compounds [7], mostly by inhibition of fatty acid synthase [8,9]. However, sea-buckthorn seeds and berries are rich in FA [10], which constitute an important percentage of the sea-buckthorn seed oil [5]. It is expected that various FA would contribute to the cellular effects reported in sea-buckthorn-oil-related studies, including effects on skin cells and in animal models.

Normal adult human skin contains a variable dysplastic cell population, which gradually increases with sun exposure [11,12], mostly following UV exposure. These cells are characterized by atypical nuclei and disorganized growth, leading to precancerous skin lesions [13]. Evidence demonstrates that UVA irradiation of dysplastic keratinocytes has detrimental effects in the first few hours of exposure, but long-term, it activates cell protection and survival mechanisms [14], aggravating their malignant potential. Additionally, malignancy was previously shown to be aggravated by alterations in cellular lipid metabolism [15,16] to favor cell survival and proliferation.

Given the paradoxical involvement of FA in health and disease, we investigated whether sea-buckthorn seed oil has regenerative properties for skin cells, in basal conditions as well as under UVA radiation, and if this effect is the same, regardless of the dysplastic nature of the cells. The expression of CD36/SR-B2, a fatty acid translocator, which favors the uptake of fatty acids from the extracellular environment, was also assessed in relationship to UVA exposure.

2. Material and Methods

2.1. Cell Lines and Cell Treatments

Normal human epidermal cells (HEKa-ATCC PCS 200-011) and dysplastic keratinocytes (DOK-ECACC) were cultivated in standard cell culture conditions (37°C, 5% CO_2) according to manufacturer instructions regarding cell culture media and supplements. The sea-buckthorn oil was a cold-pressed, commercially available product of Romanian origin and stored as 1/10 DMSO solution. Further dilutions were made with complete cell culture medium and appropriate controls containing a comparable dilution of DMSO. Cells were exposed to UVA with a UV-365 nm lamp (VL-340 BLB model—Vilber Lourmat, France) at a light intensity of 381 $\mu W/cm^2$, for 30 min, in a laminar flow hood, as previously described [17].

2.2. Sea-Buckthorn Seed Oil Fatty Acid Composition

Targeted quantification of fatty acids was carried out by liquid chromatography coupled with tandem mass spectrometry (LC-MS/MS). Analyses were performed on a triple quadrupole mass spectrometer model API3200 (Sciex) coupled with an Infinity 1260 binary pump (Agilent) and autosampler. Analyst software version 1.5.2 was used for data acquisition and processing. After testing several stationary phases, chromatographic separation was achieved on a Phenomenex Luna pentafluorophenyl (PFP2) column (100 mm × 2 mm, 3 µm, 100 Å) using a mobile phase composed of water and acetonitrile at a flow rate of 0.3 mL/min. Seed oil was dissolved in ethanol at 1 mg/mL, and 3 µL of the solution were injected in the LC-MS/MS system. The mass spectrometer was operated in negative electrospray ionization (ESI). Acquisitions were carried out in multiple reaction monitoring (MRM) mode using the specific traces of each fatty acid (see Supplementary information Table S1). A general screening of the seed oil volatile constituents was performed by gas chromatography–mass spectrometry (GC/MS). A Perkin Elmer CLARUS 680 gas chromatograph (equipped with an ELITE 5 MS column (1,4-bis (dimethylsiloxy)) phenylene dimethyl polysiloxane stationary phase, 30 m, 0.25 mm ID, 0.25 µm film thickness, eluted with helium at 1 mL/min), connected to a Clarus SQ8T quadrupole, was used for this purpose. For analysis, 1 µg of seed oil solutions prepared at 50 mg/mL in ethanol were injected in split mode (40:1). Compound identification was achieved by searching the obtained mass spectra in the NIST and Wiley libraries.

2.3. Cell Proliferation and Toxicity Assays

Cytotoxicity was assessed by cellular lactate dehydrogenase (LDH)release (CytoTox 96 Non-Radioactive Cytotoxicity Assay, Promega, Madison, WI, USA). Specifically, 10,000 cells were seeded in triplicate overnight in 96-well plates and incubated the next day with serial dilutions of stock solution for an additional 72 h. Two controls were included—a negative control (cell culture medium only) and a positive control (addition of Cell Lysis Reagent 10x, Promega, 45 min prior to LDH detection). For background subtraction, additional triplicates of cell-free wells were incubated with tested solutions. For LDH analysis, 50 µL of supernatant were collected from each well and incubated with assay reagent for 30 min in the dark. After the addition of stop solution, absorbance was read at 490 nm by using a microplate reader Anthos Zenyth 3100 (Wals, Austria). Cytotoxicity was assessed as a percentage of the positive control, according to the formula cytotoxicity = 100*(Sample OD − background OD)/(average positive control − average background).

Proliferation was assessed by MTS assay (CellTiter 96 AQueous One Solution Reagent, Promega, Madison, WI USA). Specifically, 10,000 cells were seeded in triplicates overnight in 96-well plates and incubated the next day with cell culture medium and/or serial dilutions of stock solution for 72 h. A positive control (non-treated cells) was included. For background subtraction, additional triplicates of cell-free wells were incubated with tested solutions. On the day of the reading, the cell media was removed, and 100 µL of fresh medium and 20 µL of MTS reagent were added to each well. The plate was incubated at 37 °C for 3 h in a humidified, 5% CO_2 atmosphere. Absorbance was read at 490 nm by using a microplate reader Anthos Zenyth 3100 (Wals, Austria). Proliferation was assessed as a percentage of the control: % of proliferation = 100*(sample OD − background OD)/(average control − average control background).

Oil Red staining: Cells were fixed in 3.7% formaldehyde for 30 min to 1 h, washed with water, and then incubated with 60% isopropanol for 5 min. Oil Red O Stock solution (Sigma-Aldrich, St Louis, MO, USA) was reconstituted with 100% isopropanol. Oil Red O Working solution was prepared 15 min before staining by mixing three parts of Oil Red O Stock solution and two parts of water, and then the solution was filtered through Whatman No.1 filter paper. The cells were stained with Oil Red O Working solution for 10 min at room temperature and afterward washed 2–5 times with water until no excess stain was seen. DAPI staining can be performed after this step for 10 min, at room temperature, and protected from light. The red lipid droplets were visualized by using fluorescent microscopy with a Nikon TI (Nikon, Tokyo, Japan) inverted fluorescence microscope.

Real-time impedance readings: Cell adhesion and cell proliferation were assessed using RTCA DP platform (Agilent Technologies, Santa Clara, CA, USA). Cells were pre-irradiated with UVA for 30 min as previously described [17], and then they were trypsinized and seeded in E-16 plates at a density of 20,000 cells/well, with or without the cell medium, and supplemented or not with sea-buckthorn oil 1/8000. Readings were collected every 5 min for 24 h. Cell index at 2 h (at plateau) was used for statistical analysis (One-Way Anova, Dunnett multiple comparison, where data were compared to control. * $p < 0.05$, ** $p < 0.01$, *** $p < 0.001$, **** $p < 0.0001$)

Scratch-wound assay: Cells were seeded in a 35 mm glass-bottom dish and grown to confluence in normal cell culture conditions. A scratch was performed with a 200 µL pipette tip, with debris washed and cells further incubated in cell medium supplemented with 1/8000 sea-buckthorn oil for 24 h, in Nikon Biostation IM. Images were acquired with 20× Ph objective every 20 min, and data were analyzed with NIS-Elements BR (Nikon Tokyo, Japan).

2.4. Evaluation of the Expression CD36

Immunofluorescence (IF): Cells were grown on coverslips fixed with 4% formaldehyde for 5 min, rinsed in phosphate buffer saline (PBS), permeabilized in 0.1%Triton-X 100 and in 0.5% BSA for 10 min and incubated for 2 h with the primary antibody (anti-CD36 ThermoFisher PA1-16813, 1:100) at room temperature. After 3 × 5 min washes in PBS, cells were incubated with the secondary antibody (goat anti-rabbit Oregon Green 488, Invitrogen 011038, 1:2000 in PBS), and the nuclei were counterstained with DAPI. Image acquisition was performed with a Leica TCS SP8 white light laser confocal microscope.

Western blotting (WB): Cells were lysed in RIPA buffer with 1% protease inhibitor cocktail (P8340 Sigma), centrifuged for 10 min at 11,000 rpm (Ohaus R5510), and the supernatant boiled for 10 min (1:1 v/v) in Laemmli two times. Then, 40 µg of protein were loaded on each well, migrated in 10% SDS-PAGE gel for 2 h at 20 mA/gel and transferred onto a polyvinylidene fluoride (PVDF) membrane (BioRad) (1 h, 100 V). The membrane was incubated overnight in primary antibodies (anti-CD36 AF2519, R&D Systems, anti-GAPDH PA1-987, ThermoFisher), washed three times in TBS-T 0.5% and one time in TBS the next day and incubated for 1 h at room temperature (RT) in secondary antibodies (chicken-anti goat sc2953, SantaCruz, goat-anti rabbit 92680011, LiCor). Image acquisition was performed using a c-Digit scanner (LI-COR).

3. Results

3.1. Biochemical Composition of Sea-Buckthorn Seed Oil

Considering the important role of polyunsaturated fatty acids in skin growth and protection, we conducted a few experiments in order to estimate the composition of the tested sea-buckthorn seed oil. Linoleic acid was the main component (28.5% of the total fatty acid content), followed by palmitic acid (24.4%), linolenic acid (19.7%), oleic acid (12.6%) and palmitoleic acid (9.2%). Only small amounts of myristic and stearic acid were found in the tested oil (2.3 and 3.2%, respectively). A general screening of the volatile constituents of seed oil was also performed by using gas chromatography–mass spectrometry (GC/MS). Based on the total peak area, fatty acids represented 61% of the volatile compounds, with the other main components being sitosterol (12.4%), vitamin E (6.2%), α- and β-amyrin (2.14 and 3.3%, respectively) and fucosterol (1.96%) (Figure 1). The distribution of fatty acids was similar to that assessed by LC/MS.

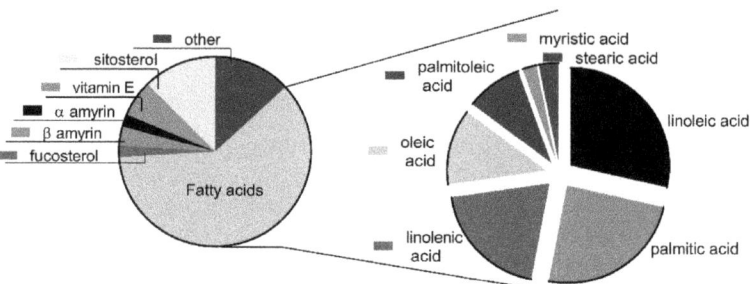

Figure 1. The chemical composition of the volatile fraction of sea-buckthorn seed oil, as assessed by gas chromatography–mass spectrometry.

3.2. The Sea-Buckthorn Seed Oil Showed Pro-Proliferative Effects at Low Concentrations

We tested the effect of sea-buckthorn seed oil on viability of normal and dysplastic skin cells using serial dilutions starting at 1/2000 (v/v in complete cell medium). The starting concentration was chosen following previous experiments, in which higher concentrations were cytotoxic for both cell types (data not shown). Further dilutions showed no cytotoxicity when reported on non-treated controls. Cell viability increased with subsequent dilution up to 1/8000, and then it started to decrease for both cell types (Figure 2). As a result, this concentration was selected for further tests.

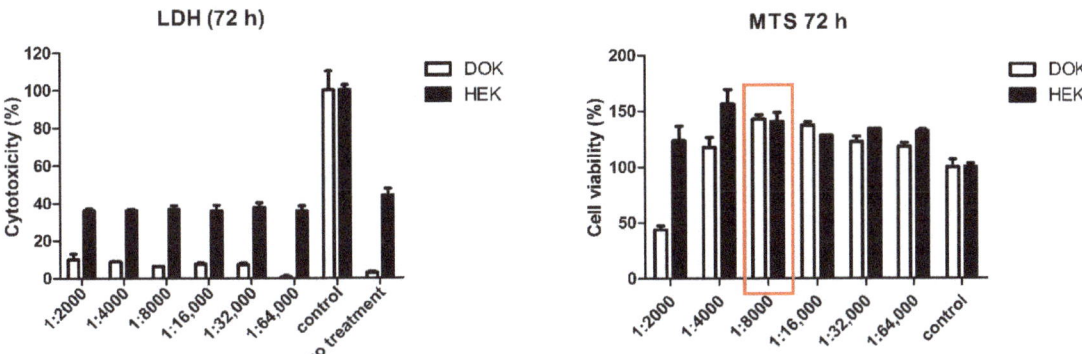

Figure 2. Assessment of toxicity of sea-buckthorn seed oil. Normal human keratinocytes (HEK) and dysplastic keratinocytes were seeded at a density of 10,000 cells/well in 96 well plates and treated for three days with the indicated dilutions of sea-buckthorn seed oil. Cytotoxicity was assessed by lactate dehydrogenate (LDH) release in the cell medium and viability by MTS assay. LDH control is represented by the lysis control (100% mortality). The MTS control was represented by cells maintained in standard cell culture conditions. The highest non-toxic and pro-proliferative concentrations (highlighted in red) were chosen for further tests. Bars represent average of triplicates, calculated as percentage to control.

3.3. Sea-Buckthorn Seed Oil Inhibits Cell Migration of Dysplastic Keratinocytes

Next, in real-time microscopy we assessed the ability of cells to proliferate and migrate in a scratch-wound assay, following 24 h treatment with sea-buckthorn oil at 1/8000 dilution. After 24 h, both treated and untreated dysplastic cells failed to migrate and close the denuded area, and the oil treatment impaired migration even further (Figure 3). Normal keratinocytes were also less effective at closing the gap in the presence of diluted sea-buckthorn oil, but the effect was less impaired than that of dysplastic cells.

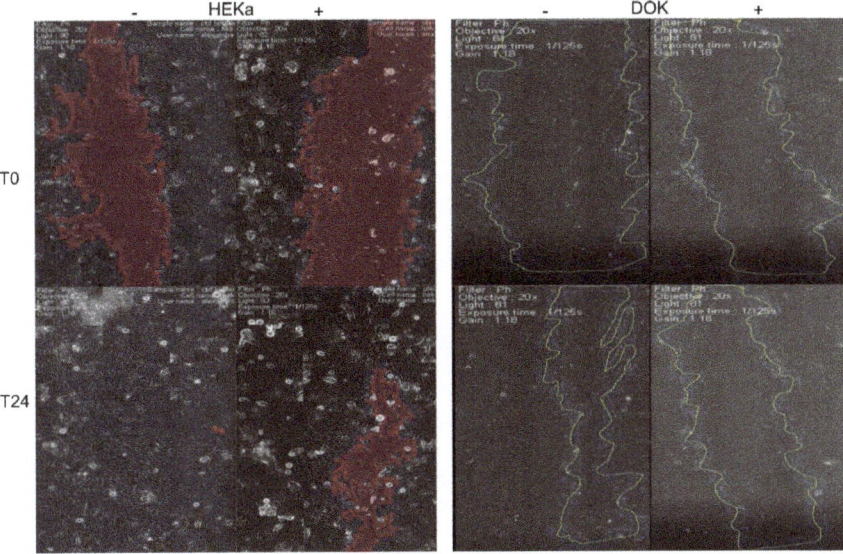

Figure 3. Real-time assessment of cell migration and proliferation of normal and dysplastic keratinocytes, treated (+) with sea-buckthorn seed oil. Treated cells (both normal and dysplastic) were less efficient in covering the denudated area. The effect was more prominent for dysplastic cells.

To this point, we noticed that there is a contrast between the effects of sea-buckthorn seed oil on cell proliferation versus cell migration, which might indicate a possible deleterious effect of such treatment on the migration of epidermis cell populations. We wanted to further confirm these findings and address other literature-reported effects of sea-buckthorn oil, such as protection against UVA irradiation and use of a real-time assessment of cell proliferation.

3.4. Treatment with Sea-Buckthorn Oil Following UVA Irradiation Does Not Mitigate the Deleterious Effect on Dysplastic Cells

As sea-buckthorn oil is reported to have protective effects against irradiation, we tested the effect of UVA irradiation on normal and dysplastic keratinocytes adherence using a real-time impedance reading system. This investigation allowed for the quantification of cell adherence (e.g., required for re-adhesion of daughter-cells after cell division) and of cell proliferation by calculation of doubling times using the xCELLigence platform (Figure 4). Consistent with videomicroscopy observations, oil treatment impairs cell adhesion and fails to mitigate UVA irradiation effects. Doubling times analysis confirmed MTS data regarding stimulation of cell viability with the selected dilution of sea-buckthorn seed oil. Notably, oil treatment on irradiated cells significantly decreased doubling times, which translates into increased proliferation rate of cells.

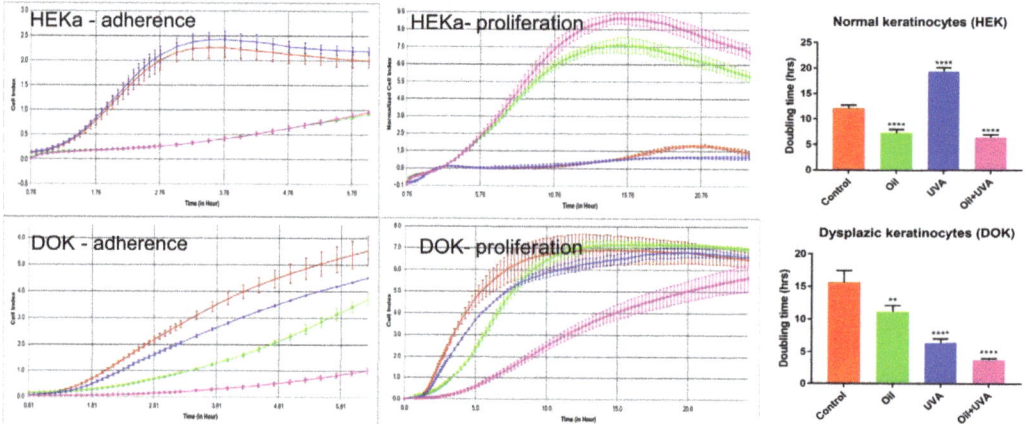

Figure 4. Cell adhesion and proliferation of normal and dysplastic keratinocytes, treated with sea-buckthorn seed oil, in the presence or absence of UVA irradiation. Each point on graphs represents the average cell index of triplicates, recorded every 15 min for 24 h. Bars represent average of triplicates with SD. One-Way Anova was used to assess statistical significance (** $p < 0.01$, **** $p < 0.0001$).

3.5. UVA Irradiation Does Not Affect Uptake of Lipids into Normal and Dysplastic Keratinocytes

Next, we tested whether irradiation affects oil uptake into cells. Keratinocytes use lipids to seal the epidermis from the outer environment by deposition of sphingolipids in the extracellular space [18]; therefore, a normal degree of lipid inclusion is to be expected in non-treated cells. Both normal and dysplastic cells uptake presented increased lipid load following oil treatment. However, unlike normal cells, where only some cells are loaded with lipid inclusions, all dysplastic cells have a degree of lipid load. Irradiation did not significantly affect the upload of lipids in both normal and dysplastic cells, but dysplastic cells showed a more uniform lipid uptake (Figure 5).

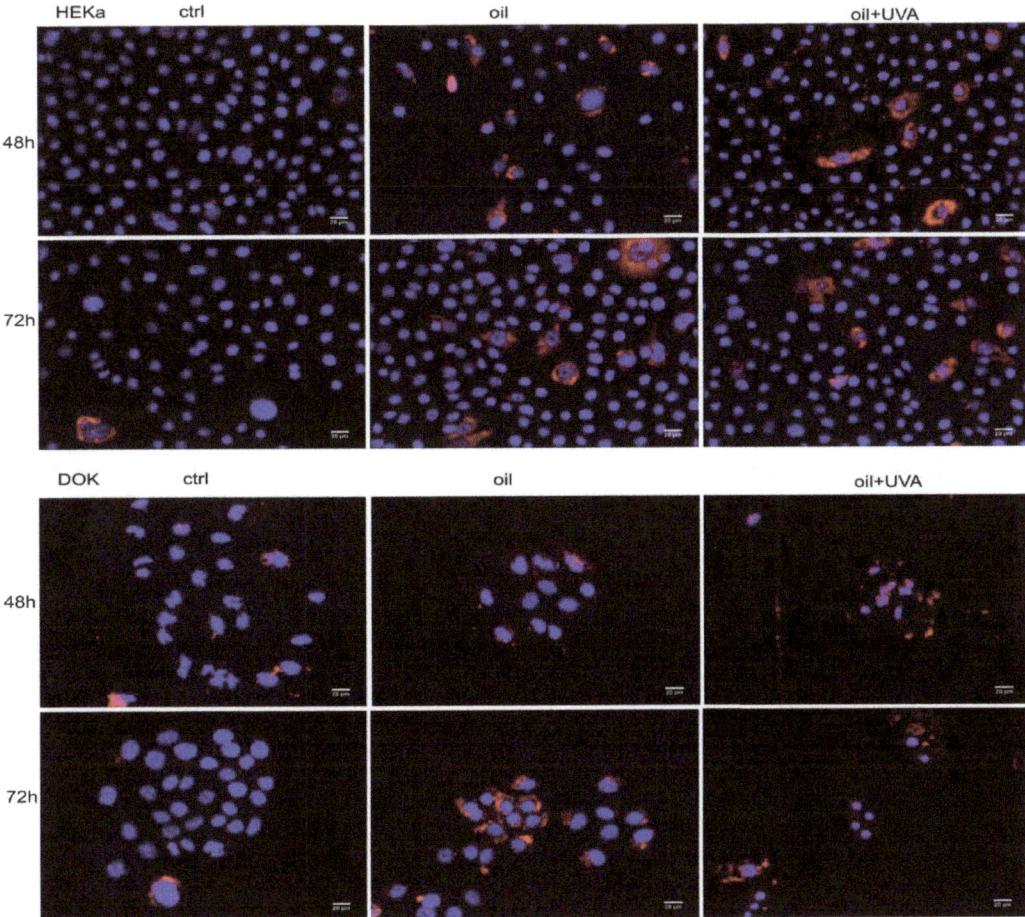

Figure 5. Oil uptake in irradiated and non-irradiated cells. Irradiated and non-irradiated cells were treated with sea-buckthorn seed oil (dilution 1/8000) for the indicated periods of time. Non-treated, non-irradiated cells were used as controls. Lipid inclusions were stained with Oil Red O.

3.6. The Fatty Acid Translocator CD36 Is Expressed in Dysplastic, but Not Normal Keratinocytes

Long-chain FA used by cells to synthesize phospholipids and sphingolipids do not easily diffuse through cell membranes and are more efficiently up-taken with the help of fatty acid translocators, such as CD36/SR-B2. Furthermore, CD36/SR-B2 was shown to be involved in the tumorigenesis of aggressive, metastatic cancers (reviewed in [19]). Using two different methods, we investigated the expression of CD36 in normal and dysplastic keratinocytes following UVA irradiation. The expression of CD36 in normal keratinocytes is undetectable in both IF (data not shown) and WB, and it appears to be slightly induced by irradiation. In contrast, dysplastic keratinocytes express a stronger signal for CD36, in both control and irradiated cells (Figure 6).

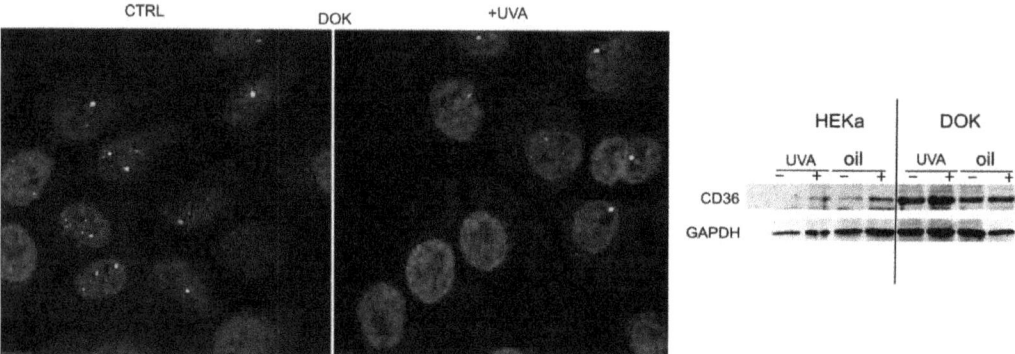

Figure 6. CD36 expression in normal (HEKa) and dysplastic (DOK) keratinocytes after UVA irradiation. Expression of CD36 in both HEKa and DOK cells was assessed by confocal immunofluorescence and confirmed by Western blot. In basal conditions, CD36 expression in normal keratinocytes is undetectable with the selected methods. Its expression increases in dysplastic cells, as well as following UVA irradiation.

4. Discussion

Our manuscript compares the effect of sea-buckthorn seed oil on normal and dysplastic human keratinocytes, starting from the premise that normal skin contains a mixture of both cells, whose proportion changes with age. It was demonstrated that sea-buckthorn fatty acids have the ability to improve the post-inflammatory response resulting from deleterious UV exposure. Moreover, they could alleviate the effects of sun burns, support regenerative processes of the skin and appease irritation [5]. UVA exposure was reported to affect these cell populations differently in terms of migration and proliferation. It was previously demonstrated that dysplastic cells are less able to spread across a denuded area than normal keratinocytes, and were more affected than the latter by UVA treatment [17]. In terms of cell proliferation, UVA exposure induced cell-cycle arrest for normal keratinocytes [20,21]; this outcome, reviewed in [22], may lead to an increased doubling time of a cell population, a finding which also was observed in our real-time, impedance-reading experiments. Dysplastic cells do not exhibit this protective effect; they are more prone to proliferate under UV irradiation, and the seed-oil treatment further aggravates this noxious behavior.

One putative mechanism for increased dysplastic cell proliferation following seed-il treatment could be CD36-mediated lipid uptake. Fatty acid transporters, including CD36, are overexpressed in tissues with an increased fatty acid metabolism [23]. FA are able to activate peroxisome proliferator-activated receptors (PPARs) [24], transcription factors which further activate gene transcription of CD36 [25]. It was previously shown that tumor cells modify their lipid metabolism [15,16] to favor cell survival and proliferation. A study by Pascual et al. revealed that CD36+ cells react to dietary lipids and rely on lipid metabolism for metastatic potential. In their study, CD44 bright cells isolated from human oral carcinomas exerted a distinctive ability to overexpress both the fatty acid receptor CD36 and lipid metabolism genes, thus accelerating the initiation of metastasis [26].

Various studies in the literature shed light on the potential relationship between an impaired lipid metabolism and different skin conditions, but the extent to which fatty acid transporters are involved in directing fatty acids to keratinocytes, altering the fate of lipid metabolism, remains an open question [23]. As far as the current literature goes, normal keratinocytes do not require CD36 for their metabolism; it is only transiently expressed in pathological circumstances such as wounds [27], infectious [28] and autoimmune [29,30] cutaneous diseases and tumor-related pathologies [31]. A stable CD36 expression can be a driver for increased lipid metabolism, which can fuel a possible malignant transformation.

5. Conclusions

Plant-derived bioactive compounds or mixtures have gradually become a hot topic in recent years, as a growing body of data points to their beneficial effects. However, these effects can vary from cell type to cell type. Here, we showed that, although sea-buckthorn seed oil has been associated with skin health and protection against irradiation, it also stimulates proliferation of dysplastic cells, while impairing the ability of both normal and dysplastic cells for wound-healing. We also investigated the expression of CD36, a fatty acid translocator, on normal and dysplastic keratinocytes, and we found that UVA exposure increases its expression, which could hold functional significance for further progression towards malignancy.

Supplementary Materials: The following are available online at https://www.mdpi.com/article/10.3390/jpm11040278/s1, Table S1: Optimized parameters for fatty acids mass spectrometric detection.

Author Contributions: M.D., A.C.V., E.C., I.D.P., S.M., L.A. and I.T. performed cell culture-based experiments; I.T. and G.M. performed chromatographic and mass-spectrometry analysis; L.C.C. performed confocal microscopy data acquisition, interpretation and report; A.-M.E. designed the study; A.-M.E., C.T. and M.E.H. designed the study and critically read the manuscript; A.-M.E., M.D. and A.C.V. wrote the manuscript; A.-M.E. was the project Administrator; C.T. was responsible for funding acquisition. All authors have read and agreed to the published version of the manuscript.

Funding: This work was partially funded by Ministry of Research and Innovation grant: COP A 1.2.3., ID:P_40_197/2016 and PN 19.29.01.04.

Acknowledgments: The graphical abstract was created with BioRender.com.

Conflicts of Interest: The authors have no conflict of interest to declare.

References

1. Ekor, M. The growing use of herbal medicines: Issues relating to adverse reactions and challenges in monitoring safety. *Front. Pharmacol.* **2014**, *4*, 177. [CrossRef]
2. Rashrash, M.; Schommer, J.C.; Brown, L.M. Prevalence and Predictors of Herbal Medicine Use Among Adults in the United States. *J. Patient Exp.* **2017**, *4*, 108–113. [CrossRef] [PubMed]
3. Gęgotek, A.; Jastrząb, A.; Jarocka-Karpowicz, I.; Muszyńska, M.; Skrzydlewska, E. The Effect of Sea Buckthorn (Hippophae rhamnoides L.) Seed Oil on UV-Induced Changes in Lipid Metabolism of Human Skin Cells. *Antioxidants* **2018**, *7*, 110. [CrossRef] [PubMed]
4. Olas, B.; Skalski, B.; Ulanowska, K. The Anticancer Activity of Sea Buckthorn [Elaeagnus rhamnoides (L.) A. Nelson]. *Front. Pharmacol.* **2018**, *9*, 232. [CrossRef] [PubMed]
5. Zielińska, A.; Nowak, I. Abundance of active ingredients in sea-buckthorn oil. *Lipids Health Dis.* **2017**, *16*, 95. [CrossRef]
6. Bala, M.; Gupta, M.; Saini, M.; Abdin, M.Z.; Prasad, J. Sea Buckthorn Leaf Extract Protects Jejunum and Bone Marrow of 60 Cobalt-Gamma-Irradiated Mice by Regulating Apoptosis and Tissue Regeneration. *Evid. Based Complement Altern Med.* **2015**, *2015*, 1–10. [CrossRef]
7. Yasukawa, K.; Kitanaka, S.; Kawata, K.; Goto, K. Anti-tumor promoters phenolics and triterpenoid from Hippophae rhamnoides. *Fitoterapia* **2009**, *80*, 164–167. [CrossRef] [PubMed]
8. Brusselmans, K.; Vrolix, R.; Verhoeven, G.; Swinnen, J.V. Induction of Cancer Cell Apoptosis by Flavonoids Is Associated with Their Ability to Inhibit Fatty Acid Synthase Activity. *J. Biol. Chem.* **2005**, *280*, 5636–5645. [CrossRef]
9. Wang, Y.; Nie, F.; Ouyang, J.; Wang, X.; Ma, X. Inhibitory effects of sea buckthorn procyanidins on fatty acid synthase and MDA-MB-231 cells. *Tumour Biol.* **2014**, *35*, 9563–9569. [CrossRef] [PubMed]
10. Fatima, T.; Snyder, C.L.; Schroeder, W.R.; Cram, D.; Datla, R.; Wishart, D.; Weselake, R.J.; Krishna, P. Fatty Acid Composition of Developing Sea Buckthorn (Hippophae rhamnoides L.) Berry and the Transcriptome of the Mature Seed. *PLoS ONE* **2012**, *7*, e34099. [CrossRef] [PubMed]
11. Krouse, R.S.; Alberts, D.S.; Prasad, A.R.; Bartels, H.; Yozwiak, M.; Liu, Y.; Bartels, P.H. Progression of skin lesions from normal skin to squamous cell carcinoma. *Anal. Quant. Cytol. Histol.* **2009**, *31*, 17–25. [PubMed]
12. Berman, B.; Cockerell, C.J. Pathobiology of actinic keratosis: Ultraviolet-dependent keratinocyte proliferation. *J. Am. Acad. Dermatol.* **2013**, *68*, S10–S19. [CrossRef]
13. Ratushny, V.; Gober, M.D.; Hick, R.; Ridky, T.W.; Seykora, J.T. From keratinocyte to cancer: The pathogenesis and modeling of cutaneous squamous cell carcinoma. *J Clin Investig.* **2012**, *122*, 464–472. [CrossRef] [PubMed]
14. Nechifor, M.T.; Niculițe, C.M.; Urs, A.O.; Regalia, T.; Mocanu, M.; Popescu, A.; Manda, G.; Dinu, D.; Leabu, M. UVA Irradiation of Dysplastic Keratinocytes: Oxidative Damage versus Antioxidant Defense. *Int. J. Mol. Sci.* **2012**, *13*, 16718–16736. [CrossRef] [PubMed]

15. Baenke, F.; Peck, B.; Miess, H.; Schulze, A. Hooked on fat: The role of lipid synthesis in cancer metabolism and tumour development. *Dis. Model Mech.* **2013**, *6*, 1353–1363. [CrossRef] [PubMed]
16. Röhrig, F.; Schulze, A. The multifaceted roles of fatty acid synthesis in cancer. *Nat. Rev. Cancer* **2016**, *16*, 732–749. [CrossRef]
17. Niculiţe, C.M.; Nechifor, M.T.; Urs, A.O.; Olariu, L.; Ceafalan, L.C.; Leabu, M. Keratinocyte Motility Is Affected by UVA Radiation-A Comparison between Normal and Dysplastic Cells. *Int. J. Mol. Sci.* **2018**, *19*, 1700. [CrossRef] [PubMed]
18. Sigruener, A.; Tarabin, V.; Paragh, G.; Liebisch, G.; Koehler, T.; Farwick, M.; Schmitz, G. Effects of sphingoid bases on the sphingolipidome in early keratinocyte differentiation. *Exp. Dermatol.* **2013**, *22*, 677–679. [CrossRef]
19. Enciu, A.-M.; Radu, E.; Popescu, I.D.; Hinescu, M.E.; Ceafalan, L.C. Targeting CD36 as Biomarker for Metastasis Prognostic: How Far from Translation into Clinical Practice? *Biomed. Res. Int.* **2018**, *2018*, 1–12. [CrossRef]
20. Maeda, T.; Hanna, A.N.; Sim, A.B.; Chua, P.P.; Chong, M.T.; Tron, V.A. GADD45 Regulates G2/M Arrest, DNA Repair, and Cell Death in Keratinocytes Following Ultraviolet Exposure. *J. Investig. Dermatol.* **2002**, *119*, 22–26. [CrossRef]
21. Farrell, A.W.; Halliday, G.M.; Lyons, J.G. Brahma deficiency in keratinocytes promotes UV carcinogenesis by accelerating the escape from cell cycle arrest and the formation of DNA photolesions. *J. Dermatol. Sci.* **2018**, *92*, 254–263. [CrossRef] [PubMed]
22. Gao, Y. The Role of p21 in Apoptosis, Proliferation, Cell Cycle Arrest, and Antioxidant Activity in UVB-Irradiated Human HaCaT Keratinocytes. *Med. Sci. Monit. Basic Res.* **2015**, *21*, 86–95. [CrossRef] [PubMed]
23. Lin, M.-H.; Khnykin, D. Fatty acid transporters in skin development, function and disease. *Biochim. Biophys. Acta Mol. Cell Biol. Lipids* **2014**, *1841*, 362–368. [CrossRef] [PubMed]
24. Varga, T.; Czimmerer, Z.; Nagy, L. PPARs are a unique set of fatty acid regulated transcription factors controlling both lipid metabolism and inflammation. *Biochim. Biophys. Acta Mol. Basis Dis.* **2011**, *1812*, 1007–1022. [CrossRef] [PubMed]
25. Sato, O.; Kuriki, C.; Fukui, Y.; Motojima, K. Dual Promoter Structure of Mouse and Human Fatty Acid Translocase/CD36 Genes and Unique Transcriptional Activation by Peroxisome Proliferator-activated Receptor α and γ Ligands. *J. Biol. Chem.* **2002**, *277*, 15703–15711. [CrossRef]
26. Pascual, G.; Avgustinova, A.; Mejetta, S.; Martín, M.; Castellanos, A.; Attolini, C.S.; Berenguer, A.; Prats, N.; Toll, A.; Hueto, J.A.; et al. Targeting metastasis-initiating cells through the fatty acid receptor CD36. *Nature* **2017**, *541*, 41–45. [CrossRef]
27. Simon, M.; Juhász, I.; Herlyn, M.; Hunyadi, J. Thrombospondin receptor (CD36) expression of human keratinocytes during wound healing in a SCID mouse/human skin repair model. *J. Dermatol.* **1996**, *23*, 305–309. [CrossRef] [PubMed]
28. Grange, P.A.; Chéreau, C.; Raingeaud, J.; Nicco, C.; Weill, B.; Dupin, N.; Batteux, F. Production of superoxide anions by keratinocytes initiates, P. acnes-induced inflammation of the skin. *PLoS Pathog.* **2009**, *5*, e1000527. [CrossRef]
29. Das, D.; Anand, V.; Khandpur, S.; Sharma, V.K.; Sharma, A. T helper type 1 polarizing γδ T cells and Scavenger receptors contribute to the pathogenesis of Pemphigus vulgaris. *Immunology* **2018**, *153*, 97–104. [CrossRef]
30. Bumiller-Bini, V.; Cipolla, G.A.; Spadoni, M.B.; Augusto, D.G.; Petzl-Erler, M.L.; Beltrame, M.H.; Boldt, A.B. Condemned or Not to Die? Gene Polymorphisms Associated with Cell Death in Pemphigus Foliaceus. *Front. Immunol.* **2019**, *10*, 2416. [CrossRef]
31. Allen, M.H.; Barker, J.N.W.N.; MacDonald, D.M. Keratinocyte expression of CD36 antigen in benign and malignant epidermal cell-derived tumours. *J. Cutan. Pathol.* **1991**, *18*, 198–203. [CrossRef] [PubMed]

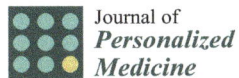

Article

Serum Sialylation Changes in Actinic Keratosis and Cutaneous Squamous Cell Carcinoma Patients

Mircea Tampa [1,2], Ilinca Nicolae [2,*], Cristina Iulia Mitran [3], Madalina Irina Mitran [3], Cosmin Ene [4], Clara Matei [1], Simona Roxana Georgescu [1,2,*] and Corina Daniela Ene [5,6]

[1] Department of Dermatology, 'Carol Davila' University of Medicine and Pharmacy, 020021 Bucharest, Romania; tampa_mircea@yahoo.com (M.T.); matei_clara@yahoo.com (C.M.)
[2] Department of Dermatology, 'Victor Babes' Clinical Hospital for Infectious Diseases, 030303 Bucharest, Romania
[3] Department of Microbiology, 'Carol Davila' University of Medicine and Pharmacy, 020021 Bucharest, Romania; cristina.iulia.mitran@gmail.com (C.I.M.); madalina.irina.mitran@gmail.com (M.I.M.)
[4] Departments of Urology, 'Carol Davila' University of Medicine and Pharmacy, 020021 Bucharest, Romania; cosmin85_ene@yahoo.com
[5] Department of Nephrology, 'Carol Davila' Nephrology Hospital, 010731 Bucharest, Romania; koranik85@yahoo.com
[6] Departments of Nephrology, 'Carol Davila' University of Medicine and Pharmacy, 020021 Bucharest, Romania
* Correspondence: drnicolaei@yahoo.ro (I.N.); srg.dermatology@gmail.com (S.R.G.)

Abstract: Cutaneous squamous cell carcinoma (cSCC), a malignant proliferation of the cutaneous epithelium, is the second most common skin cancer after basal cell carcinoma (BCC). Unlike BCC, cSCC exhibits a greater aggressiveness and the ability to metastasize to any organ in the body. Chronic inflammation and immunosuppression are important processes linked to the development of cSCC. The tumor can occur de novo or from the histological transformation of preexisting actinic keratoses (AK). Malignant cells exhibit a higher amount of sialic acid in their membranes than normal cells, and changes in the amount, type, or linkage of sialic acid in malignant cell glycoconjugates are related to tumor progression and metastasis. The aim of our study was to investigate the sialyation in patients with cSCC and patients with AK. We have determined the serum levels of total sialic acid (TSA), lipid-bound sialic acid (LSA), beta-galactoside 2,6-sialyltransferase I (ST6GalI), and neuraminidase 3 (NEU3) in 40 patients with cSCC, 28 patients with AK, and 40 healthy subjects. Data analysis indicated a significant increase in serum levels of TSA ($p < 0.001$), LSA ($p < 0.001$), ST6GalI ($p < 0.001$), and NEU3 ($p < 0.001$) in the cSCC group compared to the control group, whereas in patients with AK only the serum level of TSA was significantly higher compared to the control group ($p < 0.001$). When the cSCC and AK groups were compared, significant differences between the serum levels of TSA ($p < 0.001$), LSA ($p < 0.001$), ST6GalI ($p < 0.001$) and NEU3 ($p < 0.001$) were found. The rate of synthesis of sialoglycoconjugates and their rate of enzymatic degradation, expressed by the ST6GalI/NEU3 ratio, is 1.64 times lower in the cSCC group compared to the control group ($p < 0.01$) and 1.53 times lower compared to the AK group ($p < 0.01$). The tumor diameter, depth of invasion, and Ki67 were associated with higher levels of TSA and LSA. These results indicate an aberrant sialylation in cSCC that correlates with tumor aggressiveness.

Keywords: cSCC; AK; sialylation; sialyltransferase; sialidase

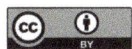

1. Introduction

Cutaneous squamous cell carcinoma (cSCC) together with basal cell carcinoma (BCC) represent the most frequent non-melanoma skin cancers [1]. Unlike BCC, cSCC may exhibit an aggressive behavior with a great ability to metastasize to any organ in the body. The most important risk factors associated with cSCC are sun exposure, fair skin phototype, age (mainly diagnosed in middle-aged and older adults), certain beta human papillomavirus

(HPV) types [2], and immunosuppression [2,3]. It is well known that cSCC arises on damaged skin, on sites characterized by chronic inflammation such as scars or burns [4]. Sun-exposed keratinocytes produce a wide range of molecules (e.g., inflammatory cytokines, chemokines, growth factors, etc.) that induce increased vascular permeability and the recruitment of immune cells such as neutrophils, macrophages, etc. However, UV radiation leads to the depletion of Langerhans cells in the epidermis [5]. UV radiation promotes the formation of an inflammatory milieu that contributes to skin carcinogenesis [6]. Chronic inflammation is a cofactor for tumor development and induces local immunosuppression facilitating tumor invasiveness and metastasis. Immunocompromised individuals have a 65- to 250-fold increased risk of developing a cSCC [4,7]. Regarding HPV infection, several studies suggest the role of beta HPV types in the pathogenesis of cSCC [4,8–10]. Beta HPV DNA has been identified in cSCC samples and antibodies against HPV have been detected in the serum of cSCC patients [4]. The main factors predicting a poor outcome are depth of invasion higher than 2 mm, a low degree of differentiation, location in high-risk areas (face, ear, hands, feet, genitalia), perineural involvement, and the presence of multiple tumors [11–13]. cSCC can occur de novo or from the histological transformation of preexisting actinic keratoses (AK), which represent the intradermal proliferation of dysplastic keratinocytes and display potential for malignant transformation into non-melanoma skin cancer, giving rise especially to SCC [14,15].

Carcinogenesis is frequently associated with abnormal sialylation of glycoproteins and glycolipids as a consequence of changes in the activity of sialyltransferases and sialidases [16–19]. Sialic acids are negatively charged sugars that commonly are coupled to the terminal carbohydrate chains of glycoproteins and glycolipids [20]. Aberrant expression of sialic acid plays a crucial role in tumor aggressivity by promoting cell proliferation, cell-cell interaction, cell migration, angiogenesis, and tumor metastasis [17,19,21–23]. Total serum sialic acid (TSA) and lipid-bound sialic acid (LSA) are significantly elevated in skin cancers [18,24]. Hypersilalylation influences immune cell responses. Sialic acid-binding receptors such as Siglecs modulate the activity of immune cells in the tumor microenvironment, leading to an abnormal inflammatory response [25]. Siglecs are involved in tumor progression and immune evasion, for example, engagement of Siglec-9 or Siglec-E on neutrophils prevents neutrophil-mediated killing of malignant cells [26].

Sialylation is a process mainly governed by sialyltransferases and sialidases [27]. The transfer of sialic acids is modulated by sialyltransferases, a group of glycosyltransferases divided into four families: β-galactoside α2,3-sialyltransferases (ST3Gal-I-VI), β-galactoside α2,6-sialyltransferases (ST6Gal-I and -II), GalNAc α2,6-sialyltransferases (ST6GalNAc-I-VI), and α2,8-sialyltransferases (ST8Sia-I-VI) [28]. During cell differentiation and neoplastic transformation, the expression of sialyltransferases undergoes substantial alterations resulting in phenotypic changes [27–30]. Sialyltransferases are well known as crucial modulators of several important processes such as cell-cell communication, cell-matrix interaction, cell adhesion, cell signaling, and trafficking [29]. Sialidases, or neuraminidases, are glycohydrolytic enzymes that catalyze the hydrolysis of α−glycosidically linked sialic acid residues from carbohydrate groups of glycoproteins and glycolipids [31]. To date, four types of human sialidases have been identified: NEU1, NEU2, NEU3, and NEU4 [32]. In cancer, the alteration of sialidase activity was associated with cell proliferation, invasion, and metastasis [33].

We have previously investigated sialoglycoconjugate abnormalities and anti-ganglioside immune response as possible mechanisms involved in oncogenesis (cutaneous melanoma [23], clear cell renal cell carcinoma [34]), autoimmune diseases (systemic lupus erythematosus, lupus nephritis [35]), and diabetes [36]. Increased sialylation in melanoma cells could represent an event associated with the progression of cutaneous melanoma [17]. Sialoglycoconjugates may promote processes that are involved in the modulation of host immune and inflammatory responses [37]. Sialylation, manifested as the overexpression of TSA, LSA, and orosomucoid, has been shown to be an early, well-expressed event in the initial stages of clear cell renal cell carcinoma [34]. In the medical literature, there are few studies that have analyzed sialylation in cSCC and AK [29,38–40]. Therefore, the data are scarce and inconclusive. The aim of our study is to investigate the sialyation in patients with cSCC and patients with AK and find reliable serum parameters useful in the diagnosis of cSCC. To achieve these goals, we have investigated both the levels of sialic acid (TSA and LSA) and the levels of the enzymes involved in its metabolism (ST6GalI and NEU3). In addition, we have analyzed the relationship between the studied parameters and the histological characteristics of the tumor (diameter, depth of invasion, Ki67, and ulceration).

2. Materials and Methods

2.1. Study Participants

We have conducted a study on 40 consecutive patients with cSCC, 28 consecutive patients with AK and 40 healthy subjects as controls, with skin phototypes I–IV. The patients and controls were matched by age and sex. In the control group, we included healthy subjects who addressed the dermatology clinic for disorders such as skin tags or nevi, disorders that do not interfere with our determinations. In all cases, the diagnosis was confirmed histopathologically. Informed consent was obtained from all study participants. The procedures and experiments were conducted according to the Declaration of Helsinki. The study protocol was approved by the Ethics Committee of the Victor Babes Infectious and Tropical Diseases Hospital (3/10.03.2018).

2.2. Histopathological Examination

The tissue samples were fixed in 10% formalin and the method of paraffin embedding was used. For microscopic examination, hematoxylin–eosin stain (HE) was performed (Figures 1 and 2). We have determined the tumor diameter, depth of invasion, and the presence of ulceration. Depth of invasion was calculated as the perpendicular distance between the basement membrane and the deepest point of the infiltrative zone of the tumor according to the recommendations from the 8th Edition of the AJCC [41]. The values were expressed as millimeters.

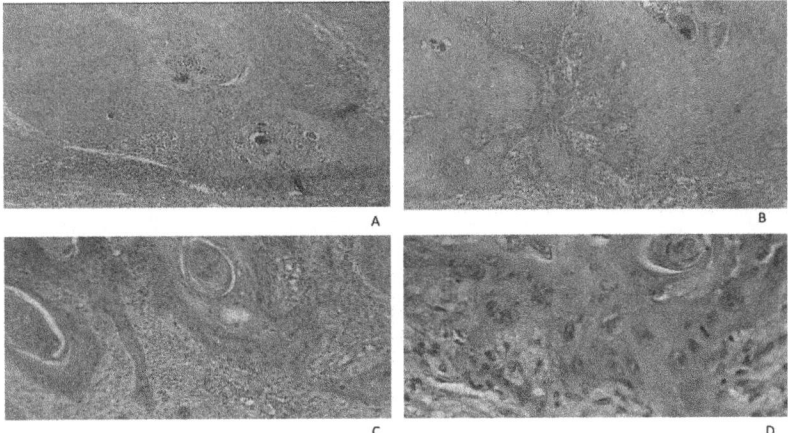

Figure 1. Histopathological examination of cSCC. (**A**) Cell proliferation with giant nuclei and nuclear polymorphism (HE, ×40). (**B**) Proliferation of squamous cells which extend into the deeper layers of the skin, abundant inflammatory infiltrate (HE, ×40). (**C**) Massive inflammatory infiltrate distributed throughout the tumor mass and disseminated tumor cells with giant nuclei (HE, ×40). (**D**) Proliferation of squamous cells with nuclear pleomorphism and nuclear abnormalities and abundant inflammatory infiltrate (HE, ×90).

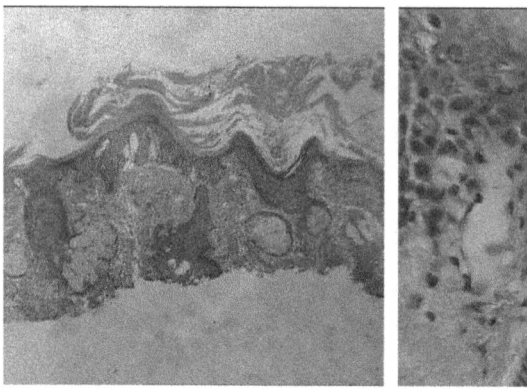

Figure 2. Histopathological examination of AK. (**A**) Disorganized growth, which disrupts differentiation (HE, ×10). (**B**) Dysplasia of basal keratinocytes (HE, ×90).

The Ki-67 antigen is a marker for cell proliferation and is widely used as a cancer activity marker [42]. We used the VECTASTAIN ABC KIT (PK-6101), specifically designed for immunohistochemical staining of tissues. The kit contains biotinylated IgG that was used to bind to the primary anti-Ki67 antibody. The cSCC samples were divided into three subgroups according to the Ki67 index as follows: low < 25%, intermediate 25–75%, and high > 75%.

2.3. Laboratory Determinations

Blood samples were drawn from the patients and controls enrolled in the study, under basal conditions using a holder-vacutainer system. The blood samples were centrifuged at 3000× g for ten minutes and the supernatant was frozen at −80 °C. The hemolyzed or lactescent samples were rejected.

The serum levels of sialic acid were determined using resorcinol-chlorohydric acid. Blue chromophore was extracted with n-butyl/n-butanol acetate and the optical density was measured at 580 nm with the Sigma reactive (SIALICQ Kit) and the BS3000 analyzer (SINNOWA Medical Science and Technology, Nanjing, China). The results were expressed as mg/dL.

The determination of lipid-bound sialic acid (LSA) levels was performed as follows: 50 µL serum was diluted with 150 µL of cold distilled water. There was added 3 mL of chloroform:methanol (v/v) 2:1, at 4 °C. The extraction and partition were made after adding 0.5 mL of cold distilled water. After separating the phases by centrifugation, sialic acid was titred with resorcinol-chlorhidric acid.

The serum levels of beta-galactoside 2,6-sialyltransferase I (ST6GalI) (E.C.2.4.99.1) were assessed by ELISA method-sandwich variant (IBL. Co., Ltd., 27762 kit, Okayama, Japan) using a Tecan analyzer (Männedorf, Switzerland). The method is sensible (0.20 ng/mL), reproducible (95–97%), both intra-assay coefficient of variation (CV) and inter-assay CV are less than 15%. It has large limits of detection (1.09–70 ng/mL). The technique uses two kinds of highly specific antibodies. The colorimetric evaluation of the final product was made at a wavelength of 450 nm. The concentration of ST6GalI in the samples was determined by comparing the optical density of the samples to the standard curve. The results were expressed as ng/mL serum.

The serum levels of human sialidase-3 (NEU3) (E.C.3.2.1.18) were assessed by ELISA method-sandwich variant (Mybiosource. Cat. No:MBS 9368355) using a Tecan analyzer (Männedorf, Switzerland). The method is sensible (0.1ng/mL), reproducible (95–97%), both intra-assay CV and inter-assay CV are less than 15%. It has large limits of detection (0.25 ng/mL–8 ng/mL). The colorimetric evaluation of the final product was made at a wavelength of 450 nm. The concentration of NEU3 in the samples was determined by comparing the optical density of the samples to the standard curve. The results were expressed as ng/mL serum.

2.4. Statistical Analysis

Triple comparison of the groups was performed using Kruskal–Wallis test and the Dunn post hoc test and pairwise comparison of the groups was performed using Mann–Whitney U test, according to the data distribution (evaluated by Kolmogorov–Smirnov test). The relationship between pairs of two parameters was assessed by Spearman's correlation coefficient, according to the data distribution. We chose a significance level (p) of 0.05 (5%) and a confidence interval of 95% for hypothesis testing.

3. Results

Descriptive data of the study participants and the characteristics of the tumors are presented in Table 1.

Table 1. Clinical data of the study participants and tumor characteristics.

	cSCC Group (n = 40)	AK Group (n = 28)	Control Group (n = 40)
Patient characteristics			
Female/male	16/24	12/16	18/22
Age (years)	56.6 ± 10.8	55.8 ± 8.5	54.6 ± 9.3
BMI (kg/m^2)	23.6 ± 1.7	22.4 ± 1.4	22.1 ± 1.9
Skin phototypes I-II/III-IV	16/24	15/13	22/18
Exposure/non-exposure to UV	34/6	24/4	32/8
Tumor characteristics			
Tumor diameter <2 cm/>2 cm	28/12	28/0	-
Depth of invasion <4 mm/>4 mm	23/17	-	-
Ki67 index: <25%/25–75%/>75%	15/14/11	-	-
Lesion ulceration - Present/absent	23/17	1/27	-

cSCC—cutaneous squamous cell carcinoma; AK—actinic keratosis.

The serum levels of TSA and LSA were higher in the cSCC group compared to the controls. In the AK group, only the TSA levels were higher compared to the control group. In addition, there were significant differences between the cSCC and AK groups. The serum levels of ST6GalI and NEU3 were higher in the cSCC group and AK group compared to the controls, the differences were statistically significant only when we compared cSCC patients to the control group. In addition, there were significant differences between the cSCC and AK groups (Table 2, Figure 3).

The rate of synthesis of sialoglycoconjugates and their rate of enzymatic degradation, expressed by the ST6GalI/NEU3 ratio, is 1.64 times lower in the cSCC group compared to the control group ($p < 0.01$) and 1.53 times lower compared to the AK group ($p < 0.01$).

There were statistically significant positive correlations between the serum levels of TSA and LSA and the tumor characteristics (diameter, depth of invasion, and Ki67 index) (Table 3). There were also statistically significant positive correlations between the serum levels of ST6GalI and the tumor characteristics (diameter and Ki67 index) (Table 3).

Table 2. The serum levels of TSA, LSA, ST6GalI, and NEU3 in the studied groups expressed as the mean ± standard deviation.

Parameter	cSCC Group (n = 40, A)	AK Group (n = 28, B)	Control Group (n = 40, C)	p *	p **
TSA (mg/dL)	86.26 ± 8.58	56.41 ± 4.27	49.71 ± 3.56	$p < 0.01$	A vs. B: <0.001 A vs. C: <0.001 B vs. C: <0.001
LSA (mg/dL)	36.59 ± 7.14	18.92 ± 0.56	18.77 ± 0.49	$p < 0.01$	A vs. B: <0.001 A vs. C: <0.001 B vs. C: 0.79
ST6GalI (ng/mL)	49.06 ± 10.02	24.62 ± 3.71	22.31 ± 2.90	$p < 0.01$	A vs. B: <0.001 A vs. C: <0.001 B vs. C: 0.052
NEU3 (ng/mL)	7.64 ± 4.22	2.32 ± 1.16	2.27 ± 1.01	$p < 0.01$	A vs. B: <0.001 A vs. C: <0.001 B vs. C: 0.89

cSCC—cutaneous squamous cell carcinoma; AK—actinic keratosis; TSA—total sialic acid; LSA—lipid-bound sialic acid; ST6GalI—beta-galactoside 2,6-sialyltransferase I; NEU3—neuraminidase 3; p-significance level, p *—triple comparison of the groups, p **—pairwise comparison of the groups.

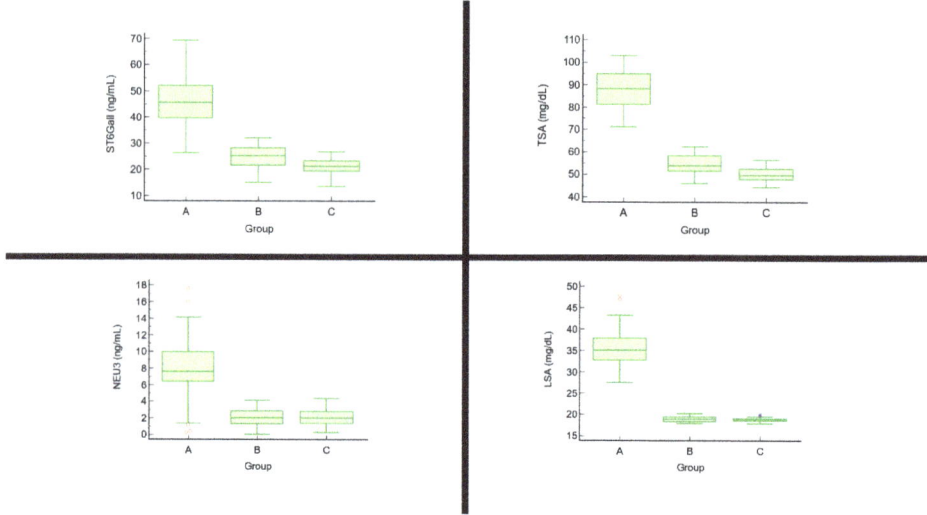

Figure 3. The serum levels of TSA, LSA, ST6GalI, and NEU3 in the studied groups (A = cSCC group, B = AK group, C = control group).

Table 3. Correlations between the serum levels of TSA, LSA, ST6GalI, and NEU3 and histological features of cSCC.

Parameter	TSA		LSA		ST6GalI		NEU3	
	rho	p	rho	p	rho	p	rho	p
Diameter	0.63	<0.001 *	0.58	<0.010 *	0.78	0.01 *	0.58	0.07
Depth of invasion	0.39	0.02 *	0.46	0.01 *	0.29	0.13	0.46	0.11
Ki67	0.34	0.04 *	0.66	0.01 *	0.25	0.82	0.26	0.102
Ulceration	0.12	0.29	−0.02	0.78	0.33	0.42	0.47	0.03 *

cSCC—cutaneous squamous cell carcinoma; TSA—total sialic acid; LSA—lipid-bound sialic acid; ST6GalI—beta-galactoside 2,6-sialyltransferase I; NEU3—neuraminidase 3; Ki67—proliferative index; rho—correlation coefficient; p—significance level. *—statistically significant.

4. Discussion

The pathogenesis of cSCC is complex and includes numerous intrinsic and extrinsic factors [43–45]. Carcinogenesis is a multistep process involving many cells, mediators, and signaling pathways [46,47]. In carcinogenesis, significant structural changes have been described regarding the carbohydrates in the structure of glycoproteins and glycolipids such as a high number of polylactosaminnoglycan chains, multiple branching of asparagine-linked glycans, and increased sialylation [33]. Sialic acid is the outermost monosaccharide unit in the glycan chains of glycolipids and glycoproteins [48] and is ubiquitously distributed in the human body being involved in both physiological and pathological processes. Sialic acid participates in physiological processes such as the transport of positively charged compounds or conformational changes of glycoproteins on cell membranes and mediates cell–cell interactions [21,49]. Elevated levels of sialic acid are associated with resistance to apoptosis and altered cell interactions, promoting cell survival and migration [50]. Abnormal activity of the enzymes involved in sialic acid metabolism or abnormal expression of their corresponding genes leads to aberrant sialylation of glycoproteins or glycolipids [51]. Malignant cell surface glycoproteins and glycolipids display a modified sialic acid composition [39]. Changes in the structure of these glycoproteins and glycolipids may impair processes such as cell recognition, adhesion, or antigenicity. Thus, nowadays sialylation is regarded as one of the major features of the malignant process [21,49]. Aberrant sialylation is the main cancer-associated change of glycosylation process [52,53]. Therefore, it has been suggested that the serum levels of sialic acid and enzymes of sialic acid metabolism may be useful markers in monitoring cancer patients [49]. Parmar et al. have shown higher serum levels of sialic acid in patients with head and neck SCC compared to the control group [38]. Vural et al. have detected increased serum TSA levels in patients with actinic keratoses compared to controls. When they compared the serum TSA levels between AK patients and BCC patients, no differences were obtained [39]. In the current study, we have also detected higher serum levels of TSA in the patient groups compared to controls. However, the serum levels of LSA were significantly higher only when we compared cSCC patients to the control group. In cSCC patients, we have identified higher serum levels of both TSA and LSA compared to AK patients. These results indicate that biochemical changes in glycoproteins start at an early stage of tumorigenesis. High serum levels of LSA are indicative of a premalignant change. Krishnan et al. have shown a positive correlation between TSA level and the grade of dysplasia in patients with oral leukoplakia, but no specific changes regarding LSA levels and the grade of epithelial dysplasia [54].

In various types of cancer, alteration in sialyltransferase activity has been observed [55,56]. ST6GalI seems to be the major sialyltransferase that is overexpressed in malignant tumors [57]. ST6GALI is upregulated in several cancers such as breast, ovarian, and pancreatic neoplasms, being involved in tumor aggressiveness and metastasis [27,57]. Recent studies have demonstrated the role of ST6GALI in the malignant phenotype (growth, survival, angiogenesis, apoptosis, invasion, resistance to cell stress, chemoresistance). Increased ST6GAL1 activity is determined by genetic instability and epigenetic, transcriptional, and posttranslational factors [27,30].

Although there are several studies that identified overexpression of ST6GalI in advanced disease [58,59], a study evaluating patients with oral SCC (OSCC) has revealed ST6GalI overexpression in the early stages of the disease [60]. In line with this, recently, Mehta et al. have analyzed mRNA expression of a group of sialyltransferases, including ST3GALI, ST3GALII, ST3GALIII, ST3GALIV, ST3GALVI, ST6GALI, and the plasma membrane-associated sialidase NEU3, and found down-regulation of these transcripts in OSCC samples compared to adjacent healthy tissue. In normal tissue, they observed increased mRNA levels of sialyltransferases and sialidase NEU3. These results may indicate that alterations of glycosylation are very early events during carcinogenesis. Probably in fact, in the adjacent tumor tissue, although macroscopically normal, a population of cells with early genetic changes is present. The authors also demonstrated that elevated mRNA levels of ST3GALII and ST3GALIII may be prognostic markers in OSCC [61].

We have detected higher serum levels of ST6GalI in cSCC patients compared to controls, whereas there were no significant differences between AK patients and controls. The soluble form of ST6GalI, possibly secreted by SCC cells, may participate in cancer progression and metastasis. This finding is supported by a previous study that showed high immunohistochemical expression of ST3GalI and ST6GalI in cutaneous epithelial lesions including keratoacanthoma, AK, BCC, and SCC. These results suggest that sialyltransferases are deregulated in skin tumors. No significant differences were found between SCC and AK samples [29]. In our study, we have found higher serum levels of ST6GalI in cSCC compared to AK. These findings show that AK and cSCC have a different pattern of sialylation that is related to tumor behavior. Only a small number of AK suffer malignant transformation [62].

Plzak et al. found that poorly differentiated SCCs are positive for 2,6-linked NeuNAc, whereas differentiated SCCs express 2,3-linked-NeuNAc [63]. The cleavage of 2,6-linked NeuNAc by sialidases allows tumor cells to be recognized by Gal-3, a useful prognostic marker in head and neck SCC. It has been shown that 2,6-NeuNAc is a more potent masking compound than 2,3-NeuNAc with regard to the binding of Gal-3 [63,64]. Melanoma is a very aggressive tumor [65] and a recent study has highlighted the role of ST3GALI in melanoma metastasis [50]. Inhibition of enzyme activity is associated with decreased invasion capacity of melanoma cells and reduced ability to hematogenously disseminate. In this process, the ST3GALI–AXL axis may have a role, where the receptor tyrosine kinase AXL represents the key effector of the ST3GALI pro-invasive function. Modulation of the ST3GAL1–AXL axis may represent a target in melanoma treatment [50].

The plasma membrane-associated sialidase NEU3 is upregulated in various types of cancer including renal, colon and prostate neoplasms [66–68]. In malignant tumors, NEU3 promotes cell survival, migration, and adhesion [69]. NEU3 induces carcinogenesis primarily by altering cell signaling at the cell surface [22]. Recent data have revealed that NEU3 modulates transmembrane signaling through the interaction with various molecules such as caveolin-1, Rac-1, integrin β4, and epidermal growth factor receptor (EGFR) [33]. In colon neoplasms, NEU3 mediates tumor cell proliferation through integrin-mediated signaling, depending on the extracellular matrix. Therefore, NEU3 produces increased adhesion to laminin, promoting cell proliferation and decreased adhesion to fibronectin [70]. On the other hand, in renal cancer, increased levels of NEU3 mRNA have been identified in association with high levels of IL-6, a cytokine that acts as an activator of NEU3, and in turn, NEU3 drives IL-6-mediated signaling via the PI3K/Akt pathway leading to a malignant phenotype characterized by reduced apoptosis and increased cell mobility [67].

Hata et al. suggested that the serum levels of NEU3 are correlated with serum gangliosides, which have been detected in patients with neoplasms [22]. It seems that NEU3 is released from the cell surface in response to the accumulation of gangliosides in serum. It should be noted that NEU3 is an important enzyme for ganglioside degradation [22]. NEU3 acts on gangliosides that are located on the same cell membrane (cis-activity) or on the membrane of neighboring cells (trans-activity), regulating the interactions between cells [71]. The overexpression of *NEU3* and *GD3* synthase genes has been reported in cutaneous melanoma. NEU3 and GM1 and GM2 synthases, involved in ganglioside metabolism, were associated with melanoma cell proliferation and invasion [72]. NEU3 regulates transmembrane signaling through the modulation of ganglioside catabolism. NEU3 hydrolyzes polysialic acid-containing gangliosides to GM1 ganglioside and is involved in the increase in GM1 levels [73]. In addition, in some instances, gangliosides are not efficiently hydrolyzed by plasma membrane sialidases and this explains why gangliosides may accumulate [72].

In our study, we have found higher serum levels of NEU3 in cSCC patients when compared to the control group and as well as when compared to AK patients. The results were similar between AK patients and the control group. The study by Shiga et al. has revealed that mRNA levels of NEU3 are upregulated in head and neck SCC with lymph nodes metastases compared to normal cells. In addition, the study has shown that NEU3 stimulates cell mobility and invasion. NEU3 increases the phosphorylation of EGFR, which may lead to ERK activation and subsequent release of metalloproteinases (MMP-2 and MMP-9) that promote cell invasion [40]. It has also been shown that NEU3 modulates the phosphorylation of EGFR and its dimerization in HeLa cells, activating the Ras cascade, which will promote cell survival [69].

The results of the present study show that there is an altered degradation rate of sialoglycoconjugates in cSCC patients compared to AK and control groups. Hypersialylation and increased glycoconjugate catabolism are features of patients with cSCC compared to AK patients and controls. Our study has revealed that the ST6GalI/NEU3 ratio is significantly altered in patients with cSCC and could represent a potential molecular target in these patients.

This is necessary to determine markers for SCC diagnosis and management [74]. In our study, the tumor diameter, depth of invasion, and Ki67 were associated with higher levels of TSA and LSA. Inal et al. also found increased levels of LSA that correlated with tumor size in patients with head and neck SCC [75]. There was no correlation between NEU3 and tumor aggressiveness. As mentioned above, NEU3 plays an important role in tumor invasion and metastasis, but metastasis in cSCC is very rare. In line with this, in head and neck SCC, NEU3 has been associated especially with lymph node metastasis [40]

These results support the role of these compounds in tumor progression and invasiveness. A potential role of sialidases as therapeutical targets in the management of cancer has been highlighted. For example, oseltamivir phosphate, an extensively used anti-influenza drug and a viral sialidase inhibitor, targets human NEU1 showing encouraging results in preventing tumor cell metastasis [76,77] The inhibition of NEU1 expression by oseltamivir phosphate leads to overexpression of E-cadherin and downregulation of N-cadherin expression, which may limit the ability of cells to metastasize and increase their sensitivity of antineoplastic drugs [78].

Monitoring serum levels of total sialic acid, lipid-bound sialic acid, sialyltransferases, and sialidases in correlation with tumor characteristics may have useful clinical applications for the diagnosis of cSCC. Future research is required to find reliable markers for the management of cSCC.

5. Conclusions

The current study reveals aberrant sialylation in cSCC patients, but not in AK patients. We have found a significant increase in serum levels of TSA, LSA, ST6GalI, and NEU3 in the cSCC group compared to the control group, whereas in patients with AK only the serum level of TSA was significantly higher compared to the control group. When the cSCC and AK groups were compared, significant differences between the serum levels of TSA, LSA, ST6GalI, and NEU3 were found. In conclusion, the serum ST6GalI/NEU3 level may represent a potential molecular factor to distinguish cSCC patients from non-cancer patients, pending further validation. Further studies are needed to understand sialylation-related changes in cSCC, supporting further improvements in the diagnostic and treatment approach.

Author Contributions: All authors have equally contributed to the writing and editing of the manuscript. Conceptualization, C.D.E. and I.N.; methodology, I.N.; software, C.D.E.; validation, C.D.E., I.N., S.R.G. and C.E.; formal analysis, I.N. and C.E.; investigation, C.D.E.; resources, M.T., S.R.G. and C.M.; data curation, C.D.E. and S.R.G.; writing—original draft preparation, C.D.E., C.I.M. and M.I.M.; writing—review and editing, C.D.E., C.M. and M.T.; visualization, S.R.G., C.I.M., M.I.M. and C.M.; supervision, S.R.G., I.N. and M.T. All authors have read and agreed to the published version of the manuscript.

Funding: The article processing charges were funded by Carol Davila University of Medicine and Pharmacy.

Institutional Review Board Statement: The study was conducted according to the guidelines of the Declaration of Helsinki, and approved by the Ethics Committee of the "Victor Babeş" Clinical Hospital for Infectious Diseases, Bucharest (3/10.03.2018).

Informed Consent Statement: Informed consent was obtained from all subjects involved in the study.

Data Availability Statement: The data presented in this study are available on request from the corresponding author.

Conflicts of Interest: The authors declare no conflict of interest.

References

1. Jones, O.T.; Ranmuthu, C.K.I.; Hall, P.N.; Funston, G.; Walter, F.M. Recognising Skin Cancer in Primary Care. *Adv. Ther.* **2020**, *37*, 603–616. [CrossRef] [PubMed]
2. Rollison, D.E.; Viarisio, D.; Amorrortu, R.P.; Gheit, T.; Tommasino, M. An Emerging Issue in Oncogenic Virology: The Role of Beta Human Papillomavirus Types in the Development of Cutaneous Squamous Cell Carcinoma. *J. Virol.* **2019**, *93*, e01003-18. [CrossRef] [PubMed]
3. Que, S.K.T.; Zwald, F.O.; Schmults, C.D. Cutaneous Squamous Cell Carcinoma. *J. Am. Acad. Dermatol.* **2018**, *78*, 237–247. [CrossRef] [PubMed]
4. Tampa, M.; Mitran, C.I.; Mitran, M.I.; Nicolae, I.; Dumitru, A.; Matei, C.; Manolescu, L.; Popa, G.L.; Caruntu, C.; Georgescu, S.R. The Role of Beta HPV Types and HPV-Associated Inflammatory Processes in Cutaneous Squamous Cell Carcinoma. *J. Immunol. Res.* **2020**, *2020*, 5701639. [CrossRef] [PubMed]
5. Cela, E.M.; Paz, M.L.; Leoni, J.; Maglio, D.H.G. Immune System Modulation Produced by Ultraviolet Radiation. *Immunoreg. Asp. Immunother.* **2018**, *103*. [CrossRef]
6. Kim, I.; He, Y.-Y. Ultraviolet Radiation-Induced Non-Melanoma Skin Cancer: Regulation of DNA Damage Repair and Inflammation. *Genes Dis.* **2014**, *1*, 188–198. [CrossRef]
7. Tufaro, A.P.; Chuang, J.C.-M.; Prasad, N.; Chuang, A.; Chuang, T.C.; Fischer, A.C. Molecular Markers in Cutaneous Squamous Cell Carcinoma. *Int. J. Surg. Oncol.* **2011**, *2011*, 231475. [CrossRef]
8. Wang, J.; Aldabagh, B.; Yu, J.; Arron, S.T. Role of human papillomavirus in cutaneous squamous cell carcinoma: A meta-analysis. *J. Am. Acad. Dermatol.* **2014**, *70*, 621–629. [CrossRef]
9. Chahoud, J.; Semaan, A.; Chen, Y.; Cao, M.; Rieber, A.G.; Rady, P.; Tyring, S.K. Association between β-Genus Human Papillomavirus and Cutaneous Squamous Cell Carcinoma in Immunocompetent Individuals—A Meta-Analysis. *JAMA Dermatol.* **2016**, *152*, 1354–1364. [CrossRef]
10. Hampras, S.S.; Reed, R.A.; Bezalel, S.; Cameron, M.; Cherpelis, B.; Fenske, N.; Sondak, V.K.; Messina, J.; Tommasino, M.; Gheit, T. Cutaneous Human Papillomavirus Infection and Development of Subsequent Squamous Cell Carcinoma of the Skin. *J. Skin Cancer* **2016**, *2016*, 1368103. [CrossRef]
11. Burton, K.A.; Ashack, K.A.; Khachemoune, A. Cutaneous Squamous Cell Carcinoma: A Review of High-Risk and Metastatic Disease. *Am. J. Clin. Dermatol.* **2016**, *17*, 491–508. [CrossRef]
12. Endo, Y.; Tanioka, M.; Miyachi, Y. Prognostic Factors in Cutaneous Squamous Cell Carcinoma: Is Patient Delay in Hospital Visit a Predictor of Survival? *ISRN Dermatol.* **2011**, *2011*, 285289. [CrossRef] [PubMed]
13. Brantsch, K.D.; Meisner, C.; Schönfisch, B.; Trilling, B.; Wehner-Caroli, J.; Röcken, M.; Breuninger, H. Analysis of Risk Factors Determining Prognosis of Cutaneous Squamous-Cell Carcinoma: A Prospective Study. *Lancet Oncol.* **2008**, *9*, 713–720. [CrossRef]
14. Reinehr, C.P.H.; Bakos, R.M. Actinic Keratoses: Review of Clinical, Dermoscopic, and Therapeutic Aspects. *Anais Brasileiros de Dermatologia* **2019**, *94*, 637–657. [CrossRef] [PubMed]
15. Matei, C.; Tampa, M.; Ion, R.; Neagu, M.; Constantin, C. Photodynamic properties of aluminium sulphonated phthalocyanines in human displazic oral keratinocytes experimental model. *Dig. J. Nanomater. Biostruct.* **2012**, *7*, 1535–1547.
16. Vajaria, B.N.; Patel, K.R.; Begum, R.; Patel, P.S. Sialylation: An Avenue to Target Cancer Cells. *Pathol. Oncol. Res.* **2016**, *22*, 443–447. [CrossRef] [PubMed]
17. Nicolae, C.; Nicolae, I. Heterogeneity of Gangliosides in Melanocytic Tumors. *Acta Endocrinol.* **2012**, *8*, 17–26. [CrossRef]
18. Möginger, U.; Grunewald, S.; Hennig, R.; Kuo, C.-W.; Schirmeister, F.; Voth, H.; Rapp, E.; Khoo, K.-H.; Seeberger, P.H.; Simon, J.C.; et al. Alterations of the Human Skin N- and O-Glycome in Basal Cell Carcinoma and Squamous Cell Carcinoma. *Front. Oncol.* **2018**, *8*, 70. [CrossRef]
19. Dobie, C.; Skropeta, D. Insights into the Role of Sialylation in Cancer Progression and Metastasis. *Br. J. Cancer* **2021**, *124*, 76–90. [CrossRef]
20. Dall'Olio, F.; Malagolini, N.; Trinchera, M.; Chiricolo, M. Sialosignaling: Sialyltransferases as Engines of Self-Fueling Loops in Cancer Progression. *Biochim. Biophys. Acta (BBA)-Gen. Subj.* **2014**, *1840*, 2752–2764. [CrossRef]
21. Zhang, Z.; Wuhrer, M.; Holst, S. Serum Sialylation Changes in Cancer. *Glycoconj. J.* **2018**, *35*, 139–160. [CrossRef]
22. Hata, K.; Tochigi, T.; Sato, I.; Kawamura, S.; Shiozaki, K.; Wada, T.; Takahashi, K.; Moriya, S.; Yamaguchi, K.; Hosono, M.; et al. Increased Sialidase Activity in Serum of Cancer Patients: Identification of Sialidase and Inhibitor Activities in Human Serum. *Cancer Sci.* **2015**, *106*, 383–389. [CrossRef]

23. Ene, C.D.; Nicolae, I.; Mitran, C.I.; Mitran, M.I.; Matei, C.; Caruntu, A.; Caruntu, C.; Georgescu, S.R. Antiganglioside Antibodies and Inflammatory Response in Cutaneous Melanoma. *J. Immunol. Res.* **2020**, *2020*, 2491265. [CrossRef]
24. Kolasińska, E.; Przybyło, M.; Janik, M.; Lityńska, A. Towards Understanding the Role of Sialylation in Melanoma Progression. *Acta Biochim. Pol.* **2016**, *63*, 533–541. [CrossRef]
25. Rodrigues, E.; Macauley, M.S. Hypersialylation in Cancer: Modulation of Inflammation and Therapeutic Opportunities. *Cancers* **2018**, *10*, 207. [CrossRef]
26. Pearce, O.M.; Läubli, H. Sialic Acids in Cancer Biology and Immunity. *Glycobiology* **2016**, *26*, 111–128. [CrossRef]
27. Garnham, R.; Scott, E.; Livermore, K.; Munkley, J. ST6GAL1: A Key Player in Cancer. *Oncol. Lett.* **2019**, *18*, 983–989. [CrossRef] [PubMed]
28. Takashima, S.; Tsuji, S. Functional Diversity of Mammalian Sialyltransferases. *Trends Glycosci. Glycotechnol.* **2011**, *23*, 178–193. [CrossRef]
29. Ferreira, S.A.; Vasconcelos, J.L.A.; Silva, R.C.W.C.; Cavalcanti, C.L.B.; Bezerra, C.L.; Rêgo, M.J.B.M.; Beltrão, E.I.C. Expression Patterns of A2,3-Sialyltransferase I and A2,6-Sialyltransferase I in Human Cutaneous Epithelial Lesions. *Eur. J. Histochem.* **2013**, *57*, 7. [CrossRef] [PubMed]
30. Dorsett, K.A.; Marciel, M.P.; Hwang, J.; Ankenbauer, K.E.; Bhalerao, N.; Bellis, S.L. Regulation of ST6GAL1 Sialyltransferase Expression in Cancer Cells. *Glycobiology* **2021**, *31*, 530–539. [CrossRef]
31. Glanz, V.Y.; Myasoedova, V.A.; Grechko, A.V.; Orekhov, A.N. Sialidase Activity in Human Pathologies. *Eur. J. Pharmacol.* **2019**, *842*, 345–350. [CrossRef] [PubMed]
32. Miyagi, T. Aberrant Expression of Sialidase and Cancer Progression. *Proc. Jpn. Acad. Ser. B* **2008**, *84*, 407–418. [CrossRef] [PubMed]
33. Miyagi, T.; Takahashi, K.; Hata, K.; Shiozaki, K.; Yamaguchi, K. Sialidase Significance for Cancer Progression. *Glycoconj. J.* **2012**, *29*, 567–577. [CrossRef] [PubMed]
34. Ene, C.D.; Penescu, M.N.; Georgescu, S.R.; Tampa, M.; Nicolae, I. Posttranslational Modifications Pattern in Clear Cell Renal Cell Carcinoma. *Metabolites* **2020**, *11*, 10. [CrossRef] [PubMed]
35. Ene, C.D.; Georgescu, S.R.; Tampa, M.; Matei, C.; Mitran, C.I.; Mitran, M.I.; Penescu, M.N.; Nicolae, I. Cellular Response against Oxidative Stress, a Novel Insight into Lupus Nephritis Pathogenesis. *J. Pers. Med.* **2021**, *11*, 693. [CrossRef] [PubMed]
36. Ene, C.D.; Penescu, M.; Anghel, A.; Neagu, M.; Budu, V.; Nicolae, I. Monitoring Diabetic Nephropathy by Circulating Gangliosides. *J. Immunoass. Immunochem.* **2016**, *37*, 68–79. [CrossRef] [PubMed]
37. Ene, C.-D.; Penescu, M.N.; Nicolae, I. Sialoglyco-Conjugate Abnormalities, IL-6 Trans-Signaling and Anti-Ganglioside Immune Response—Potential Interferences in Lupus Nephritis Pathogenesis. *Diagnostics* **2021**, *11*, 1129. [CrossRef] [PubMed]
38. Parmar, M.; Pandhi, N.; Patel, P. Clinical Evaluation of Sialic Acid In Head and Neck Squamous Cell Carcinoma Patients and Tobacco Chewers or Smokers with No Cancer. *Biomed. Pharmacol. J.* **2017**, *10*, 2027–2033. [CrossRef]
39. Vural, P.; Canbaz, M.; Selcuki, D. Total and Lipid-Bound Sialic Acid Levels in Actinic Keratosis and Basal Cell Carcinoma. *Turk. J. Med. Sci.* **1999**, *29*, 419–424.
40. Shiga, K.; Takahashi, K.; Sato, I.; Kato, K.; Saijo, S.; Moriya, S.; Hosono, M.; Miyagi, T. Upregulation of Sialidase NEU 3 in Head and Neck Squamous Cell Carcinoma Associated with Lymph Node Metastasis. *Cancer Sci.* **2015**, *106*, 1544–1553. [CrossRef]
41. Manualul AJCC de Stadializare a Cancerului. 2018. Available online: https://www.clb.ro/manualul-ajcc-de-stadializare-a-cancerului-2018-0000176379--p343005.html (accessed on 10 July 2021).
42. Menon, S.S.; Guruvayoorappan, C.; Sakthivel, K.M.; Rasmi, R.R. Ki-67 Protein as a Tumour Proliferation Marker. *Clin. Chim. Acta* **2019**, *491*, 39–45. [CrossRef] [PubMed]
43. Georgescu, S.R.; Tampa, M.; Mitran, C.I.; Mitran, M.I.; Caruntu, C.; Caruntu, A.; Lupu, M.; Matei, C.; Constantin, C.; Neagu, M. Tumour Microenvironment in Skin Carcinogenesis. *Adv. Exp. Med. Biol.* **2020**, *1226*, 123–142. [CrossRef]
44. Ratushny, V.; Gober, M.D.; Hick, R.; Ridky, T.W.; Seykora, J.T. From Keratinocyte to Cancer: The Pathogenesis and Modeling of Cutaneous Squamous Cell Carcinoma. *J. Clin. Investig.* **2012**, *122*, 464–472. [CrossRef] [PubMed]
45. Tampa, M.; Matei, C.; Popescu, S.; Georgescu, S.-R.; Neagu, M.; Constantin, C.; Ion, R.-M. Zinc Trisulphonated Phthalocyanine Used in Photodynamic Therapy of Dysplastic Oral Keratinocytes. *Rev. Chim.* **2013**, *64*, 639–645.
46. Peters, J.M.; Gonzalez, F.J. The Evolution of Carcinogenesis. *Toxicol. Sci.* **2018**, *165*, 272–276. [CrossRef] [PubMed]
47. Georgescu, S.R.; Mitran, C.I.; Mitran, M.I.; Caruntu, C.; Sarbu, M.I.; Matei, C.; Nicolae, I.; Tocut, S.M.; Popa, M.I.; Tampa, M. New Insights in the Pathogenesis of HPV Infection and the Associated Carcinogenic Processes: The Role of Chronic Inflammation and Oxidative Stress. *J. Immunol. Res.* **2018**, *2018*, 5315816. [CrossRef] [PubMed]
48. Lima, L.R.A.; Bezerra, M.F.; Almeida, S.M.V.; Silva, L.P.B.G.; Beltrão, E.I.C.; Carvalho Júnior, L.B. Glycophenotype Evaluation in Cutaneous Tumors Using Lectins Labeled with Acridinium Ester. *Dis. Markers* **2013**, *35*, 149–154. [CrossRef] [PubMed]
49. Raval, G.; Patel, D.; Parekh, L.; Patel, J.; Shah, M.; Patel, P. Evaluation of Serum Sialic Acid, Sialyltransferase and Sialoproteins in Oral Cavity Cancer: Sialic Acid, Sialyltransferase and Sialoproteins in Oral Cavity Cancer. *Oral Dis.* **2003**, *9*, 119–128. [CrossRef]
50. Pietrobono, S.; Anichini, G.; Sala, C.; Manetti, F.; Almada, L.L.; Pepe, S.; Carr, R.M.; Paradise, B.D.; Sarkaria, J.N.; Davila, J.I.; et al. ST3GAL1 Is a Target of the SOX2-GLI1 Transcriptional Complex and Promotes Melanoma Metastasis through AXL. *Nat. Commun.* **2020**, *11*, 5865. [CrossRef]
51. Ghosh, S. *Sialic Acids and Sialoglycoconjugates in the Biology of Life, Health and Disease*; Academic Press: Cambridge, MA, USA, 2020; ISBN 0-12-816127-2.

52. Munkley, J.; Oltean, S.; Vodák, D.; Wilson, B.T.; Livermore, K.E.; Zhou, Y.; Star, E.; Floros, V.I.; Johannessen, B.; Knight, B. The Androgen Receptor Controls Expression of the Cancer-Associated STn Antigen and Cell Adhesion through Induction of ST6GalNAc1 in Prostate Cancer. *Oncotarget* **2015**, *6*, 34358. [CrossRef]
53. Munkley, J. The Role of Sialyl-Tn in Cancer. *Int. J. Mol. Sci.* **2016**, *17*, 275. [CrossRef] [PubMed]
54. Krishnan, K.; Balasundaram, S. Evaluation of Total and Lipid Bound Sialic Acid in Serum in Oral Leukoplakia. *J. Clin. Diagn Res.* **2017**, *11*, ZC25–ZC27. [CrossRef] [PubMed]
55. Nguyen, K.; Yan, Y.; Yuan, B.; Dasgupta, A.; Sun, J.; Mu, H.; Do, K.-A.; Ueno, N.T.; Andreeff, M.; Battula, V.L. ST8SIA1 Regulates Tumor Growth and Metastasis in TNBC by Activating the FAK-AKT-MTOR Signaling Pathway. *Mol. Cancer* **2018**, *17*, 2689–2701. [CrossRef] [PubMed]
56. Vajaria, B.N.; Patel, K.A.; Patel, P.S. Role of Aberrant Glycosylation Enzymes in Oral Cancer Progression. *J. Carcinog.* **2018**, *17*, 5. [CrossRef]
57. Wang, P.-H.; Lee, W.-L.; Lee, Y.-R.; Juang, C.-M.; Chen, Y.-J.; Chao, H.-T.; Tsai, Y.-C.; Yuan, C.-C. Enhanced Expression of α 2,6-Sialyltransferase ST6Gal I in Cervical Squamous Cell Carcinoma. *Gynecol. Oncol.* **2003**, *89*, 395–401. [CrossRef]
58. Bresalier, R.S.; Ho, S.B.; Schoeppner, H.L.; Kim, Y.S.; Sleisenger, M.H.; Brodt, P.; Byrd, J.C. Enhanced Sialylation of Mucin-Associated Carbohydrate Structures in Human Colon Cancer Metastasis. *Gastroenterology* **1996**, *110*, 1354–1367. [CrossRef]
59. Recchi, M.-A.; Hebbar, M.; Hornez, L.; Harduin-Lepers, A.; Peyrat, J.-P.; Delannoy, P. Multiplex Reverse Transcription Polymerase Chain Reaction Assessment of Sialyltransferase Expression in Human Breast Cancer. *Cancer Res.* **1998**, *58*, 4066–4070.
60. Fialka, F.; Gruber, R.M.; Hitt, R.; Opitz, L.; Brunner, E.; Schliephake, H.; Kramer, F.-J. CPA6, FMO2, LGI1, SIAT1 and TNC Are Differentially Expressed in Early- and Late-Stage Oral Squamous Cell Carcinoma—A Pilot Study. *Oral Oncol.* **2008**, *44*, 941–948. [CrossRef]
61. Mehta, K.A.; Patel, K.A.; Pandya, S.J.; Patel, P.S. Aberrant Sialylation Plays a Significant Role in Oral Squamous Cell Carcinoma Progression. *J. Oral Pathol. Med.* **2020**, *49*, 253–259. [CrossRef]
62. Boukamp, P. Non-Melanoma Skin Cancer: What Drives Tumor Development and Progression? *Carcinogenesis* **2005**, *26*, 1657–1667. [CrossRef]
63. Plzák, J.; Smetana, K., Jr.; Chovanec, M.; Betka, J. Glycobiology of Head and Neck Squamous Epithelia and Carcinomas. *ORL* **2005**, *67*, 61–69. [CrossRef] [PubMed]
64. Holíková, Z.; Hrdličková-Cela, E.; Plzák, J.; Smetana, K., Jr.; Betka, J.; Dvoránková, B.; Esner, M.; Wasano, K.; André, S.; Kaltner, H.; et al. Defining the Glycophenotype of Squamous Epithelia Using Plant and Mammalian Lectins. Differentiation-dependent Expression of A2, 6-and A2, 3-linked N-acetylneuraminic Acid in Squamous Epithelia and Carcinomas, and Its Differential Effect on Binding of the Endogenous Lectins Galectins-1 And-3. *Apmis* **2002**, *110*, 845–856.
65. Caruntu, C.; Mirica, A.; Roşca, A.E.; Mirica, R.; Caruntu, A.; Tampa, M.; Matei, C.; Constantin, C.; Neagu, M.; Badarau, A.I.; et al. The role of estrogens and estrogen receptors in melanoma development and progression. *Acta Endocrinol.* **2016**, *12*, 234–241. [CrossRef] [PubMed]
66. Kakugawa, Y.; Wada, T.; Yamaguchi, K.; Yamanami, H.; Ouchi, K.; Sato, I.; Miyagi, T. Up-Regulation of Plasma Membrane-Associated Ganglioside Sialidase (Neu3) in Human Colon Cancer and Its Involvement in Apoptosis Suppression. *Proc. Natl. Acad. Sci. USA* **2002**, *99*, 10718–10723. [CrossRef] [PubMed]
67. Ueno, S.; Saito, S.; Wada, T.; Yamaguchi, K.; Satoh, M.; Arai, Y.; Miyagi, T. Plasma Membrane-Associated Sialidase Is up-Regulated in Renal Cell Carcinoma and Promotes Interleukin-6-Induced Apoptosis Suppression and Cell Motility. *J. Biol. Chem.* **2006**, *281*, 7756–7764. [CrossRef]
68. Kawamura, S.; Sato, I.; Wada, T.; Yamaguchi, K.; Li, Y.; Li, D.; Zhao, X.; Ueno, S.; Aoki, H.; Tochigi, T. Plasma Membrane-Associated Sialidase (NEU3) Regulates Progression of Prostate Cancer to Androgen-Independent Growth through Modulation of Androgen Receptor Signaling. *Cell Death Differ.* **2012**, *19*, 170–179. [CrossRef]
69. Yamamoto, K.; Takahashi, K.; Shiozaki, K.; Yamaguchi, K.; Moriya, S.; Hosono, M.; Shima, H.; Miyagi, T. Potentiation of Epidermal Growth Factor-Mediated Oncogenic Transformation by Sialidase NEU3 Leading to Src Activation. *PLoS ONE* **2015**, *10*, e0120578. [CrossRef]
70. Kato, K.; Shiga, K.; Yamaguchi, K.; Hata, K.; Kobayashi, T.; Miyazaki, K.; Saijo, S.; Miyagi, T. Plasma-Membrane-Associated Sialidase (NEU3) Differentially Regulates Integrin-Mediated Cell Proliferation through Laminin-and Fibronectin-Derived Signalling. *Biochem. J.* **2006**, *394*, 647–656. [CrossRef]
71. Fanzani, A.; Zanola, A.; Faggi, F.; Papini, N.; Venerando, B.; Tettamanti, G.; Sampaolesi, M.; Monti, E. Implications for the Mammalian Sialidases in the Physiopathology of Skeletal Muscle. *Skelet. Muscle* **2012**, *2*, 23. [CrossRef]
72. Tringali, C.; Silvestri, I.; Testa, F.; Baldassari, P.; Anastasia, L.; Mortarini, R.; Anichini, A.; López-Requena, A.; Tettamanti, G.; Venerando, B. Molecular Subtyping of Metastatic Melanoma Based on Cell Ganglioside Metabolism Profiles. *BMC Cancer* **2014**, *14*, 1–14. [CrossRef]
73. Kappagantula, S.; Andrews, M.R.; Cheah, M.; Abad-Rodriguez, J.; Dotti, C.G.; Fawcett, J.W. Neu3 Sialidase-Mediated Ganglioside Conversion Is Necessary for Axon Regeneration and Is Blocked in CNS Axons. *J. Neurosci.* **2014**, *34*, 2477–2492. [CrossRef] [PubMed]
74. Tampa, M.; Mitran, M.I.; Mitran, C.I.; Sarbu, M.I.; Matei, C.; Nicolae, I.; Caruntu, A.; Tocut, S.M.; Popa, M.I.; Caruntu, C.; et al. Mediators of Inflammation—A Potential Source of Biomarkers in Oral Squamous Cell Carcinoma. *J. Immunol. Res.* **2018**, *2018*, 1061780. [CrossRef] [PubMed]

75. Inal, E.; Laçin, M.; Asal, K.; Ceylan, A.; Köybaşioğlu, A.; Ileri, F.; Uslu, S.S. The Significance of Ferritin, Lipid-Associated Sialic Acid, CEA, Squamous Cell Carcinoma (SCC) Antigen, and CYFRA 21-1 Levels in SCC of the Head and Neck. *Kulak Burun Bogaz Ihtisas Dergisi* **2004**, *12*, 23–30. [PubMed]
76. O'Shea, L.K.; Abdulkhalek, S.; Allison, S.; Neufeld, R.J.; Szewczuk, M.R. Therapeutic Targeting of Neu1 Sialidase with Oseltamivir Phosphate (Tamiflu®) Disables Cancer Cell Survival in Human Pancreatic Cancer with Acquired Chemoresistance. *OncoTargets Ther.* **2014**, *7*, 117.
77. Haxho, F.; Allison, S.; Alghamdi, F.; Brodhagen, L.; Kuta, V.E.; Abdulkhalek, S.; Neufeld, R.J.; Szewczuk, M.R. Oseltamivir Phosphate Monotherapy Ablates Tumor Neovascularization, Growth, and Metastasis in Mouse Model of Human Triple-Negative Breast Adenocarcinoma. *Breast Cancer Targets Ther.* **2014**, *6*, 191.
78. Haxho, F.; Neufeld, R.J.; Szewczuk, M.R. Neuraminidase-1: A Novel Therapeutic Target in Multistage Tumorigenesis. *Oncotarget* **2016**, *7*, 40860–40881. [CrossRef]

Review

Cannabinoids and Inflammations of the Gut-Lung-Skin Barrier

Cristian Scheau [1], Constantin Caruntu [1,2], Ioana Anca Badarau [1], Andreea-Elena Scheau [3], Anca Oana Docea [4,*], Daniela Calina [5,*] and Ana Caruntu [6,7]

1. Department of Physiology, "Carol Davila" University of Medicine and Pharmacy, 050474 Bucharest, Romania; cristian.scheau@umfcd.ro (C.S.); costin.caruntu@gmail.com (C.C.); ancab52@yahoo.com (I.A.B.)
2. Department of Dermatology, "Prof. N. Paulescu" National Institute of Diabetes, Nutrition and Metabolic Diseases, 011233 Bucharest, Romania
3. Department of Radiology and Medical Imaging, Fundeni Clinical Institute, 022328 Bucharest, Romania; andreea.ghergus@gmail.com
4. Department of Toxicology, University of Medicine and Pharmacy of Craiova, 200349 Craiova, Romania
5. Department of Clinical Pharmacy, University of Medicine and Pharmacy of Craiova, 200349 Craiova, Romania
6. Department of Oral and Maxillofacial Surgery, "Carol Davila" Central Military Emergency Hospital, 010825 Bucharest, Romania; ana.caruntu@gmail.com
7. Department of Oral and Maxillofacial Surgery, Faculty of Dental Medicine, "Titu Maiorescu" University, 031593 Bucharest, Romania
* Correspondence: ancadocea@gmail.com (A.O.D.); calinadaniela@gmail.com (D.C.)

Abstract: Recent studies have identified great similarities and interferences between the epithelial layers of the digestive tract, the airways and the cutaneous layer. The relationship between these structures seems to implicate signaling pathways, cellular components and metabolic features, and has led to the definition of a gut-lung-skin barrier. Inflammation seems to involve common features in these tissues; therefore, analyzing the similarities and differences in the modulation of its biomarkers can yield significant data promoting a better understanding of the particularities of specific signaling pathways and cellular effects. Cannabinoids are well known for a wide array of beneficial effects, including anti-inflammatory properties. This paper aims to explore the effects of natural and synthetic cannabinoids, including the components of the endocannabinoid system, in relation to the inflammation of the gut-lung-skin barrier epithelia. Recent advancements in the use of cannabinoids as anti-inflammatory substances in various disorders of the gut, lungs and skin are detailed. Some studies have reported mixed or controversial results, and these have also been addressed in our paper.

Keywords: cannabinoids; inflammation; gut-lung-skin barrier; signaling pathways; inflammatory biomarkers

1. Introduction

The epithelial lining is the first line of defense against the abundance of aggressive factors in the environment. The integer epithelium represents a mechanical barrier, while the physiological processes occurring in and between the cells contribute to dynamic and complex protection from physical, chemical and biological agents. The immune role of the epithelial layer is supported by various cells and cytokines, which show common features between the gastrointestinal tract and the pulmonary and cutaneous systems [1–3]. These similarities in role and functioning have led recent research in the direction of exploring the gut-lung-skin barrier as an entity that not only shows common elements but also interactions [4]. The cross-talk between these three regions refers to various signaling molecules which are mainly involved in local and systemic inflammation [5].

This paper focuses on the roles of cannabinoids in inflammation affecting the gut-lung-skin barrier and brings forward the similarities and distinctions in the pathophysiology of the inflammatory conditions affecting these systems. The latest advancements in the field are discussed and supported by the available in vitro and in vivo evidence in the recent literature, as well as the human studies which have been undertaken to validate the effectiveness and safety of cannabinoids in the epithelial inflammation of the gut-lung-skin barrier.

2. The Gut-Lung-Skin Barrier

The gut-lung-skin barrier is a virtual structure encompassing the epithelium of the digestive tract, the pulmonary system and the cutaneous layer. More and more often, studies cite similarities and interactions in the immune response regulated in these structures [4–6]. The recently described T helper 17 (Th17) subset of cells and their regulatory pathway provide further evidence validating the unity of the immune response and regulation in the gut-lung-skin barrier [7]. These cells are capable of producing various cytokines such as granulocyte colony-stimulating factor (G-CSF) and interleukins (ILs) -8 and -22, and trigger the synthesis of effectors producing IL-17 and interferon-gamma (IFN-γ) [8]. Furthermore, Th17 cells are involved in the interactions between the microbiota of the specific tissue and the host, regulating the immune response [8]. The most prominent cytokines involved in the protection against microbial infection are IL-17 and IL-22, which increase the release of antimicrobial peptides, neutrophil recruitment and granulopoiesis while maintaining the integrity of the epithelial layer in boundary tissues [9]. When IL-17 fails due to insufficient expression, a large variety of cutaneous, pulmonary and gastrointestinal infections may occur, accompanied by significant inflammation [10–12]. Some infectious agents such as *Staphylococcus aureus* are capable of stimulating its expression [13]. IL-22 also contributes to the immune response against various infectious diseases of the gut-lung-skin barrier and exhibits pro-inflammatory roles by enhancing the effects of tumor necrosis factor-alpha (TNF-α), and by activating various other cytokines [9,14].

However, the gut-lung-skin barrier cross-talk in inflammation is not limited to the activity of Th17 cells. The epithelial cells produce thymic stromal lymphopoietin (TSLP), a cytokine similar to IL-7, which is involved in the allergic response and is a key factor in the onset of allergic inflammation in the skin, lungs and gastrointestinal tract [15]. TSLP is considered to be a biomarker for disruptions of the epithelial integrity, and was cited as a determining and aggravating factor in a variety of allergy models, including ovalbumin (OVA)-induced asthma, atopic dermatitis and allergic diarrhea [16].

Sustained inflammatory processes in the gut-lung-skin barrier develop similar complications, regardless of the initial location of the inflammation. Among the common comorbidities are metabolic syndrome, cardiovascular events and bone loss [5,17,18]. These may be explained by the increased production of TNF-α, which is an essential mediator of chronic inflammation and is usually accompanied by IL-4, IL-6 and IL-17, increasing the risk of the aforementioned complications, as well as favoring the appearance of other metabolic conditions [5,19,20].

Because inflammation is the cornerstone of many pathological conditions, including cancer, the possible connections and interferences between inflammatory processes in different organs and systems have substantial implications. Inflammatory conditions, regardless of their substrate or location, benefit from relatively specific management, which includes one or several anti-inflammatory drugs. However, due to adverse effects and interactions, there is a growing interest in medicinal-grade natural compounds that have demonstrated their effectiveness and usually act through dedicated receptors that are widely distributed in the human body. These substances have been labeled 'phytochemicals', and some examples include capsaicin, curcumin, resveratrol and cannabinoids [21–24]. Curcumin, resveratrol, gingerol, and ginsenoside have demonstrated antioxidant and anti-inflammatory effects by modulating the MAP and NF-κB pathways, making them excellent candidates in the treatment of atopic dermatitis [25]. Multiple in vivo and in vitro studies have outlined the chemopreventive properties of whole-fruit substances in skin carcinogenesis, where carotenoids, polyphenols, flavonoids and anthocyanins have demonstrated pro-apoptotic, antiproliferative, and ROS-reducing effects in basal and squamous cell carcinoma models [26–29]. Capsaicin's effects on chemonociception were fundamental in cutaneous pathophysiology research, but its applications have extended from skin pain modulation to various local and system-wide pathologies, including malignancies [30–32]. Cannabinoids, in particular, show great promise due to the mediation of their actions by the dedicated cannabinoid receptors, which serve the activity of the endocannabinoid system but also respond to the administration of natural or synthetic cannabinoids.

3. Cannabinoids and Inflammation

Cannabinoids have been used for their anti-inflammatory properties for millennia; for instance, T'ang Shên-wei records effects such as "undoing rheumatism" or the "discharge of pus" in the 10th century A.D. work called 'Chêng-lei pên-ts'ao' [33]. An increasing number of studies explore their properties and interactions in a wide range of experimental models [34]. The chemical group of cannabinoids includes over 60 natural (phyto-) cannabinoids and over 150 artificial (synthetic) cannabinoids alongside the two well-known endocannabinoids anandamide (AEA) and 2-Arachidonoylglycerol (2-AG), and their few derivates [35,36]. Evidently, the process of testing and comparing the anti-inflammatory effects of these substances in inflammatory conditions is lengthy and complex. There are two G protein-coupled receptor (GPCRs) cannabinoid receptors activated by cannabinoids: CB1, which is mostly located in the central, peripheral and enteric nervous system, and is responsible, among others, for the psychoactive effects; and CB2, which is expressed by immune cells and some tissues, and is mostly involved in immunomodulation [37]. The two receptors exert distinct functions via specific signaling pathways, and different cannabinoids can activate them to various degrees; therefore, cannabinoids can vary in terms of effectiveness and potency [38]. While some anti-inflammatory properties were also described for CB1-specific agonists, their effects may also be carried through non-CB1-non-CB2 signaling, and their most common usage is the management of pain, in which they prove highly effective [39,40]. Conversely, CB2 receptors are mainly involved in regulating inflammation by modulating the levels of various cytokines [41]. A recent systematic review of in vivo studies regarding the anti-inflammatory effects of various cannabinoids concluded that the CB2 antagonist CBD is efficient in reducing inflammation, while CB1 agonists—such as THC—may be used for the alleviation of the associated pain [42].

Some cannabinoids are favorites in the race for the identification of the substance with the optimal anti-inflammatory actions and minimal adverse reactions. Cannabidiol (CBD) is one of the most commonly tested substances due to its lack of psychoactive effects and high potency in modulating the immune response and exerting anti-inflammatory properties in a variety of animal models [43–45]. Tetrahydrocannabinol is still tested, despite its psychoactive effects, due to its activity on the CB1 receptor which triggers specific signaling pathways in inflammation [46]. As for synthetic cannabinoids, there are multiple classes and subclasses defined by their chemical structure, which encompass a growing number of substances, developed with the intent of emulating the favorable effects while maximizing the receptor specificity and limiting side effects. These substances are agonists for CB1 and/or CB2, and usually bind to the cannabinoid receptors with higher affinity than natural compounds, showing great potential in developing new treatments [47].

The following sections explore the roles of synthetic, phyto-, and endocannabinoids in the inflammations of the gastrointestinal tract, the pulmonary apparatus and the skin.

4. Cannabinoids and Gut Inflammations

The discovery of the intestinal endocannabinoid system was encouraged by numerous reports of the beneficial effects of administering cannabinoids for various digestive tract disorders [48]. This system plays various roles in the homeostasis of the gastrointestinal tract, including the regulation of secretion, sensitivity and motility, as well as upholding the integrity of the gut epithelial barrier [48,49]. Physiological and pharmacological studies have investigated the interactions between endocannabinoids and various receptors, and have concluded that these substances may play a role in modulating intestinal inflammation and cellular proliferation [50]. These findings led to the consideration of phyto- and artificial cannabinoids as candidates for the treatment of intestinal inflammatory disorders, such as irritable bowel syndrome (IBS), inflammatory bowel disease (IBD) and Crohn's disease [51].

In the gastrointestinal tract, CB1 and CB2 receptors are located in the myenteric and submucosal neurons (mostly CB1) as well as the inflammatory and epithelial cells (mostly CB2) [52]. Besides GPCRs, cannabinoids may also bind to the transient receptor potential cation channel subfamily V member 1 (TRPV1) receptors in the capsaicin-sensitive sensory nerves located in the digestive tract wall, especially in the mucosa, muscle layers and blood vessels, but also in epithelial cells [53]. Furthermore, cannabinoids may bind to G protein-coupled receptor (GPR) type 55, which was identified in smooth muscle cells and peroxisome proliferator-activated receptor alpha (PPAR-α), located in blood vessels and smooth muscle cells, and also to GPR119, which is expressed in the digestive mucosa and enteroendocrine cells [54–56].

4.1. In Vitro Studies

An in vitro study on Caco-2 cells demonstrated that adding AEA or cannabidiol (CBD) alongside IL-17A when incubating the cell monolayers for 48 h prevents mucosal damage and the changes in the epithelial permeability associated with inflammation [57]. In a similar study using the same cell types, delta-9-tetrahydrocannabinol (THC) and CBD were also able to reduce the intestinal permeability induced by IFN-γ and TNF-α, while AEA and 2-AG enhanced the cytokine-induced permeability [58]. This leads to the conclusion that the effects are CB1-related, and that the specific agonistic effects of various cannabinoids trigger specific effects [58,59]. These findings were validated ex vivo, in inflammatory and hypoxic states, on Caco-2 cells harvested from colorectal resections [60].

Improving on this experimental model, Couch et al. tested the effects of CBD and palmitoylethanolamide (PEA) on colon explants from patients with inflammatory conditions; these cannabinoids elicit anti-inflammatory properties by preventing the increased cytokine production and reducing the intracellular signaling phosphoprotein levels [61]. The anti-inflammatory properties of phytocannabinoids have been investigated using fresh and baked *C. sativa* flowers, and it was revealed that tetrahydrocannabinolic acid (THCA) is the main active compound and is able to reduce IL-8 levels in HCT116 colon cancer cells pretreated with TNF-α at concentrations of 114–207 µg/mL, partially via the GPR55 receptor [62]. The same study further confirmed the anti-inflammatory effects on patients suffering from IBD, through COX-2 and matrix metalloproteinase (MMP)-9 mediated mechanisms, and showed that THCA exerts superior effects and less cytotoxicity than CBD on these cell lines [62].

Another important anti-inflammatory property is the maintenance of the epithelial barrier's integrity. CBD is able to preserve the mucosal integrity in Caco-2 cells at concentrations of 10^{-7} to 10^{-9} M, opposing the effects of *Clostridium difficile* toxin A in an inflammation experimental model; this activity is CB1-mediated, as the use of AM251, a CB1 antagonist, inhibited the observed effects [63]. An in vitro study on HT29 cells showed that AEA, methanandamide (mAEA), and arachidonylcyclopropylamide (ACPA) stimulate CB1-dependent wound closure even in low nanomolar concentrations [64]. These findings consolidate the hypothesis of the intrinsic protective effect of endocannabinoids against intestinal barrier disruptions.

Conversely, CB2 receptors have also been implicated in mediating the anti-inflammatory effects of β-Caryophyllene on oral mucositis, which is characterized by the decrease of TNF-α, IL-1β, IL-6 and IL-17A [65]. Furthermore, Matalon et al. showed, in their recent paper, that the synthetic CB2 agonist JWH-133 is able to reduce MMP-9 and IL-8 levels in inflamed colon biopsies from patients with IBD. These findings draw further attention to the specific involvement of the two cannabinoid receptors in the various facets of inflammation. There is extensive evidence that CB1 is normally expressed in the intestinal epithelium, while CB2 expression seems to be stimulated by inflammatory conditions, supporting its attributed role in the regulation of inflammation, cell growth and the immune response [64,66–68].

4.2. In Vivo Animal Studies

The effectiveness of cannabinoids in inflammatory diseases has been demonstrated on various animal models. Couch et al. published a comprehensive meta-analysis presenting undeniable evidence that cannabinoids prove to be effective in intestinal inflammatory conditions [69]. The disease activity index (DAI) score and levels of myeloperoxidase (MPO) activity were the criteria of choice for the measurement of the effects of various synthetic and phyto-cannabinoids.

In an in vivo murine model of IBD induced by the intracolonic administration of dinitrobenzene sulphonic acid (DNBS), cannabigerol (CBG) reduced the expression of inducible nitric oxide synthase (iNOS), as well as the levels of IL-1β, IL-10 and IFN-γ, and the activity of myeloperoxidase, while increasing the activity of superoxide dismutase [70]. CBD appears to elicited analogous effects in a parallel study [71]. Using the same experimental model, Pagano et al. noted similar effects when using a combination of fish oil, CBD and CBG [72]. The association of fish oil and CBD enhances their anti-inflammatory effects, which occur at lower doses (20 mg and 0.3–10 mg/kg, respectively) than the per se administration of the two substances; these findings were reported in mice with induced colitis, in which the combination of fish oil and CBD decreased the myeloperoxidase (MPO) activity, DAI score, intestinal permeability, and levels of IL-1β and IL-6 [73].

An additional key factor in the evolution and management of intestinal inflammations is the gut microbiome. The interactions between various microbes and the intestinal mucosa seem to play an important role in the local immune response to various conditions including IBD and Crohn's disease [74]. CBD is able to induce changes in the gut microbiota, apparently independently from its effects on local inflammation [73]. This is of interest because there is evidence that the endocannabinoid system connects the intestinal microbiome with the physiological processes occurring in the adipose tissue, through regulatory pathways [75]. Furthermore, and more importantly, it appears that the alteration of the balance between the endocannabinoid system and the microbiota can negatively impact the integrity of the intestinal barrier [76].

In vivo studies on animal models confirmed that cannabinoids protect the intestinal barrier's integrity. In this regard, the role of CB1 has been validated using a knockout mice model which showed that CB1 is responsible for the intestinal physiological response to inflammation, leading to the secretion of IgA and the regulation of intestinal permeability, among other effects [77]. Synthetic cannabinoids can further enhance these properties. Cao et al. provoked acute lesions of the gastrointestinal mucosa in rats by inducing acute pancreatitis and then showed that synthetic cannabinoid HU210, a non-selective CB agonist, reversed the morphological and serum anomalies, demonstrating its anti-inflammatory properties [78]. A later study showed that HU210 protects the intestinal mucosa in a murine model of ulcerative colitis, most likely through the toll-like receptor 4 (TLR4) and mitogen-activated protein (MAP) signaling pathways [79]. Another synthetic cannabinoid, abnormal cannabidiol, is an isomer of cannabidiol that exerts its effects via non-CB1-non-CB2 signaling and elicits protective effects against chemically induced colitis in mice, stimulating wound healing while inhibiting neutrophil recruitment [80].

4.3. Human Clinical Trials

Up to the moment of this review, limited information is available regarding the in vivo effects of cannabinoids on intestinal inflammatory conditions in humans. The outcome predictors in IBD trials usually include DAI, C-reactive protein (CRP), rapid fecal calprotectin (FC), the Mayo score and the Crohn's Disease Activity Index (CDAI), and the correct interpretation of the results relies on quality preparation for colonoscopy [81–83].

A recent paper by Kienzl et al. gathered retrospective data from patients suffering from IBD that used cannabis to alleviate symptoms [76]. Most studies included in the analysis showed that cannabis users benefited from symptom relief, improved DAI, and better quality of life. However, despite the overall good tolerance, the adverse reactions of cannabis inhalation are to be considered [76,84]. Furthermore, in one survey, patients with Crohn's disease presented a higher risk for surgery [85]. The legalization of medicinal marijuana did not affect its use in patients with IBD, despite an upward trend in the use of cannabis in the tested population throughout the previous 5 years [86].

A randomized clinical trial on healthy subjects performed by Couch et al. tested the effects of PEA and CBD on the regulation of the increased intestinal permeability induced by the pro-inflammatory effects of aspirin [87]. A dose of 600 mg of PEA and CBD, respectively, managed to prevent the increase in intestinal permeability caused by 600 mg of aspirin, evidenced by the measurement of lactulose and mannitol excretion in the urine.

Two randomized clinical trials were published by Naftali et al., in 2013 and 2017, which tested the effects of inhaled THC and oral CBD, respectively, in Crohn's disease [88,89]. While THC showed some clinical benefits, CBD failed to improve the DAI in active Crohn's disease. However, both trials received some criticism for methodological flaws, small patient groups and various other biases [69,90].

Two other randomized placebo-controlled studies studied the effects of cannabinoids in ulcerative colitis. Irving et al. tested a combination of THC and CBD capsules that were administered in increasing doses, and found that while the remission rates were similar to the placebo, the cannabinoid capsules offered subjective improvements to the patients' quality of life, despite mild to moderate side effects [91]. Naftali et al. tested the effects of inhaled THC and recorded significant improvements in the DAI, as well as decreases in the CRP and FC while registering no serious adverse effects [92].

These findings are encouraging, and the favorable in vitro results and animal studies observations warrant that further human clinical trials despite the low number of studies published to date. Furthermore, synthetic cannabinoids may demonstrate superior effectiveness and similar or fewer side effects, and could represent a major improvement in the treatment of intestinal inflammatory diseases.

5. Cannabinoids and Lung Inflammatory Conditions

Cannabis has been known for its recreational use for millennia, so it is not surprising that the effects of cannabinoid inhalation have been thoroughly documented in many studies. Though it is difficult to distinguish from concurrent chronic exposure to tobacco smoke, which is common, cannabis smoke inhalation causes some specific effects in the pulmonary system; it decreases the antimicrobial activity and cytokine production, and increases sputum production, coughing and possibly the risk of lung cancer [93,94]. Furthermore, marijuana smoke induces epithelial hyperplasia, cellular disorganization, cell atypia and fibrosis [95,96]. In vitro studies seem to confirm these findings at a cellular level, as cannabinoids have demonstrated immunosuppressive properties and profibrotic effects [97,98]. However, in vivo studies using the direct administration of pharmaceutical-grade cannabinoids have revealed benefic effects on several inflammatory conditions, inducing a decrease in the recruitment of inflammatory cells, the suppression of cytokines, and an overall improvement in mortality [99]. These anti-inflammatory and immunomodulatory properties have prompted researchers to investigate the potential of cannabinoids in the management of coronavirus disease (COVID-19) infection [100–102]. However intriguing, the risks of drug interactions and partial inhibition of the immune response seem to outweigh the potential untested benefits in this condition, and the use of these substances is not recommended in this case, according to some authors [103]. Therefore, the main application and use of cannabinoids appear to be inflammatory diseases, and there is a great interest in this topic, which has encouraged numerous studies in the field.

No cannabinoid receptors have been isolated in vivo in the epithelial cells of the lungs; however, CB1 receptors have been identified in the nerve endings of the airways [104]. Both CB1 and CB2 receptors are expressed by eosinophils, monocytes and monocyte-derived macrophages [99,105]. CB1, CB2 and TRPV1 have been identified in situ and in vitro at the protein level in airway epithelial cells; however, the impact of these findings on the biology of respiratory inflammations remains unclear [106].

5.1. In Vitro Studies

A study on A549 cells has shown that marijuana smoke causes mitochondrial damage, impairing the energetic metabolism of the cell [107]. Furthermore, using the ECV304 cell line, Sarafian et al. demonstrated that even short exposures to marijuana smoke cause an increase in reactive oxygen species (ROS) production capable of inducing necrotic cell death, and the effects seem to be mainly attributed to the gaseous phase—not the particulate phase—of the smoke [108].

However, studies focused on the direct effects of the substances isolated from plants showed controversial results. In a study on multiple human cell lines, including eosinophils and natural killer (NK) cells, both THC and CBD decreased the levels of IL-8, macrophage inflammatory protein (MIP)-1, IFN-γ and TNF-α, thus demonstrating anti-inflammatory properties [109].

The anti-inflammatory effects of cannabinoids were cited in the context of septic lung injury. The highly CB2-selective synthetic cannabinoid HU308 decreased the levels of TNF-α, IL-18, IL-1β, and NLR family pyrin domain containing 3 (NLRP3) in RAW264.7 macrophages in lipopolysaccharide (LPS)-induced inflammation, effects which were also observed in an in vivo animal model of acute lung injury (ALI) in the same study [110].

Additional studies revealed a more complex interaction between cannabinoids and the immune system. In a study on macrophages, lung fibroblasts and epithelial cells, Muthumalage et al. showed that CBD reduced the levels of IL-8, monocyte chemoattractant protein (MCP)-1 and nuclear factor-kappa B (NF-κB) activity when they were increased by an LPS-induced inflammatory state [111]. However, when co-administered with dexamethasone, CBD demonstrates antagonistic effects, possibly due to receptor competitivity and pharmacological interactions in the signaling pathways [111,112].

Cannabinoids have also demonstrated anti-angiogenic properties, with possible applications in inflammation and cancer. The synthetic cannabinoids arachidonyl-2′-chloroethylamide (ACEA) and JWH-133 are selective CB1 and, respectively, CB2 agonists which inhibit the LPS-induced production and release of vascular endothelial growth factors A and C, angiopoietins 1 and 2, and IL-6 from human lung macrophages [113].

5.2. In Vivo Animal Studies

The observational studies citing the toxic effects of marijuana smoke on the pulmonary system have prompted in vivo studies on animals to further investigate the extent of the effects. As expected, animal studies have evidenced a large variety of lung lesions, including neutrophil, lymphocyte, and macrophage infiltration, goblet cell hyperplasia, endothelial proliferation, emphysema and airway hyperresponsiveness (AHR) doubled by increased cytokines and inflammatory pathway activation [114]. Interestingly, when the cannabinoids were removed from the inhaled smoke, the alveolar inflammation and wall thickening, pneumonitis, tracheobronchial fibrosis, inflammation and sputum excess were still observed [115]. These findings prompted the need for research using *per se* cannabinoids in controlled studies.

A study investigating the effects of the synthetic cannabinoid CP55,940, a full CB1 and CB2 agonist, in C57BL6/J mice showed that the oropharyngeal instillation of the compound caused CB1 activation and the subsequent increase of TNF-α, IL-1β, IL-6, C-C Motif Chemokine Ligand 2 (CCL) 2 and 3, C-X-C motif chemokine ligand 10 (CXCL10), and various pro-inflammatory transcription factors [116].

However, the in vivo effects of cannabinoids were most commonly investigated in animal-induced inflammatory conditions, most commonly using LPS to induce ALI. The intraperitoneal administration of CBD is able to reduce TNF-α, IL-6, MCP-1 and MIP-2 in the bronchoalveolar lavage fluid (BALF), as well as being able to decrease the lung myeloperoxidase activity and the pulmonary infiltration of leukocytes [117,118]. Other cannabinoids exhibited similar effects. WIN 55,212-2, THC and AEA caused a dose-dependent decrease of TNF-α and neutrophil recruitment in BALF after intranasal administration, while PEA only decreased the TNF-α levels [119]. Conversely, pro-inflammatory effects were cited for

CBD in this animal model of ALI. The oral administration of CBD amplified the production of TNF-α, IL-5, IL-23 and G-CSF in C57BL/6 mice, while also increasing the infiltration of neutrophils and monocytes in the BALF [120].

Another animal model of lung inflammation was used by Arruza et al. to test the effects of CBD on newborn piglets with hypoxic–ischemic brain damage [121]. CBD decreased IL-1, the protein content and leukocyte infiltration in the BALF and the extravascular lung compartment; interestingly, the authors identified that the serotonin 1A (5-HT$_{1A}$) receptor participated in the mediation of these effects.

Some pulmonary anti-inflammatory effects of cannabinoids appear to be carried out through non-cannabinoid receptors. Tauber et al. showed that WIN55,212-2 causes a decrease in MMP-9 production in mice with lung inflammation induced by cigarette smoke via the extracellular signal-regulated kinase (ERK) signaling pathway consecutive to TRPV1 activation [122].

Asthma is a serious pulmonary disease with an important associated inflammatory component. Mice with ovalbumin (OVA)-induced asthma were treated with 5 mg/kg intraperitoneal CBD, and a reduction of TNF-α and ILs 4, 5, 6 and 13 was observed [123]. In the same animal model, CBD also decreased AHR and the collagen fiber content alongside a decrease of the inflammatory markers in the BALF [124]. Conversely, JWH-133 caused an increase in eosinophil migration, chemotaxis and ROS generation, aggravating the AHR [125]. Furthermore, a study using a CB2 knockout mouse model showed that CB2 activation triggers pro-inflammatory effects with increased IFN-γ production by pulmonary NK cells in the BALF [126].

Cannabinoids are also able to modulate the inflammation related to various infectious diseases. In a series of articles, Tahamtan et al. showed that the activation of CB1 and CB2 receptors by JZL184 and JWH-133, respectively, decreased the production of cytokines and the influx of cells, alleviating lung pathology in Balb/c mice infected with the respiratory syncytial virus (RSV) [127,128]. THC also exhibits anti-inflammatory properties in mice with influenza infection via CB1 and/or CB2 activation by decreasing the levels of IL-17 and IFN-γ, as well as the macrophage infiltration in the BALF; however, THC also caused immunosuppression by decreasing the recruitment of CD4+ and CD8+ T-cells and macrophages with a subsequent increase of the viral load [129,130]. THC is capable of reducing the cell proliferation and levels of IFN-γ, inhibiting the phosphatidylinositol 3-kinase/protein kinase B (PI3K/Akt) pathway and decreasing the *Staphylococcal* enterotoxin B-induced lung toxicity in C3H/HeJ mice [131]. PI3K/Akt pathway activation was also achieved in C57BL/6 mice treated with JWH-133 for paraquat-induced ALI, causing a CB2-mediated decrease of TNF-α, IL-6 and MPO activity while improving lung function [132].

JWH-133 reduces the serum and tissue levels of TNF-α, IL-6 and IL-1β in a polymicrobial sepsis model in rats while increasing the IL-10 levels [133]. Additionally, neutrophil recruitment, bacteremia and lung injury are decreased when CB2 synthetic agonist GP1a is used in septic C57BL/6J wild-type mice [134]. Other CB2 agonists, such as melilotus, exhibit similar effects in this animal model, while also decreasing neutrophils and lymphocyte infiltration and blocking NF-κβ activity [135].

Various other pulmonary disease models have been used to evaluate the efficacy of cannabinoids. A dose of 1 mg/kg of JWH-133 improves neurogenic pulmonary edema at 24 h after subarachnoid hemorrhage in rats, decreasing the MPO activity and leukocyte infiltration while improving the lung permeability and tight junction protein levels [136]. Furthermore, AEA demonstrated anti-inflammatory effects by increasing the expression of heat shock proteins (HSP) 25 and 70 in the lungs of rats injected with 1 mg/kg AEA [137]. Moreover, the oral or intraperitoneal administration of β-Caryophyllene prevents neutrophil infiltration and the decreased production of IL-12, NO, leukotriene B4 and CXCL1/keratinocytes-derived chemokine (KC) in C57Bl/6 mice with *Mycobacterium bovis*-induced pulmonary inflammation [138].

5.3. Human Clinical Trials

The usage of cannabinoids for pulmonary disorders in humans is encumbered by numerous reports of lung injury, pneumonia and respiratory depression related to recreational use, especially of synthetic cannabinoids [139–141]. The respiratory failure was assumed to be CB1-mediated via the mitogen-activated protein kinase (MAPK) pathway and aggravated by cumulative central nervous system depression; however, due to small sample sizes and high bias risks more information is needed to confirm these findings [142].

Genetic studies have shown that mutations of the Q63R variant of the CB2 receptor increase the severity of acute infections with RSV in children, confirming the role of cannabinoids in modulating the immune response and carrying on their known anti-inflammatory effects [128].

One of the few trials investigating the role of cannabinoids in lung inflammations is the recently published randomized controlled trial (RCT) on the use of lenabasum in patients with cystic fibrosis [143]. This Phase 2 trial showed fewer pulmonary exacerbations, a decrease in Immunoglobulin G and IL-8 levels, and a significant reduction in neutrophil and eosinophil infiltration in the sputum of patients taking 1 or 5 mg lenabasum daily for a month. An RCT investigating the anti-inflammatory effects of smoked cannabis in the pain and inflammation of patients with radiated lung cancer is still in Phase 1 [144].

A clinical trial published in 1973 showed that THC inhalation causes bronchodilation in healthy subjects [145]. Subsequently, several studies emerged attempting to apply these beneficial effects to patients with various inflammatory lung conditions. However, the results of the ensuing studies were not substantial. A clinical trial investigating the role of inhaled cannabis in the management of advanced chronic obstructive pulmonary disease showed no benefits in terms of lung function and exercise performance [146]. Furthermore, in their study, Gong et al. showed that the oral administration of 2 mg nabilone does not produce significant bronchodilation in asthmatic patients compared to a placebo [147]. In a previous study, THC was shown to be unsuitable for clinical use in asthma, because when it was administered in aerosols it produced bronchodilation in some asthmatic patients but caused bronchoconstriction, coughing and discomfort in others [148]. Oral THC did not show better results in asthmatic patients because it caused inconsistent bronchodilation, central nervous system effects and, in some cases, bronchoconstriction [149].

Positive results were obtained in a clinical trial testing the benefits of using a vaporizer to improve respiratory symptoms in frequent cannabis smokers [150]. This suggests that finding alternate vehicles of administration may improve the clinical results in future studies.

6. Cannabinoids and Inflammatory Skin Disorders

Phytochemicals have been increasingly employed in skin disorders as emerging data demonstrate their utility. Cannabinoids and their receptors are regarded with increasing interest for their implications in skin pathology, especially in the field of inflammatory skin disorders. While some action mechanisms are still unclear, encouraging data is becoming available as a result of a multitude of in vivo and in vitro studies investigating this topic [151]. Based on the reported anti-inflammatory properties, the application of cannabinoids has been attempted for various conditions such as acne, psoriasis, atopic dermatitis and even cancer [152]. Among the most common tested substances, CBD is preferred due to its lack of psychoactive effects, and there is evidence that it is effective in various skin inflammations, despite the incomplete understanding of its effects and interactions in molecular signaling pathways [153].

The simple and effective topical administration of cannabinoids on skin lesions is helpful not only in ensuring substance delivery to the inflammation site but also in observing local adverse effects [154]. The additional anti-aging, anti-oxidative and antitumoral effects provide supplementary benefits in the use of cannabinoids in other diseases that are associated with inflammation, including cancer [155,156]. However, many of the studies are preclinical, and there are very few trials free of bias with a large enough number of participants to be considered high-quality [157]. Nevertheless, the in vitro and animal models support further research due to the uncovered effects of cannabinoids on inflammatory cells, cytokines and signaling pathways, which are mediated to various degrees by CB receptors, depending on the affinity and effectiveness of the tested substance [156].

The cannabinoid receptors are widely dispersed in the skin. CB1 and CB2 receptors have been identified on nerve fibers, keratinocytes and mast cells [158]. CB1 was isolated in the hair follicles, while CB2 was found in sebocytes [159,160]. The intensely studied TRP channels have been identified in the sensory nerve endings, keratinocytes, endothelial cells, mast cells and dendritic cells [161,162].

6.1. In Vitro Studies

One of the key elements of the skin inflammatory process is the array of actions performed by the multitude of cytokines that are involved in the response to skin barrier disruption, but also in immunity, apoptosis, and even the development and progression of skin cancer [163–166].

An in vitro experiment in a larger study performed by Karsak et al. investigating the impact of the endocannabinoid system on allergic contact dermatitis (ACD) revealed that HaCaT keratinocytes with contact hypersensitivity conditions induced via polyinosinic:polycytidylic acid express an upregulation of CB1 and a downregulation of CB2 receptors [167]. An ensuing study by Petrosino et al., using the same experimental model, showed that PEA and AEA are upregulated in these conditions, while exogenous PEA causes a decrease of MCP-2 expression [168]. Continuing their previous work on this in vitro model, Petrosino et al. showed that CBD inhibits the production of MCP-2, but also of interleukins 6 and 8 and tumor necrosis factor-alpha (TNF-α) while increasing the endogenous levels of AEA [169].

While they are not considered to have anti-inflammatory effect per se, cannabinoids have demonstrated the ability to inhibit keratinocyte cell proliferation, thus limiting the pro-inflammatory roles of these cells [170]. Wilkinson et al. showed that THC, cannabinol (CBN), CBD and CBG inhibit the proliferation of human papillomavirus (HPV)-16 E6/E7 transformed human skin keratinocytes in an in vitro model for psoriasis [171]. The synthetic CB1 agonist ACEA inhibited the upregulation of keratins K6 and K16 in isolated human skin samples of psoriasis lesions [172].

The cannabinoids' property of decreasing pro-inflammatory cytokine concentrations was also evidenced in an in vitro study performed by Robinson et al. on mononuclear cells from the peripheral blood of dermatomyositis patients treated with ajulemic acid (AJA) [173]. In their paper, the authors cite a significantly decreased concentration of TNF-α, but also of IFN-α and -β in the cells treated with ajulemic acid compared to untreated cells. These findings further indicate that cannabinoids decrease the production of cytokines in inflammatory skin disorders.

A study on SZ95 human sebocyte cultures performed by Oláh et al. demonstrated that CBD can prevent the increase of TNF-α when sebocytes are stimulated with linoleic acid and testosterone in an in vitro acne model [174]. Furthermore, CBD also decreased the expression of IL-1β and IL-6 when the sebocytes were stimulated with lipopolysaccharides, a finding that suggests a potential positive effect of CBD in the treatment of acne vulgaris. The same study identified that the anti-inflammatory effects of CBD are mediated by the Tribbles homolog (TRIB3)-NF-κB pathway via A2a adenosine receptors, yielding important insight into the action mechanisms of cannabinoids.

The anti-inflammatory effects of cannabinoids are also extended to the inflammatory milieu of tumors, as demonstrated in an in vitro study performed by Maor et al. on Kaposi's sarcoma-associated herpesvirus-infected primary human dermal endothelial cells in an in vitro model for Kaposi sarcoma [175]. The authors reported that CBD demonstrates antiproliferative effects by blocking the expression of growth-regulated oncogenes (GRO-α), as well as of the viral G protein-coupled receptor and vascular endothelial growth factor C and its receptor. GRO-α is a chemokine involved in angiogenesis, tumorigenesis and inflammation, suggesting that the inflammatory milieu plays a role in Kaposi cancer development, and that CBD may also demonstrate anti-tumoral effects through its anti-inflammatory properties [176].

6.2. In Vivo Animal Studies

VCE-004.8, a synthetic agonist for PPAR-γ and CB2 receptors, demonstrated anti-inflammatory properties in an in vivo study on mice with bleomycin-induced scleroderma performed by del Río et al. [177]. The non-thiophilic, fully substituted CBD quinol derivative labeled VCE-004.8 decreased the expression of IL-1β and IL-13, and prevented macrophage infiltration and mast cells degranulation, thus indirectly reducing the concentration of Transforming Growth Factor-beta (TGF-β), a key factor in fibrosis development. Another study on the same experimental model, performed by Balistreri et al., showed the similar properties of another synthetic cannabinoid labeled WIN55,212-2, a full CB1 agonist that prevents dermal fibrosis by inhibiting TGF-β as well as connective tissue growth factor and platelet-derived growth factor [178]. Mast cell downregulation, alongside a decrease in IL-4 levels, was also reported in an in vivo model for ACD induced with oxazolone on Balb/c and hairless mice that were treated with a topical synthetic CB1 agonist named α-oleoyl oleylamine serinol (α-OOS) [179].

Topically applied cannabidiol has also demonstrated anti-inflammatory and analgesic effects by inhibiting cyclooxygenase and lipoxygenase, properties that were observed by Formukong et al. in an experimental model of the tetradecanoylphorbol acetate-induced erythema of mouse skin performed decades ago, a study which represented a basis for more advanced research and unlocked the potential for the application of cannabinoids in acne, ACD, dermatomyositis, and other inflammatory skin disorders [180].

A suspected yet unconfirmed consequence of the anti-inflammatory roles of cannabinoids is the decrease of tumor viability, proliferation and growth in cutaneous melanoma. Armstrong et al. studied a combination of THC and CBD in a cutaneous melanoma model on mice bearing BRAF wild-type melanoma xenografts and found that the product caused a reduction of reactive oxygen species production and caspase activation, effects that may be triggered by the anti-inflammatory effects of CBD [181]. Skin tumorigenesis is an intricate process that depends on molecules common to the inflammatory signaling pathways, entailing complex interferences induced by substances such as matrix metalloproteinases, TNF-α and IL-1 that are implicated in inflammation as well as a wide array of malignancies, including skin cancer [182–186].

The decreased expression of TNF-α and NF-κB triggered by cannabinoids noted in in vitro studies was also demonstrated in an in vivo study on the CB receptors in the inflammatory milieu of skin cancer. Zheng et al. showed that CB receptors play a role in the resistance to ultraviolet (UV) B inflammation in an in vivo model of UV-induced skin carcinogenesis, and that CB receptor deficiency correlates with an increase in the expression of TNF-α, and the activation of NF-κB and mitogen-activated protein MAP kinases [187].

6.3. Human Clinical Trials

Developing on the favorable results cited in multiple in vivo studies, Ali et al. tested the safety and efficacy of an extract cream made of cannabis seeds in healthy patients and noted significant sebum diminution and erythema reduction while noting possible skin irritation as an adverse effect [188]. A Phase 2 study ran by Botanix Pharmaceuticals evaluating a proprietary synthetic CBD-derived cannabinoid labeled BTX 1503 on more than 350 patients with acne was recently completed, but the results are not yet available [189].

Cannabinoids were clinically tested in diffuse cutaneous systemic sclerosis, in a double-blind, randomized placebo-controlled study on 42 subjects performed by Spiera et al. [190]. The authors noted that while the side effects included fatigue and vertigo, the patients receiving ajulemic acid had a significant improvement in their clinical scores, with a reduction in the expression of key genes related to inflammation on skin biopsies. Subsequently, a Phase 3 trial was launched in 2018, with an estimated 350 patients receiving either ajulemic acid in 20 mg or 5 mg concentrations, or a placebo [191].

Ajulemic acid was also tested in another Phase 2 trial conducted by Chen et al. for the effectiveness in controlling the inflammation in patients with dermatomyositis [192]. The oral administration of ajulemic acid leads to a decrease of IL-31, IFN-β and -γ, and T-helper cell inflammation, demonstrating effectiveness in the treatment of dermatomyositis skin lesions. Werth et al. developed a Phase 3 study to test the performance of ajulemic acid in dermatomyositis [193].

7. Integrative Vision on the Effects of Cannabinoids in Gut-Lung-Skin Epithelial Inflammation

In summary, in a multitude of inflammatory models located in the epithelia of the gut-lung-skin barrier, cannabinoids show similar and consistent effects. In vitro studies show that all types of cannabinoids have potent anti-inflammatory effects, mostly expressed as the ability to prevent a rise in cytokines when inflammation is produced in the cellular experimental model (Table 1). Consistently, both natural and artificial cannabinoids were able to regulate the induced increase in the expression of TNF-α, IFN-γ, Ils 1β, 6, 8 and 17A, as well as MCP-1 and 2, and various other cofactors of inflammation. Vascular and cellular proliferative factors were also suppressed, adding to the potential benefits in regulating inflammation, possibly including the processes in the tumoral microenvironment. While some controversial results were documented, there is a large number of studies supporting the positive effects of cannabinoids in inflammations of the gut-lung-skin axis, and some significant results are presented in Table 1.

The investigation of the effects of cannabinoids on animal models of various inflammatory conditions of the gut-lung-skin axis has validated the anticipated results. Cannabinoids are able to reproduce the same anti-inflammatory effects that were observed in vitro in advanced experimental in vivo models, which lead to the identification of further beneficial effects. Cannabinoids modulate cell signaling and regulate the accumulation of inflammatory cells at the site of the inflammation, while also decreasing the activity of some chemokines and the expression of pro-inflammatory proteins. All of these positive direct and indirect anti-inflammatory effects have been attributed to a wide variety of cannabinoids, and relevant studies that support these findings are listed in Table 2.

The encouraging results emerging from in vitro and animal studies have prompted the translation to human trials. However, this has been made difficult, at least in part, by legislation and the need to obtain authorization from institutions regulating the use of cannabinoids that need to enforce national, trans-national and international regulations [194]. However, multiple trials have explored the potential of cannabinoids in inflammatory diseases pertaining to the gut-lung-skin barrier. The status of these trials and the preliminary or definitive results are listed in Table 3.

Unfortunately, not all of the cannabinoids that have proven effective in in vitro conditions or on animal models have provided significant results in humans, and some even presented significant adverse effects. Nevertheless, perfecting some new artificial cannabinoids with optimal receptor affinities or associating other compounds that modulate the effects via antagonism or post-receptor regulation may lead to improved results. The higher patient acceptance of natural compounds or their derivatives may prove essential in obtaining better compliance and superior results when associating cannabinoids in inflammatory conditions, especially in a chronic setting which implies sustained treatment [195]. Further randomized placebo-controlled clinical trials are needed to support the already overwhelming evidence regarding the beneficial results of cannabinoids in inflammations of the gut-lung-skin epithelium. In Figure 1, we summarized the effects of natural or synthetic cannabinoids on several receptors implicated in decreasing the inflammation in the gut-lung-skin barrier.

Table 1. The roles of cannabinoids in inflammatory conditions of the gut-lung-skin barrier demonstrated in in vitro studies.

Cannabinoid	Impacted Molecules	Receptors/Pathway	Experimental Model	Study
AEA and CBD	IL-17A inflammatory effects (↓)	Mostly CB2, possibly PPAR-γ-mediated effects	Confluent Caco-2 cell monolayers	Harvey et al. [57]
THC and CBD	IFN-γ and TNF-α-induced permeability (↓)	CB1-mediated effects	Confluent Caco-2 cell monolayers	Alhamoruni et al. [58]
AEA and 2-AG	IFN-γ and TNF-α-induced permeability (↑)	CB1-mediated effects	Confluent Caco-2 cell monolayers	Alhamoruni et al. [58]
AEA	IL-6, IL-8 (↓)	CB1-mediated effects, possibly TRPV1 modulation	Caco-2 cell monolayers	Karwad et al. [60]
CBD and PEA	prevents production of CREB, JNK, STAT5	CB2, TRPV1 (CBD) PPAR-α (PEA)	Caco-2 cells	Couch et al. [61]
CBD and THCA	IL-8 (↓)	partially GPR55-mediated (THCA)	HCT116, HT29, and Caco-2 colon cells	Nallathambi et al. [62]
BPC	TNF-α, IL-1β, IL-6, IL-17A (↓) IL-13 (↑)	CB2-mediated STAT-3 downregulation	Human gingival fibroblasts and mucosa epithelial cells	Picciolo et al. [65]
CBD	IL-6, G-CSF, CXCL1 (↓) IL-8, GM-CSF, CXCL2 (↑)	Unspecified, possibly CB2-mediated	Normal bronchial cells treated with TNF-α	Muthumalage et al. [111]
CBD	MCP-1 (↓)	NF-κB inhibition	BEAS-2B, U937, and HFL-1 cells	Muthumalage et al. [111]
ACEA and JWH-133	VEGF-A, VEGF-C, Ang1, and Ang2 (↓)	CB1 (ACEA) CB2 (JWH-133)	Human lung macrophages	Staiano et al. [113]
AJA	TNF-α, IFN-α and β (↓)	Unspecified, possibly CB2-mediated	Peripheral blood mononuclear cells from dermatomyositis patients	Robinson et al. [173]
PEA	MCP-2 (↓)	"Entourage" effect on TRPV1 ligands (AEA and OEA)	HaCaT keratinocytes treated with polyinosinic:polycytidylic acid	Petrosino et al. [168]
CBD	MCP-2, IL-6, IL-8, TNF-α (↓)	CB2-mediated as well as through TRPV1 activation/desensitization	HaCaT keratinocytes treated with polyinosinic:polycytidylic acid	Petrosino et al. [169]
THC, CBN, CBD, and CBG	Keratinocytes (inhibits proliferation)	Predominantly mediated by PPAR-γ	HPV-16 E6/E7 transformed human skin keratinocytes	Wilkinson et al. [171]
ACEA	keratinocytes (inhibits proliferation)	CB1-mediated signaling	Isolated human skin samples of psoriasis lesions	Ramot et al. [172]
CBD	GRO-α, vGPCR, VEGF-C, VEGFR-3 (↓)	Unspecified, possibly mediated by multiple receptors (CB1, CB2, TRPVs, and/or GPRs)	Kaposi's sarcoma-associated herpesvirus-infected primary human dermal endothelial cells	Maor et al. [175]

Table 1. *Cont.*

Cannabinoid	Impacted Molecules	Receptors/Pathway	Experimental Model	Study
CBD	TNF-α, IL-1β, IL-6 (↓)	A2a adenosine receptor-cAMP-TRIB3-NF-κB pathway	SZ95 human sebocytes cultures	Oláh et al. [174]

(↓) = decrease in expression and/or concentration; (↑) = increase in expression and/or concentration; TRPV = transient receptor potential channel; BPC = β-Caryophyllene; OEA = oleoylethanolamide; GPR = G-coupled protein receptor.

Table 2. The roles of cannabinoids in inflammatory conditions of the gut-lung-skin barrier evidenced in vivo studies.

Cannabinoid	Impacted Molecules	Receptors/Pathway	Experimental Model	Study
CBG	IL-1β, IL-10, IFN-γ, iNOS expression, MPO activity (↓)	CB2 and possibly TRPV4-mediated	Murine colitis induced by DNBS	Borrelli et al. [70]
CBD	IL-1β, IL-10, iNOS expression (↓)	Unspecified, possibly CB2-mediated	Murine colitis induced by DNBS	Borrelli et al. [71]
CBD and CBG combined with fish oil	IL-1β, MPO activity (↓)	Possibly by regulating endocannabinoids and their derivates	Murine colitis induced by DNBS	Pagano et al. [72]
CBD combined with fish oil	IL-1β, IL-6, MPO activity (↓) IL-10 (↑)	Unspecified	DSS model of murine colitis	Silvestri et al. [73]
Abn-CBD	MPO activity (↓)	Non-CB1/2, possibly GPR18 and GPR55	TNBS-induced colitis in CD1 mice	Krohn et al. [80]
HU210	IL-1β, IL-6, IL-17, TNF-α, MPO activity (↓)	TLR4/MAPK signaling pathway	DSS model of murine colitis	Lin et al. [79]
HU210	IL-6, chemokine KC (↓)	CB1/2 receptor agonism	Gastric mucosa inflammation secondary to acute pancreatitis in rats	Cao et al. [78]
CBD	IL-6, TNF-α, MCP-1, MIP-2, MPO activity (↓)	Non-CB1/2, possibly through the adenosine A2A receptor	Lipopolysaccharide-induced acute lung injury in mice	Ribeiro et al. [117,118]
WIN 55,212-2, PEA and THC	TNF-α (↓)	Partially CB2-mediated	Lipopolysaccharide-induced acute lung injury in mice	Beryshev et al. [119]
CBD	IL-5, IL-23, G-CSF, TNF-α (↑)	Increased activation of NFAT and Ca²⁺ signaling	Lipopolysaccharide-induced acute lung injury in mice	Karmaus et al. [120]
CBD	IL-1 and total protein content (↓)	5-HT1A receptor	Lung inflammation induced by brain ischemia in newborn piglets	Arruza et al. [121]
WIN55,212-2	MMP-9 (↓)	ERK1/2 signaling pathway	Lung inflammation in mice exposed to cigarette smoke	Tauber et al. [122]

Table 2. Cont.

Cannabinoid	Impacted Molecules	Receptors/Pathway	Experimental Model	Study
CBD	IL-4, IL-5, IL-13, IL-6, and TNF-α (↓)	CB1/2-mediated	Ovalbumin-induced asthma in mice	Vuolo et al. [123,124]
JWH-133	CD11b surface expression/adhesion, ROS production (↑)	CB2-mediated	Ovalbumin-induced asthma in mice	Frei et al. [125]
JWH-133 combined with JZL184	IFN-γ, MIP-1α (↓) IL-10 (↑)	CB1 (JZL184) CB2 (JWH-133)	Lung inflammation in RSV infection in mice	Tahamtan et al. [127,128]
THC	IFN-γ (↓)	PI3K/Akt pathway signaling inhibition	Murine model of lung injury caused by SEB	Rao et al. [131]
JWH-133	IL-6, TNF-α, MPO activity (↓) SOD activity (↑)	CB2-mediated activation of PI3K/Akt pathway signaling	Lung ischemia-reperfusion injury model in mice	Zeng et al. [132]
JWH-133	IL-1β, IL-6, TNF-α, caspase-3 (↓) IL-10 (↑)	NF-κB signaling inhibition	Mice with CLP-induced sepsis	Çakır et al. [133]
GP1a	IL-6, chemokine KC, MIP-2 (↓)	CB2-mediated	Mice with CLP-induced sepsis	Tschöp et al. [134]
M. suaveolens	IL-1β, IL-6, TNF-α, VEGF (↓) IL-4, IL-10 (↑)	NF-κB signaling inhibition	Mice with CLP-induced sepsis	Liu et al. [135]
JWH-133	MPO activity (↓)	CB2-mediated	Murine model of NPE after subarachnoid hemorrhage	Fujii et al. [136]
BPC and GP1a	IL-12, chemokine KC, leukotriene B4, NO (↓)	CB2-mediated	Mycobacterium bovis-induced pulmonary inflammation	Andrade-Silva et al. [138]
Possible unspecified agonist *	TNF-α, NF-κB and MAP kinases * (↓)	CB1 and CB2-mediated NF-κB and MAP/ERK signaling	Murine UV-induced skin carcinogenesis	Zheng et al. [187]
VCE-004.8	IL-1β and IL-13. Prevention of macrophages infiltration and mast cells degranulation. Indirectly decreased TGF-β	PPAR-γ and CB2-mediated SMAD-signaling transcriptional activity modulation	Mice with bleomycin-induced scleroderma	del Rio et al. [177]
WIN55,212-2	TGF-β, CTGF, and PDGF (↓)	Non-CB1, non-CB2 mediated downregulation of PDGF/TGFβ signaling pathways	Mice with bleomycin-induced scleroderma	Balistreri et al. [178]

Table 2. *Cont.*

Cannabinoid	Impacted Molecules	Receptors/Pathway	Experimental Model	Study
α-OOS	Mast cells degranulation and IL-4 (↓)	"Entourage" effect on CB1 with possible PPAR-γ and GPR55 involvement	Oxazolone induced atopic dermatitis in Balb/c and hairless mice	Kim et al. [179]
CBD	Arachidonate (↑) and prostaglandins (↓)	Increased PLA$_2$ activity and inhibition of cyclooxygenase and lipoxygenase	Tetradecanoylphorbol acetate-induced erythema of mouse skin	Formukong et al. [180]
CBD	ROS production and caspase activation (↓)	Undetermined anti-inflammatory pathway *. TRIB3-Akt/mTOR signaling pathway	Mice bearing BRAF wild-type melanoma xenografts	Armstrong et al. [181]

* Hypothesized, yet to be demonstrated; (↓) = decrease in expression and/or concentration; (↑) = increase in expression and/or concentration; CLP = cecal ligation and puncture; DNBS = 2,4-dinitrobenzene sulphonic acid; DSS = dextran sulphate sodium; PLA$_2$ = phospholipase A$_2$; MDA = malondialdehyde; MPO = myeloperoxidase; mTOR = mammalian target of rapamycin; NFAT = nuclear factor of activated T cells; NPE = neurogenic pulmonary edema; TNBS = trinitrobenzene sulfonic acid; RSV = respiratory syncytial virus; SEB = taphylococcal enterotoxin B; SOD = superoxide dismutase.

Table 3. Human trials evaluating the safety and efficacy of cannabinoids in inflammatory conditions of the gut-lung-skin barrier.

Cannabinoid	Effects	Inflammatory Condition	Clinical Trial Stage	Study
PEA and CBD	Decreased intestinal permeability	Aspirin-induced intestinal inflammation	Phase 1	Couch et al. [87]
THC	Decreased CDAI and CRP Increased quality of life	Crohn's disease	Phase 1	Naftali et al. [88]
CBD	No beneficial effects	Crohn's disease	Phase 2	Naftali et al. [89]
CBD	Minor improvements in rectal bleeding and endoscopic scores. Increased quality of life	Ulcerative colitis	Phase 2	Irving et al. [91]
THC	Decreased DAI and endoscopic score	Ulcerative colitis	Phase 1	Naftali et al. [92]
Lenabasum	Decreased IgG, IL-8, exacerbations, and lymphocyte infiltration	Cystic fibrosis	Phase 2	Chmiel et al. [143]
Cannabis (high CBD/low THC)	*Results pending*	Pain and Inflammation in Lung Cancer	Phase 1	Martinez et al. [144]
Cannabis (high CBD/low THC)	No clinical positive or negative effects	Chronic obstructive pulmonary disease	Phase 2	Abdallah et al. [146]
Nabilone	No significant bronchodilation	Asthma	Phase 1	Gong et al. [147]

Table 3. Cont.

Cannabinoid	Effects	Inflammatory Condition	Clinical Trial Stage	Study
THC	Antagonistic effects on bronchodilation. Irritating effect on airways	Asthma	Phase 1	Tashkin et al. [148]
THC	Mild bronchodilation effect. Significant psychoactive effects	Asthma	Phase 1	Abboud et al. [149]
Cannabis seeds mixture	Decreased erythema	Acne	Phase 1	Ali et al. [188]
BTX 1503	Results pending	Acne	Phase 2	Botanix Pharmaceuticals [189]
AJA	Decreased expression of key genes related to inflammation	Cutaneous systemic sclerosis	Phase 2	Spiera et al. [190]
AJA	Decreased IL-31, IFN-β and γ, and T-helper cell inflammation	Dermatomyositis	Phase 2	Chen et al. [192]
AJA	Initiated study	Cutaneous systemic sclerosis	Phase 3	Burstein et al. [191]
AJA	Developed study protocol	Dermatomyositis	Phase 3	Werth et al. [193]

CDAI = Crohn's disease activity index; CRP = C-reactive protein; DAI = disease activity index; IgG = immunoglobulin G.

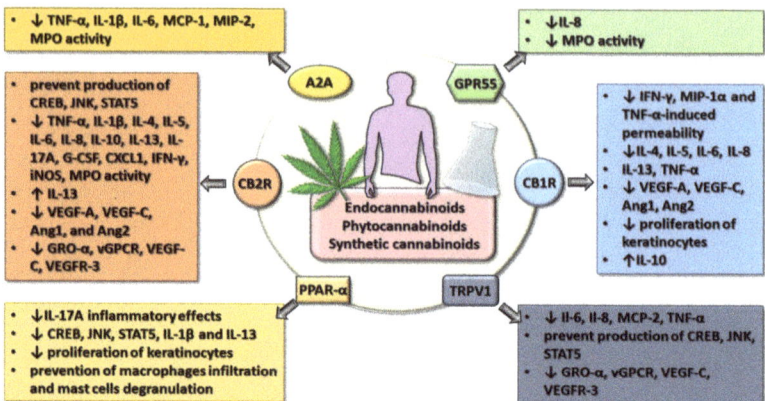

Figure 1. The summarization of the main effects of endocannabinoids, as well as natural and synthetic cannabinoids on several receptors promoting the decrease of inflammation in the gut-lung-skin barrier. (↓) = decrease in expression and/or concentration; (↑) = increase in expression and/or concentration.

8. Conclusions

The epithelia of the gastrointestinal tract, the pulmonary system and the cutaneous membrane share common features in regard to physiology, molecular signaling, and cell activity in pathological conditions. Furthermore, recent data suggest that the gut-lung-skin barrier exhibits cross-talk involving various cells and cytokines, and responds in a similar way to epithelial disruption and local inflammation. This unitary behavior is also evidenced in the response to cannabinoids, a large class of compounds with well-known anti-inflammatory properties. A large number of in vitro and in vivo animal studies have shown promising results in either reducing or preventing inflammation in experimental models involving the elements of the gut-lung-skin barrier. Human studies have shown mixed results, with some cannabinoids either being ineffective or not tolerable in the treatment of specific inflammatory conditions. The reasons for treatment failure or intolerance may be revealed by translating the observations regarding the effects of cannabinoids on inflammation between studies involving specific elements of the gut-lung-skin barrier. The success that some of the clinical trials have achieved is encouraging and warrants further studies that will undoubtedly clarify the definitive role of cannabinoids in epithelial inflammation.

Author Contributions: Conceptualization, C.S., C.C., A.C.; writing—original draft preparation, C.S., C.C., I.A.B., A.-E.S., A.O.D., D.C., A.C.; writing—review and editing, C.S., A.O.D., D.C., A.C. All authors have read and agreed to the published version of the manuscript.

Funding: This research was funded by a grant of the Romanian Ministry of Research and Innovation, CCCDI-UEFISCDI [project number 61PCCDI/2018 PN-III-P1-1.2-PCCDI-2017-0341], within PNCDI-III.

Institutional Review Board Statement: Not applicable.

Informed Consent Statement: Not applicable.

Data Availability Statement: Not applicable.

Conflicts of Interest: The authors declare no conflict of interest.

References

1. Stanke, F. The Contribution of the Airway Epithelial Cell to Host Defense. *Mediat. Inflamm.* **2015**, *2015*, 463016. [CrossRef] [PubMed]
2. Hornef, M.W.; Normark, S.; Henriques-Normark, B.; Rhen, M. Bacterial evasion of innate defense at epithelial linings. *Chem. Immunol. Allergy* **2005**, *86*, 72–98. [CrossRef] [PubMed]

3. Wan, L.Y.; Chen, Z.J.; Shah, N.P.; El-Nezami, H. Modulation of Intestinal Epithelial Defense Responses by Probiotic Bacteria. *Crit. Rev. Food Sci. Nutr.* **2016**, *56*, 2628–2641. [CrossRef] [PubMed]
4. Zhu, T.H.; Zhu, T.R.; Tran, K.A.; Sivamani, R.K.; Shi, V.Y. Epithelial barrier dysfunctions in atopic dermatitis: A skin-gut-lung model linking microbiome alteration and immune dysregulation. *Br. J. Dermatol.* **2018**, *179*, 570–581. [CrossRef]
5. Uluçkan, Ö.; Wagner, E.F. Chronic systemic inflammation originating from epithelial tissues. *FEBS J.* **2017**, *284*, 505–516. [CrossRef]
6. Wang, H.; Liu, J.S.; Peng, S.H.; Deng, X.Y.; Zhu, D.M.; Javidiparsijani, S.; Wang, G.R.; Li, D.Q.; Li, L.X.; Wang, Y.C.; et al. Gut-lung crosstalk in pulmonary involvement with inflammatory bowel diseases. *World J. Gastroenterol.* **2013**, *19*, 6794–6804. [CrossRef]
7. Weaver, C.T.; Hatton, R.D.; Mangan, P.R.; Harrington, L.E. IL-17 family cytokines and the expanding diversity of effector T cell lineages. *Annu. Rev. Immunol.* **2007**, *25*, 821–852. [CrossRef]
8. Weaver, C.T.; Elson, C.O.; Fouser, L.A.; Kolls, J.K. The Th17 pathway and inflammatory diseases of the intestines, lungs, and skin. *Annu. Rev. Pathol.* **2013**, *8*, 477–512. [CrossRef]
9. Eyerich, K.; Dimartino, V.; Cavani, A. IL-17 and IL-22 in immunity: Driving protection and pathology. *Eur. J. Immunol.* **2017**, *47*, 607–614. [CrossRef]
10. Puel, A.; Cypowyj, S.; Bustamante, J.; Wright, J.F.; Liu, L.; Lim, H.K.; Migaud, M.; Israel, L.; Chrabieh, M.; Audry, M.; et al. Chronic mucocutaneous candidiasis in humans with inborn errors of interleukin-17 immunity. *Science* **2011**, *332*, 65–68. [CrossRef]
11. O'Connor, W., Jr.; Kamanaka, M.; Booth, C.J.; Town, T.; Nakae, S.; Iwakura, Y.; Kolls, J.K.; Flavell, R.A. A protective function for interleukin 17A in T cell-mediated intestinal inflammation. *Nat. Immunol.* **2009**, *10*, 603–609. [CrossRef]
12. Isailovic, N.; Daigo, K.; Mantovani, A.; Selmi, C. Interleukin-17 and innate immunity in infections and chronic inflammation. *J. Autoimmun.* **2015**, *60*, 1–11. [CrossRef]
13. Eyerich, K.; Pennino, D.; Scarponi, C.; Foerster, S.; Nasorri, F.; Behrendt, H.; Ring, J.; Traidl-Hoffmann, C.; Albanesi, C.; Cavani, A. IL-17 in atopic eczema: Linking allergen-specific adaptive and microbial-triggered innate immune response. *J. Allergy Clin. Immunol.* **2009**, *123*, 59–66.e54. [CrossRef]
14. Aujla, S.J.; Kolls, J.K. IL-22: A critical mediator in mucosal host defense. *J. Mol. Med.* **2009**, *87*, 451–454. [CrossRef]
15. Blázquez, A.B.; Mayer, L.; Berin, M.C. Thymic stromal lymphopoietin is required for gastrointestinal allergy but not oral tolerance. *Gastroenterology* **2010**, *139*, 1301–1309. [CrossRef]
16. Luo, J.; Li, Y.; Gong, R. The mechanism of atopic march may be the 'social' event of cells and molecules (Review). *Int. J. Mol. Med.* **2010**, *26*, 779–785. [CrossRef]
17. Schett, G.; Elewaut, D.; McInnes, I.B.; Dayer, J.M.; Neurath, M.F. How cytokine networks fuel inflammation: Toward a cytokine-based disease taxonomy. *Nat. Med.* **2013**, *19*, 822–824. [CrossRef]
18. Zhang, Y.; Zeng, X.; Lu, H.; Li, Y.; Ji, H. Association between Interleukin-8-251A/T polymorphism and gastric cancer susceptibility: A meta-analysis based on 5286 cases and 8000 controls. *Int. J. Clin. Exp. Med.* **2015**, *8*, 22393–22402.
19. Albareda, M.; Ravella, A.; Castelló, M.; Saborit, S.; Peramiquel, L.; Vila, L. Metabolic syndrome and its components in patients with psoriasis. *Springerplus* **2014**, *3*, 612. [CrossRef]
20. Andersen, N.N.; Jess, T. Risk of cardiovascular disease in inflammatory bowel disease. *World J. Gastrointest. Pathophysiol.* **2014**, *5*, 359–365. [CrossRef]
21. Scheau, C.; Mihai, L.G.; Bădărău, I.A.; Caruntu, C. Emerging applications of some important natural compounds in the field of oncology. *Farmacia* **2020**, *68*, 8. [CrossRef]
22. Calina, D.; Buga, A.M.; Mitroi, M.; Buha, A.; Caruntu, C.; Scheau, C.; Bouyahya, A.; El Omari, N.; El Menyiy, N.; Docea, A.O. The Treatment of Cognitive, Behavioural and Motor Impairments from Brain Injury and Neurodegenerative Diseases through Cannabinoid System Modulation-Evidence from In Vivo Studies. *J. Clin. Med.* **2020**, *9*, 2395. [CrossRef]
23. Ilie, M.A.; Caruntu, C.; Tampa, M.; Georgescu, S.R.; Matei, C.; Negrei, C.; Ion, R.M.; Constantin, C.; Neagu, M.; Boda, D. Capsaicin: Physicochemical properties, cutaneous reactions and potential applications in painful and inflammatory conditions (Review). *Exp. Ther. Med.* **2019**, *18*, 916–925. [CrossRef]
24. Salehi, B.; Calina, D.; Docea, A.O.; Koirala, N.; Aryal, S.; Lombardo, D.; Pasqua, L.; Taheri, Y.; Marina Salgado Castillo, C.; Martorell, M.; et al. Curcumin's Nanomedicine Formulations for Therapeutic Application in Neurological Diseases. *J. Clin. Med.* **2020**, *9*, 430. [CrossRef]
25. Sharma, S.; Naura, A.S. Potential of phytochemicals as immune-regulatory compounds in atopic diseases: A review. *Biochem. Pharmacol.* **2020**, 113790. [CrossRef]
26. Mintie, C.A.; Singh, C.K.; Ahmad, N. Whole Fruit Phytochemicals Combating Skin Damage and Carcinogenesis. *Transl. Oncol.* **2019**, *13*, 146–156. [CrossRef]
27. Kim, J.E.; Lee, K.W. Molecular Targets of Phytochemicals for Skin Inflammation. *Curr. Pharm. Des.* **2018**, *24*, 1533–1550. [CrossRef]
28. Salehi, B.; Sharifi-Rad, J.; Cappellini, F.; Reiner, Ž.; Zorzan, D.; Imran, M.; Sener, B.; Kilic, M.; El-Shazly, M.; Fahmy, N.M.; et al. The Therapeutic Potential of Anthocyanins: Current Approaches Based on Their Molecular Mechanism of Action. *Front. Pharmacol.* **2020**, *11*, 1300. [CrossRef]
29. Salehi, B.; Quispe, C.; Chamkhi, I.; El Omari, N.; Balahbib, A.; Sharifi-Rad, J.; Bouyahya, A.; Akram, M.; Iqbal, M.; Docea, A.O.; et al. Pharmacological Properties of Chalcones: A Review of Preclinical Including Molecular Mechanisms and Clinical Evidence. *Front. Pharmacol.* **2020**, *11*, 592654. [CrossRef]
30. Makara, G.B. Superficial and deep chemonociception: Differential inhibition by pretreatment with capsaicin. *Acta Physiol. Acad. Sci. Hung.* **1970**, *38*, 393–399.

31. Georgescu, S.R.; Sarbu, M.I.; Matei, C.; Ilie, M.A.; Caruntu, C.; Constantin, C.; Neagu, M.; Tampa, M. Capsaicin: Friend or Foe in Skin Cancer and Other Related Malignancies? *Nutrients* **2017**, *9*, 1365. [CrossRef] [PubMed]
32. Scheau, C.; Badarau, I.A.; Caruntu, C.; Mihai, G.L.; Didilescu, A.C.; Constantin, C.; Neagu, M. Capsaicin: Effects on the Pathogenesis of Hepatocellular Carcinoma. *Molecules* **2019**, *24*, 2350. [CrossRef] [PubMed]
33. Rubin, V. *Cannabis and Culture*; De Gruyter Mouton: Berlin, Germany, 1975.
34. Zurier, R.B.; Burstein, S.H. Cannabinoids, inflammation, and fibrosis. *FASEB J.* **2016**, *30*, 3682–3689. [CrossRef] [PubMed]
35. Pertwee, R.G. The pharmacology of cannabinoid receptors and their ligands: An overview. *Int. J. Obes.* **2006**, *30*, S13–S18. [CrossRef]
36. Walsh, K.B.; Andersen, H.K. Molecular Pharmacology of Synthetic Cannabinoids: Delineating CB1 Receptor-Mediated Cell Signaling. *Int. J. Mol. Sci.* **2020**, *21*, 6115. [CrossRef]
37. Zou, S.; Kumar, U. Cannabinoid Receptors and the Endocannabinoid System: Signaling and Function in the Central Nervous System. *Int. J. Mol. Sci.* **2018**, *19*, 833. [CrossRef]
38. Demuth, D.G.; Molleman, A. Cannabinoid signalling. *Life Sci.* **2006**, *78*, 549–563. [CrossRef]
39. Thapa, D.; Cairns, E.A.; Szczesniak, A.M.; Toguri, J.T.; Caldwell, M.D.; Kelly, M.E.M. The Cannabinoids Δ(8)THC, CBD, and HU-308 Act via Distinct Receptors to Reduce Corneal Pain and Inflammation. *Cannabis Cannabinoid Res.* **2018**, *3*, 11–20. [CrossRef]
40. Britch, S.C.; Goodman, A.G.; Wiley, J.L.; Pondelick, A.M.; Craft, R.M. Antinociceptive and Immune Effects of Delta-9-Tetrahydrocannabinol or Cannabidiol in Male Versus Female Rats with Persistent Inflammatory Pain. *J. Pharmacol. Exp. Ther.* **2020**, *373*, 416–428. [CrossRef]
41. Lunn, C.A.; Fine, J.S.; Rojas-Triana, A.; Jackson, J.V.; Fan, X.; Kung, T.T.; Gonsiorek, W.; Schwarz, M.A.; Lavey, B.; Kozlowski, J.A.; et al. A novel cannabinoid peripheral cannabinoid receptor-selective inverse agonist blocks leukocyte recruitment in vivo. *J. Pharmacol. Exp. Ther.* **2006**, *316*, 780–788. [CrossRef]
42. Henshaw, F.R.; Dewsbury, L.S.; Lim, C.K.; Steiner, G.Z. The Effects of Cannabinoids on Pro- and Anti-Inflammatory Cytokines: A Systematic Review of In Vivo Studies. *Cannabis Cannabinoid Res.* **2021**. [CrossRef]
43. Costa, B.; Trovato, A.E.; Comelli, F.; Giagnoni, G.; Colleoni, M. The non-psychoactive cannabis constituent cannabidiol is an orally effective therapeutic agent in rat chronic inflammatory and neuropathic pain. *Eur. J. Pharmacol.* **2007**, *556*, 75–83. [CrossRef]
44. Costa, B.; Colleoni, M.; Conti, S.; Parolaro, D.; Franke, C.; Trovato, A.E.; Giagnoni, G. Oral anti-inflammatory activity of cannabidiol, a non-psychoactive constituent of cannabis, in acute carrageenan-induced inflammation in the rat paw. *Naunyn Schmiedebergs Arch. Pharmacol.* **2004**, *369*, 294–299. [CrossRef]
45. Sumariwalla, P.F.; Gallily, R.; Tchilibon, S.; Fride, E.; Mechoulam, R.; Feldmann, M. A novel synthetic, nonpsychoactive cannabinoid acid (HU-320) with antiinflammatory properties in murine collagen-induced arthritis. *Arthritis Rheum.* **2004**, *50*, 985–998. [CrossRef]
46. Buchweitz, J.P.; Karmaus, P.W.; Williams, K.J.; Harkema, J.R.; Kaminski, N.E. Targeted deletion of cannabinoid receptors CB1 and CB2 produced enhanced inflammatory responses to influenza A/PR/8/34 in the absence and presence of Delta9-tetrahydrocannabinol. *J. Leukoc. Biol.* **2008**, *83*, 785–796. [CrossRef]
47. An, D.; Peigneur, S.; Hendrickx, L.A.; Tytgat, J. Targeting Cannabinoid Receptors: Current Status and Prospects of Natural Products. *Int. J. Mol. Sci.* **2020**, *21*, 5064. [CrossRef]
48. Hasenoehrl, C.; Taschler, U.; Storr, M.; Schicho, R. The gastrointestinal tract—A central organ of cannabinoid signaling in health and disease. *Neurogastroenterol. Motil. Off. J. Eur. Gastrointest. Motil. Soc.* **2016**, *28*, 1765–1780. [CrossRef]
49. Uranga, J.A.; Vera, G.; Abalo, R. Cannabinoid pharmacology and therapy in gut disorders. *Biochem. Pharmacol.* **2018**, *157*, 134–147. [CrossRef]
50. Izzo, A.A.; Sharkey, K.A. Cannabinoids and the gut: New developments and emerging concepts. *Pharmacol. Ther.* **2010**, *126*, 21–38. [CrossRef]
51. Goyal, H.; Singla, U.; Gupta, U.; May, E. Role of cannabis in digestive disorders. *Eur. J. Gastroenterol. Hepatol.* **2017**, *29*, 135–143. [CrossRef]
52. Camilleri, M. Cannabinoids and gastrointestinal motility: Pharmacology, clinical effects, and potential therapeutics in humans. *Neurogastroenterol. Motil.* **2018**, *30*, e13370. [CrossRef] [PubMed]
53. Peng, J.; Li, Y.J. The vanilloid receptor TRPV1: Role in cardiovascular and gastrointestinal protection. *Eur. J. Pharmacol.* **2010**, *627*, 1–7. [CrossRef] [PubMed]
54. Overton, H.A.; Fyfe, M.C.; Reynet, C. GPR119, a novel G protein-coupled receptor target for the treatment of type 2 diabetes and obesity. *Br. J. Pharmacol.* **2008**, *153* (Suppl. 1), S76–S81. [CrossRef] [PubMed]
55. Galiazzo, G.; Giancola, F.; Stanzani, A.; Fracassi, F.; Bernardini, C.; Forni, M.; Pietra, M.; Chiocchetti, R. Localization of cannabinoid receptors CB1, CB2, GPR55, and PPARα in the canine gastrointestinal tract. *Histochem. Cell Biol.* **2018**, *150*, 187–205. [CrossRef]
56. Brown, A.J. Novel cannabinoid receptors. *Br. J. Pharmacol.* **2007**, *152*, 567–575. [CrossRef]
57. Harvey, B.S.; Sia, T.C.; Wattchow, D.A.; Smid, S.D. Interleukin 17A evoked mucosal damage is attenuated by cannabidiol and anandamide in a human colonic explant model. *Cytokine* **2014**, *65*, 236–244. [CrossRef]
58. Alhamoruni, A.; Wright, K.L.; Larvin, M.; O'Sullivan, S.E. Cannabinoids mediate opposing effects on inflammation-induced intestinal permeability. *Br. J. Pharmacol.* **2012**, *165*, 2598–2610. [CrossRef]
59. Alhamoruni, A.; Lee, A.C.; Wright, K.L.; Larvin, M.; O'Sullivan, S.E. Pharmacological effects of cannabinoids on the Caco-2 cell culture model of intestinal permeability. *J. Pharmacol. Exp. Ther.* **2010**, *335*, 92–102. [CrossRef]

60. Karwad, M.A.; Couch, D.G.; Theophilidou, E.; Sarmad, S.; Barrett, D.A.; Larvin, M.; Wright, K.L.; Lund, J.N.; O'Sullivan, S.E. The role of CB(1) in intestinal permeability and inflammation. *FASEB J.* **2017**, *31*, 3267–3277. [CrossRef]
61. Couch, D.G.; Tasker, C.; Theophilidou, E.; Lund, J.N.; O'Sullivan, S.E. Cannabidiol and palmitoylethanolamide are anti-inflammatory in the acutely inflamed human colon. *Clin. Sci.* **2017**, *131*, 2611–2626. [CrossRef]
62. Nallathambi, R.; Mazuz, M.; Ion, A.; Selvaraj, G.; Weininger, S.; Fridlender, M.; Nasser, A.; Sagee, O.; Kumari, P.; Nemichenizer, D.; et al. Anti-Inflammatory Activity in Colon Models Is Derived from Δ9-Tetrahydrocannabinolic Acid That Interacts with Additional Compounds in Cannabis Extracts. *Cannabis Cannabinoid Res.* **2017**, *2*, 167–182. [CrossRef]
63. Gigli, S.; Seguella, L.; Pesce, M.; Bruzzese, E.; D'Alessandro, A.; Cuomo, R.; Steardo, L.; Sarnelli, G.; Esposito, G. Cannabidiol restores intestinal barrier dysfunction and inhibits the apoptotic process induced by *Clostridium difficile* toxin A in Caco-2 cells. *United Eur. Gastroenterol. J.* **2017**, *5*, 1108–1115. [CrossRef]
64. Wright, K.; Rooney, N.; Feeney, M.; Tate, J.; Robertson, D.; Welham, M.; Ward, S. Differential expression of cannabinoid receptors in the human colon: Cannabinoids promote epithelial wound healing. *Gastroenterology* **2005**, *129*, 437–453. [CrossRef]
65. Picciolo, G.; Pallio, G.; Altavilla, D.; Vaccaro, M.; Oteri, G.; Irrera, N.; Squadrito, F. β-Caryophyllene Reduces the Inflammatory Phenotype of Periodontal Cells by Targeting CB2 Receptors. *Biomedicines* **2020**, *8*, 164. [CrossRef]
66. Podolsky, D.K. Inflammatory bowel disease. *N. Engl. J. Med.* **2002**, *347*, 417–429. [CrossRef]
67. Ihenetu, K.; Molleman, A.; Parsons, M.E.; Whelan, C.J. Inhibition of interleukin-8 release in the human colonic epithelial cell line HT-29 by cannabinoids. *Eur. J. Pharmacol.* **2003**, *458*, 207–215. [CrossRef]
68. Ligresti, A.; Bisogno, T.; Matias, I.; De Petrocellis, L.; Cascio, M.G.; Cosenza, V.; D'Argenio, G.; Scaglione, G.; Bifulco, M.; Sorrentini, I.; et al. Possible endocannabinoid control of colorectal cancer growth. *Gastroenterology* **2003**, *125*, 677–687. [CrossRef]
69. Couch, D.G.; Maudslay, H.; Doleman, B.; Lund, J.N.; O'Sullivan, S.E. The Use of Cannabinoids in Colitis: A Systematic Review and Meta-Analysis. *Inflamm. Bowel Dis.* **2018**, *24*, 680–697. [CrossRef]
70. Borrelli, F.; Fasolino, I.; Romano, B.; Capasso, R.; Maiello, F.; Coppola, D.; Orlando, P.; Battista, G.; Pagano, E.; Di Marzo, V.; et al. Beneficial effect of the non-psychotropic plant cannabinoid cannabigerol on experimental inflammatory bowel disease. *Biochem. Pharmacol.* **2013**, *85*, 1306–1316. [CrossRef]
71. Borrelli, F.; Aviello, G.; Romano, B.; Orlando, P.; Capasso, R.; Maiello, F.; Guadagno, F.; Petrosino, S.; Capasso, F.; Di Marzo, V.; et al. Cannabidiol, a safe and non-psychotropic ingredient of the marijuana plant *Cannabis sativa*, is protective in a murine model of colitis. *J. Mol. Med.* **2009**, *87*, 1111–1121. [CrossRef]
72. Pagano, E.; Iannotti, F.A.; Piscitelli, F.; Romano, B.; Lucariello, G.; Venneri, T.; Di Marzo, V.; Izzo, A.A.; Borrelli, F. Efficacy of combined therapy with fish oil and phytocannabinoids in murine intestinal inflammation. *Phytother. Res.* **2021**, *35*, 517–529. [CrossRef]
73. Silvestri, C.; Pagano, E.; Lacroix, S.; Venneri, T.; Cristiano, C.; Calignano, A.; Parisi, O.A.; Izzo, A.A.; Di Marzo, V.; Borrelli, F. Fish Oil, Cannabidiol and the Gut Microbiota: An Investigation in a Murine Model of Colitis. *Front. Pharmacol.* **2020**, *11*, 585096. [CrossRef]
74. Manichanh, C.; Borruel, N.; Casellas, F.; Guarner, F. The gut microbiota in IBD. *Nat. Rev. Gastroenterol. Hepatol.* **2012**, *9*, 599–608. [CrossRef]
75. Muccioli, G.G.; Naslain, D.; Bäckhed, F.; Reigstad, C.S.; Lambert, D.M.; Delzenne, N.M.; Cani, P.D. The endocannabinoid system links gut microbiota to adipogenesis. *Mol. Syst. Biol.* **2010**, *6*, 392. [CrossRef]
76. Kienzl, M.; Storr, M.; Schicho, R. Cannabinoids and Opioids in the Treatment of Inflammatory Bowel Diseases. *Clin. Transl. Gastroenterol.* **2020**, *11*, e00120. [CrossRef]
77. Zoppi, S.; Madrigal, J.L.; Pérez-Nievas, B.G.; Marín-Jiménez, I.; Caso, J.R.; Alou, L.; García-Bueno, B.; Colón, A.; Manzanares, J.; Gómez-Lus, M.L.; et al. Endogenous cannabinoid system regulates intestinal barrier function in vivo through cannabinoid type 1 receptor activation. *Am. J. Physiol. Gastrointest. Liver Physiol.* **2012**, *302*, G565–G571. [CrossRef]
78. Cao, M.H.; Li, Y.Y.; Xu, J.; Feng, Y.J.; Lin, X.H.; Li, K.; Han, T.; Chen, C.J. Cannabinoid HU210 protects isolated rat stomach against impairment caused by serum of rats with experimental acute pancreatitis. *PLoS ONE* **2012**, *7*, e52921. [CrossRef]
79. Lin, S.; Li, Y.; Shen, L.; Zhang, R.; Yang, L.; Li, M.; Li, K.; Fichna, J. The Anti-Inflammatory Effect and Intestinal Barrier Protection of HU210 Differentially Depend on TLR4 Signaling in Dextran Sulfate Sodium-Induced Murine Colitis. *Dig. Dis. Sci.* **2017**, *62*, 372–386. [CrossRef]
80. Krohn, R.M.; Parsons, S.A.; Fichna, J.; Patel, K.D.; Yates, R.M.; Sharkey, K.A.; Storr, M.A. Abnormal cannabidiol attenuates experimental colitis in mice, promotes wound healing and inhibits neutrophil recruitment. *J. Inflamm.* **2016**, *13*, 21. [CrossRef]
81. Negreanu, L.; Voiosu, T.; State, M.; Mateescu, R.B. Quality of colonoscopy preparation in patients with inflammatory bowel disease: Retrospective analysis of 348 colonoscopies. *J. Int. Med. Res.* **2020**, *48*. [CrossRef]
82. Negreanu, L.; Voiosu, T.; State, M.; Voiosu, A.; Bengus, A.; Mateescu, B.R. Endoscopy in inflammatory bowel disease: From guidelines to real life. *Ther. Adv. Gastroenterol.* **2019**, *12*. [CrossRef]
83. Voiosu, T.; Benguş, A.; Dinu, R.; Voiosu, A.M.; Bălănescu, P.; Băicuş, C.; Diculescu, M.; Voiosu, R.; Mateescu, B. Rapid fecal calprotectin level assessment and the SIBDQ score can accurately detect active mucosal inflammation in IBD patients in clinical remission: A prospective study. *J. Gastrointest. Liver Dis.* **2014**, *23*, 273–278. [CrossRef] [PubMed]
84. Phatak, U.P.; Rojas-Velasquez, D.; Porto, A.; Pashankar, D.S. Prevalence and Patterns of Marijuana Use in Young Adults With Inflammatory Bowel Disease. *J. Pediatr. Gastroenterol. Nutr.* **2017**, *64*, 261–264. [CrossRef] [PubMed]

85. Storr, M.; Devlin, S.; Kaplan, G.G.; Panaccione, R.; Andrews, C.N. Cannabis use provides symptom relief in patients with inflammatory bowel disease but is associated with worse disease prognosis in patients with Crohn's disease. *Inflamm. Bowel Dis.* **2014**, *20*, 472–480. [CrossRef] [PubMed]
86. Merker, A.M.; Riaz, M.; Friedman, S.; Allegretti, J.R.; Korzenik, J. Legalization of Medicinal Marijuana Has Minimal Impact on Use Patterns in Patients with Inflammatory Bowel Disease. *Inflamm. Bowel Dis.* **2018**, *24*, 2309–2314. [CrossRef] [PubMed]
87. Couch, D.G.; Cook, H.; Ortori, C.; Barrett, D.; Lund, J.N.; O'Sullivan, S.E. Palmitoylethanolamide and Cannabidiol Prevent Inflammation-induced Hyperpermeability of the Human Gut In Vitro and In Vivo—A Randomized, Placebo-controlled, Double-blind Controlled Trial. *Inflamm. Bowel Dis.* **2019**, *25*, 1006–1018. [CrossRef] [PubMed]
88. Naftali, T.; Bar-Lev Schleider, L.; Dotan, I.; Lansky, E.P.; Sklerovsky Benjaminov, F.; Konikoff, F.M. Cannabis induces a clinical response in patients with Crohn's disease: A prospective placebo-controlled study. *Clin. Gastroenterol. Hepatol.* **2013**, *11*, 1276–1280.e1. [CrossRef]
89. Naftali, T.; Mechulam, R.; Marii, A.; Gabay, G.; Stein, A.; Bronshtain, M.; Laish, I.; Benjaminov, F.; Konikoff, F.M. Low-Dose Cannabidiol Is Safe but Not Effective in the Treatment for Crohn's Disease, a Randomized Controlled Trial. *Dig. Dis. Sci.* **2017**, *62*, 1615–1620. [CrossRef]
90. Kafil, T.S.; Nguyen, T.M.; MacDonald, J.K.; Chande, N. Cannabis for the treatment of Crohn's disease. *Cochrane Database Syst. Rev.* **2018**, *11*, CD012853. [CrossRef]
91. Irving, P.M.; Iqbal, T.; Nwokolo, C.; Subramanian, S.; Bloom, S.; Prasad, N.; Hart, A.; Murray, C.; Lindsay, J.O.; Taylor, A.; et al. A Randomized, Double-blind, Placebo-controlled, Parallel-group, Pilot Study of Cannabidiol-rich Botanical Extract in the Symptomatic Treatment of Ulcerative Colitis. *Inflamm. Bowel Dis.* **2018**, *24*, 714–724. [CrossRef]
92. Naftali, T.; Benjaminov, F.; Lish, I. Cannabis induces clinical and endoscopic improvement in moderately active ulcerative colitis. *J. Crohns Colitis* **2018**, *12*, S306. [CrossRef]
93. Tashkin, D.P.; Roth, M.D. Pulmonary effects of inhaled cannabis smoke. *Am. J. Drug Alcohol Abus.* **2019**, *45*, 596–609. [CrossRef]
94. Yayan, J.; Rasche, K. Damaging Effects of Cannabis Use on the Lungs. *Adv. Exp. Med. Biol.* **2016**, *952*, 31–34. [CrossRef]
95. Fligiel, S.E.; Beals, T.F.; Tashkin, D.P.; Paule, M.G.; Scallet, A.C.; Ali, S.F.; Bailey, J.R.; Slikker, W., Jr. Marijuana exposure and pulmonary alterations in primates. *Pharmacol. Biochem. Behav.* **1991**, *40*, 637–642. [CrossRef]
96. Gong, H., Jr.; Fligiel, S.; Tashkin, D.P.; Barbers, R.G. Tracheobronchial changes in habitual, heavy smokers of marijuana with and without tobacco. *Am. Rev. Respir. Dis.* **1987**, *136*, 142–149. [CrossRef] [PubMed]
97. Burstein, S.; Hunter, S.A.; Latham, V.; Mechoulam, R.; Melchior, D.L.; Renzulli, L.; Tefft, R.E., Jr. Prostaglandins and cannabis XV. Comparison of enantiomeric cannabinoids in stimulating prostaglandin synthesis in fibroblasts. *Life Sci.* **1986**, *39*, 1813–1823. [CrossRef]
98. Roth, M.D.; Whittaker, K.; Salehi, K.; Tashkin, D.P.; Baldwin, G.C. Mechanisms for impaired effector function in alveolar macrophages from marijuana and cocaine smokers. *J. Neuroimmunol.* **2004**, *147*, 82–86. [CrossRef]
99. Turcotte, C.; Blanchet, M.R.; Laviolette, M.; Flamand, N. Impact of Cannabis, Cannabinoids, and Endocannabinoids in the Lungs. *Front. Pharmacol.* **2016**, *7*, 317. [CrossRef]
100. Esposito, G.; Pesce, M.; Seguella, L.; Sanseverino, W.; Lu, J.; Corpetti, C.; Sarnelli, G. The potential of cannabidiol in the COVID-19 pandemic. *Br. J. Pharmacol.* **2020**, *177*, 4967–4970. [CrossRef]
101. Raj, V.; Park, J.G.; Cho, K.H.; Choi, P.; Kim, T.; Ham, J.; Lee, J. Assessment of antiviral potencies of cannabinoids against SARS-CoV-2 using computational and in vitro approaches. *Int. J. Biol. Macromol.* **2021**, *168*, 474–485. [CrossRef]
102. Costiniuk, C.T.; Jenabian, M.A. Acute inflammation and pathogenesis of SARS-CoV-2 infection: Cannabidiol as a potential anti-inflammatory treatment? *Cytokine Growth Factor Rev.* **2020**, *53*, 63–65. [CrossRef]
103. Brown, J.D. Cannabidiol as prophylaxis for SARS-CoV-2 and COVID-19? Unfounded claims versus potential risks of medications during the pandemic. *Res. Soc. Adm. Pharm.* **2021**, *17*, 2053. [CrossRef]
104. Calignano, A.; Kátona, I.; Désarnaud, F.; Giuffrida, A.; La Rana, G.; Mackie, K.; Freund, T.F.; Piomelli, D. Bidirectional control of airway responsiveness by endogenous cannabinoids. *Nature* **2000**, *408*, 96–101. [CrossRef]
105. Bozkurt, T.E. Endocannabinoid System in the Airways. *Molecules* **2019**, *24*, 4626. [CrossRef]
106. Fantauzzi, M.F.; Aguiar, J.A.; Tremblay, B.J.-M.; Yanagihara, T.; Chandiramohan, A.; Revill, S.; Ryu, M.H.; Carlsten, C.; Ask, K.; Stämpfli, M.; et al. Expression of the endocannabinoid system in the human airway epithelial cells—Impact of sex and chronic respiratory disease status. *bioRxiv* **2020**. [CrossRef]
107. Sarafian, T.A.; Habib, N.; Oldham, M.; Seeram, N.; Lee, R.P.; Lin, L.; Tashkin, D.P.; Roth, M.D. Inhaled marijuana smoke disrupts mitochondrial energetics in pulmonary epithelial cells in vivo. *Am. J. Physiol. Lung Cell. Mol. Physiol.* **2006**, *290*, L1202–L1209. [CrossRef]
108. Sarafian, T.A.; Magallanes, J.A.; Shau, H.; Tashkin, D.; Roth, M.D. Oxidative stress produced by marijuana smoke. An adverse effect enhanced by cannabinoids. *Am. J. Respir. Cell Mol. Biol.* **1999**, *20*, 1286–1293. [CrossRef]
109. Srivastava, M.D.; Srivastava, B.I.; Brouhard, B. Delta9 tetrahydrocannabinol and cannabidiol alter cytokine production by human immune cells. *Immunopharmacology* **1998**, *40*, 179–185. [CrossRef]
110. Liu, A.P.; Yuan, Q.H.; Zhang, B.; Yang, L.; He, Q.W.; Chen, K.; Liu, Q.S.; Li, Z.; Zhan, J. Cannabinoid receptor 2 activation alleviates septic lung injury by promoting autophagy via inhibition of inflammatory mediator release. *Cell. Signal.* **2020**, *69*, 109556. [CrossRef]

111. Muthumalage, T.; Rahman, I. Cannabidiol differentially regulates basal and LPS-induced inflammatory responses in macrophages, lung epithelial cells, and fibroblasts. *Toxicol. Appl. Pharmacol.* **2019**, *382*, 114713. [CrossRef]
112. Adcock, I.M.; Caramori, G. Cross-talk between pro-inflammatory transcription factors and glucocorticoids. *Immunol. Cell Biol.* **2001**, *79*, 376–384. [CrossRef] [PubMed]
113. Staiano, R.I.; Loffredo, S.; Borriello, F.; Iannotti, F.A.; Piscitelli, F.; Orlando, P.; Secondo, A.; Granata, F.; Lepore, M.T.; Fiorelli, A.; et al. Human lung-resident macrophages express CB1 and CB2 receptors whose activation inhibits the release of angiogenic and lymphangiogenic factors. *J. Leukoc. Biol.* **2016**, *99*, 531–540. [CrossRef] [PubMed]
114. Helyes, Z.; Kemény, Á.; Csekő, K.; Szőke, É.; Elekes, K.; Mester, M.; Sándor, K.; Perkecz, A.; Kereskai, L.; Márk, L.; et al. Marijuana smoke induces severe pulmonary hyperresponsiveness, inflammation, and emphysema in a predictive mouse model not via CB1 receptor activation. *Am. J. Physiol. Lung Cell. Mol. Physiol.* **2017**, *313*, L267–L277. [CrossRef] [PubMed]
115. Kleinman, M.T.; Arechavala, R.J.; Herman, D.; Shi, J.; Hasen, I.; Ting, A.; Dai, W.; Carreno, J.; Chavez, J.; Zhao, L.; et al. E-cigarette or Vaping Product Use-Associated Lung Injury Produced in an Animal Model from Electronic Cigarette Vapor Exposure Without Tetrahydrocannabinol or Vitamin E Oil. *J. Am. Heart Assoc.* **2020**, *9*, e017368. [CrossRef] [PubMed]
116. Zawatsky, C.N.; Abdalla, J.; Cinar, R. Synthetic cannabinoids induce acute lung inflammation via cannabinoid receptor 1 activation. *ERJ Open Res.* **2020**, *6*. [CrossRef]
117. Ribeiro, A.; Almeida, V.I.; Costola-de-Souza, C.; Ferraz-de-Paula, V.; Pinheiro, M.L.; Vitoretti, L.B.; Gimenes-Junior, J.A.; Akamine, A.T.; Crippa, J.A.; Tavares-de-Lima, W.; et al. Cannabidiol improves lung function and inflammation in mice submitted to LPS-induced acute lung injury. *Immunopharmacol. Immunotoxicol.* **2015**, *37*, 35–41. [CrossRef]
118. Ribeiro, A.; Ferraz-de-Paula, V.; Pinheiro, M.L.; Vitoretti, L.B.; Mariano-Souza, D.P.; Quinteiro-Filho, W.M.; Akamine, A.T.; Almeida, V.I.; Quevedo, J.; Dal-Pizzol, F.; et al. Cannabidiol, a non-psychotropic plant-derived cannabinoid, decreases inflammation in a murine model of acute lung injury: Role for the adenosine A(2A) receptor. *Eur. J. Pharmacol.* **2012**, *678*, 78–85. [CrossRef]
119. Berdyshev, E.; Boichot, E.; Corbel, M.; Germain, N.; Lagente, V. Effects of cannabinoid receptor ligands on LPS-induced pulmonary inflammation in mice. *Life Sci.* **1998**, *63*, PL125–PL129. [CrossRef]
120. Karmaus, P.W.; Wagner, J.G.; Harkema, J.R.; Kaminski, N.E.; Kaplan, B.L. Cannabidiol (CBD) enhances lipopolysaccharide (LPS)-induced pulmonary inflammation in C57BL/6 mice. *J. Immunotoxicol.* **2013**, *10*, 321–328. [CrossRef]
121. Arruza, L.; Pazos, M.R.; Mohammed, N.; Escribano, N.; Lafuente, H.; Santos, M.; Alvarez-Díaz, F.J.; Hind, W.; Martínez-Orgado, J. Cannabidiol reduces lung injury induced by hypoxic-ischemic brain damage in newborn piglets. *Pediatr. Res.* **2017**, *82*, 79–86. [CrossRef]
122. Tauber, S.; Paulsen, K.; Wolf, S.; Synwoldt, P.; Pahl, A.; Schneider-Stock, R.; Ullrich, O. Regulation of MMP-9 by a WIN-binding site in the monocyte-macrophage system independent from cannabinoid receptors. *PLoS ONE* **2012**, *7*, e48272. [CrossRef]
123. Vuolo, F.; Petronilho, F.; Sonai, B.; Ritter, C.; Hallak, J.E.; Zuardi, A.W.; Crippa, J.A.; Dal-Pizzol, F. Evaluation of Serum Cytokines Levels and the Role of Cannabidiol Treatment in Animal Model of Asthma. *Mediat. Inflamm.* **2015**, *2015*, 538670. [CrossRef]
124. Vuolo, F.; Abreu, S.C.; Michels, M.; Xisto, D.G.; Blanco, N.G.; Hallak, J.E.; Zuardi, A.W.; Crippa, J.A.; Reis, C.; Bahl, M.; et al. Cannabidiol reduces airway inflammation and fibrosis in experimental allergic asthma. *Eur. J. Pharmacol.* **2019**, *843*, 251–259. [CrossRef]
125. Frei, R.B.; Luschnig, P.; Parzmair, G.P.; Peinhaupt, M.; Schranz, S.; Fauland, A.; Wheelock, C.E.; Heinemann, A.; Sturm, E.M. Cannabinoid receptor 2 augments eosinophil responsiveness and aggravates allergen-induced pulmonary inflammation in mice. *Allergy* **2016**, *71*, 944–956. [CrossRef]
126. Ferrini, M.E.; Hong, S.; Stierle, A.; Stierle, D.; Stella, N.; Roberts, K.; Jaffar, Z. CB2 receptors regulate natural killer cells that limit allergic airway inflammation in a murine model of asthma. *Allergy* **2017**, *72*, 937–947. [CrossRef]
127. Tahamtan, A.; Tavakoli-Yaraki, M.; Shadab, A.; Rezaei, F.; Marashi, S.M.; Shokri, F.; Mokhatri-Azad, T.; Salimi, V. The Role of Cannabinoid Receptor 1 in the Immunopathology of Respiratory Syncytial Virus. *Viral Immunol.* **2018**, *31*, 292–298. [CrossRef]
128. Tahamtan, A.; Samieipoor, Y.; Nayeri, F.S.; Rahbarimanesh, A.A.; Izadi, A.; Rashidi-Nezhad, A.; Tavakoli-Yaraki, M.; Farahmand, M.; Bont, L.; Shokri, F.; et al. Effects of cannabinoid receptor type 2 in respiratory syncytial virus infection in human subjects and mice. *Virulence* **2018**, *9*, 217–230. [CrossRef]
129. Karmaus, P.W.; Chen, W.; Crawford, R.; Kaplan, B.L.; Kaminski, N.E. Δ9-tetrahydrocannabinol impairs the inflammatory response to influenza infection: Role of antigen-presenting cells and the cannabinoid receptors 1 and 2. *Toxicol. Sci.* **2013**, *131*, 419–433. [CrossRef]
130. Buchweitz, J.P.; Karmaus, P.W.; Harkema, J.R.; Williams, K.J.; Kaminski, N.E. Modulation of airway responses to influenza A/PR/8/34 by Delta9-tetrahydrocannabinol in C57BL/6 mice. *J. Pharmacol. Exp. Ther.* **2007**, *323*, 675–683. [CrossRef]
131. Rao, R.; Nagarkatti, P.S.; Nagarkatti, M. Δ(9) Tetrahydrocannabinol attenuates Staphylococcal enterotoxin B-induced inflammatory lung injury and prevents mortality in mice by modulation of miR-17-92 cluster and induction of T-regulatory cells. *Br. J. Pharmacol.* **2015**, *172*, 1792–1806. [CrossRef]
132. Zeng, J.; Li, X.; Cheng, Y.; Ke, B.; Wang, R. Activation of cannabinoid receptor type 2 reduces lung ischemia reperfusion injury through PI3K/Akt pathway. *Int. J. Clin. Exp. Pathol.* **2019**, *12*, 4096–4105.
133. Çakır, M.; Tekin, S.; Okan, A.; Çakan, P.; Doğanyiğit, Z. The ameliorating effect of cannabinoid type 2 receptor activation on brain, lung, liver and heart damage in cecal ligation and puncture-induced sepsis model in rats. *Int. Immunopharmacol.* **2020**, *78*, 105978. [CrossRef]

134. Tschöp, J.; Kasten, K.R.; Nogueiras, R.; Goetzman, H.S.; Cave, C.M.; England, L.G.; Dattilo, J.; Lentsch, A.B.; Tschöp, M.H.; Caldwell, C.C. The cannabinoid receptor 2 is critical for the host response to sepsis. *J. Immunol.* **2009**, *183*, 499–505. [CrossRef]
135. Liu, M.W.; Su, M.X.; Wang, Y.H.; Wei, W.; Qin, L.F.; Liu, X.; Tian, M.L.; Qian, C.Y. Effect of melilotus extract on lung injury by upregulating the expression of cannabinoid CB2 receptors in septic rats. *BMC Complement. Altern. Med.* **2014**, *14*, 94. [CrossRef]
136. Fujii, M.; Sherchan, P.; Soejima, Y.; Doycheva, D.; Zhao, D.; Zhang, J.H. Cannabinoid Receptor Type 2 Agonist Attenuates Acute Neurogenic Pulmonary Edema by Preventing Neutrophil Migration after Subarachnoid Hemorrhage in Rats. *Acta Neurochir. Suppl.* **2016**, *121*, 135–139. [CrossRef]
137. Kopczyńska, B.; Sulejczak, D.; Wełniak-Kamińska, M.; Gietka, A.; Grieb, P. Anandamide enhances expression of heat shock proteins Hsp70 and Hsp25 in rat lungs. *Eur. J. Pharmacol.* **2011**, *668*, 257–263. [CrossRef]
138. Andrade-Silva, M.; Correa, L.B.; Candéa, A.L.; Cavalher-Machado, S.C.; Barbosa, H.S.; Rosas, E.C.; Henriques, M.G. The cannabinoid 2 receptor agonist β-caryophyllene modulates the inflammatory reaction induced by Mycobacterium bovis BCG by inhibiting neutrophil migration. *Inflamm. Res.* **2016**, *65*, 869–879. [CrossRef]
139. Conuel, E.J.; Chieng, H.C.; Fantauzzi, J.; Pokhrel, K.; Goldman, C.; Smith, T.C.; Tiwari, A.; Chopra, A.; Judson, M.A. Cannabinoid Oil Vaping-Associated Lung Injury and its Radiographic Appearance. *Am. J. Med.* **2020**, *133*, 865–867. [CrossRef]
140. Öcal, N.; Doğan, D.; Çiçek, A.F.; Yücel, O.; Tozkoparan, E. Acute Eosinophilic Pneumonia with Respiratory Failure Induced by Synthetic Cannabinoid Inhalation. *Balk. Med. J.* **2016**, *33*, 688–690. [CrossRef]
141. Alhadi, S.; Tiwari, A.; Vohra, R.; Gerona, R.; Acharya, J.; Bilello, K. High times, low sats: Diffuse pulmonary infiltrates associated with chronic synthetic cannabinoid use. *J. Med. Toxicol.* **2013**, *9*, 199–206. [CrossRef]
142. Alon, M.H.; Saint-Fleur, M.O. Synthetic cannabinoid induced acute respiratory depression: Case series and literature review. *Respir. Med. Case Rep.* **2017**, *22*, 137–141. [CrossRef]
143. Chmiel, J.F.; Flume, P.; Downey, D.G.; Dozor, A.J.; Colombo, C.; Mazurek, H.; Sapiejka, E.; Rachel, M.; Constantine, S.; Conley, B.; et al. Safety and efficacy of lenabasum in a phase 2 randomized, placebo-controlled trial in adults with cystic fibrosis. *J. Cyst. Fibros.* **2021**, *20*, 78–85. [CrossRef]
144. Investigation of Cannabis for Pain and Inflammation in Lung Cancer. Available online: https://ClinicalTrials.gov/show/NCT0 2675842 (accessed on 3 April 2021).
145. Tashkin, D.P.; Shapiro, B.J.; Frank, I.M. Acute pulmonary physiologic effects of smoked marijuana and oral (Delta)9 -tetrahydrocannabinol in healthy young men. *N. Engl. J. Med.* **1973**, *289*, 336–341. [CrossRef]
146. Abdallah, S.J.; Smith, B.M.; Ware, M.A.; Moore, M.; Li, P.Z.; Bourbeau, J.; Jensen, D. Effect of Vaporized Cannabis on Exertional Breathlessness and Exercise Endurance in Advanced Chronic Obstructive Pulmonary Disease. A Randomized Controlled Trial. *Ann. Am. Thorac. Soc.* **2018**, *15*, 1146–1158. [CrossRef]
147. Gong, H., Jr.; Tashkin, D.P.; Calvarese, B. Comparison of bronchial effects of nabilone and terbutaline in healthy and asthmatic subjects. *J. Clin. Pharmacol.* **1983**, *23*, 127–133. [CrossRef]
148. Tashkin, D.P.; Reiss, S.; Shapiro, B.J.; Calvarese, B.; Olsen, J.L.; Lodge, J.W. Bronchial effects of aerosolized delta 9-tetrahydrocannabinol in healthy and asthmatic subjects. *Am. Rev. Respir. Dis.* **1977**, *115*, 57–65. [CrossRef]
149. Abboud, R.T.; Sanders, H.D. Effect of oral administration of delta-tetrahydrocannabinol on airway mechanics in normal and asthmatic subjects. *Chest* **1976**, *70*, 480–485. [CrossRef]
150. Van Dam, N.T.; Earleywine, M. Pulmonary function in cannabis users: Support for a clinical trial of the vaporizer. *Int. J. Drug Policy* **2010**, *21*, 511–513. [CrossRef]
151. Scheau, C.; Badarau, I.A.; Mihai, G.L.; Scheau, A.-E.; Costache, D.O.; Constantin, C.; Calina, D.; Caruntu, C.; Costache, R.S.; Caruntu, A. Cannabinoids in the pathophysiology of skin inflammation. *Molecules* **2020**, *25*, 652. [CrossRef]
152. Sheriff, T.; Lin, M.J.; Dubin, D.; Khorasani, H. The potential role of cannabinoids in dermatology. *J. Dermatol. Treat.* **2020**, *31*, 839–845. [CrossRef]
153. Baswan, S.M.; Klosner, A.E.; Glynn, K.; Rajgopal, A.; Malik, K.; Yim, S.; Stern, N. Therapeutic Potential of Cannabidiol (CBD) for Skin Health and Disorders. *Clin. Cosmet. Investig. Dermatol.* **2020**, *13*, 927–942. [CrossRef]
154. Cintosun, A.; Lara-Corrales, I.; Pope, E. Mechanisms of Cannabinoids and Potential Applicability to Skin Diseases. *Clin. Drug Investig.* **2020**, *40*, 293–304. [CrossRef]
155. Zagórska-Dziok, M.; Bujak, T.; Ziemlewska, A.; Nizioł-Łukaszewska, Z. Positive Effect of *Cannabis sativa* L. Herb Extracts on Skin Cells and Assessment of Cannabinoid-Based Hydrogels Properties. *Molecules* **2021**, *26*, 802. [CrossRef]
156. Eagleston, L.R.M.; Kalani, N.K.; Patel, R.R.; Flaten, H.K.; Dunnick, C.A.; Dellavalle, R.P. Cannabinoids in dermatology: A scoping review. *Dermatol. Online J.* **2018**, *24*, 1.
157. Nickles, M.A.; Lio, P.A. Cannabinoids in Dermatology: Hope or Hype? *Cannabis Cannabinoid Res.* **2020**, *5*, 279–282. [CrossRef]
158. Bíró, T.; Tóth, B.I.; Haskó, G.; Paus, R.; Pacher, P. The endocannabinoid system of the skin in health and disease: Novel perspectives and therapeutic opportunities. *Trends Pharmacol. Sci.* **2009**, *30*, 411–420. [CrossRef]
159. Dobrosi, N.; Tóth, B.I.; Nagy, G.; Dózsa, A.; Géczy, T.; Nagy, L.; Zouboulis, C.C.; Paus, R.; Kovács, L.; Bíró, T. Endocannabinoids enhance lipid synthesis and apoptosis of human sebocytes via cannabinoid receptor-2-mediated signaling. *FASEB J.* **2008**, *22*, 3685–3695. [CrossRef]
160. Telek, A.; Bíró, T.; Bodó, E.; Tóth, B.I.; Borbíró, I.; Kunos, G.; Paus, R. Inhibition of human hair follicle growth by endo- and exocannabinoids. *FASEB J.* **2007**, *21*, 3534–3541. [CrossRef]
161. Tóth, B.I.; Oláh, A.; Szöllősi, A.G.; Bíró, T. TRP channels in the skin. *Br. J. Pharmacol.* **2014**, *171*, 2568–2581. [CrossRef]

162. Gouin, O.; L'Herondelle, K.; Lebonvallet, N.; Le Gall-Ianotto, C.; Sakka, M.; Buhé, V.; Plée-Gautier, E.; Carré, J.L.; Lefeuvre, L.; Misery, L.; et al. TRPV1 and TRPA1 in cutaneous neurogenic and chronic inflammation: Pro-inflammatory response induced by their activation and their sensitization. *Protein Cell* **2017**, *8*, 644–661. [CrossRef] [PubMed]
163. Hänel, K.H.; Cornelissen, C.; Lüscher, B.; Baron, J.M. Cytokines and the skin barrier. *Int. J. Mol. Sci.* **2013**, *14*, 6720–6745. [CrossRef]
164. Zaalberg, A.; Moradi Tuchayi, S.; Ameri, A.H.; Ngo, K.H.; Cunningham, T.J.; Eliane, J.-P.; Livneh, M.; Horn, T.D.; Rosman, I.S.; Musiek, A.; et al. Chronic Inflammation Promotes Skin Carcinogenesis in Cancer-Prone Discoid Lupus Erythematosus. *J. Investig. Dermatol.* **2019**, *139*, 62–70. [CrossRef]
165. Solomon, I.; Voiculescu, V.M.; Caruntu, C.; Lupu, M.; Popa, A.; Ilie, M.A.; Albulescu, R.; Caruntu, A.; Tanase, C.; Constantin, C.; et al. Neuroendocrine Factors and Head and Neck Squamous Cell Carcinoma: An Affair to Remember. *Dis. Markers* **2018**, *2018*, 9787831. [CrossRef]
166. Ion, A.; Popa, I.M.; Papagheorghe, L.M.; Lisievici, C.; Lupu, M.; Voiculescu, V.; Caruntu, C.; Boda, D. Proteomic Approaches to Biomarker Discovery in Cutaneous T-Cell Lymphoma. *Dis. Markers* **2016**, *2016*, 9602472. [CrossRef]
167. Karsak, M.; Gaffal, E.; Date, R.; Wang-Eckhardt, L.; Rehnelt, J.; Petrosino, S.; Starowicz, K.; Steuder, R.; Schlicker, E.; Cravatt, B.; et al. Attenuation of Allergic Contact Dermatitis Through the Endocannabinoid System. *Science* **2007**, *316*, 1494–1497. [CrossRef]
168. Petrosino, S.; Cristino, L.; Karsak, M.; Gaffal, E.; Ueda, N.; Tüting, T.; Bisogno, T.; De Filippis, D.; D'Amico, A.; Saturnino, C.; et al. Protective role of palmitoylethanolamide in contact allergic dermatitis. *Allergy* **2010**, *65*, 698–711. [CrossRef]
169. Petrosino, S.; Verde, R.; Vaia, M.; Allara, M.; Iuvone, T.; Di Marzo, V. Anti-inflammatory Properties of Cannabidiol, a Nonpsychotropic Cannabinoid, in Experimental Allergic Contact Dermatitis. *J. Pharm. Exp.* **2018**, *365*, 652–663. [CrossRef]
170. Rio, C.D.; Millan, E.; Garcia, V.; Appendino, G.; DeMesa, J.; Munoz, E. The endocannabinoid system of the skin. A potential approach for the treatment of skin disorders. *Biochem. Pharmacol.* **2018**, *157*, 122–133. [CrossRef]
171. Wilkinson, J.D.; Williamson, E.M. Cannabinoids inhibit human keratinocyte proliferation through a non-CB1/CB2 mechanism and have a potential therapeutic value in the treatment of psoriasis. *J. Dermatol. Sci.* **2007**, *45*, 87–92. [CrossRef]
172. Ramot, Y.; Sugawara, K.; Zakany, N.; Toth, B.I.; Biro, T.; Paus, R. A novel control of human keratin expression: Cannabinoid receptor 1-mediated signaling down-regulates the expression of keratins K6 and K16 in human keratinocytes in vitro and in situ. *PeerJ* **2013**, *1*, e40. [CrossRef]
173. Robinson, E.S.; Alves, P.; Bashir, M.M.; Zeidi, M.; Feng, R.; Werth, V.P. Cannabinoid Reduces Inflammatory Cytokines, Tumor Necrosis Factor-alpha, and Type I Interferons in Dermatomyositis In Vitro. *J. Investig. Dermatol.* **2017**, *137*, 2445–2447. [CrossRef]
174. Oláh, A.; Tóth, B.I.; Borbíró, I.; Sugawara, K.; Szöllõsi, A.G.; Czifra, G.; Pál, B.; Ambrus, L.; Kloepper, J.; Camera, E.; et al. Cannabidiol exerts sebostatic and antiinflammatory effects on human sebocytes. *J. Clin. Investig.* **2014**, *124*, 3713–3724. [CrossRef]
175. Maor, Y.; Yu, J.; Kuzontkoski, P.M.; Dezube, B.J.; Zhang, X.; Groopman, J.E. Cannabinoid inhibits growth and induces programmed cell death in kaposi sarcoma-associated herpesvirus-infected endothelium. *Genes Cancer* **2012**, *3*, 512–520. [CrossRef]
176. Bechara, C.; Chai, H.; Lin, P.H.; Yao, Q.; Chen, C. Growth related oncogene-alpha (GRO-alpha): Roles in atherosclerosis, angiogenesis and other inflammatory conditions. *Med. Sci. Monit.* **2007**, *13*, Ra87–Ra90.
177. Del Rio, C.; Navarrete, C.; Collado, J.A.; Bellido, M.L.; Gomez-Canas, M.; Pazos, M.R.; Fernandez-Ruiz, J.; Pollastro, F.; Appendino, G.; Calzado, M.A.; et al. The cannabinoid quinol VCE-004.8 alleviates bleomycin-induced scleroderma and exerts potent antifibrotic effects through peroxisome proliferator-activated receptor-gamma and CB2 pathways. *Sci. Rep.* **2016**, *6*, 21703. [CrossRef]
178. Balistreri, E.; Garcia-Gonzalez, E.; Selvi, E.; Akhmetshina, A.; Palumbo, K.; Lorenzini, S.; Maggio, R.; Lucattelli, M.; Galeazzi, M.; Distler, J.W. The cannabinoid WIN55, 212–2 abrogates dermal fibrosis in scleroderma bleomycin model. *Ann. Rheum. Dis.* **2011**, *70*, 695–699. [CrossRef]
179. Kim, H.J.; Kim, B.; Park, B.M.; Jeon, J.E.; Lee, S.H.; Mann, S.; Ahn, S.K.; Hong, S.P.; Jeong, S.K. Topical cannabinoid receptor 1 agonist attenuates the cutaneous inflammatory responses in oxazolone-induced atopic dermatitis model. *Int. J. Dermatol.* **2015**, *54*, e401–e408. [CrossRef]
180. Formukong, E.A.; Evans, A.T.; Evans, F.J. Analgesic and antiinflammatory activity of constituents of *Cannabis sativa* L. *Inflammation* **1988**, *12*, 361–371. [CrossRef]
181. Armstrong, J.L.; Hill, D.S.; McKee, C.S.; Hernandez-Tiedra, S.; Lorente, M.; Lopez-Valero, I.; Eleni Anagnostou, M.; Babatunde, F.; Corazzari, M.; Redfern, C.P.F.; et al. Exploiting cannabinoid-induced cytotoxic autophagy to drive melanoma cell death. *J. Investig. Dermatol.* **2015**, *135*, 1629–1637. [CrossRef]
182. Calenic, B.; Greabu, M.; Caruntu, C.; Tanase, C.; Battino, M. Oral keratinocyte stem/progenitor cells: Specific markers, molecular signaling pathways and potential uses. *Periodontology* **2015**, *69*, 68–82. [CrossRef]
183. Lupu, M.; Caruntu, C.; Ghita, M.A.; Voiculescu, V.; Voiculescu, S.; Rosca, A.E.; Caruntu, A.; Moraru, L.; Popa, I.M.; Calenic, B.; et al. Gene Expression and Proteome Analysis as Sources of Biomarkers in Basal Cell Carcinoma. *Dis. Markers* **2016**, *2016*, 9831237. [CrossRef] [PubMed]
184. Voiculescu, V.; Calenic, B.; Ghita, M.; Lupu, M.; Caruntu, A.; Moraru, L.; Voiculescu, S.; Ion, A.; Greabu, M.; Ishkitiev, N.; et al. From Normal Skin to Squamous Cell Carcinoma: A Quest for Novel Biomarkers. *Dis. Markers* **2016**, *2016*, 4517492. [CrossRef]
185. Tampa, M.; Caruntu, C.; Mitran, M.; Mitran, C.; Sarbu, I.; Rusu, L.C.; Matei, C.; Constantin, C.; Neagu, M.; Georgescu, S.R. Markers of Oral Lichen Planus Malignant Transformation. *Dis. Markers* **2018**, *2018*, 1959506. [CrossRef] [PubMed]

186. Scheau, C.; Badarau, I.A.; Costache, R.; Caruntu, C.; Mihai, G.L.; Didilescu, A.C.; Constantin, C.; Neagu, M. The Role of Matrix Metalloproteinases in the Epithelial-Mesenchymal Transition of Hepatocellular Carcinoma. *Anal. Cell. Pathol.* **2019**, *2019*, 9423907. [CrossRef] [PubMed]
187. Zheng, D.; Bode, A.M.; Zhao, Q.; Cho, Y.Y.; Zhu, F.; Ma, W.Y.; Dong, Z. The cannabinoid receptors are required for ultraviolet-induced inflammation and skin cancer development. *Cancer Res.* **2008**, *68*, 3992–3998. [CrossRef] [PubMed]
188. Ali, A.; Akhtar, N. The safety and efficacy of 3% Cannabis seeds extract cream for reduction of human cheek skin sebum and erythema content. *Pak. J. Pharm. Sci.* **2015**, *28*, 1389–1395. [PubMed]
189. Evaluation of BTX 1503 in Patients with Moderate to Severe Acne Vulgaris. Available online: https://clinicaltrials.gov/ct2/show/NCT03573518 (accessed on 10 January 2020).
190. Spiera, R.; Hummers, L.; Chung, L.; Frech, T.; Domsic, R.; Furst, D.; Gordon, J.; Mayes, M.; Simms, R.; Constantine, S.; et al. OP0126 A phase 2 study of safety and efficacy of anabasum (JBT-101) in systemic sclerosis. *Ann. Rheum. Dis.* **2017**, *76*, 105. [CrossRef]
191. Burstein, S.H. Ajulemic acid: Potential treatment for chronic inflammation. *Pharmacol. Res. Perspect.* **2018**, *6*, e00394. [CrossRef]
192. Chen, K.; Zeidi, M.; Reddy, N.; White, B.; Werth, V. Fri0307 lenabasum, a cannabinoid type 2 receptor agonist, reduces cd4 cell populations and downregulates type 1 and 2 interferon activities in lesional dermatomyositis skin. *Ann. Rheum. Dis.* **2019**, *78*, 835. [CrossRef]
193. Werth, V.; Oddis, C.V.; Lundberg, I.E.; Fiorentino, D.; Cornwall, C.; Dgetluck, N.; Constantine, S.; White, B. Sat0303 design of phase 3 study of lenabasum for the treatment of dermatomyositis. *Ann. Rheum. Dis.* **2019**, *78*, 1228. [CrossRef]
194. Dariš, B.; Tancer Verboten, M.; Knez, Ž.; Ferk, P. Cannabinoids in cancer treatment: Therapeutic potential and legislation. *Bosn. J. Basic Med. Sci. Udruz. Basicnih Med. Znan.* **2019**, *19*, 14–23. [CrossRef]
195. Jin, J.; Sklar, G.E.; Min Sen Oh, V.; Chuen Li, S. Factors affecting therapeutic compliance: A review from the patient's perspective. *Ther. Clin. Risk Manag.* **2008**, *4*, 269–286. [CrossRef]

MDPI
St. Alban-Anlage 66
4052 Basel
Switzerland
Tel. +41 61 683 77 34
Fax +41 61 302 89 18
www.mdpi.com

Journal of Personalized Medicine Editorial Office
E-mail: jpm@mdpi.com
www.mdpi.com/journal/jpm

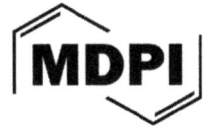

www.ingramcontent.com/pod-product-compliance
Lightning Source LLC
LaVergne TN
LVHW070455100526
838202LV00014B/1728